Endocrine Neoplasms

Cancer Treatment and Research

Steven T. Rosen, M.D., *Series Editor*

Robert H. Lurie Cancer Center

Northwestern University Medical School

Endocrine Neoplasms

edited by

ANDREW ARNOLD, M.D.
Massachusetts General Hospital
Harvard Medical School
Boston, Massachusetts

1997 **KLUWER ACADEMIC PUBLISHERS**
BOSTON / DORDRECHT / LONDON

Distributors for North America:
Kluwer Academic Publishers
101 Philip Drive
Assinippi Park
Norwell, Massachusetts 02061 USA

Distributors for all other countries:
Kluwer Academic Publishers Group
Distribution Centre
Post Office Box 322
3300 AH Dordrecht, THE NETHERLANDS

RC280
.E55
E533
1997

Library of Congress Cataloging-in-Publication Data
Endocrine neoplasms / edited by Andrew Arnold.
    p. cm. – (Cancer treatment and research; v. 62)
    Includes bibliographical references and index.
    ISBN 0-7923-4354-9 (alk. paper)
    1. Endocrine glands – Cancer. I. Arnold, Andrew. II. Series.
    [DNLM: 1. Endocrine Gland Neoplasms.
    W1 CA693 v. 62 1997 / WK 140 E558 1997]
    RC280.E55E533   1997
    616.99′44 – dc21
    DNLM/DLC
    for Library of Congress

96-49030
CIP

Contents

List of Contributors

Andrew Arnold, M.D.
Chief, Laboratory of Endocrine Oncology
Massachusetts General Hospital
Associate Professor of Medicine
Harvard Medical School
Jackson 1021
Boston, MA 02114, USA

George P. Chrousos, M.D.
Developmental Endocrinology Branch
NIH Clinical Center, Bldg. 10, Rm. 10N262
9000 Rockville Pike
Bethesda, MD 20892, USA

Giovanni Cizza, M.D.
Developmental Endocrinology Branch
NIH Clinical Center, Bldg. 10, Rm. 10N262
9000 Rockville Pike
Bethesda, MD 20892, USA

Gilbert J. Cote, Ph.D.
Section of Endocrinology
University of Texas M.D. Anderson Cancer Center
1515 Holcombe Blvd., Box 15
Houston, TX 77030, USA

Leon Fogelfeld, M.D.
Division of Endocrinology and Metabolism
Michael Reese Hospital
2929 S. Ellis Avenue
Chicago, IL 60616, USA

Isaac R. Francis, M.D.
Department of Internal Medicine and Department of Radiology
University of Michigan Medical Center
1500 E. Medical Center Drive
Ann Arbor, MI 48109-0028, USA

Robert F. Gagel, M.D.
Professor and Chief, Section of Endocrinology
University of Texas M.D. Anderson Cancer Center
1515 Holcombe Blvd., Box 15
Houston, TX 77030, USA

David Goltzman, M.D.
Calcium Research Laboratory
Royal Victoria Hospital and Department of Medicine
McGill University
687 Pine Ave. West, Room H4.67
Montreal, QC H3A 1A1, Canada

Stefan K.G. Grebe, M.D.
Visiting Scientist
Endocrine Research Unit
Division of Endocrinology and Internal Medicine
Mayo Clinic
200 First Street S.W.
Rochester, MN 55905, USA

Milton D. Gross, M.D.
Division of Nuclear Medicine
Department of Veterans Affairs Medical Center
2215 Fuller Road
Ann Arbor, MI 48105, USA

Ian D. Hay, M.B., Ph.D.
Professor of Medicine
Mayo Medical School
Consultant in Endocrinology and Internal Medicine
Mayo Clinic and Foundation
200 First Street S.W.
Rochester, MN 55905, USA

Janet E. Henderson, Ph.D.
Lady Davis Institute
S.M.B.D. Jewish General Hospital and Department of Medicine
McGill University
3755 Cote Ste. Catherine Rd.
Montreal, QC H3T 1E2, Canada

L.J. Hofland, Ph.D.
Department of Internal Medicine III
University Hospital Dijkzigt
Dr. Molewaterplein 40
3015 GD Rotterdam, The Netherlands

Robert T. Jensen, M.D.
Digestive Diseases Branch, NIDDK
National Institutes of Health
Bldg. 10, Room 9C-103
10 Center Dr. MSC 1804
Bethesda, MD 20892-1804, USA

Laurence Katznelson, M.D.
Instructor in Medicine
Neuroendocrine Unit, BUL457B
Massachusetts General Hospital
Boston, MA 02114, USA

Anne Klibanski, M.D.
Chief, Neuroendocrine Unit
Associate Professor of Medicine
Massachusetts General Hospital, BUL457B
Boston, MA 02114, USA

Richard T. Kloos, M.D.
Fellow in Nuclear Medicine
Division of Nuclear Medicine
University of Michigan Medical Center
1500 E. Medical Center Drive
B1G412 Box 28
Ann Arbor, MI 48109-0028, USA

Melvyn Korobkin, M.D.
Department of Internal Medicine and Department of Radiology
University of Michigan Medical Center
1500 E. Medical Center Drive
Ann Arbor, MI 48109-0028, USA

S.W.J. Lamberts, M.D.
Department of Internal Medicine III
University Hospital Dijkzigt
Dr. Molewaterplein 40
3015 GD Rotterdam, The Netherlands

Ana C. Latronico, M.D.
Developmental Endocrinology Branch
NIH Clinical Center, Bldg. 10, Rm. 10N262
9000 Rockville Pike
Bethesda, MD 20892, USA

Shlomo Melmed, M.D.
Division of Endocrinology and Metabolism
Cedars-Sinai Medical Center
8700 Beverly Blvd., B-131
Los Angeles, CA 90048-1865, USA

Mark E. Molitch, M.D.
Center for Endocrinology, Metabolism and Molecular Medicine
Northwestern University Medical School, Tarry 15-731
303 E. Chicago Avenue
Chicago, IL 60611, USA

Kerstin Sandelin, M.D., Ph.D.
Department of Surgery
Karolinska Hospital
S-171 76 Stockholm, Sweden

Arthur B. Schneider, M.D., Ph.D.
University of Illinois College of Medicine
Section of Endocrinology (M/C 640)
1819 W. Polk Street
Chicago, IL 60612, USA

F. John Service, M.D., Ph.D.
Division of Endocrinology and Metabolism
Mayo Clinic
200 First Street, SW
Rochester, MN 55905, USA

Brahm Shapiro, M.B., Ch.B., Ph.D.
Professor of Internal Medicine
Division of Nuclear Medicine
Department of Veterans Affairs Medical Center
2215 Fuller Road
Ann Arbor, MI 48105, USA

Ilan Shimon, M.D.
Division of Endocrinology and Metabolism
Cedars-Sinai Medical Center
8700 Beverly Blvd.
Los Angeles, CA 90048-1865, USA

Shonni J. Silverberg, M.D.
Associate Professor of Clinical Medicine
Department of Medicine
College of Physicians & Surgeons
Columbia University
630 W. 168th Street
New York, NY 10032, USA

Britt Skogseid, M.D.
Endocrine Oncology Unit
Department of Internal Medicine
University Hospital
S-751 85 Uppsala, Sweden

Peter J. Snyder, M.D.
611 Clinical Research Building
University of Pennsylvania School of Medicine
415 Curie Boulevard
Philadelphia, PA 19104-6149, USA

Pamela M. Thomas, M.D.
Department of Pediatrics
University of Michigan Medical Center
MSRB III, Room 8220A, Box 0646
1150 West Medical Center Drive
Ann Arbor, MI 48109, USA

Norman W. Thompson, M.D.
Professor of Surgery
Chief, Division of Endocrine Surgery
University of Michigan Medical Center
1500 E. Medical Center Drive
Room TC-2920D, Box 0331
Ann Arbor, MI 48109-0331, USA

William F. Young, Jr., M.D.
Associate Professor of Medicine
Endocrinology, Hypertension & Internal Medicine
Mayo Clinic and Mayo Foundation
Mayo Medical School
200 First Street S.W.
Rochester, MN 55905, USA

Preface

Andrew Arnold

The past several years have been a time of intense excitement and have brought major advances in the understanding and treatment of endocrine neoplasms. This is therefore an excellent point at which to undertake a broad-based overview of the state of the art in endocrine neoplasia for the *Cancer Treatment and Research* series. Because of the wide and interdisciplinary readership of this series, our aim for each chapter has been to provide ample background for those not highly familiar with the topic, while emphasizing the most recent advances. Furthermore, the chapters have been written with the clinician in mind, whether she or he is an oncologist, endocrinologist, surgeon, generalist, pathologist, or radiologist. As such, the authors' mission has been to focus on clinically relevant issues and to present the scientific basis of current or potential future advances in a manner easily digestible to the nonexpert.

Endocrine tumors often cause problems for the patient by virtue of their hormonal activity, which may frequently (but certainly not always) overshadow the adverse consequences related to their mass per se. In fact, it is important to keep in mind that endocrine tumors can manifest two biologically separable but often intertwined properties, namely, increased cell mass and abnormal hormonal function. These need not go hand in hand, and their distinction has definite clinical relevance in, for example, the increasingly recognized problem of incidentally discovered adrenal or pituitary masses. Endocrine tumors can also pose relatively unique problems to the clinician and pathologist because the histopathologic distinction between benign and malignant neoplasia may not be straightforward, and there can be wide variability in the clinical aggressiveness of even a clearly malignant or metastatic tumor. Therefore, depending on the specific situation, therapy may be most appropriately directed against the tumor cell mass, its hormonal activity, or the secondary consequences of either.

The organization of this volume reflects both the organ-specific and more generalized aspects of endocrine tumorigenesis. Some chapters are focused on tumors of specific endocrine glands, for example, the pituitary, parathyroid, thyroid, and adrenal glands. More general themes in pathogenesis, diagnosis, and treatment are also addressed, for example, in chapters on radiation-induced tumors, somatostatin analogs and receptors, persistent hyper-insulinemic hypoglycemia of infancy, and paraneoplastic hypercalcemia. Finally, special issues of importance to the understanding and management of the familial endocrine tumor syndromes MEN-I and MEN-II are separately discussed. Certainly, there are other topics that could have reasonably been included in this volume, but space constraints mandated a degree of arbitrary selectivity.

I would like to express my most sincere gratitude to each of the contributors for providing such timely reviews of new information in a manner designed to appeal to the interdisciplinary readership of the *Cancer Treatment and Research* series. Finally, the administrative assistance of Ms. Helen Basilesco and Ms. Kate Vallan in my office, and Ms. Rose Antonelli at Kluwer Academic Publishers, is gratefully acknowledged as is the production assistance of Ms. Stephanie Granai at Kluwer.

1. Growth hormone– and growth-hormone–releasing hormone–producing tumors

Ilan Shimon and Shlomo Melmed

Acromegaly, a clinical syndrome of disordered somatic growth and proportion, is usually caused by the unrestrained secretion of growth hormone (GH) by a pituitary adenoma and rarely may result from GH-releasing hormone (GHRH) secretion by an extrapituitary tumor. The disease was first described more than a century ago and was the earliest pituitary disorder to be recognized. The clinical features of acromegaly are caused by elevated GH and insulin-like growth factor-I (IGF-I) levels.

Physiology of the GHRH–GH–IGF–I axis

The human GH gene, located on the long arm of chromosome 17 [1], codes for a 22-kD single-chain polypeptide hormone containing 191 amino acids. Approximately 10% of pituitary GH is secreted as a 20-kD variant lacking amino acids 32–46 [2,3], probably arising as a result of an alternate splicing mechanism. The GH gene is expressed and the hormone synthesized, stored, and secreted by somatotrope cells. These acidophilic cells comprise 40–50% of pituitary cells and are located in the lateral wings of the gland. GH secretion is pulsatile, with undetectable basal levels occuring between peaks and maximum GH secretory peaks detected within 1 hour of deep-sleep onset. GHRH, a 44-amino acid hypothalamic hormone, binds to specific receptors on somatotrope cells, increases intracellular cyclic AMP, and selectively stimulates transcription of GH mRNA [4] and GH secretory pulses [5].

IGF-I, the target hormone of GH, participates in feedback regulation of GH by inhibiting both GH mRNA expression and GH secretion [6]. Somatostatin secreted from the hypothalamus suppresses basal GH secretion without altering GH mRNA levels [7]. Somatostatin appears to be the primary regulator of GH pulses in response to physiologic stimuli. Estrogens enhance GH secretion, glucocorticoid excess suppresses its release, and in hypothyroidism the GH response to GHRH and insulin-induced hypoglycemia is blunted. Thyrotropin-releasing hormone (TRH) does not stimulate GH secretion in normal subjects but induces GH release in patients with acromegaly.

Andrew Arnold (ed.) ENDOCRINE NEOPLASMS. 1997. Kluwer Academic Publishers. ISBN 0-7923-4354-9.
All rights reserved.

The liver contains the highest concentrations of GH receptors, but other tissues also express these receptors, which may circulate as soluble GH binding proteins (GHBPs). These 60-kD circulating receptor fragments are identical to the extracellular domain of the hepatic receptor [8] and bind half of circulating GH. They prolong GH plasma half-life by decreasing the GH metabolic clearance rate and also inhibit GH binding to surface receptors by ligand competition [9]. GH acts both directly, via its own receptors, and indirectly, via IGF-I, a 70 amino-acid protein, on peripheral target tissues. Longitudinal bone growth–promoting actions on epiphyseal growth-plate chondrocytes are probably stimulated indirectly by GH through local as well as hepatic-derived circulating IGF-I. GH itself has chronic anti-insulin effects, resulting in glucose intolerance, and the hormone increases muscle volume and lean body mass, and significantly decreases body fat when administered to GH-deficient adults [10].

Plasma IGF-I is associated with specific IGF binding proteins (IGFBPs). Six structurally distinct IGFBPs have been cloned, and IGFBP-III is the most abundant in adult circulation. Serum IGFBP-III levels correlate with IGF-I levels and appear to be GH responsive, that is, they double in acromegaly and are reduced in hypopituitarism. In contrast, IGFBP-I levels are elevated in hypopituitarism and decreased in acromegaly, probably reflecting their dependence on circulating insulin and somatostatin levels.

Molecular pathogenesis of somatotrope adenomas

Using chromosomal inactivation analysis, the monoclonality of GH-cell pituitary adenomas was confirmed in female patients heterozygous for variant alleles of hypoxanthine phosphoribosyltransferase and phosphoglycerate kinase [11]. This observation suggests that a somatic somatotrope cell mutation gives rise to clonal expansion and tumor formation. The G proteins are a group of guanosine triphosphate (GTP)–binding proteins that are involved in transmembrane signal transduction and the regulation of adenylyl cyclase. A subset of GH-secreting human pituitary adenomas with constitutive activation of Gs-α protein, persistent activation of adenylyl cyclase, and high levels of intracellular cyclic AMP was described [12]. As GHRH signaling is mediated by cyclic AMP, this G-protein activation bypasses the somatotrope requirement for GHRH-receptor activation and leads to sustained constitutive GH hypersecretion. These tumors harbor somatic point mutations in two sites, arginine 201 replaced by cysteine or histidine, and glutamine 227 replaced with arginine (Table 1), which activate the Gs-α protein by inhibiting its intrinsic GTPase activity and convert it into an oncogene (*gsp*) [13].

These activating *gsp* somatic mutations are present in up to 40% of GH-secreting adenomas and, compared with nonmutant tumors, the *gsp*-bearing adenomas are smaller, have mildly lower GH levels and enhanced intratumoral cyclic AMP, and do not respond briskly to GHRH [14]. More-

2

Table 1. Somatic Gs-α mutations in somatotrope adenomas: Cyclic AMP is enhanced in tumors bearing these mutations

		Adenylyl cyclase (pmol cAMP/mg/min)		Encoded amino acids	
		Tumor	Basal	Codon 201	Codon 227
Group 1	1	13		Arg	Gln
	2	6		Arg	Gln
	3	16		Arg	Gln
	4	43		Arg	Gln
Group 2	5	170		Arg (2)/Cys (3)	Gln
	6	480		Arg (0)/His (4)	Gln
	7	190		Arg (0)/Cys (3)	Gln
	8	180		Arg	Gln (0)/Arg (3)

Arg = arginine, Gln = glutamine, Cys = cysteine, His = histidine.
Adapted from Landis et al. [13], with permission.

over, similar somatic mutations in codon 201 of the Gs-α were identified in various tissues of patients with McCune-Albright syndrome, including GH-producing pituitary adenomas [15]. Recently, the phosphorylated and, hence, activated cyclic AMP-regulated factor CREB was implicated as the bio-chemical intermediate in the mechanism by which cyclic AMP stimulates somatotrope proliferation in GH-secreting pituitary adenomas [16]. Further-more, in a study of sporadic pituitary adenomas, allelic deletions involving chromosome 11 were found in a few GH-producing tumors [17].

Thus, there is intriguing evidence for both an activating as well as an inactivating mutation in acromegaly. GHRH may also act as a pituitary trophic factor. It induces somatotrope DNA synthesis [18], and patients har-boring ectopic GHRH-secreting tumors may also develop pituitary adenomas. Recently, an autocrine or paracrine mechanism of GHRH action on somatotrope proliferation has been suggested by the finding of GHRH gene expression in GH-secreting adenomas themselves [19].

Etiology of acromegaly

Benign pituitary adenoma accounts for over 98% of patients with acromegaly (Table 2). GH-secreting adenomas are relatively rare, with a prevalence of 40–70 cases per million and an annual incidence of three to four new cases per million (Table 3). These sellar adenomas are epithelial tumors that derive from and consist of adenohypophyseal cells. Pure somatotrope tumors exclu-sively producing GH occur in 60% of these cases. These tumors are either slow (densely granulated, as seen on electron microscopy) or rapidly growing (sparsely granulated). The former tumors contain large amounts of stored GH and lead to an insidious clinical progression over many years. Sparsely granu-

Table 2. Etiology of acromegaly

Excess GH secretion
Pituitary
    Densely or sparsely granulated GH-cell adenoma
    Mixed GH-cell and PRL-cell adenoma
    Mammosomatotroph cell adenoma
    Acidophil stem-cell adenoma
    Plurihormonal adenoma
    GH-cell carcinoma
    Empty sella
Ectopic pituitary tumors
    Sphenoid or parapharyngeal sinus
Extrapituitary tumor
    Pancreas, carcinoid, lung, ovary, breast
Excess GHRH secretion
Central
    Hypothalamic hamartoma
Peripheral
    Carcinoid tumor, pancreatic-cell tumor, small-cell lung cancer,
      adrenal adenoma, pheochromocytoma
Excess growth-factor secretion or action
    Acromegaloidism
Miscellaneous
    McCune-Albright syndrome
    Multiple endocrine neoplasia

GH = growth hormone; GHRH = growth hormone–releasing hormone; PRL = prolactin.
Adapted from Melmed [42], with permission.

Table 3. Worldwide epidemiology of acromegaly

Annual incidence: 3–4 per million
Population prevalence: 40–70 per million
Mean age at death, ca. 60 years
Mortality
    2–3 × expected rate
    Primarily vascular and malignant disorders

Data from Molitch [31], Bengtsson et al. [34], Rajasoorya et al. [35], and Bates et al. [51].

lated adenomas are locally invasive and are usually associated with suprasellar extension. Mixed GH-cell and prolactin (PRL)-cell adenomas [20] (bimorphous tumors, 25%) cause acromegaly associated with moderately elevated serum PRL levels. In contrast, monomorphous mammosomatotrope cell adenomas (10%) arise from a single cell expressing both GH and PRL, and are believed to be related to the more primitive acidophil stem cells.

Clinical features of acromegaly may also occur in patients with either monomorphous or plurimorphous plurihormonal tumors that express GH with any combination of PRL, thyroid-stimulating hormone (TSH), adreno-corticotrophic hormone (ACTH), or α-subunit [21]. GH-cell adenoma causing scromegaly is a well-documented component of the autosomal dominant multiple endocrine neoplasia-I (MEN-I) syndrome (including hyperpara-thyroidism, pancreatic islet-cell tumors, and pituitary adenomas) and has been diagnosed in several patients with sporadic McCune-Albright syndrome (polyostotic fibrous dysplasia, cutaneous pigmentation, precocious puberty, and hypersecretory polyendocrinopathy, including acromegaly).

In rare cases acromegaly may be caused by ectopic somatotrope cell adenoma arising in pituitary tissue remnants in the sphenoid or para-pharyngeal sinuses [22], reflecting the embryologic origin of the adeno-hypophysis from Rathke's pouch. GH-cell pituitary carcinomas with well-documented extracranial metastases are exceedingly rare, aggressive, and rap-idly growing tumors [23,24]. Their clinical presentation is initially similar to that of a benign adenoma, and malignancy is diagnosed when distant meta-static tumor is found. Rarely a functional metastasis may account for clinical hypersomatotrphism [24].

Ectopic GH-secreting tumor with clinical evidence of acromegaly, GH gene expression by the tumor tissue, marked arteriovenous gradient in GH levels across the ectopic source, and a rapid fall of GH and IGF-I after tumor resection have been documented in a single patient with a GH-producing pancreatic islet-cell tumor [25]. In several other tumors, including lung, breast, and gastric carcinomas, and bronchial carcinoids, GH immunoreactivity was demonstrated. However, in these cases clinically excessive GH secretion was not proven and no evidence of acromegaly was demonstrated.

Somatotrope hyperplasia is difficult to differentiate histologically from a GH-producing adenoma and usually is associated with acromegaly due to stimulation by ectopic GHRH-secreting tumors. This rare cause of acromegaly, indistinguishable clinically from acromegaly due to a pituitary adenoma, has been reported in patients with bronchial carcinoid tumors [26] (50–60% of patients with GHRH-secreting tumors), pancreatic islet-cell tu-mors [27], and small-cell lung cancers (see Table 2), and also adrenal adenomas, pheochromocytomas, medullary thyroid, endometrial, and breast cancers have rarely been described to express GHRH and to cause acromegaly. The structure of GHRH was originally elucidated from extracts of pancreatic islet-cell tumors removed from patients with this syndrome. Some ectopic tumors may secrete GHRH with reduced biologic activity due to chemical modifications of the hormone, while others synthesize GH but se-crete it inefficiently. GHRH-producing tumors may also contain somatostatin. Some patients with GHRH-secreting pancreatic tumors have hyperpara-thyroidism or familial disease suggestive of MEN-I syndrome.

Eutopic hypothalamic GHRH-secreting tumors, including hamartomas, choristomas, gliomas, and ganglioneuromas, may directly induce pituitary somatotrope hyperplasia or adenoma and resultant acromegaly [28,29]. Rarely, a clearly acromegalic patient will be encountered with acromegaloidism, presenting as acromegaly without demonstrable pituitary or extrapituitary tumor. GH and IGF-I levels are not elevated, and some of these patients may produce an erythroprogenitor growth factor, distinguishable from other growth factors [30] and demonstrated by bioassay techniques.

Clinical presentation (Table 4)

Acromegaly is insidious, and the mean delay from disease onset until diagnosis is estimated to be 8–10 years [31]. Rarely, excess GH secretion preceeds epiphyseal closure of the long bones in children, resulting in gigantism. About one quarter of acromegalic patients are found to harbor microadenomas (diameter <10 mm), while most patients have macroadenomas, many of them with parasellar invasion at the time of diagnosis [32]. Headaches are common, and visual-field defects and hypopituitarism occurring secondary to the large tumor mass correlate well with tumor size. Hyperprolactinemia is found in about one third of patients, and in most cases is caused by cosecretion of PRL with GH by the tumor (mixed somatotrope-lactotrope tumor, mammosomatotrope or plurihormonal adenomas). However, immunohistochemical staining for PRL is observed in the majority of somatotrope adenomas. Pituitary stalk compression by large GH-cell macroadenomas may also lead to hyperprolactinemia. Amenorrhea or impotence are common, and galactorrhea may be present even in patients with normal PRL levels, when elevated GH levels behave as an apparent agonist for PRL receptors in the breast.

Acral and soft-tissue overgrowth results in increased hand, foot, and heel-pad thickness, with increased shoe or glove size, and ring tightening. Skeletal overgrowth leads to mandibular enlargement with prognathism, frontal bossing, characteristic coarse facial features with wide spacing of the teeth, and a large, fleshy nose. Patients present with voice deepening, arthropathy, kyphosis, carpal tunnel syndrome, proximal muscle weakness and fatigue, oily skin, hyperhidrosis, acanthosis nigricans, skin tags, and depression. Generalized visceromegaly with enlargement of the tongue, thyroid, salivary glands, heart, and soft organs occur commonly.

Cardiovascular disease occurs in about a third of patients and consists of coronary heart disease, cardiomyopathy with arrhythmias, left ventricular hypertrophy, decreased diastolic function, and hypertension. Upper airway obstruction, diagnosed in 70% of male and 25% of female acromegalic patients [33], has been attributed to macroglossia and laryngeal soft-tissue overgrowth. Sleep apnea occurs in about 60% of patients, and a third of them, in fact, harbor central sleep apnea [33]. Patients with central sleep apnea have significantly higher GH and IGF-I levels than those with obstructive sleep apnea.

GH is a major peripheral antagonist of insulin, and glucose intolerance is

Table 4. Risks of long-term exposure to elevated growth hormone

Arthropathy
  Unrelated to age of onset or to GH levels
  Usually occurs with long duration
  Reversibility
    Rapid symptomatic improvement
    Irreversibility of bone and cartilage lesions
Neuropathy
  Peripheral nerves
    Intermittent anesthesias, paresthesias
    Sensorimotor polyneuropathy
  Reversibility
    Onion bulbs (whorls) do not regress
Cardiovascular disease
  Cardiomyopathy
    LV diastolic function decreased
    LV mass increased; arrhythmias
    Fibrous connective tissue hyperplasia
  Hypertension
    Exacerbates cardiomyopathy
  Reversibility
    May progress, even with normalized GH
Respiratory disease
  Upper-airway obstruction
    Soft-tissue overgrowth
  Reversibility
    Improves with reduction in GH
Malignancy
  Increased risk
  Increased soft-tissue polyps
  Reversibility
    Effect of therapy on risk unknown
Carbohydrate intolerance
  25% diabetes
  Reversibility
    Improves with reduced GH

LV = left ventricular; GH = growth hormone.
Adapted from the Acromegaly Therapy Consensus Development Panel [49], with permission.

present in about 50% of patients. Frank diabetes is diagnosed in 25% of patients, and most of these have a family history of diabetes. Metabolic disturbances as hypertriglyceridemia or hypercalciuria are found frequently in acromegaly.

In children, GH hypersecretion is associated with pituitary gigantism. In up to 20% of these cases McCune-Albright syndrome is diagnosed with somatotrope hyperplasia, or less often with a pituitary adenoma.

Increased overall mortality in acromegaly, about threefold higher in male patients, has been reported [31,34] due to cardiovascular and cerebrovascular disorders, malignancy, and respiratory disease (Table 5). Survival of these

Table 5. Acromegaly: Causes of death

Cardiovascular	38–62%
Respiratory	0–25%
Malignancy	9–25%

Compiled from, Nabarro [32], Bengtsson [34], Bates [51], and Rajasoorya [35].

Table 6. Survival determinants in 151 acromegalic patients

Last known growth hormone	$p < 0.0001$
Hypertension	$p < 0.02$
Cardiac disease	$p < 0.03$
Symptom duration	$p < 0.04$

Adapted from Rajasoorya et al. [35], with permission.

Table 7. Common cancers in 1041 acromegalic male patients without evidence of cancer at diagnosis

1190 males
↓
1041 → 149 (18% prevalent gastrointestinal cancer

	Cancers	Expected	O/E
All	116	72	1.6
Colon	13	4.2	3.1
Esophagus	7	2.3	3.1
Stomach	4	1.6	2.5
Melanoma	3	0.9	3.3

O/E = observed/expected.
Adapted from Ron et al. [38], with permission.

patients is reduced an average of 10 years compared with the non-acromegalic population [35] and correlates negatively with higher levels of GH at diagnosis ($p < 0.001$; Table 6). Other important determinants of mortality are the presence of cardiovascular disease at diagnosis ($p < 0.03$), diabetes mellitus ($p < 0.03$), and hypertension ($p < 0.02$) [35]. In fact, patients with cardiac disease already present at the time of diagnosis of acromegaly do not survive longer than 14 years [35], and only 30% of acromegalic patients who already have diabetes at diagnosis appear to survive more than 20 years.

Acromegaly increases the risk of malignancy and tissue polyps. This may be associated with the role of the GH–IGF-I axis in pathways that regulate cellular proliferation of both malignant and normal cells [36]. In contrast, hypophysectomy appears to protect against neoplasia in both animal models as well as in several earlier human studies. About 10% of patients develop a malignancy, most commonly colonic, gastric, and esophageal adenocarcinomas [37,38], occurring in acromegalic patients with a two- to threefold increase, and melanoma (Table 7). Adenomatous colonic polyps are present in up to one third of acromegalic patients [39,40]. Colonoscopy is helpful in the diagnosis of these premalignant lesions and differentiates them from the hypertrophic mucosal folds occasionally found in these patients.

Diagnosis of acromegaly

The clinical diagnosis is usually clear cut in long-standing cases but may be difficult in the early stages of the disease. The biochemical diagnosis of acromegaly is based on the demonstration of excess GH and IGF-I secretion with failure to suppress circulating GH levels by a glucose load. Random serum GH measurements are not helpful in the diagnosis of GH hypersecretion because of the pulsatile nature of pituitary GH release and its relatively short circulating half-life (about 22 minutes). Therefore, integrated measurements over time (at least every 20 minutes) are required. In addition, GH levels may also be elevated in uncontrolled diabetes, malnutrition, anorexia nervosa, cirrhosis, renal failure, and states of physical and emotional stress. Many laboratories consider 5 µg/l the upper limit of normal basal morning GH levels, using radioimmunoassay (RIA), but this criterion is no longer acceptable. Normal subjects have basal values ranging between 0.25 and 0.7 µg/l, which are below the sensitivity of most GH RIAs, and the probability of acromegaly is high if morning levels are higher than 10 µg/l.

A random GH level is not an absolute criterion for the diagnosis or exclusion of acromegaly and correlates poorly with disease severity. Accordingly, random morning levels are not cost effective for screening. When GH is sampled every 5 minutes, levels are undetectable in about half of samples collected from healthy individuals, while in acromegaly all samples collected over 24 hours contain detectable GH levels (>2 µg/l) [41]. GH immunoradiometric assays (IRMAs), employing a double monoclonal antibody sandwich system, are now widely used because of their sensitivity and accuracy, compared with RIAs. These new IRMAs indicate normal integrated GH levels of less than 0.5 µg/l.

Oral glucose tolerance test (OGTT)

This classic method is essential to establish the diagnosis of active acromegaly. Oral glucose load (50–100 g; after overnight fasting) normally suppresses GH levels to <1 µg/l within 1–2 hours, but acromegalic patients do not show this suppression [42], and 20% of patients have a paradoxic rise after 30–60 minutes. This dynamic test is also useful in monitoring the response to therapy.

9

IGF-I levels

Serum IGF-I levels are invariably high in acromegaly [43], correlate well with 24-hour GH secretion, and correlate better with the clinical manifestations of hypersomatotropism than single random GH measurements [44,45]. IGF-I clearance from the circulation takes hours (half-life 12–15 hours in association with the IGFBP-3 complex), and its levels do not fluctuate during the course of the day and are not affected by stress or physical exercise. Thus, single elevated IGF-I level measured by a commercial RIA is highly specific for diagnosing acromegaly and may also be helpful in monitoring the progress of therapy. IGF-I levels reach a plateau when GH is above 40 µg/l, and at higher GH concentrations the IGF-I increase is not linear. IGF-I levels are affected by nutritional status, age, and estrogens. Pregnancy and late puberty are associated with elevated levels, while values are normally low in infants and elderly subjects.

IGFBPs

IGFBP-III levels correlate well with IGF-I levels and are significantly elevated in acromegaly [46], even in patients with normal GH suppression in response to glucose. The utility of IGFBP-III as a sensitive diagnostic test of acromegaly needs confirmation. IGFBP-I levels are low in acromegaly, are inversely correlated with GH levels, and may be useful in determining responses to therapy [47].

TRH and gonadotropin-releasing hormone (GnRH) tests

In 50% of acromegalic patients, intravenous administration of TRH [48] or GnRH increases GH levels, unlike normal subjects, who have no induced GH response. GH response to TRH may indicate the presence of adenomatous tissue after unsuccessful trans-sphenoidal surgery. However, this test is not specific, because TRH may also stimulate GH release in renal failure, liver disease, anorexia nervosa, and depression.

The recommended strategy for diagnosis and subsequent post-therapy monitoring of acromegaly is to measure plasma IGF-I level and the GH response to OGTT [49].

Differential diagnosis of acromegaly (Fig. 1)

Magnetic resonance imaging (MRI) of the pituitary, with the paramagnetic contrast agent gadolinium, should identify the GH-secreting adenoma in patients with pituitary acromegaly. True acromegaly with normal GH and IGF-I levels and no evidence for extrapituitary tumor probably represents

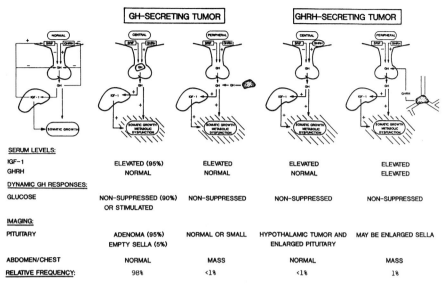

	GH-SECRETING TUMOR		GHRH-SECRETING TUMOR	
	CENTRAL	PERIPHERAL	CENTRAL	PERIPHERAL
SERUM LEVELS:				
IGF-1	ELEVATED (95%)	ELEVATED	ELEVATED	ELEVATED
GHRH	NORMAL	NORMAL	NORMAL	ELEVATED
DYNAMIC GH RESPONSES:				
GLUCOSE	NON-SUPPRESSED (90%) OR STIMULATED	NON-SUPPRESSED	NON-SUPPRESSED	NON-SUPPRESSED
IMAGING:				
PITUITARY	ADENOMA (95%) EMPTY SELLA (5%)	NORMAL OR SMALL	HYPOTHALAMIC TUMOR AND ENLARGED PITUITARY	MAY BE ENLARGED SELLA
ABDOMEN/CHEST	NORMAL	MASS	NORMAL	MASS
RELATIVE FREQUENCY:	98%	<1%	<1%	1%

Figure 1. Differential diagnosis of acromegaly. (Adapted from Melmed [42], with permission.)

'burned out' acromegaly associated with an infarcted previously active pituitary adenoma.

If tumor is not evident, the rare possibility of ectopic secretion of GHRH with somatotrope hyperplasia should be considered. An enlarged pituitary is, however, often found on MRI of patients with ectopic GHRH-secreting tumors. Excess GHRH secretion leading to pituitary hyperplasia may result in subsequent somatotrope adenoma formation. Imaging of the hypothalamic region is mandatory to exclude the presence of hypothalamic GHRH-secreting tumor. Plasma GHRH levels are usually elevated as much as 3–10 ng/ml in patients with peripleral GHRH-secreting tumors [50] compared with barely measurable concentrations (<30 pg/ml) in patients with pituitary acromegaly. However, hypothalamic GHRH-secreting tumors do not raise peripheral GHRH leves because excess eutopic hypothalamic GHRH is probably secreted into the hypophyseal portal system.

Unique clinical features and biochemical markers related to carcinoid syndrome (respiratory wheezing, flushing), islet-cell tumors (peptic ulcers and hypergastrinemia, hypoglycemia, and hyperinsulinemia), or small-cell lung cancer (hypercortisolism) may be associated with extrapituitary acromegaly and should be an indication for localization of a secreting tumor by abdominal [computed tomography (CT), MRI, arteriography, endoscopic ultrasound] or chest (x-ray, CT, bronchoscopy) imaging. Radiolabeled octreotide scan may be helpful to visualize ectopic GHRH-producing tumors or their metastases, as has been demonstrated in somatostatin receptor–positive endocrine tumors, including carcinoid tumors.

11

Treatment

Long-term exposure to high levels of GH and IGF-I reduces the quality of life by causing chronic pain, discomfort, and disfigurement, and shortens life expectancy. In addition, large pituitary tumors may compress and destroy adjacent structures and result in visual decompensation and hypopituitarism. Thus, to improve patient outcome the disease should be diagnosed early and medical intervention undertaken [51], even in the presence of mild GH excess with minimal signs and symptoms. The source of excess GH secretion should be identified, and the goal of management is either to remove it or suppress its activity. Effective treatment should restore soft-tissue overgrowth, and the other classic symptoms and biochemical derangements should be ameliorated. GH (after a glucose load) and IGF-I levels should ideally be normalized, and the pituitary tumor should be selectively resected or shrunken with preservation of residual anterior pituitary function. Criteria for biochemical cure of acromegaly include GH reduction to <1 µg/l after glucose load and IGF-I normalization [49]. Furthermore, restored circadian rhythm and appropriate responses of GH to provocative stimuli, including arginine, L-dopa, and exercise, should ideally be achieved to ensure that acromegaly is cured. Unfortunately, none of the three therapeutic modes currently available — surgery, irradiation, and medical treatment — alone fulfills all these comprehensive biochemical criteria, and acromegaly has in many patients been 'controlled' but not 'cured.'

Surgical management

Well-localized GH-secreting pituitary adenoma should be resected by an experienced neurosurgeon using a selective trans-sphenoidal surgical approach [52–55]. This procedure has yielded high success rates at major neurosurgical centers, with the use of accurate MRI localization, microinstrumentation, and sophisticated head-immobilization techniques. Residual pituitary function is usually preserved after resection of well-encapsulated tumors with no extrasellar extension. A transfrontal pituitary operation is rarely reserved for patients harboring large tumors with suprasellar extension or contiguity with blood vessels or the optic tract. Signs of preoperative tumor compression and compromised trophic hormone secretion are often restored by surgery. Soft-tissue swelling and metabolic dysfunction start improving immediately after successful tumor resection, GH levels usually return to normal within 1 hour, and IGF-I levels are normalized after 1 week but may remain elevated for several months, even when GH levels are in remission. In contrast to soft-tissue swelling, the hard-tissue changes induced by the acromegaly are irreversible.

Precise interpretation of surgical results in acromegaly is difficult, because most reports do not provide results of postglucose GH levels or IGF-I measurements. In addition, long-term data are often not reported in these series.

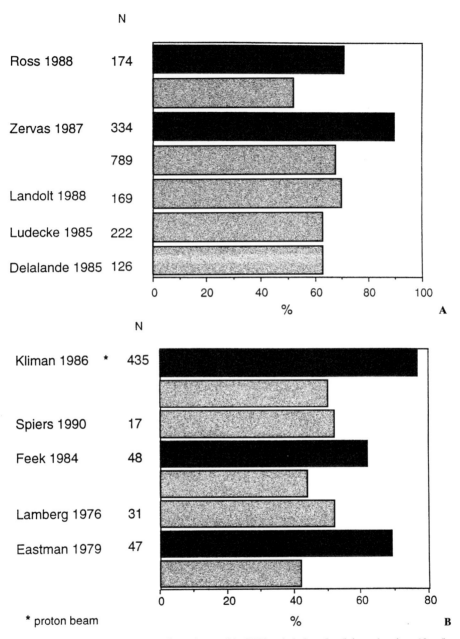

Figure 2. Percentage of acromegalic patients with GH levels below 5 μg/l (gray bars) or 10 μg/l (black bars) in different series (**A**) after trans-sphenoidal surgery and (**B**) 10 years after radio-therapy. (Adapted from Melmed et al. [56], with permission.)

In patients with intrasellar microadenomas, 72% had postglucose GH levels of <2μg/l (81% had basal levels of <5μg/l) in the early postoperative period [53], while only 50% of all-sized macroadenomas had GH levels <2μg/l after glucose load [53]. In most large surgical series, 60% of acromegalic patients had postoperative random GH levels <5μg/l [52–56] (Fig. 2A), and the success rate was significantly lower for macroadenomas. However, many patients with postoperative random GH levels of <5μg/l had increased IGF-I levels, or increased GH secretion when retested a year or more after the operation. Acromegaly may recur several years after surgery in 5–10% of operated patients despite normal dynamic GH shortly after the operation. This probably reflects the incomplete resection of the tumor, and if residual tumor is documented by MRI, reoperation is indicated with less favorable results than for primary resection.

Postoperative anterior pituitary failure and the need for lifelong hormonal replacement is found in up to 15% of patients [52,53], and the risk is increased in patients operated for large invasive tumors. Permanent diabetes insipidus occurs in 2.6% of patients [52], and other complications, including cerebrospinal fluid rhinorrhea, meningitis, and central nervous system damage, are rare. A mortality rate of about 1% or less may be encountered in association with resection of large invasive tumors.

The therapy of choice for ectopic acromegaly is surgical removal of GHRH- or GH-producing tumors if feasible and after accurate localization of the secreting tumor [57]. Cure is achieved when GHRH, GH, and IGF-I are normalized, together with GH suppressibility to glucose. Alternative therapeutic strategies are used in patients with inoperable metastatic disease (i.e., lung cancer), including pituitary surgery (ineffective in most GHRH-producing tumors) and octreotide administration (see later).

Radiotherapy

External-beam irradiation for acromegaly should be considered as adjuvant therapy when surgery or medical therapy has failed to control the disease. Maximal tumor irradiation with minimal normal tissue damage are achieved with precise MRI tumor localization, highly reproducible simulation, and isocentral rotational techniques. Conventional x-irradiation, proton beam (heavy-particle) therapy (performed in a limited number of centers), and gamma-knife excision (available in a few centers) can be used. The conventional megavoltage radiotherapy generated by cobalt-60 and linear accelerators is the common method of treatment. The recommended total dose is 4500–5000 rad given over 5–6 weeks in treatment fractions not exceeding 180 rad/day [57]. In addition to a high rate of late complications, the slow rate of response is the main disadvantage of radiotherapy, and many patients continue to be exposed to unacceptably high levels of circulating GH and IGF-I for several years after irradiation. Thus, radiotherapy is an inappropriate option for young patients with progressive physical deformities. The reduction in GH levels is more rapid with proton-beam therapy (the recommended dose is 15,000 rad), compared with conventional radiotherapy, and hormone levels begin falling gradually during the first year after treatment. GH levels drop to less than 10 µg/l after 5–10 years, and values <5 µg/l are encountered 10–15 years after treatment, with up to 77% of patients falling below 5 µg/l after 15 years [58–60] (Fig. 2B). Tumor growth is arrested, and over 95% of GH-cell adenomas shrink and headaches improve [58,61].

Proton-beam therapy is contraindicated in patients with suprasellar extension of their tumors because the optic tract can be exposed to the radiation field. Stereotactic ablation of GH-secreting adenomas by gamma-knife radiosurgery is highly promising but is performed only in specialized centers, and long-term results are not yet available. About half of acromegalic patients receiving radiotherapy develop hypopituitarism within 10 years after treatment [58], and the incidence increases thereafter. Hypocortisolism and hypogonadism are the common trophic hormone deficits (40–50%), and isolated hypothyroidism occurs in 10% of irradiated patients. Thus, many patients will require replacement of gonadal steroids, hydrocortisone, and thyroid hormone. Other postirradiation complications, including cranial-nerve palsies, vision loss, memory deficits, and cerebral necrosis, are very rare and are usually associated with larger doses than currently recommended. Secondary brain tumors occuring within the radiation field following treatment have been reported in 1.3–1.7% of irradiated patients during the first 10 years after therapy [62,63]. These include astrocytoma, glioma, meningioma, and rarely meningeal sarcoma [62,63]. The relative risk of developing such a second tumor has been estimated as 9–16 times greater than that of the normal population.

Medical treatment

Bromocriptine. Bromocriptine, an ergot-derivative dopamine agonist, suppresses GH secretion by neoplastic somatotropes and has therefore been used as a primary or adjuvant therapy for acromegaly, in combination with octreotide or irradiation, or before surgery. Usually patients require up to 20–30 mg/day, higher than the dose required to suppress PRL secretion in patients with prolactinoma. In addition, the duration of GH suppression is shorter in acromegaly, compared with the effect on PRL in prolactinoma, necessitating three to four daily doses instead of two. Among 549 patients from 31 different series treated with bromocriptine, random GH levels decreased to <10 µg/l in 53% and to <5 µg/l in 20% [64]. IGF-I levels were normalized in 10% of treated patients, and the drug resulted in minimal tumor shrinkage in less than 20% of patients. However, the majority of patients in this retrospective analysis experienced subjective clinical improvement while taking the drug, including decreased soft-tissue swelling, fatigue, perspiration, and headache. Thus, it has been suggested that bromocriptine may have a beneficial peripheral effect by impairing GH bioactivity unrelated to the direct effect on somatotrope secretion.

Bromocriptine does not reduce GHRH levels in patients with GHRH-producing tumors and fails to significantly lower serum GH and IGF-I levels in most of these patients. At the initiation of therapy, bromocriptine may cause gastointestinal upset, nausea, postural hypotension, and dizziness. Most of these side effects resolve with continued drug use. Other side effects, including nasal suffiness, depression, nightmares, and hallucinations, are reversible after decreasing the drug dose.

Octreotide. The somatostatin analog, octreotide, inhibits GH secretion with at least 40-fold greater potency than the naturally occuring hypothalamic somatostatin, but with only mild suppressive effect on insulin secretion. This eight amino-acid analog is relatively resistant to enzymatic degradation, with a circulating half-life of approximately 2 hours after subcutaneous injection, compared with the short duration of action of human somatostatin (serum half-life, about 3 minutes). Furthermore, rebound GH hypersecretion seen following somatostatin infusion is not encountered after octreotide, and prolonged use of the analog is not associated with desensitization. Cultured GH-secreting tumor cells respond in a qualitatively normal way to somatostatin, and this inhibitory effect is mediated via specific membrane receptors on the tumor cells [65]. Circulating GH suppression after octreotide administration closely correlates with the density of somatostatin receptors on the tumor tissue removed [66] and with the presence of receptors demonstrated by radiolabeled octreotide scan [67]. Acute lowering of GH levels in response to a test dose of octreotide was demonstrated only in patients with pituitary uptake of the labeled analog, while patients who do not respond to octreotide do not have visible in vivo receptors. Recently, expression of somatostatin receptor subtypes 2 and 5 was demonstrated in GH-secreting tumors [68,69].

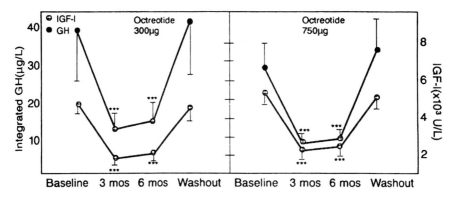

Figure 3. Effect of low-dose (100 µg every 8 hours, n = 50) and high-dose octreotide (250 µg every 8 hours, n = 54) on integrated GH and IGF-I levels in acromegalic patients treated with subcutaneous octreotide for 6 months. ***p < 0.001 versus baseline. (Adapted from Ezzat et al. [71], with permission.)

Octreotide exerts its GH-suppression effect predominantly through these receptor subtypes.

A single subcutaneous injection of 50–100 µg octreotide suppresses GH secretion for 4–6 hours [70] (Fig. 3). The drug is administered in three daily injections (100–200 µg each), and the daily dose can be increased up to 1500 µg. A long-acting formulation of somatostatin analog (Sandostatin LAR) that produces slow release of octreotide from microspheres is currently under clinical investigation, and has shown comparable GH suppression in acromegalic patients for as long as 6 weeks after a single 30-mg intramuscular injection. Octreotide administered subcutaneously every 8 hours significantly suppresses GH levels in over 90% of acromegalic patients [71] (see Fig. 3), decreasing the integrated GH levels over 5 hours after injection to <5 µg/l in 50% of patients, and to <2 µg/l in 25%.

Octreotide normalizes IGF-I levels in 47% of patients treated worldwide [56]. In patients treated for microadenomas, integrated GH and IGF-I levels are almost invariably normalized [71], while the drug is less effective in larger adenomas (Table 8). In a recent multicenter follow-up of 103 acromegalic

Table 8. Factors influencing biochemical and clinical responsiveness to octreotide in acromegaly

Dose
Delivery mode
Duration
Disease severity
  Baseline GH and IGF-I
  Tumor size

GH = growth hormone; IGF-I = insulin-like growth factor I.

Table 9. Comparison of treatment modalities for acromegaly: Success rates and complications

	Trans-sphenoidal surgery		Radiotherapy	Bromocriptine	Octreotide
	Microadenoma	Macroadenoma			
GH <5 µg/l	80%	50–60%	77% (15 yr)	20%	65%
GH <2 µg/l	70%	40%	n.d.	n.d.	40%
Normal IGF-I	~50%*		n.d.	10%	50%
Tumor shrinkage	>95%	70%	95%	10%	50%
Disadvantages		Recurrence 5–10%	Late response	Low efficacy	3 s.c. injections/day
		Persistent GH↑ 40%			
Complications					
New hypopituitarism	15%		>50%	No	No
Other	Diabetes insipidus 2.6%		Neurological deficits	Nausea, dizziness	Asymptomatic gallstones

n.d. = no data; GH = growth hormone; IGF-I = insulin-like growth factor I.
ª Data derived from our experience.
Data summarized from Fahlbusch et al. [53], Eastman et al. [58], Jaffe et al. [64], Ezzat [71], and Newman et al. [72].

patients receiving long-term octreotide treatment, GH levels 2 hours after analog injection were $\leq 5 \mu g/l$ in 65% of patients and $\leq 2 \mu g/l$ in 40% [72] (Table 9). IGF-I concentrations decrease to normal in 56% of patients [72]. Significant tumor shrinkage, as assessed by MRI or CT scan, occurs in up to 50% of patients [71]. This effect on tumor size is evident within the first 3 months and is reversible if treatment is stopped. Over 70% of patients experience rapid and marked improvement in many signs and symptoms within several days [71], including soft tissue swelling, hyperhidrosis, headache, arthralgia, and paresthesias.

Combined therapy with bromocriptine and octreotide induces an additive suppression of GH and IGF-I compared with separate administration of similar doses of either drug [73]. Sleep apnea responds dramatically to long-term octreotide treatment [74]. However, this improvement is independent of the biochemical response of GH or IGF-I to the drug administration, and it does not differ in patients who are in biochemical remission or in those who do not achieve this remission. In patients with left ventricular hypertrophy, treatment with a somatostatin analog results in a rapid decrease of left ventricular mass within weeks, associated with reductions of GH and IGF-I levels [75]. However, the biochemical remission often does not cure the hypertension commonly seen in acromegaly.

Octreotide also suppresses hypersecretion of ectopic GHRH-producing tumors, while decreasing the secretion of GH by the pituitary, and can be used to treat this unusual form of acromegaly. However, GHRH suppression is incomplete and transient, and the drug acts both at the pituitary level and on the GHRH-secreting tumor. Octretotide improves the clinical and biochemical manifestations of acromegaly in these patients [76], and rarely inhibits the primary and metastatic carcinoid tumor growth. Symptoms due to other hypersecreted hormones (i.e., gastrin) can be ameliorated.

Table 10. Octreotide side effects

Gallbladder
    Asymptomatic gallstones or sludge
Gastrointestinal
    Diarrhea
    Nausea
    Abdominal discomfort
Glucose levels
    Hypoglycemia
    Hyperglycemia

Thyroid function
    Hypothyroidism
Cardiac
    Sinus bradycardia

Other adverse events
    Pain on injection
    Headache

Octreotide treatment is indicated in acromegalic patients who have inadequately responded to surgery or bromocriptine, or cannot be treated by these modalities; to control acromegaly after radiotherapy, as clinical improvement is delayed; and to control severe symptoms, including headaches and sleep apnea, before trans-sphenoidal adenomectomy.

Side effects (Table 10). Octreotide is well tolerated in most patients. Most side effects are related to the suppression of gastrointestinal motility and secretion by the drug, and are often short lived [49]. They include nausea, mild malabsorption, loose stools, abdominal discomfort, and flatulence in one third of the patients. Mild glucose intolerance may occur due to transient suppression of insulin secretion, but insulin requirements in diabetic acromegalics are dramatically reduced while receiving octreotide. The most significant side effect relates to the gallbladder. Octreotide attenuates postprandial gallbladder contractility and delays emptying, and up to 40% of long-term treated patients in the United States develop asymptomatic cholesterol gallstones or sludge [72], usually during the first year of treatment. The incidence of gallstones is geographically variable, with higher rates observed in China, Australia, and the United Kingdom. Other side effects include asymptomatic bradycardia, headache, hypothyroxinemia, and local pain at the injection site.

Management strategy (Fig. 4)

Trans-sphenoidal surgery is the primary therapeutic option in pituitary acromegaly, both for invasive and noninvasive adenomas. In addition, octreotide may be used as the initial treatment in selected patients. Preoperative octreotide is commonly tried in patients harboring large invasive macroadenomas to shrink the tumor and to improve the postsurgical outcome. If GH and IGF-I levels have normalized after surgery, no additional treatment is needed. If surgical therapy fails to achieve biochemical remission, medical management with bromocriptine and/or octreotide should be initiated. Sellar radiotherapy is selected if medical treatment does not normalize GH or IGF-I. Octreotide treatment should be instituted to control symptoms and to prevent further tissue damage until radiation becomes effective. In the case of recurrent disease, octreotide is the best therapeutic option for immediate relief of symptoms and reduction of GH hypersecretion. For elderly asymptomatic patients, no therapy may be indicated, and for elderly patients experiencing morbidity, octreotide is the preferred treatment [49].

Follow-up

The criteria for biochemical cure are suppressed GH of $<1\,\mu g/l$ after glucose load and normal IGF-I levels, and patients should be followed quarterly after treatment to achieve these goals of therapy. However, even 'cured'

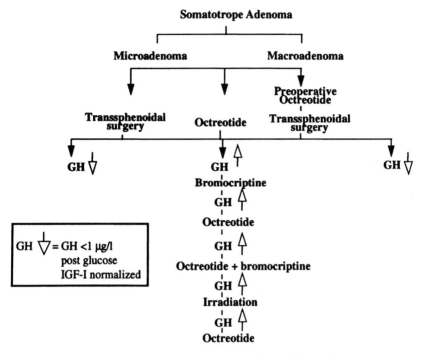

Figure 4. Management strategy for acromegaly caused by a pituitary adenoma.

acromegalic patients usually have abnormal patterns of GH secretion and experience most of their secretion as detectable basal GH and not during pulses, as do normal subjects. To monitor residual anterior pituitary function, hormone evaluation should be performed semiannually, and MRI should be repeated every year in the first years following successful therapy. Semiannual visual field assessment by perimetry is mandatory in acromegalic patients with residual tumor, in those treated with octreotide or bromocriptine, and in patients requiring hormone replacement. Frequent colonoscopic examination is recommended in patients over 50 years old, and rheumatologic, dental, and cardiac evaluations are included in the follow-up.

Future developments

Novel somatostatin analogs with longer acting formulations and delivery systems are currently being developed [77]. Other peptide preparations include GH analogs behaving as antagonists. Transgenic mice expressing high levels of a mutated bovine GH gene are dwarf and secrete low levels of IGF-I [78]. This analog acts as a functional antagonist to the action of endogenous GH at the receptor level. This may serve as a model for the future development of human GH agonists or antagonists that, hopefully, will block the adverse effects of

20

GH hypersecretion in acromegaly. In addition, GHRH antagonist administration blocks GHRH activity in the pituitary and hypothalamus, and prevents GH secretion and somatic growth in immature animals. These advances will provide the treating physician with new nonsurgical therapies for neuroendocrine control of acromegaly.

References

1. Miller WL, Eberhardt NL. 1983. Structure and evaluation of growth hormone gene family. Endocr Rev 4:97–130.
2. Lewis UJ, Bonewald LF, Lewis VJ. 1980. The 20,000-dalton variant of human growth hormone: Location of the amino acid deletions. Biochem Biophys Res Commun 92:511–516.
3. Baumann G. Growth hormone heterogeneity: Genes, isohormones, variants, and binding proteins. 1991. Endocr Rev 12:235–251.
4. Barinaga M, Yamanoto G, Rivier G, Vale W, Evans R, Rosenfeld MG. 1983. Transcriptional regulation of growth hormone gene expression by growth hormone-releasing factor. Nature 306:84–86.
5. Fukata J, Diamond DJ, Martin JB. 1985. Effects of rat growth hormone (rGH)-releasing factor and somatostatin on the release and synthesis of rGH in dispersed pituitary cells. Endocrinology 117:457–467.
6. Yamashita S, Weiss M, Melmed S. 1986. Insulin-growth factor I regulates growth hormone secretion and messenger ribonucleic acid levels in human pituitary tumor cells. J Clin Endocrinol Metab 63:730–735.
7. Herman V, Weiss M, Becker D, Melmed S. 1990. Hypothalamic hormonal regulation of human growth harmane gene expression in somatotroph adenoma cell cultures. Endocr Pathol 1:236–244.
8. Leung DW, Spencer SA, Cachianes G, Hammonds RG, Collins C, Henzel WG, Barnard R, Waters MJ, Wood EI. 1987. Growth hormone receptor and serum binding protein: Purification, cloning and expression. Nature 330:537–543.
9. Mannor DA, Winer LM, Shaw MA, Baumann G. 1991. Plasma growth hormone (GH)-binding proteins: Effect on GH binding to receptors and GH action. J Clin Endocrinol Metab 73:30–34.
10. Salomon F, Cuneo RC, Hesp R, Sonksen PH. 1989. The effects of treatment with recombinant human growth hormone on body composition and metabolism in adults with growth hormone deficiency. N Engl J Med 321:1797–1803.
11. Herman V, Fagin J, Gonsky R, Kovacs K, Melmed S. 1990. Clonal origin of pituitary adenomas. J Clin Endocrinol Metab 71:1427–1433.
12. Vallar L, Spada A, Giannattasio G. 1987. Altered Gs and adenylate cyclase activity in human GH-secreting pituitary adenomas. Nature 330:566–568.
13. Landis CA, Masters SB, Spada A, Pace AM, Bourne HR, Vallar L. 1989. GTPase inhibiting mutations activate the α chain of Gs and stimulate adenylyl cyclase in human pituitary tumours. Nature 340:692–696.
14. Landis CA, Harsh G, Lyons J, Davis RL, McCormick F, Bourne HR. 1990. Clinical characteristics of acromegalic patients whose pituitary tumors contain mutant Gs protein. J Clin Endocrinol Metab 71:1416–1420.
15. Weinstein LS, Shenker A, Gejman PV, Merino MJ, Friedman E, Spiegel AM. 1991. Activating mutations of the stimulatory G protein in the McCune-Albright syndrome. N Engl J Med 325:1688–1695.
16. Bertherat J, Chanson P, Montminy M. 1995. The cyclic adenosine 3′,5′-monophosphate-responsive factor CREB is constitutively activated in human somatotroph adenomas. Mol Endocrinol 9:777–783.

21

17. Thakker RV, Pook MA, Wooding C, Boscaro M, Scanarini M, Clayton RN. 1993. Association of somatotrophinomas with loss of alleles on chromosome 11 and with gsp mutations. J Clin Invest 91:2815–2821.

18. Billestrup N, Swanson LW, Vale W. 1986. Growth hormone-releasing factor stimulates proliferation of somatotrophs in vitro. Proc Natl Acad Sci USA 83:6854–6857.

19. Joubert (Bression) D, Benlot C, Lagoguey A, Garnier P, Brandi AM, Gautron JP, Legrand JC, Peillon F. 1989. Normal and growth hormone (GH)-secreting adenomatous human pituitaries release somatostatin and GH-releasing hormone. J Clin Endocrinol Metab 68:572–577.

20. Lloyd RV, Cano M, Chandler WF, Barkan AL, Horvath E, Kovacs K. 1989. Human growth hormone and prolactin secreting pituitary adenomas analyzed by in situ hybridization. Am J Pathol 134:605–613.

21. Kovacs K, Horvath E, Asa SL, Stefaneanu L, Sano T. 1989. Pituitary cells producing more than one hormone. Trends Endocrinol Metab 1:104–107.

22. Rasmussen P, Lindholm J. 1979. Ectopic pituitary adenomas. Clin Endocrinol 11:69–74.

23. Mountcastle RB, Roof BS, Mayfield RK, Mordes DB, Sagel J, Biggs PJ, Rawe SE. 1989. Case report: Pituitary adenocarcinoma in an acromegalic patient: Response to bromocriptine and pituitary testing: A review of the literature on 36 cases of pituitary carcinoma. Am J Med Sci 298:109–118.

24. Greenman Y, Woolf P, Congilio J, O'Mara R, Pei L, Said JW, Melmed S. 1996. Remission of acromegaly caused by pituitary carcinoma after surgical excision of growth hormone secreting metastasis detected by 111-indium pentetreotide scan. J Clin Endocrinol Metab, in press.

25. Melmed S, Ezrin C, Kovacs K, Goodman RS, Frohman LA. 1985. Acromegaly due to secretion of growth hormone by an ectopic pancreatic islet-cell tumor. N Engl J Med 312:9–17.

26. Scheithauer BW, Carpenter PC, Bloch B, Brazeau P. 1984. Ectopic secretion of a growth hormone-releasing factor. Report of a case of acromegaly with bronchial carcinoid tumor. Am J Med 76:605–615.

27. Schulte HM, Benker G, Windeck R, Olbricht T, Reinwein D. 1985. Failure to respond to growth hormone releasing hormone (GHRH) in acromegaly due to a GHRH secreting pancreatic tumor: Dynamics of multiple endocrine testing. J Clin Endocrinol Metab 61:585–587.

28. Asa SL, Scheithauer BW, Bilbao JM, Horvath E, Ryan N, Kovacs K, Randall RV, Laws ER Jr, Singer W, Linfoot JA, Thorner MO, Vale W. 1984. A case for hypothalamic acromegaly: A clinicopathological study of six patients with hypothalamic gangliocytomas producing growth hormone-releasing factor. J Clin Endocrinol Metab 58:796–803.

29. Asa SL, Bilbao JM, Kovacs K, Linfoot JA. 1980. Hypothalamic neuronal hamartoma associated with pituitary growth hormone cell adenoma and acromegaly. Acta Neuropathol 53:231–234.

30. Ashcraft MW, Hartzband PI, Van Herle AJ, Bersch N, Golde DW. 1983. A unique growth factor in patients with acromegaloidism. J Clin Endocrinol Metab 57:272–276.

31. Molitch ME. 1992. Clinical manifestations of acromegaly. Endocrinol Metab Clin North Am 21:597–614.

32. Nabarro JDN. 1987. Acromegaly. Clin Endocrinol 26:481–512.

33. Grunstein RR, Ho KY, Sullivan CE. 1991. Sleep apnea in acromegaly. Ann Intern Med 115:527–532.

34. Bengtsson B-A, Eden S, Ernest I, Oden A, Sjogren B. 1988. Epidemiology and long-term survival in acromegaly. Acta Med Scand 223:327–335.

35. Rajasoorya C, Holdaway MI, Wrightson P, Scott DJ, Ibbertson HK. 1994. Determinants of clinical outcome and survival in acromegaly. Clin Endocrinol 41:95–102.

36. Ezzat S, Melmed S. 1991. Are patients with acromegaly at increased risk for neoplasia? J Clin Endocrinol Metab 72:245–2249.

37. Ituarte EA, Petrini J, Hershman JM. 1984. Acromegaly and colon cancer. Ann Intern Med 101:627–628.

38. Ron E, Gridley G, Hrubec Z, Page W, Arora S, Fraumeni JJ. 1991. Acromegaly and gastrointestinal cancer. Cancer 68:1673–1677.
39. Klein I, Parveen G, Gavaler JS, Vanthiel DH. 1982. Colonic polyps in patients with acromegaly. Ann Intern Med 97:27–30.
40. Ezzat S, Storm C, Melmed S. 1991. Colon polyps in acromegaly. Ann Intern Med 114:754–758.
41. Hartman ML, Veldhuis JD, Vance ML, Faria AC, Furlanetto RW, Thorner MO. 1990. Somatotropin pulse frequency and basal concentrations are increased in acromegaly and are reduced by successful therapy. J Clin Endocrinol Metab 70:1375–1384.
42. Melmed S. 1990. Acromegaly. N Engl J Med 322:966–977.
43. Clemmons DR, Van Wyk JJ, Ridgway EC, Kliman B, Kjellberg RN, Underwood KE. 1979. Evaluation of acromegaly by radioimmunoassay of somatomedin-C. N Engl J Med 301:1138–1142.
44. Rieu M, Girard F, Bricaire H, Binoux M. 1982. The importance of insulin-like growth factor (somatomedin) measurements in the diagnosis and surveillance of acromegaly. J Clin Endocrinol Metab 55:147–153.
45. Chang-DeMoranville BM, Jackson IM. 1992. Diagnosis and endocrine testing in acromegaly. Endocrinol Metab Clin North Am 21:649–668.
46. Grinspoon S, Clemmons D, Swearingen B, Klibanski A. 1995. Serum insulin-like growth factor-binding protein-3 levels in the diagnosis of acromegaly. J Clin Endocrinol Metab 80:927–932.
47. Ezzat S, Ren S, Braunstein GD, Melmed S. 1991. Octreotide stimulates insulin-like growth factor binding protein-1 (IGFBP-1) levels in acromegaly. J Clin Endocrinol Metab 73:441–443.
48. Irie M, Tsushima T. 1972. Increase of serum growth hormone concentration following thyrotropin-releasing hormone injection in patients with acromegaly or gigantism. J Clin Endocrinol Metab 35:97–100.
49. Acromegaly Therapy Consensus Development Panel. 1994. Consensus statement: Benefits versus risks of medical therapy for acromegaly. Am J Med 97:468–473.
50. Frohman LA. 1984. Ectopic hormone production by tumors. Clin Neuroendocr Perspect 3:201–224.
51. Bates AS, Van't Hoff W, Jones JM, Clayton RN. 1993. An audit of outcome of treatment in acromegaly. Q J Med 86:293–299.
52. Ross DA, Wilson CB. 1988. Results of transsphenoidal microsurgery for growth hormone-secreting pituitary adenomas in a series of 214 patients. J Neurosurg 68:854–867.
53. Fahlbusch R, Honegger J, Buchfelder M. 1992. Surgical management of acromegaly. Endocrinol Metab Clin North Am 21:669–692.
54. Tindall GT, Oyesiku NM, Watts NB, Clark RV, Christy JH, Adams DA. 1993. Transsphenoidal adenomectomy for growth hormone-secreting pituitary adenomas in acromegaly: Outcome analysis and determinants of failure. J Neurosurg 78:205–215.
55. Zervas NT. 1987. Multicenter surgical results in acromegaly. In Ludecke DK, Tolis G, eds. Growth Hormone, Growth Factors, and Acromegaly. New York: Raven Press, p 253.
56. Melmed S, Ho K, Thorner M, Klibanski A, Reichlin S. 1995. Recent advances in pathogenesis, diagnosis and management of acromegaly. J Clin Endocrinol Metab 80:3395–3402.
57. Faglia G, Arosio M, Bazzoni N. 1992. Ectopic acromegaly. Endocrinol Metab Clin North Am 21:575–595.
58. Eastman RC, Gorden P, Glatstein E, Roth J. 1992. Radiation therapy of acromegaly. Endocrinol Metab Clin North Am 21:693–712.
59. Eastman RC, Gorden P, Roth J. 1979. Conventional supervoltage irradiation is an effective treatment for acromegaly. J Clin Endocrinol Metab 48:931–940.
60. Gorden P, Glatstein E, Oldfield E, Roth J. 1987. Conventional supervoltage radiation in the treatment of acromegaly. In Robbins RJ, Melmed S, eds. Acromegaly. A Century of Scientific and Clinical Progress. New York: Plenum, pp 211–228.

61. Dowsett RJ, Fowble B, Sergott RC, Savino PJ, Bosley TM, Snyder PJ, Gennarelli TA. 1990. Results of radiotherapy in the treatment of acromegaly: Lack of ophthalmologic complications. Int J Radiat Oncol Biol Phys 19:453–459.
62. Brada M, Ford D, Ashley S, Bliss JM, Crowley S, Mason M, Rajan B, Traish D. 1992. Risk of second brain tumour after conservative surgery and radiotherapy for pituitary adenoma. Br Med J 304:1343–1346.
63. Tsang RW, Laperriere NJ, Simpson WJ, Brierley J, Panzarella T, Smyth HS. 1993. Glioma arising after radiation therapy for pituitary adenoma. Cancer 72:2227–2233.
64. Jaffe CA, Barkan AL. 1992. Treatment of acromegaly with dopamine agonists. Endocrinol Metab Clin North Am 21:713–735.
65. Reubi JC, Landolt AM. 1984. High density of somatostatin receptors in pituitary tumors from acromegalic patients. J Clin Endocrinol Metab 59:1148–1151.
66. Reubi JC, Landolt AM. 1989. The growth hormone responses to octreotide in acromegaly correlate with adenoma somatostatin receptor status. J Clin Endocrinol Metab 68:844–850.
67. Ur E, Mather SJ, Bomanji J, Ellison D, Britton KE, Grossman AB, Wass JAH, Besser GM. 1992. Pituitary imaging using a labelled somatostatin analogue in acromegaly. Clin Endocrinol 36:147–150.
68. Greenman Y, Melmed S. 1994. Heterogeneous expression of two somatostatin receptor subtypes in pituitary tumors. J Clin Endocrinol Metab 78:398–403.
69. Greenman Y, Melmed S. 1994. Expression of three somatostatin receptor subtypes in pituitary adenomas: Evidence for preferential SSTR5 expression in the mammosomatotroph lineage. J Clin Endocrinol Metab 79:724–729.
70. Lamberts SWJ. 1988. The role of somatostatin in the regulation of anterior pituitary hormone secretion and the use of its analogs in the treatment of human pituitary tumors. Endocr Rev 9:417–436.
71. Ezzat S, Snyder PJ, Young WF, Boyajy LD, Newman C, Klibanski A, Molitch ME, Boyd AE, Sheeler L, Cook DM, Malarkey WB, Jackson I, Lee Vance M, Thorner MO, Barkan A, Frohman LA, Melmed S. 1992. Octreotide treatment of acromegaly: A randomized, multicenter study. Ann Intern Med 117:711–718.
72. Newman CB, Melmed S, Snyder PJ, Yound WF, Boyajy LD, Levy R, Stewart WN, Klibanski A, Molitch ME, Gagel RF, Boyd AE, Sheeler L, Cook D, Malarkey WB, Jackson IMD, Lee Vance M, Thorner MO, Ho PJ, Jaffe CA, Frohman LA, Kleinberg DL. 1995. Safety and efficacy of long term octreotide therapy of acromegaly: Results of a multicenter trial in 103 patients — a clinical research center study. J Clin Endocrinol Metab 80:2768–2775.
73. Lamberts SWJ, Zweens M, Verschoor L, del Pozo E. 1986. A comparison among the growth hormone-lowering effects in acromegaly of the somatostatin analog SMS 201-995, bromocriptine, and the combination of both drugs. J Clin Endocrinol Metab 63:16–20.
74. Grunstein RR, Ho KY, Sullivan CE. 1994. Effect of octreotide, a somatostatin analog, on sleep apnea in patients with acromegaly. Ann Intern Med 121:478–483.
75. Lim MJ, Barkan AL, Buda AJ. 1992. Rapid reduction of left ventricular hypertrophy in acromegaly after suppression of growth hormone hypersecretion. Ann Intern Med 117:719–726.
76. von Werder K, Losa M, Muller OA, Schweiberer L, Fahlbusch R, del Poso E. 1984. Treatment of metastasing GRH-producing tumor with a long-acting somatostatin analogue. Lancet 2:282–283.
77. Flogstad AK, Halse J, Haldorsen T, Lancranjan I, Marbach P, Bruns C, Jervell J. 1995. Sandostatin LAR in acromegalic patients: A dose-range study. J Clin Endocrinol Metab 80:3601–3607.
78. Chen WY, Chen N, Yun J, Wagner TE, Kopchick JJ. 1994. In vitro and in vivo studies of antagonistic effects of human growth hormone analogs. J Biol Chem 269:15892–15897.

24

2. Adrenocorticotrophic hormone–dependent Cushing's syndrome

Giovanni Cizza and George P. Chrousos

Cushing's syndrome is the state that results from prolonged exposure of tissues to excess glucocorticoids. At the beginning of the century, Harvey Cushing recognized that Cushing's syndrome could result from tumors arising from either the anterior pituitary (basophilic adenomata) or the adrenal cortex [1,2]. This observation set the basis for our current classification of Cushing's syndrome into adrenocorticotrophic hormone (ACTH)-dependent and ACTH-independent forms. The former, in addition to pituitary adenomas, includes nonpituitary tumors that secrete ACTH (ectopic ACTH syndrome) or, rarely, corticotropin-releasing hormone (CRH; ectopic CRH syndrome). In the early 1950s, when glucocorticoids were first employed in the treatment of rheumatoid arthritis, the iatrogenic form of Cushing's syndrome appeared. As the use of glucocorticoids was extended to many immunological, hematologic, renal, and other diseases, the prevalence of exogenous Cushing's syndrome far exceeded that of the endogenous forms. More recently, factitious use of glucocorticoids was also reported [3].

Clinical presentation

Cushing's syndrome is a multisystem disorder. The typical clinical presentation of Cushing's syndrome results primarily from excess glucocorticoids (hypercortisolism) and, to a lesser extent, from excess mineralocorticoids (hypermineralocorticoidism) and/or adrenal androgens (hyperandrogenism). One of the earliest signs in virtually all patients with Cushing's syndrome is obesity, while in growing children this is combined with deceleration or arrest of growth [4,5]. The accumulation of visceral fat in patients with Cushing's syndrome, a result of excess cortisol and insulin secretion, is associated with the full expression of metabolic syndrome X (hyperlipidemia, hypertension, insulin resistance) and its long-term sequelae.

Etiology: definition

Endogenous Cushing's syndrome can result either from ACTH or CRH excess of pituitary or ectopic tumor origin, or from autonomous cortisol hyper-

Andrew Arnold (ed.) ENDOCRINE NEOPLASMS. 1997. Kluwer Academic Publishers. ISBN 0-7923-4354-9.

secretion by cortisol-secreting adrenal benign or malignant tumors or by 'micronodular' or 'massively macronodular' adrenals (Table 1). Endogenous Cushing's syndrome is rare, with an overall incidence of approximately two to four new cases per million of population per year, and has a female to male preponderance (9:1). ACTH-dependent Cushing's syndrome accounts for about 85% of endogenous cases. In the great majority of these cases (80%), the cause is autonomous pituitary ACTH secretion, referred to as Cushing's disease. In the remaining 20% the source of ACTH secretion is ectopic. Ectopic CRH production causing Cushing's syndrome has also been described in a number of case reports [6,7].

The molecular pathophysiology of ACTH-secreting tumors, either in the pituitary or ectopically, remains elusive. Unlike the case of growth hormone–secreting adenomas, abnormalities of the G-proteins are not frequent in corticotropinomas; however, approximately 50% of these tumors overexpress the p53 tumor suppressor gene, possibly as a result of neutralizing mutations of this gene [8]. The possibility of activating/oncogenic somatic mutations of the CRH receptor and/or the vasopressin V1β receptor genes is currently under investigation, while a somatic frame-shift mutation of the glucocorticoid receptor gene was recently described in a large corticotropinoma [9]. Familial ACTH-dependent Cushing's syndrome can be seen within the context of multiple endocrine neoplasia.

Table 1. Classification of hypercortisolism

Physiologic states
  Stress
  Pregnancy
  Chronic strenuous excercise
  Malnutrition
Pathophysiologic states
  Cushing's syndrome
    ACTH dependent (85%)
      Pituitary adenoma (80%) (rarely MEN-I)
      Ectopic ACTH (20%) (rarely MEN-I, MEN-II)
      Ectopic CRH (rare)
    ACTH independent (15%)
      Adrenal adenoma (rarely MEN-I, McCune-Albright syndrome)
      Adrenal carcinoma
      Micronodular adrenal disease (rare)
      Massive macronodular adrenal disease (rare)
  Psychiatric states
      Melancholic depression (pseudo-Cushing's)
      Obsessive-compulsive disorder
      Chronic active alcoholism (pseudo-Cushing's)
      Panic disorder
      Anorexia nervosa
      Narcotic withdrawal
  Complicated diabetes mellitus
  Glucocorticoid resistance

MEN-I, II = Multiple endocrine neoplasia I, II.

Diagnosis and differential diagnosis

Despite major recent advances, the diagnosis and differential diagnosis of Cushing's syndrome continues to challenge the diagnostic skills of physicians [10]. The goal of the clinician should be to identify individuals with Cushing's syndrome and to differentiate its causes as early in the course of the disease as possible, so as to avoid the chronic complications of hypercortisolism.

Once there is clinical suspicion of Cushing's syndrome, the first step is the biochemical documentation of endogenous hypercortisolism. This step can usually be accomplished by outpatient tests. Measurement of 24-hour urinary free cortisol (UFC) and/or 17-hydroxysteroid excretion and the 1-mg overnight dexamethasone suppression test are used for this purpose.

Twenty-four hour UFC excretion remains constant throughout life when normalized per square meter of body surface area, obviating the need of using age-specific normal values in children or obese subjects [11]. When assays for UFC excretion are not available, measurement of urinary 24-hour 17-hydroxysteroids can be of help. These compounds include all cortisol metabolites with a 17-dihydroxyacetone side chain and thus give an indirect measure of the rate of cortisol secretion. Correction is required, however, for urinary creatinine excretion because size and adiposity influence their daily production.

Determination of 24-hour UFC excretion is the best screening test available for documentation of endogenous hypercortisolism [12]. Values consistently in excess of 300 μg/day are virtually diagnostic of Cushing's syndrome. Assuming complete collections have been performed, there are virtually no false-negative results. False-positive results, however, may be obtained in several non-Cushing's hypercortisolemic states (see Table 1). In these states, however, rarely are the levels of UFC higher than 300 μg per day.

The overnight 1-mg dexamethasone suppression test is a simple screening procedure for hypercortisolism [13]. The test has a low incidence of false-normal suppression (less than 3%). However, the incidence of false-positive results is significantly high (approximately 20–30%). In children, the dose of dexamethasone that should be employed is 15 μg/kg body weight.

Cushing's syndrome is generally excluded if the response to the single-dose dexamethasone suppression test and the 24-hour UFC or 17-hydroxysteroid excretion are normal. One should bear in mind, however, that cortisol hypersecretion may be intermittent and periodic in 5–10% of patients with Cushing's syndrome of any etiology. Documenting loss of diurnal variation of plasma cortisol would support the diagnosis of Cushing's syndrome and vice versa. The same is true for loss of stress-induced activation of the hypothalamic-pituitary-adrenal (HPA) axis in Cushing's syndrome. More than a single morning and evening blood draws increase the value of the test, because a significant variability of cortisol levels may be present. Similarly, isolated plasma ACTH determinations are of limited value, especially because there is significant overlap between the ACTH levels in Cushing's patients and those in normal subjects. On the other hand, plasma ACTH measurements can be quite useful in providing an early distinction between ACTH-dependent and ACTH-independent sourses.

Distinguishing Cushing's syndrome from pseudo-Cushing states

The clinical and biochemical presentation of mild hypercortisolism in Cushing's syndrome if often indistinguishable from that seen in pseudo-Cushing states, such as depression or chronic active alcoholism (see Table 1) [14,15]. A hyperactive/hyper-responsive hypothalamic CRH neuron is central to the hypercortisolism of pseudo-Cushing states in the context of a pituitary-adrenal axis that is otherwise appropriately, albeit not fully, restrained by negative cortisol feedback [16]. In contrast, the hypercortisolism of Cushing's syndrome, regardless of the classification, feeds back negatively on the hypothalamus and completely suppresses hypothalamic CRH secretion. These concepts form the basis for the tests used in the differential diagnosis of mild hypercortisolism. Thus, most patients with Cushing's syndrome (80–90%) show inadequate suppression to low-dose (0.5 mg every 6 hours for 2 days) dexamethasone and do not respond to insulin-induced hypoglycemia, in contrast to the normal responses of depressed and other pseudo-Cushing patients. In addition, patients with Cushing's disease (85%) have a 'normal' or exaggerated ACTH response to CRH, whereas patients with depression (75%) show a blunted response. Whether these three tests, however, are considered individually or taken in combination, their diagnostic accuracy in the differential diagnosis of mild hypercortisolism does not exceed 80%.

Recently, we combined dexamethasone suppression (0.5 mg every 6 hours for 2 days) and the ovine (o) CRH stimulation test to optimize the ability of oCRH to distinguish between the hypercortisolism of Cushing's disease and pseudo-Cushing's states (Table 2) [17]. In the latter, the pituitary corticotroph is appropriately restrained by glucocorticoid feedback and does not respond to CRH, whereas in the former the corticotroph tumor is resistant to this dose of dexamethasone and responds to CRH. Thus, the dexamethasone/CRH test achieves nearly 100% specificity, sensitivity, and diagnostic accuracy. This test should be reserved, however, for those borderline/mildly hypercortisolemic patients who have already failed to suppress to 1 mg of overnight dexamethasone and who the clinician suspects as having Cushing's disease. The criterion used for the diagnosis of Cushing's disease is a 15-minute cortisol level of >38 nmol/l (1.4 µg/dl) after the CRH injection.

Another strategy, which is always helpful in diagnosing or ruling out Cushing's syndrome, is to closely monitor the patient over the course of a few months. While true hypercortisolism will persist and cause further symptomatology, the hypercortisolism of pseudo-Cushing's states will be frequently corrected spontaneously with effective antidepressant treatment or abstinence from alcohol.

Table 2. Combined dexamethasone suppression–oCRH test

Method	Give dexamethasone 0.5 mg every 6 hours for 2 days before injecting ovine (o) CRH. Last dexamethasone administration at midnight. Next morning at 8 AM, CRH 1 μg/kg body weight is given iv over 1 minute. Draw blood for plasma cortisol 15 minutes after CRH injection.
Response	Cushing disease is likely if plasma cortisol after CRH is >1.4 μg/dl.
Uses	To distinguish pseudo-Cushing's from Cushing's syndrome in patients with mild hypercortisolism.
Problems	CRH is a new agent, not yet commercially available. Human CRH is not as good a diagnostic test as oCRH.

Differential diagnosis of Cushing's syndrome

Once the diagnosis of endogenous Cushing's syndrome has been established, the next challenge is to establish the specific cause [10,18]. Generally, a relatively acute onset of symptoms with rapid progression and associated hypokalemic alkalosis point toward an ectopic ACTH source. In most of the cases, however, accurate differential diagnosis can only be achieved by the combination of dynamic endocrine testing of the integrity of the feedback of the HPA axis, and imaging techniques used mainly to examine the size and shape of the pituitary and adrenal glands and to localize ectopic ACTH- or CRH-secreting tumors (see Table 2). It is essential that dynamic adrenal testing is performed while the patient is clearly hypercortisolemic. This always needs to be documented at the time of testing to avoid mistakes. For this purpose, all adrenal-blocking agents should be discontinued for at least 6 weeks prior to testing.

Morning measurement of plasma ACTH concentrations simultaneously with plasma cortisol would distinguish ACTH-dependent from ACTH-independent Cushing's syndrome. Plasma ACTH concentrations are normal or elevated in Cushing's disease and the ectopic ACTH and CRH syndrome. There is significant differential diagnosis value in the degree elevation of circulating ACTH concentrations, because patients with the ectopic ACTH syndrome frequently have greater plasma ACTH levels than those with Cushing's disease. Interestingly, in many of these patients ACTH immunoreactivity consists primarily of larger precursor molecules [19]. Thus, specific measurement of ACTH precursors, if available, may provide a better marker of the ectopic ACTH syndrome. Circulating ACTH is typically suppressed/undetectable in adrenal cortisol–secreting tumors, micronodular adrenal disease, and autonomously functioning massive macronodular adrenals. If ectopic CRH secretion is suspected to be the cause of Cushing's syndrome, detection of elevated CRH concentrations in the circulation (>50 pg/ml) is helpful.

CRH stimulation test. Most patients with Cushing's disease respond to oCRH with increases in plasma ACTH and cortisol, while patients with ectopic

ACTH production do not [20]. Recently, new criteria were developed for the interpretation of the morning oCRH test that maximize simplicity and cost effectiveness without compromising diagnostic accuracy [21]. The best cortisol criterion suggestive of Cushing's disease is a mean increase at 30 and 45 minutes of >20% above mean basal values at −5 and 0 minutes (91% sensitivity and 88% specificity). Similarly, an increase in mean ACTH concentrations at 15 and 30 minutes after oCRH of at least 35% above the mean basal values achieves a sensitivity of 91% and a specificity of nearly 100%. Indeed, while all patients with ectopic ACTH secretion appear to have a <35% increase in ACTH, the probability of Cushing's disease remains high at all levels of responses, suggesting that, in the absence of a discrete lesion on pituitary imaging, it is prudent to perform a second test (e.g., the high-dose dexamethasone suppression test or bilateral inferior petrosal sinus sampling) to confirm the diagnosis. The oCRH test is rapidly superceding the classic tests of dexamethasone suppression and metyrapone stimulation because it is simple, brief, reliable, and economical.

Standard low-dose high-dose dexamethasone suppression test. This test was developed by Grant Liddle [22] and has been used extensively for differentiating Cushing's disease from the ectopic ACTH syndrome. In patients with Cushing's disease, the abnormal corticotrophs are sensitive to glucocorticoid inhibition only at a high dose of dexamethasone (2.0 mg every 6 hours for 2 days). In contrast, patients with the ectopic ACTH syndrome or cortisol-secreting adrenal tumors usually fail to respond to a dose of 8 mg per day. The classic Liddle criterion for a positive response consistent with Cushing's disease is a >50% drop in 17-hydroxysteroid excretion on day 2 of high-dose dexamethasone treatment (80% diagnostic accuracy). The diagnostic accuracy of the test, however, increases to 86% by measuring both UFC and 17-hydroxysteroid excretion and by requiring greater suppression of both steroids (>64% and >90%, respectively, for 100% specificity) [23].

Overnight 8-mg dexamethasone suppression test. A simple, reliable, and inexpensive alternative to the Liddle dexamethasone suppression test is the overnight 8-mg dexamethasone suppression test. The advantages are its outpatient administration and the avoidance of errors due to incomplete urine collection. The diagnostic accuracy of this overnight test may be similar to that of the standard Liddle dexamethasone suppression test [24,25].

Metyrapone testing. This is a relatively simple test but is not as reliable as the dexamethasone suppression test due to its high variability. It is rapidly becoming obsolete but remains an option in cases where all the other tests mentioned here have failed to provide an unequivocal diagnosis.

Imaging evaluation. Bilateral enlargement of the adrenal gland with preservation of a relatively normal overall glandular configuration is observed in both

Cushing's disease and ectopic ACTH production. Approximately 10–15% of patients with ACTH-dependent Cushing's syndrome demonstrate bilateral nodules (macronodular hyperplasia) [26].

Computed tomography (CT) and magnetic resonance imaging (MRI) scans have largely superceded the need for iodocholesterol scan in the evaluation of patients with Cushing's syndrome. The iodocholesterol scan can occasionally be useful in distiguishing between ACTH-dependent (bilateral uptake) and ACTH-independent (unilateral uptake) macronodular adrenals or in localizing ectopic adrenal tissue (adrenal rest) or an adrenal remnant causing recurrent hypercortisolism after bilateral adrenalectomy [27].

Pituitary. The large majority of pituitary ACTH-secreting tumors are microadenomas with a diameter of <10 mm. MRI scanning is the imaging procedure of choice to visualize pituitary adenomas. Pituitary adenomas are usually best demonstrated on coronal T1-weighted images as foci of reduced signal intensity within the pituitary gland. On unenhanced scans, however, ACTH-producing adenomas are detected in only 40% of patients with Cushing's disease [28]. An additional 15–20% of microadenomas are visualized with injection of contrast material (gadolinium-DTPA) and a repeat T1-weighted coronal scan immediately after the injection (combined MRI sensitivity 55–60%). Unlike the normal pituitary gland and its stalk, pituitary microadenomas do not enhance after the contrast injection and appear as foci of reduced signal intensity.

CT scanning with infusion of contrast demonstrates microadenomas in <20% of patients with bona fide lesions on subsequent surgery. Thus, pituitary CT should be performed only to demonstrate bony anatomy prior to transsphenoidal surgery.

Ectopic tumors. The association of Cushing's syndrome with carcinoma was recognized first in 1928. Since then there have been many reports of neoplasms able to produce a biologically active ACTH that can induce Cushing's syndrome (Table 3). About 60% of these tumors are located in the chest and are lung tumors, especially small-cell carcinomas (8%), and bronchial carcinoids. In the abdomen, carcinomas of the endocrine pancreas and pheochromocytomas are also reported. Medullary carcinoma of the thyroid is responsible in 5% of cases. Adenocarcinoma of the stomach, exocrine carcinoma of the pancreas, anorectal carcinoma, prostatic cancer, uterine small-cell carcinoma, and clear-cell sarcoma of the kidney have all been associated with this condition. A few cases of CRH-producing tumors have also been reported [5,6].

Clinically this condition can be associated with rapid-onset hypertension, hypokalemia, glucose intolerance, and hyperpigmentation. In cases of small-cell tumor of the lung, extremely rapid clinical progression associated with anorexia, weight loss, and hypokalemic alkalosis are suggestive of the diagnosis of ectopic ACTH syndrome. In most cases, plasma ACTH is usually more

Table 3. Tumors causing the ectopic ACTH syndrome

Location	Frequency (%)
Thorax	
Oat-cell carcinoma	50
Thymic carcinoid	10
Bronchial carcinoid	5
Abdomen and pelvis	
Pancreatic islet-cell tumor	10
Pheochromocytoma	5
Ovarian tumors	2
Prostatic carcinoma	<2
Cervical carcinoma	<2
Gastric carcinoid	<2
Gallbladder carcinoma	<2
Head and neck	
Medullary carcinoma of the thyroid	5
Parathyroid carcinoma	<2
Parotic carcinoma	<2
Uncertain primary site	5

elevated than in Cushing's disease, there is no response to oCRH, and there is nonsuppressibility to high doses of dexamethasone. ACTH chromatography and assays of the POMC molecule have some utility, when available. If suppression and/or stimulation tests are suggestive of ectopic ACTH production in a patient with Cushing's syndrome, imaging studies of the chest and abdomen should be undertaken. ACTH-producing thymic carcinoids and pheochromocytomas are generally apparent by CT at the initial presentation of the patient [29,30]. Patients with a negative CT should undergo MRI of the chest and abdomen using T2-weighted and STIR sequences in which carcinoid tumors and pheochromocytomas demonstrate high signal intensity [31]. There are still a significant number of small ectopic tumors, most frequently bronchial carcinoids, that elude CT and MRI detection [32]. In these cases, follow-ups with MRI of the chest at 3–6 month intervals are indicated. In some cases, a body scan following injection of the radiolabeled somatostatin analogue, octreotide, might be helpful in detecting occult carcinoids.

Catheterization studies. Distinguishing Cushing's disease from the ectopic ACTH syndrome frequently presents a major diagnostic challenge. Both pituitary microadenomas and ectopic ACTH-secreting tumors may be radiologically occult and may have similar clinical and laboratory features. Bilateral inferior petrosal venous sinus and peripheral vein catheterization with simultaneous collection of samples for measurement of ACTH is one of the most specific tests available to localize the source of ACTH production [33].

Venous blood from the anterior pituitary drains into the cavernous sinus and subsequently into the superior and inferior petrosal sinuses (Fig. 1, upper panel). Catheters are led into each inferior petrosal sinus via the ipsilateral

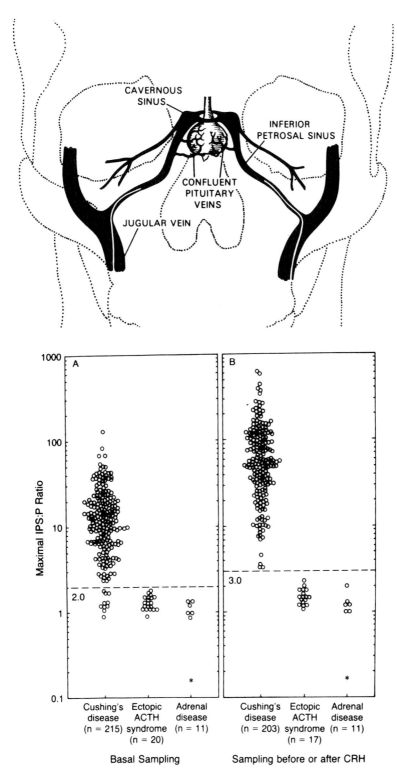

Figure 1. **Top**: Catheter placement for bilateral simultaneous blood sampling of the inferior petrosal sinuses. (From Oldfield et al. [41], p 100, with permission.) **Bottom**: Maximal ratio of ACTH concentration in plasma from either petrosal sinuses and a peripheral vein at baseline (**A**) and after administration of oCRH (**B**). (From Oldfield EH et al. [33], p 897, with permission.)

femoral vein. Samples for measurement of plasma ACTH are collected from each inferior petrosal sinus and a peripheral vein both before and after infection of 1 μg/kg body weight of oCRH. Patients with the ectopic ACTH syndrome have no ACTH concentration gradient between either inferior petrosal sinus and the peripheral sample (see Fig. 1, lower panel) [33]. A ratio ≥2.0 in basal ACTH samples between either or both of the inferior petrosal sinuses and a peripheral vein is highly suggestive of Cushing's disease (95% sensitivity, 100% specificity). Stimulation with CRH during the procedure, with the resulting secretion of ACTH, increases the sensitivity of BIPSS for detecting corticotroph adenomas to almost 100%, when the peak ACTH central to peripheral ratio is ≥3.0 (see Fig. 1, lower panel). Petrosal sinus sampling must be performed bilaterally and simultaneously, because the sensitivity of the test decreases to <70% with unilateral catheterization.

BIPSS is technically difficult and, like all invasive procedures, can never be risk free, even in the most experienced hands [34]. It should be reserved only for (a) patients with classic Cushing's syndrome, strong suspicion of a pituitary origin, and negative or equivocal MRI of the pituitary, and (b) patients with positive pituitary MRI but equivocal suppression and stimulation tests. In the former group, BIPSS unequivocally distinguishes ACTH-secreting pituitary adenomas from pituitary-simulating lung and thymic carcinoid tumors and provides lateralization data of potential value to the surgeon. In the latter group, BIPSS excludes the possibility of a pituitary incidentaloma, which can be visualized on MRI in as many as 10% of young women.

Cushing's syndrome with unusual laboratory results

Periodic Cushing's syndrome. Occasionally, cortisol production in Cushing's syndrome may not be constantly increased but may fluctuate in a 'periodic' infradian pattern, ranging in length from days to months. This relatively rare phenomenon of periodic, cyclic, or episodic hormonogenesis has been described in patients with Cushing's disease [35], the ectopic ACTH syndrome (bronchial carcinoids were involved in half of the reported cases), and cortisol-secreting adrenal tumors or micronodular adrenal disease [36].

Biochemically, patients with periodic hormonogenesis may have consistently normal 24-hour UFC and paradoxically 'normal' responses to dexamethasone in the presence of clinical stigmata of Cushing's syndrome. In such patients, several weekly 24-hour UFC determinations for a period of 3–6 months may be necessary to establish the diagnosis.

Occult ectopic ACTH syndrome. The occult ectopic ACTH syndrome has gained increasing recognition. This syndrome can mimic the clinical and biochemical picture of Cushing's disease. Despite extensive localization studies, the tumor frequently eludes detection. The use of the BIPSS test in patients with the occult ectopic ACTH syndrome is the best possible mean to ascertain the diagnosis. The absence of a central to peripheral ACTH gradient before and after administration of oCRH rules out Cushing's disease [33]. In the search for the tumor, special emphasis should be placed on the lungs, thymus, pancreas, adrenal medulla, and thyroid because most described ectopic ACTH-secreting tumors have been found in these organs (see Table 2). Thymic vein sampling for measurement of ACTH concentrations can be of help in localizing the tumor to the thorax, but not necessarily the thymus [37]. The presence of a concentration gradient in the thymic vein versus the systemic venous circulation is compatible with a thymic or lung carcinoid.

Cushing's syndrome in pregnancy. In normal pregnancy, a small progressive rise in plasma ACTH and a two- to threefold increase in plasma total and free cortisol occur. Twenty-four hour UFC excretion is also elevated above non-pregnant levels, especially between the 34th and 40th weeks of gestation (90–350 μg/day). In the latter part of pregnancy, IR-CRH of placental origin is detected in plasma, with levels reaching up to 10,000 pg/ml [38]. Because plasma cortisol is poorly suppressed in response to dexamethasone in normal pregnancy, the diagnosis of mild or early Cushing's syndrome may be difficult to ascertain [39]. Transient pregnancy-related and limited Cushing's syndrome cases have been described. Their etiology is unknown; however, deficiency of CRH-binding protein might explain the pregnancy-limited expression.

Treatment

Cushing's disease

The treatment of choice for Cushing's disease is selective trans-sphenoidal microadenomectomy, a procedure with a cure rate approaching 95% on the first exploration, and the added advantage of eventually normal anterior pituitary function [40]. The neurosurgeon always explores the entire pituitary gland to find the microadenoma responsible for the disease. If such an adenoma cannot be found during trans-sphenoidal exploration, the surgeon may perform a hemihypophysectomy on the site of a lateral IPS ACTH gradient >1.5. This approach has proved successful in 80–85% of cases [41]. Failure of surgery at the first exploration may be followed by a repeat procedure with a 50–60% chance of cure [42]. Success is defined as a drop of serum cortisol and/or UFC to an undetectable level in the immediate postoperative period. A successful outcome can also be predicted by a lack of cortisol response to oCRH when the test is performed 7–10 days after surgery [43]. Hemihypophysectomy on the side of lateralization of the ACTH gradient in the inferior petrosal sinuses is successful in 80–85% of patients in whom the surgeon fails to identify the tumor during trans-sphenoidal exploration [44].

The next line of therapy is pituitary irradiation with 4500–5000 rad delivered over a period of 6 weeks. In association with mitotane (o p′DDD), a remission rate of about 80% can be expected in the first year [45]. This can increase further in the second year, but the sustained remission rate after discontinuing mitotane therapy drops significantly to about 50–70% of patients. Mitotane can be discontinued after 1 year if UFC has normalized. It can be reinitiated if hypercortisolemia recurs. By 3 years 80–90% of patients will have achieved biochemical remission of Cushing's syndrome and will no longer need mitotane because the effects of irradiation become established. If mitotane therapy is not tolerated by or fails to cure the patient, the final line of treatment is bilateral adrenalectomy [45]. This procedure is uniformly effective at the expense, however, of a significant surgical mortality rate of approximately 2%, a commitment for hormone replacement for life, and a significant risk (10–15%) for subsequent development of Nelson's syndrome [46].

Ectopic ACTH

Once the source of ectopic ACTH is identified, the appropriate therapeutic intervention is surgical resection. With regard to the bronchial carcinoids, which are by far the most common tumors producing the ectopic ACTH syndrome, lung lobectomy may be sufficient to cure the patient. Carcinoids, however, should not be considered benign. They may be extremely slow growing but have the potential for both local invasion and distant metastases [47,48]. If surgical cure is impossible, blockade of steroidogenesis is indicated and combination chemotherapy and/or radiation therapy may be administered.

Adrenal blockade is also indicated for the treatment of ACTH-secreting occult tumors, at least until they surface or are treated surgically. Ketoconazole is the most useful agent. It blocks adrenal steroidogenesis at several levels, the most important being the 20–22 desmolase step, which catalyzes the conversion of cholesterol to pregnenolone, thus avoiding the accumulation of steroid biosynthesis intermediates that can cause or worsen hypertension and/or hirsutism. Reversible side effects, including elevations of hepatic transaminases and gastrointestinal irritation, may occur and may be dose limiting. In this case, metyrapone can be added to achieve normocortisolemia. Other blocking agents that may be used alone or in combination with ketoconazole and/or metyrapone include aminoglutethimide and trilostane [49]. Repeat searches for the tumor should be untertaken every 6–12 months. Bilateral adrenalectomy should be considered in developing children in whom ketoconazole and other medications may interfere with growth and pubertal progression.

Glucocorticoid replacement

Glucocorticoid replacement should be started after a successful pituitary adenomectomy or complete resection of an ACTH-secreting ectopic or a unilateral cortisol-producing adrenal tumor. This is because in those patients the HPA axis is suppressed by chronic exposure to excess glucocorticoids and fails to function for several months after the removal of glucocorticoid inhibition [50]. Hydrocortisone should be replaced at a rate of 12–15 mg/m²/day by mouth with appropriate increases in minor stress (twofold) and major stress (10-fold) for appropriate lengths of time, usually 48 hours. Recovery of the suppressed HPA axis can be monitored with a short ACTH test every 3 months [43]. When the 30-minute plasma cortisol exceeds 18 µg/dl, hydrocortisone can be discontinued. After a bilateral adrenalectomy, corticosteroid replacement will be necessary for life and includes both glucocorticoids and mineralocorticoids.

Summary

Excess endogenous glucocorticoid production, whether ACTH dependent or ACTH independent, results in the classic clinical and biochemical picture of Cushing's syndrome. The diagnosis requires the demonstration of an increased cortisol secretion rate, best achieved by using the 24-hour UFC corrected for body surface area as an index. In mild cases, distinction from the hypercortisolism of pseudo-Cushing states may be difficult. A dexamethasone/oCRH test or close monitoring of the patient for a few months may be helpful. A discrete pituitary lesion on imaging and a standard oCRH test with results consistent with such a lesion are sufficient to proceed to trans-sphenoidal surgery. If no visible pituitary adenoma is present or if the oCRH test is equivocal, bilateral simultaneous inferior petrosal sinus sampling with oCRH administration is necessary to distinguish between a pituitary and an ectopic source. Surgical ablation is the treatment of choice for all types of Cushing's syndrome. In the 5% of cases with Cushing's disease in whom trans-sphenoidal surgery fails and in the 5% of cases in whom the disease recurs, repeat trans-sphenoidal surgery or radiation therapy in association with mitotane treatment may be pursued. Bilateral adrenalectomy effectively cures hypercortisolism if resection of the ACTH-secreting tumor is unsuccessful and radiation/medical therapy fails.

References

1. Cushing H. 1912. The Pituitary Body and its Disorders. Philadelphia: JB Lippincott, p 219.
2. Cushing H. 1932. The basophil adenomas of the pituitary body and their clinical manifestations (pituitary basophilism). Bull John Hopkins Hosp 50:137–195.
3. Cizza G, Nieman LK, Doppman JL, Passaro FS, Czerwiec FS, Chrousos GP, Cutler GB. 1996. Factitious Cushing syndrome. J Clin Endocrinol Metab 81:3573–3577.
4. Magiakou MA, Mastorakos G, Oldfield EA, Gomez MT, Doppman JL, Cutler GB Jr, Nieman LK, Chrousos GP. 1994. Cushing syndrome in children and adolescents: Presentation, diagnosis and therapy. N Engl J Med 331:629–636.

5. Magiakou MA, Mastorakos G, Chrousos GP. 1994. Final stature in patients with endogenous Cushing syndrome. J Clin Endocrinol Metab 79:1082–1085.

6. Carey RM, Varna SK, Drake CR, Thorner MO, Kovacs K, Rivier J, Vale W. 1984. Ectopic secretion of corticotropin-releasing factor as a cause of Cushing's syndrome. N Engl J Med 311:13–20.

7. Auchus RJ, Mastorakos G, Friedman TC, Chrousos GP. 1994. Corticotropin releasing hormone production by a small cell carcinoma in a patient with ACTH-dependent Cushing syndrome. J Endocrinol Invest 17:447–452.

8. Buckley N, Bates AS, Broome JC, Strange RC, Perrett CW, Burke CW, Clayton RN. 1994. P53 protein accumulates in Cushing's adenomas and invasive non-functional adenomas. J Clin Endocrinol Metab 79:1518–1521.

9. Karl M, Von Wichert G, Kempter E, Katz DA, Reincke M, Monig H, Ali IU, Stratakis CA, Oldfield EH, Chrousos GP, Schulte HM. 1996. Nelson's syndrome associated with a somatic frame shift mutation in the glucocorticoid receptor gene. J Clin Endocrinol Metab 81:124–129.

10. Tsigos C, Chrousos GP. 1995. Cushing's syndrome. Curr Opin Endocrinol Diabetes 2:203–213.

11. Gomez MT, Malozowski S, Winterer J, Chrousos GP. 1991. Urinary free cortisol values in normal children and adolescents. J Pediatr 118:256–258.

12. Contreras LN, Hanes S, Tyrrell JB. 1986. Urinary free cortisol in the assessment of pituitary-adrenal function. Utility of 24-hour and spot determinations. J Clin Endocrinol Metab 62:965–969.

13. Pavlatos FC, Smilo RP, Forsham PH. 1965. A rapid screening test for Cushing's syndrome. JAMA 193:720–723.

14. Tsigos C, Chrousos GP. 1994. Physiology of the hypothalamic pituitary-adrenal axis in health and dysregulation in psychiatric and autoimmune disorders. Endocrinol Metab Clin 23:451–466.

15. Tsigos C, Chrousos GP. 1995. Stress, endocrine manifestations and diseases. In Cooper GL, ed. Handbook of Stress Medicine. Boca Raton, FL: CRC Press, pp 61–65.

16. Gold PW, Loriaux DL, Roy A, Kling MA, Calabrese JR, Kellner CH, Nieman LK, Post RM, Pickar D, Gallucci W, Avgerinos P, Paul S, Oldfield EH, Cutler GB Jr, Chrousos GP. 1986. Responses to corticotropin-releasing hormone in the hypercortisolism of depression and Cushing's disease: Pathophysiologic and diagnostic implications. N Engl J Med 314:1329–1335.

17. Yanovski JA, Cutler GB Jr, Chrousos GP, Nieman LK. 1993. Corticotropin-releasing hormone stimulation following low dose dexamethasone administration. A new test to distinguish Cushing's syndrome from pseudo-Cushing's states. JAMA 269:2232–2238.

18. Orth DN. 1991. Differential diagnosis of Cushing's syndrome. N Engl J Med 325:957.

19. White A, Clark AJL. 1993. The cellular and molecular basis of the ectopic ACTH syndrome. Clin Endocrinol 39:131–141.

20. Chrousos GP, Schulte HM, Oldfield EH, Gold PW, Cutler GB Jr, Loriaux DL. 1984. The corticotropin-releasing factor stimulation test: An aid in the evaluation of patients with Cushing's syndrome. N Engl J Med 310:622–627.

21. Nieman LK, Oldfield EH, Wesley R, Chrousos GP, Loriaux DX, Cutler GB Jr. 1993. A simplified morning ovine corticotropin-releasing hormone stimulation test for the differential diagnosis of ACTH dependent Cushing's syndrome. J Clin Endocrinol Metab 77:1308–1312.

22. Liddle GW. 1960. Tests of pituitary-adrenal suppressibility in the diagnosis of Cushing's syndrome. J Clin Endocrinol Metab 20:1539–1561.

23. Flack MR, Oldfield EH, Cutler GB Jr, Nieman LK, Loriaux DX. 1991. Urine free cortisol in the high-dose dexamethasone suppression test for the differential diagnosis of the Cushing syndrome. Ann Intern Med 116:211–217.

24. Tyrell JB, Findling JW, Aron DC, Fitzgerald PA, Forsham PH. 1986. An overnight high-dose dexamethasone suppression test for rapid differential diagnosis of Cushing's syndrome. Ann Intern Med 104:180–186.

25. Dichek HL, Nieman LK, Oldfield EH, Pass HI, Malley JD, Cutler GB Jr. 1994. A comparison of the standard high dose dexamethasone suppression test and the overnight 8-mg dexamethasone suppression test for the differential diagnosis of adrenocorticotropin-dependent Cushing's syndrome. J Clin Endocrinol Metab 78:418–422.
26. Doppman JF, Reinig JW, Dwyer A, Frank JA, Loriaux DL, Keiser H, Norton JA. 1987. Differentiation of adrenal masses by magnetic resonance imaging. Surgery 102:1018–1026.
27. Rufini V, Salentnich I, Troncone L. 1992. Radiocholesterol scintigraphy in Cushing's syndrome. Rays 17:40–48.
28. Doppman JL, Frank JA, Dwyer AJ, Oldfield EH, Miller DL, Nieman LK, Chrousos GP, Cutler GB Jr, Loriaux DL. 1988. Gadolinium-DTPA enhanced imaging of ACTH-secreting microadenomas of the pituitary gland: Correlation of MR appearance with surgical findings. J Comput Assist Tomogr 12:728–735.
29. Doppman JL, Nieman L, Miller DL, Pass HI, Chung R, Cutler GB Jr, Schaaf M, Chrousos GP, Norton JA, Zirrsman HA, Oldfield EH, Loriaux DL. Ectopic adrenocorticotropic hormone syndrome: Localization studies in 28 patients. Radiology 172:115–124.
30. Leinung MC, Young WF Jr, Whitaker MD, Scheithauer BW, Tvastek VF, Kvols LK. 1990. Diagnosis of corticotropin-producing bronchial carcinoid tumors causing Cushing's syndrome. Mayo Clin Proc 65:1314–1321.
31. Doppman JL, Pass HI, Nieman LK, Findling TW, Dwyer AJ, Fenerstein IM, Ling A, Travis WD, Cutler GB Jr, Chrousos GP, Loriaux DL. 1991. Detection of ACTH-producing bronchial carcinoid tumors: MR imaging vs. CT. Am J Radiol 156:39–43.
32. Limper AH, Carpenter PC, Scheithauser B, Staats BA. 1992. The Cushing syndrome induced by bronchial carcinoid tumors. Ann Intern Med 117:209–214.
33. Oldfield EH, Doppman JL, Nieman LK, Chrousos GP, Miller DL, Katz DA, Culter GB Jr, Loriaux DL. 1991. Petrosal sinus sampling with and without corticotropin-releasing hormone for the differential diagnosis of Cushing's syndrome. N Engl J Med 325:897–905.
34. Miller DL, Doppman JL, Peterman SB, Nieman LK, Oldfield EH, Chang R. 1992. Neurologic complications of petrosal sinus sampling. Radiology 185:143–147.
35. Vagnucci AH, Evans E. 1986. Cushing's disease with intermittent hypercortisolism. Am J Med 80:83–88.
36. Sakiyama R, Ashcraft MW, Van Herle AJ. 1984. Cyclic Cushing's syndrome. Am J Med 77:944–946.
37. Doppman JL, Pass HI, Nieman LK, Miller DL, Chang R, Cutler GB, Chrousos GP, Jaffe GS, Norton JA. 1992. Corticotropin-secreting carcinoid tumors of the thymus: Diagnostic unreliability of thymic venous sampling. Radiology 184:71–74.
38. Sasaki A, Shinkawa O, Margioris AN, et al. 1987. Immunoreactive corticotropin-releasing hormone in human plasma during pregnancy, labor and delivery. J Clin Endocrinol Metab 64:224–229.
39. Buescher MA, McClamrock HD, Adashi EY. 1992. Cushing syndrome in pregnancy. Obstet Gynecol 79:130–137.
40. Mampalam TJ, Tyrrell JB, Wilson CB. 1988. Transphenoidal microsurgery for Cushing's disease. A report of 216 cases. Ann Intern Med 109:487–493.
41. Oldfield EH, Chrousos GP, Schulte HM, Loriaux DL, Schaaf M, Doppman J. 1985. Preoperative lateralization of ACTH-secreting pituitary microadenomas by bilateral and simultaneous inferior petrosal venous sinus sampling. N Engl J Med 312:100–103.
42. Ram Z, Nieman LK, Cutler GB Jr, Chrousos GP, Doppman J, Oldfield EH. 1994. Early repeat surgery for persistent Cushing's disease. J Neurosurg 80:37–45.
43. Avgerinos PC, Chrousos GP, Nieman LK, Oldfield EH, Loriaux DL, Cutler GB Jr. 1987. The corticotropin-releasing hormone test in the postoperative evaluation of patients with Cushing's syndrome. J Clin Endocrinol Metab 65:906–913.
44. Luton JP, Mahoudeau JA, Bouchard P, Thieblot P, Hautecouverture M, Simon D, Laudat MH, Touitou Y, Bricaire H. 1979. Treatment of Cushing's disease by o,p'DDD. Survey of 62 cases. N Engl J Med 300:459–464.

45. Zeiger MA, Fraker DL, Pass HI, Nieman LK, Cutler GB, Chrousos GP, Norton JA. 1993. Effective reversibility of the signs and symptoms of hypercortisolism by bilateral adrenalectomy. Surgery 114:1138–1143.

46. Nelson DH, Meakin JW, Thorn GW. 1960. ACTH-producing pituitary tumors following adrenalectomy for Cushing's syndrome. Ann Intern Med 52:560–569.

47. Davila DG, Dunn WF, Tazelaar HD, Pairolero PC. 1993. Bronchial carcinoid tumors. Mayo Clinic Proc 68:795–803.

48. Doppman JL, Nieman LK, Cutler GB Jr, Chrousos GP, Fraker DL, Norton JA, Jensen RT. 1994. Adrenocorticotropin hormone-secreting islet cell tumors: Are they always malignant? Radiology 190:59–64.

49. Miller JW, Crapo L. 1993. The medical treatment of Cushing's syndrome. Endocr Rev 14:443–458.

50. Doherty G, Nieman LK, Cutler GB Jr, Chrousos GP, Norton J. 1990. Time to recovery of the hypothalamic-pituitary-adrenal axis after curative resection of adrenal tumors in patients with Cushing's syndrome. Surgery 108:1085–1090.

3. Prolactinomas

Laurence Katznelson and Anne Klibanski

Prolactin is a peptide hormone secreted by the anterior pituitary gland. A specific cell type, the lactotroph, is responsible for prolactin biosynthesis and secretion. The only established role of prolactin is to initiate and maintain lactation. Prolactin levels rise progressively with pregnancy and peak at term (100–300 µg/l) [1]. Lactation begins when estradiol levels fall at parturition. The nursing stimulus effectively promotes acute prolactin release via afferent spinal neural pathways and, within 20–30 minutes of nursing, prolactin levels increase 60-fold [2]. With established nursing, nipple stimulation itself elicits progressively less prolactin release, and in the weeks following initiation of lactation both basal and nursing-stimulated prolactin pulses decrease [2]. Within 4–6 months postpartum, basal prolactin levels are normal without a nursing-induced rise, despite continued lactation.

Pathologic hyperprolactinemia is defined as a persistently elevated serum prolactin value in a nongravid state and is a frequent cause of anovulation and infertility in women. The syndrome of amenorrhea-galactorrhea is the classic sequelae of hyperprolactinemia; however, there is a spectrum of clinical manifestations described in both women and men.

Causes of hyperprolactinemia

The clinical approach to a patient with hyperprolactinemia requires an understanding of normal prolactin physiology. Fluctuations in prolactin levels may occur in several physiologic states, and serum concentrations may reach the upper limit of normal or may become slightly elevated in these situations. It is therefore important to review key physiologic aspects of prolactin regulation. Prolactin is secreted in a pulsatile fashion with 4–14 pulses per day (60% occur during sleep) [3]. The amplitude of pulses is highly variable between individuals, with peak levels occurring during the late hours of sleep. Prolactin pulsatility is not associated with any specific stage of sleep. A number of studies have suggested that prolactin varies during the menstrual cycle, although the precise nature of this relationship remains unclear. In such studies, prolactin levels were found to be significantly higher during the ovulatory and

Andrew Arnold (ed.) ENDOCRINE NEOPLASMS. 1997. Kluwer Academic Publishers. ISBN 0-7923-4354-9.
All rights reserved.

luteal phases, particularly at midcycle, and this is possibly attributable to increased circulating estradiol levels [4]. Abrupt rises in serum prolactin occur within an hour of eating in normal individuals but not in individuals with prolactinomas. The protein component of meals appears to be the main stimulus to prolactin secretion [5].

Prolactin rises during stress, including physical exertion, surgery, sexual intercourse, insulin hypoglycemia, and seizures. The significance of these alterations during stress is not known. Nipple stimulation, chest-wall trauma or surgery, and herpes zoster infection of the breast may result in increased prolactin levels [6]. Mean levels of prolactin are slightly higher in premenopausal women than men, probably due to a direct effect of estrogen on pituitary prolactin secretion. Some studies suggest that there is a progressive decline in prolactin levels in women with age, particularly after menopause [7]. This is likely due to postmenopausal estrogen deficiency. Therefore, the approach to a mildly elevated prolactin level should include a careful review of the clinical situation in which the sample was drawn, such as the proximity to a meal, time of day, and phase of the menstrual cycle.

There are multiple pathologic causes of hyperprolactinemia. Like other pituitary hormones, prolactin secretion is controlled by dual inhibitory and stimulatory factors (Fig. 1). However, in contrast to other pituitary hormones, prolactin secretion is predominantly under tonic inhibitory control. Dopamine, the main physiologic inhibitor of prolactin secretion, is transported from the hypothalamus to the pituitary gland via the hypophyseal stalk circulation to directly inhibit the lactotroph cells from synthesizing and secreting prolactin [8]. Therefore, damage to the hypothalamus or the hypophyseal stalk, for example, tumor compression (both pituitary and nonpituitary lesions), infiltrative disorders, trauma, surgery, or radiation scarring, can impede normal dopaminergic inhibitory control, resulting in hyperprolactinemia.

Pharmacologic causes of hyperprolactinemia are often mediated through alterations of dopamine secretion or effect. Antihypertensive drugs, such as reserpine and alpha-methyldopa, cause moderate hyperprolactinemia by dopamine depletion in the tuberoinfundibular neurons. Psychotropic agents are a frequent cause of hyperprolactinemia [9]. Phenothiazines and haloperidol may cause prolactin release via blockade of dopamine receptors. Tricyclic antidepressants may cause modest hyperprolactinemia in up to one fourth of patients. Psychotropic agents that affect the serotonergic axis, such as fluoxetine (Prozac), may also cause hyperprolactinemia. Calcium-channel blockers such as verapamil may increase prolactin levels, although the underlying mechanism is largely unknown. Prolactin elevations have been seen in subjects undergoing therapy with angiotensin-converting enzyme inhibitors such as enalopril. Chronic opiate use, cocaine abuse, and therapy with H_2 antagonists such as cimetidine have been associated with hyperprolactinemia, possibly through stimulatory mechanisms. Typically, hyperprolactinemia associated with medication use causes an increase in serum prolactin to levels of $<100\,\mu g/l$.

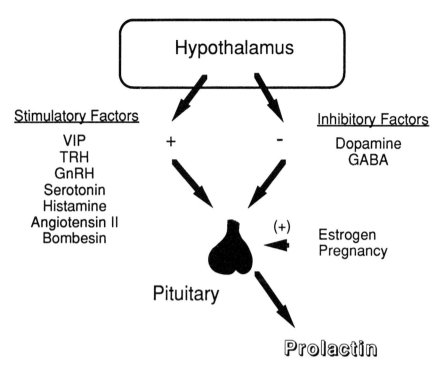

Figure 1. Regulation of prolactin secretion. Prolactin release is under tonic inhibition by dopamine, the most important prolactin inhibiting factor. Prolactin release is stimulated by a number of factors, including thyroid-releasing hormone (TRH) and estrogen.

Stimulatory factors also regulate prolactin secretion. These substances may act directly on the pituitary or may act indirectly by means of dopaminergic blockade or depletion at the level of the hypothalamus. Estrogens are highly important physiologic stimulators of prolactin release and are responsible for the elevation in prolactin levels with gestation [10]. Chronic exposure to estrogens results in an increase in lactotroph number and size (i.e., 'pregnancy cells'), and the pituitary volume normally increases during pregnancy due to lactotroph hyperplasia [11]. In nongravid individuals, estrogen therapy may lead to increases in prolactin levels, such as that seen in pregnancy. However, estrogen concentrations in typical oral contraceptive agents (i.e., 35 µg ethinyl estradiol) are not associated with hyperprolactinemia, and there is no evidence that postmenopausal estrogen replacement causes elevations in serum prolactin. Thyrotropin-releasing hormone (TRH) also stimulates prolactin secretion [12]. Although the physiologic role of TRH in prolactin secretion is unclear, prolactin levels may be elevated in primary hypothyroidism, presumably due to TRH stimulation and/or hypothyroid-induced changes in dopaminergic tone. Gonadotropin-releasing hormone (GnRH) may have stimulatory properties, and administration of GnRH induces the acute release of prolactin in normally cycling women and hypogonadal patients [13]. However, the role of GnRH in the normal physiologic control of prolactin secretion is unknown.

Other causes of hyperprolactinemia include chronic renal disease, probably because of altered metabolism or clearance of prolactin or decreases in dopaminergic tone [14]. Hemodialysis usually does not reverse the hyperprolactinemia. Liver disease has also been associated with hyperprolactinemia.

Prolactin-secreting pituitary adenomas are a frequent cause of pathologic hyperprolactinemia. Prolactinomas are the most common type of pituitary tumor and may account for as many as 40–50% of all pituitary tumors [15]. Hyperprolactinemia may be detected in as many as 40% of patients with acromegaly and has been reported in patients with Cushing's disease. The presence of acromegaly and Cushing's disease should be evaluated in hyperprolactinemic patients with suggestive clinical manifestations. This is particularly true in young women with acromegaly who have not had the disease for a sufficient duration to have acral changes and whose first manifestation of acromegaly may be hyperprolactinemia-associated reproductive disease.

Clinical presentation

The clinical signs and symptoms of hyperprolactinemia are due to both the biochemical effects of hyperprolactinemia and the local complications of tumors responsible for the elevated prolactin level (Table 1).

Manifestations of hyperprolactinemia

Hyperprolactinemia is a common cause of amenorrhea, and approximately 20% of women with secondary amenorrhea have elevated prolactin levels [16]. Women with hyperprolactinemia may have more subtle abnormalities in gonadal function, including oligomenorrhea or luteal-phase insufficiency. A

Table 1. Symptoms associated with hyperprolactinemia

Hypogonadism
  Amenorrhea
  Oligomenorrhea
  Infertility
  Impotence
  Decreased libido
Galactorrhea
Hirsutism, acne
Headaches
Mass effect (if macroprolactinoma)
  Visual loss
  Cranial neuropathies
  Hypopituitarism
  Temporal lobe seizures

subset of infertile women has been described with mild hyperprolactinemia in whom fertility was restored with bromocriptine therapy. In addition, subjects with primary amenorrhea and delayed puberty have been found to have hyperprolactinemia as the etiology of their clinical symptoms [17].

Galactorrhea is present in up to 25% of parous women with regular menses and normal serum prolactin levels. However, subjects with 'idiopathic' galactorrhea, defined as the presence of normal prolactin levels, may demonstrate intermittent hyperprolactinemia. In a recent study, 8 of 9 normoprolactinemic women with galactorrhea had elevated levels of prolactin during sleep [18]. In addition, several studies have shown that infertile, normoprolactinemic women with luteal-phase defects may show improved luteal function and/or fertility following the administration of dopamine agonist therapy [18]. Therefore, unrecognized hyperprolactinemia may occur in a subset of subjects with presumed normoprolactinemic galactorrhea and luteal-phase defects. A single prolactin value determined during the day may not rule out the presence of a pathologic hyperprolactinemic state and multiple determinations, particularly in the periovulatory phase of the menstrual cycle, may be necessary to make this diagnosis.

Hypogonadism is frequently found in patients with hyperprolactinemia. In women, hypogonadism and its associated estrogen deficiency includes abnormal menstrual function, dry vaginal mucosa and dyspareunia, and diminished libido. Men may present with decreased libido, impotence, infertility due to oligospermia, and gynecomastia due to the associated testosterone deficiency. Galactorrhea is rare in hyperprolactinemic men, and this is likely due to the lack of estrogen priming of the breast. There are multiple potential mechanisms underlying the induction of hypogonadism by hyperprolactinemia, which may take place at several levels. Hypogonadism is frequently associated with decreased or inappropriately normal luteinizing hormone (LH) and follicle-stimulating hormone (FSH) levels relative to the state of estrogen deficiency, consistent with central hypogonadism. Prolactin, probably via alterations in dopamine inhibitory tone, decreases hypothalamic GnRH secretion with a resultant suppressive effect on spontaneous LH release [19]. The restoration of ovulatory menstrual periods in hyperprolactinemic women with pulsatile exogenous GnRH administration further suggests that suppression of endogenous GnRH is the key mechanism underlying hypogonadism in women [20]. In addition, prolactin may modulate androgen secretion at the level of both the adrenal gland and ovary, resulting in increased secretion of dehydroepiandrosterone sulfate and testosterone [21]. Therefore, altered ratios of estrogens and androgens may further result in abnormal gonadal function, with evidence of clinical hyperandrogenism (e.g., hirsutism).

If the underlying etiology of the hyperprolactinemia is a pituitary macroadenoma or a large nonpituitary mass, the lesion could cause compression of the normal, adjacent pituitary gland, with a resultant decrease in gonadotroph function. Mass effects from the tumor could also lead to visual compromise from compression of the optic chiasm, cranial nerve palsies via extension laterally into the cavernous sinus, headaches, and, potentially, seizures. Patients with hyperprolactinemia often describe headaches, which appear to be out of proportion to the size of the underlying tumor. Hyperprolactinemic patients without demonstrable tumors on scan may also suffer from headaches, which may diminish or subside completely following institution of therapy.

Hyperprolactinemia is also associated with both trabecular and cortical osteopenia. Hyperprolactinemic women may have trabecular osteopenia, with

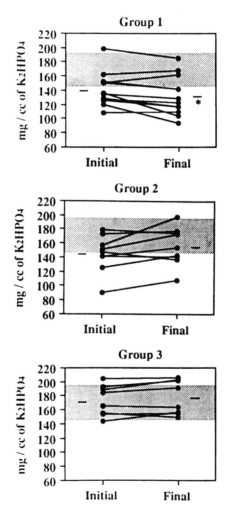

Figure 2. Initial and final trabecular bone mineral density in women with hyperprolactinemia. Group 1 refers to women amenorrheic throughout the study (N = 12), Group 2 refers to women with resumption of menses with treatment after study entry (N = 9), and Group 3 refers to women with hyperprolactinemia and normal menses (N = 8). The shaded area represents the mean ±1.0 SD of bone density in 41 normal women. *p = 0.04 compared with initial mean bone density. (Reprinted with permission from Biller et al. [24].)

spinal bone density ranging from 10% to 25% below normal [22,23]. The etiology of this decrease in bone density appears to be due to the hypogonadism resulting from the hyperprolactinemic state, and not to the prolactin per se [22]. Figure 2 shows the progressive nature of spinal bone mineral density loss associated with hyperprolactinemia [24]. Group 1 refers to women with amenorrhea throughout the study, group 2 refers to women with normalization of menses after study entry, and group 3 refers to women with normal menses before and during the study. The amenorrheic women with hyperprolactinemic had decreased mean spinal bone density values, and over a mean 1.8 years spinal bone mineral density progressively decreased in this hyperprolactinemic group. Resumption of menses following therapy was associated with an increase in bone mineral density. This study and others have shown that the bone density in such patients may increase concomitant with normalization of prolactin levels with therapy; however, the bone density typically still remains lower than that of normal control subjects. Of importance, hyperprolactinemia in eumenorrheic women is not associated with bone loss and is therefore not an indication for therapy in this patient group.

Approach to an elevated prolactin value

The approach to an elevated prolactin value should include careful consideration of the presence of physiologic causes of hyperprolactinemia. The prolactin level should be repeated in a nonstimulated state, and if possible we recommend measuring a morning prolactin level after an overnight fast in a nonstressed state. For example, prolactin may be secreted to a modest degree following a breast exam, so a mild increase in prolactin levels after such an exam warrants a repeat prolactin determination. A mildly elevated prolactin level determined after a meal should clearly be repeated.

Substantial elevations in prolactin, $>150 \mu g/l$, in a nongravid state are usually indicative of a prolactin-secreting pituitary tumor. In an actively secreting lactotroph tumor, there is an excellent correlation between radiographic estimates of tumor size and prolactin levels, and, therefore, very high levels of prolactin are associated with larger tumors. Prolactinomas are classified as microadenomas (<10 mm) and macroadenomas (>10 mm). Therefore, the presence of a substantial elevation in serum prolactin in association with a pituitary lesion >10 mm by radiographic imaging supports the diagnosis of a macroprolactinoma. A significant discrepancy between tumor volume and the degree of hyperprolactinemia should raise the suspicion of a 'clinically nonfunctioning pituitary tumor' or a sella lesion of nonpituitary origin.

The majority of women with prolactinomas have microadenomas. This is in contrast to men, in whom the majority of tumors are macroadenomas. This may be due to the fact that women may present earlier for evaluation then men because of complaints of menstrual disturbances.

Modest levels of prolactin elevation (e.g., 25–100 µg/l) may be associated with a number of diagnoses. All etiologies of hyperprolactinemia should be excluded before a tumor is considered. Pregnancy, primary hypothyroidism, liver disease, and chronic renal disease should be excluded. A careful history of medication use should be obtained.

One diagnostic problem is the evaluation of patients with psychiatric disease who are receiving phenothiazines and are found to have an elevated prolactin level. Women with these medications often describe menstrual abnormalities and modest hyperprolactinemia is often the culprit. We recommend a magnetic resonance imaging (MRI) scan for patients whose prolactin levels are >100 µg/l and assume that levels under this value are consistent with neuroleptic administration. This strategy is based on the finding that the majority of patients receiving neuroleptics with modest prolactin elevations have no evidence of a pituitary abnormality on scan. However, if patients with prolactin levels <100 µg/l have any complaints suggestive of local mass effects or other pituitary hypersecretory or hyposecretory syndromes, then imaging studies should be performed.

When an elevated serum prolactin level is not associated with a clear secondary cause, a pituitary radiographic scan should be performed to rule out the presence of either a prolactin-secreting pituitary tumor or other lesions. In addition, as described later, it is important to distinguish microprolactinomas from macroprolactinomas. If the scan shows normal sellar and extrasellar contents and there is no clear secondary cause of the hyperprolactinemia, then the diagnosis of idiopathic hyperprolactinemia is made. These cases may represent occult microprolactinomas with an anatomic lesion beyond the sensitivity of the scanning technique.

Management

Treatment is dependent on the etiology of hyperprolactinemia, its associated clinical symptoms, and anatomic considerations. If the above-mentioned evaluation suggests the presence of a prolactinoma, then the goals of therapy are to suppress excessive prolactin secretion, and to reduce or stabilize tumor size and restore normal physiologic anterior pituitary function. There are four available treatment options: no therapy with close observation, medical therapy with a dopamine agonist, and, rarely, surgery or radiation. Determination of the appropriate treatment option for a patient is individual and takes into account the presence of mass effect, biochemical consequences of the hyperprolactinemia, and personal preferences.

Therapeutic considerations

Tumor size. A very important therapeutic consideration is the size of the prolactinoma. Patients are stratified into those who have microprolactinomas

(<10 mm) and those with macroprolactinomas (>10 mm). Microprolactinomas are typically intrasellar and are not associated with evidence of local mass effects. In addition, studies investigating the natural history of such tumors have shown that in the majority of cases, prolactin elevations usually remain stable and, in some cases, spontaneously normalize. The degree of prolactin elevation is a prognostic factor for spontaneous resolution. In one study with 41 patients with idiopathic hyperprolactinemia followed for 5.5 years, 67% of patients whose initial prolactin values were <57 μg/l had normalization of prolaction [25]. In contrast, none of the patients with initial prolactin values >60 μg/l normalized. In another study of 38 patients with untreated microprolactinomas followed for an average of 50.5 months, 36.6% had an increase, 55.3% had a spontaneous decrease, and 13.1% had no change in prolactin levels [26]. A prospective study in untreated hyperprolactinemic women showed that patients with normal initial menstrual function were more likely to have normalization of prolactin values, whereas patients with oligomenorrhea or amenorrhea were more likely to have no change or increases in prolactin values [27]. Therefore, basal menstrual function is an important variable in predicting the progression of the prolactin level, and prolactin levels may spontaneously normalize.

Another important feature of the natural history of microprolactinomas is that the majority of such tumors do not increase in size. In one study of 43 patients with presumed microadenomas with a mean follow-up of 5.4 years, only 2 patients showed evidence of tumor progression [28]. In a prospective study by Schlechte et al. [27], 27 women were followed for an average of 5.2 years. Of 14 women with normal radiographic studies at baseline, 4 developed evidence of an adenoma, although none of these subjects developed a macroadenoma. Of the 13 women with evidence of a tumor at baseline, only 2 showed worsening of radiographic findings. This study suggests that although radiologic evidence of tumor growth may occur in up to 22% of cases, it is rarely accompanied by clinical symptoms. However, patients with microprolactinomas who demonstrate an increase in tumor size during follow-up without therapy should be seriously considered for medical therapy.

All patients with macroprolactinomas should undergo therapy. In contrast, because microprolactinomas tend to enlarge rarely and slowly, the presence of a microprolactinoma alone without other indications does not in itself necessitate therapy. From the standpoint of size alone, it is reasonable to withhold therapy on microprolactinomas and follow closely with serial examinations and radiographic imaging.

Biochemical consequences of hyperprolactinemia. The presence of hypogonadism is a second important therapeutic consideration. Hyperprolactinemia-induced hypogonadism may lead to several important clinical symptoms and findings. It is often associated with fatigue, diminished libido, and dyspareunia. Men with hyperprolactinemia often describe decreased libido and erectile dysfunction. Hypogonadal symptoms are reversible with therapy in the majority of cases.

Amenorrhea and oligomenorrhea are associated with an increased risk of osteoporosis [22,23]. As many of these women are young when diagnosed, hypogonadism may lead to long-term osteoporosis with a significantly increased risk of fracture. Cortical and trabecular bone density may increase following therapy of the hyperprolactinemia with resumption of menses. Therefore, the risk of osteoporosis associated with hyperprolactinemia is significant and may be, at least in part, reversible with therapy. Therefore, hypogonadism in the presence of hyperprolactinemia is a clear indication for therapy.

Hyperprolactinemia may lead to ovulatory disorders and luteal-phase defects, resulting in infertility [18]. If an elevated prolactin level is found in a woman desiring fertility, then therapy should be instituted. Prolactin may modulate androgen secretion in the adrenal gland and ovary, resulting in increased secretion of androgens, including testosterone and dehydroepiandrosterone sulfate [21]. Hyperandrogenism may result in hirsutism, oily skin, and an acneiform rash. In some hyperprolactinemic individuals, androgen excess may be particularly bothersome and require therapy.

Galactorrhea. Galactorrhea affects as many as 30% of women with hyperprolactinemia. Although galactorrhea in itself is not an absolute indication for therapy, if the degree of galactorrhea is significantly bothersome to the patient, then it is reasonable to initiate therapy.

Headaches. Headaches are frequently a result of the expanding tumor mass, and therefore therapy with a decrease in tumor size will lead to improvement in the headaches. Many subjects with hyperprolactinemia without a large mass describe headaches that are out of proportion to the tumor size. Headaches may lead to the need for therapy in certain individuals.

Management options

Medical therapy. Almost all patients with hyperprolactinemia due to pituitary disease can be effectively treated medically with a dopamine agonist. Bromocriptine (Parlodel), the most frequently used dopamine agonist, lowers serum prolactin in patients with pituitary tumors and all other causes of hyperprolactinemia. Bromocriptine has been the primary medical therapy for hyperprolactinemic disorders for approximately two decades. Bromocriptine normalizes prolactin levels and leads to resumption of ovulatory function and menses in 80–90% of patients [29]. Therefore, bromocriptine is very effective in decreasing prolactin levels and in both normalizing reproductive function and reversing galactorrhea. In some patients, return of menstrual function is accompanied by prolactin levels that are significantly reduced but not normal. This suggests that in some patients reduction but not normalization of prolactin levels may be sufficient for return of gonadal function. Bromocriptine is also useful in treating galactorrhea in patients with normoprolactinemic galactorrhea.

The effects of bromocriptine are rapid in onset (1–2 hours), but normalization may take weeks. Discontinuation of the drug is typically followed by a return of hyperprolactinemia to basal values. Acute bromocriptine side effects, including nausea, headache, dizziness, nasal congestion, and constipation, may occur and may be dose limiting. Gastrointestinal side effects may be minimized by starting with a very low dose at night, for example, 1.25 mg ($^{1}/_{2}$ tablet) with a snack, and increasing by 1.25 mg over 4- to 5-day intervals as tolerated. This is continued until a dose that normalizes prolactin levels is reached. The rate of dose escalation is dictated by the clinical situation, such as the presence of mass effects. Side effects, particularly gastrointestinal, usually improve with either continuing the medication at the same dose or by temporarily reducing the dose. If patients stop taking the medication for a few days, therapy should be reinstituted at a lower dose because these side effects may return. Chronic therapy may result in side effects, including painless cold-sensitive digital vasospasm, alcohol intolerance, and dyskinesia. Psychiatric and affective reactions include fatigue, depression, insomnia, and anxiety, and have been reported as well as the precipitation of acute psychosis.

Bromocriptine will result in significant tumor shrinkage in up to 75% of patients with macroadenomas. Tumor-size reduction may occur early, in weeks, or over many months. This is frequently accompanied by improvement in visual-field abnormalities and pituitary function. Visual-field deficits have been reported to improve within hours of institution of medical therapy. Of 27 such patients treated with bromocriptine, 64% had a reduction in tumor volume of at least 50% [30]. The fall in prolactin level does not always correlate with reduction in tumor size. Medical therapy represents the initial option for patients with macroprolactinomas because of the low cure rates with surgery in such patients.

In contrast to what is seen in women, the majority of men with diagnosed prolactinomas have macroadenomas. In men with hyperprolactinemia-induced hypogonadism and normal residual pituitary function, it may take 3–6 months for testosterone levels to increase and normal sexual function to be restored after prolactin levels normalize.

In order to reduce the gastrointestinal side effects, bromocriptine has recently been administered intravaginally. Reductions in prolactin similar to that attained by oral bromocriptine have been achieved with the intravaginal route [31,32]. However, long-term patient compliance has not been demonstrated.

Pergolide (Permax) is a dopamine agonist approved by the U.S. Food and Drug Administration for the treatment of Parkinson's disease. Although not approved for use in the management of hyperprolactinemia. pergolide may be efficacious in reducing prolactin levels in patients with hyperprolactinemia [33].

There are other dopamine agonists under investigation, including the long-acting preparations, bromocriptine mesylate (Parlodel LAR) and cabergoline. Cabergoline is an ergoline derivative with selective, potent and long-lasting dopaminergic properties and has been shown to be highly effective in the management of hyperprolactinemia. Because of the ease of administration of cabergoline (once or twice a week) and its improved side-effect profile relative to bromocriptine, patients have a high rate of compliance. Administration of cabergoline to patients with microprolactinomas results in normalization of prolactin levels in 95% of cases [34]. In a recent study, the administration of cabergoline to 15 patients with macroprolactinomas resulted in a decrease in tumor size in 73%, a decrease in prolactin levels in 94%, and normalization of prolactin in 73% of subjects [35]. Cabergoline appears to be better tolerated than bromocriptine and may play an important role in the management of patients resistant to or intolerant of bromocriptine [36].

Surgery. Although surgery is not a primary mode of management for patients with prolactinomas, it may be indicated in several settings. These include large tumors with visual-field deficits unresponsive to bromocriptine, inability to tolerate bromocriptine due to side effects, and cystic tumors that do not to respond to medical therapy. The presence of apoplexy is another important indication for surgery because of the necessity to evacuate the hemorrhage. A trans-sphenoidal approach is almost exclusively used. When performed by experienced surgeons, the major morbidity rate is negligible. The mortality rate is <0.27% and the major morbidity rate is <3% [37].

Surgical efficacy is clearly a function of the experience of the neurosurgeon. However, even in experienced hands, postoperative cure as defined by a normal serum prolactin level is found in approximately 71% of patients with microprolactinomas and 32% of patients with macroprolactinomas [29]. An important concern is the significant recurrence rate following initial prolactin value normalization. The recurrence rates for microprolactinomas and macroprolactinomas may be as high as 39% and 80%, respectively, up to 5 years after surgery [38].

Radiation therapy. Conventional radiotherapy (4500–5000 rads) or, rarely, proton-beam therapy may be indicated in patients with larger tumors in whom definitive therapy is desired but who are unable to tolerate chronic medical therapy. Given the long delay between therapy and normalization of prolactin levels, medical therapy is typically required for years.

Pregnancy and prolactinomas

Many women with hyperprolactinemia present with infertility, and bromocriptine is typically used to normalize prolactin levels and to allow normal ovulation to occur. Because of estrogen-stimulated lactotroph

52

hyperplasia, there is concern in patients with prolactinomas that the high estrogen levels may lead to lactotroph stimulation and tumor growth, with resulting local complications, including visual-field deficits, headaches, and diabetes insipidus. Molitch [39] reviewed the data on pregnancy outcomes in hyperprolactinemic patients. Clinically significant tumor enlargement (headaches or visual deficits or both) has been described in only up to 5.5% of patients with microprolactinomas. Therefore, in patients with microprolactinomas it is reasonable to discontinue the bromocriptine after pregnancy is established. These patients should be followed carefully during pregnancy, with serial visual-field monitoring.

In contrast, 15.5–35.7% of patients with macroadenomas are at risk for clinically significant tumor enlargement during any trimester. We do not recommend trans-sphenoidal resection of the macroadenomas prior to conception because surgical resection does not prevent symptomatic enlargement during pregnancy. If there is no evidence of local mass effects after pregnancy is established, then bromocriptine may be discontinued. The decision to reinstitute therapy depends on the development of clinical symptoms, not the serum prolactin levels, because prolactin levels increase markedly during normal pregnancy. If a complication caused by tumor growth does occur, it is rapidly reversible with the reinstinution of bromocriptine, which is then continued through term. A large international experience with bromocriptine and pregnancy suggests that bromocriptine therapy does not result in complications for the fetus [40].

Breast feeding after delivery appears to be safe in prolactinoma patients not receiving bromocriptine. In a patient with a prolactinoma, the suckling stimulus does not elicit an increase in the prolactin concentration or significant tumor growth. However, patients with macroadenomas should continue to be followed closely, and the decision to institute therapy is dependent on tumor size and clinical symptoms.

References

1. Rigg LA, Lein A, Yen SS. 1977. Pattern of increase in circulating prolactin levels during human gestation. Am J Obstet Gynecol 129:454–456.
2. Noel GL, Suh HK, Frantz AG. 1974. Prolactin release during nursing and breast stimulation in postpartum and nonpostpartum subjects. J Clin Endocrinol Metab 38:413–423.
3. Veldhuis JD, Johnson ML. 1988. Operating characteristics of the hypothalamo-pituitary-gonadal axis in men: Circadian, ultradian, and pulsatile release of prolactin and its temporal coupling with luteinizing hormone. J Clin Endocrinol Metab 67:116–123.
4. Franchimont P, Dourcy C, Legros JJ, Reuter A, Vrindts-Gevaert Y, Van-Cauwenberge JR, Gaspard U. 1976. Prolactin levels during the menstrual cycle. Clin Endocrinol 5:643–650.
5. Carlson HE. 1989. Prolactin stimulation by protein is mediated by amino acids in humans. J Clin Endocrinol Metab 69:7–14.
6. Boyd AE, Spare S, Bower B, Reichlin S. 1978. Neurogenic galactorrhea-amenorrhea. J Clin Endocrinol Metab 47:1374–1377.
7. Vekemans M, Robyn C. 1975. Influence of age on serum prolactin levels in women and men. Br Med J 4:738–739.

8. Leblanc H, Lachelin GC, Abu-Fadil S, Yen SS. 1976. Effects of dopamine infusion on pituitary hormone secretion in humans. J Clin Endocrinol Metab 43:668–674.

9. Rivera JL, Lal S, Ettigi P, Hontela S, Muller HF, Friesen HG. 1976. Effect of acute and chronic neuroleptic therapy on serum prolactin levels in men and women of different age groups. Clin Endocrinol 5:273–282.

10. Raymond V, Beaulieu M, Labrie F, Boissier J. 1978. Potent antidopaminergic activity of estradiol at the pituitary level on prolactin release. Science 200:1173–1175.

11. Scheithauer BW, Sano T, Kovacs KT, Young WF Jr, Ryan N, Randall RV. 1990. The pituitary gland in pregnancy: A clinicopathologic and immunohistochemical study of 69 cases. Mayo Clin Proc 65:461–474.

12. Bowers CY, Friesen HG, Hwang P, Guyda HJ, Folkers K. 1971. Prolactin and thyrotropin release in man by synthetic pyroglutamyl-histidyl-prolinamide. Biochem Biophys Res Commun 45:1033–1041.

13. Casper RF, Yen SS. 1981. Simultaneous pulsatile release of prolactin and luteinizing hormone induced by luteinzing hormone-releasing factor agonist. J Clin Endocrinol Metab 52:934–936.

14. Cowden EA, Ratcliffe WA, Ratcliffe JG, Dobbie JW, Kennedy AC. 1978. Hyperprolactinaemia in renal disease. Clin Endocrinol 9:241–248.

15. Klibanski A, Zervas NT. 1991. Diagnosis and management of hormone-secreting pituitary adenomas. N Engl J Med 324:822–831.

16. Franks S, Murray MA, Jequier AM, Steele SJ, Nabarro JD, Jacobs HS. 1975. Incidence and significance of hyperprolactinaemia in women with amenorrhea. Clin Endocrinol 4:597–607.

17. Patton ML, Woolf PD. 1983. Hyperprolactinemia and delayed puberty: A report of three cases and their response to therapy. Pediatrics 71:572–575.

18. Asukai K, Uemura T, Minaguchi H. 1993. Occult hyperprolactinemia in infertile women. Fertil Steril 60:423–427.

19. Park SK, Keenan MW, Selmanoff M. 1993. Graded hyperprolactinemia first suppresses LH pulse frequency and then pulse amplitude in castrated male rats. Neuroendocrinology 58:448–453.

20. Polson DW, Sagle M, Mason HD, Adams J, Jacobs HS, Franks S. 1986. Ovulation and normal luteal function during LHRH treatment of women with hyperprolactinaemic amenorrhoea. Clin Endocrinol 24:531–537.

21. Lobo RA, Kletzky OA, Kaptein EM, Goebelsmann U. 1980. Prolactin modulation of dehydroepiandrosterone sulfate secretion. Am J Obstet Gynecol 138:632–636.

22. Klibanski A, Biller BM, Rosenthal DI, Schoenfeld DA, Saxe V. 1988. Effects of prolactin and estrogen deficiency in amenorrheic bone loss. J Clin Endocrinol Metab 67:124–130.

23. Koppelman MC, Kurtz DW, Morrish KA, Bou E, Susser JK, Shapiro JR, Loriaux DL. 1984. Vertebral body bone mineral content in hyperprolactinemic women. J Clin Endocrinol Metab 59:1050–1053.

24. Biller BM, Baum HB, Rosenthal DI, Saxe VC, Charpie PM, Klibanski A. 1992. Progressive trabecular osteopenia in women with hyperprolactinemic amenorrhea. J Clin Endocrinol Metab 75:692–697.

25. Martin TL, Kim M, Malarkey WB. 1985. The natural history of idiopathic hyperprolactinemia. J Clin Endocrinol Metab 60:855–858.

26. Sisam DA, Sheehan JP, Sheeler LR. 1987. The natural history of untreated microprolactinomas. Fertil Steril 48:67–71.

27. Schlechte J, Dolan K, Sherman B, Chapler F, Luciano A. 1989. The natural history of untreated hyperprolactinemia: A prospective analysis. J Clin Endocrinol Metab 68:412–418.

28. March CM, Kletzky OA, Davajan V, Teal J, Weiss M, Apuzzo ML, Marrs RP, Mishell DR Jr. 1981. Longitudinal evaluation of patients with untreated prolactin-secreting pituitary adenomas. Am J Obstet Gynecol 139:835–844.

29. Molitch ME. 1992. Pathologic hyperprolactinemia. Endocrinol Metab Clin North Am 21:877–901.

30. Molitch ME, Elton RL, Blackwell RE, Caldwell B, Chang RJ, Jaffe R, Joplin G, Robbins RJ, Tyson J, Thorner MO. 1985. Bromocriptine as primary therapy for prolactin-secreting

macroadenomas: Results of a prospective multicenter study. J Clin Endocrinol Metab 60:698–705.

31. Kletzky OA, Vermesh M. 1989. Effectiveness of vaginal bromocriptine in treating women with hyperprolactinemia. Fertil Steril 51:269–272.

32. Vermesh M, Fossum GT, Kletzky OA. 1988. Vaginal bromocriptine: Pharmacology and effect on serum prolactin in normal women. Obstet Gynecol 72:693–698.

33. Kletzky OA, Borenstein R, Mileikowsky GN. 1986. Pergolide and bromocriptine for the treatment of patients with hyperprolactinemia. Am J Obstet Gynecol 154:431–435.

34. Webster J, Piscitelli G, Polli A, DAlberton A, Falsetti L, Ferrari C, Fioretti P, Giordano G, Lhermite M, Ciccarelli E. 1992. Dose-dependent suppression of serum prolactin by cabergoline in hyperprolactinaemia: A placebo controlled, double blind, multicentre study. European Multicentre Cabergoline Dose-Fiding Study Group. Clin Endocrinol 37:534–541.

35. Biller BMK, Molitch ME, Vance ML, Cannistraro KB, Davis KR, Simons JA, Schoenfelder JR, Klibanski A. 1996. Treatment of prolactin-secreting macroadenomas with the once-weekly dopamine agonist cabergoline. J Clin Endocrinol Metab, in press.

36. Webster J, Piscitelli G, Polli A, Ferrari CI, Ismail I, Scanlon MF. 1994. A comparison of cabergoline and bromocriptine in the treatment of hyperprolactinemic amenorrhea. Cabergoline Comparative Study Group. N Engl J Med 331:904–909.

37. Zervas NT. 1984. Surgical results in pituitary adenomas: Results of an international study. In Black PM, ed. Secretory Tumors of the Pituitary Gland. New York: Raven, pp 377–385.

38. Serri O, Rasio E, Beauregard H, Hardy J, Somma M. 1983. Recurrence of hyperprolactinemia after selective transsphenoidal adenomectomy in women with prolactinoma. N Engl J Med 309:280–283.

39. Molitch ME. 1985. Pregnancy and the hyperprolactinemic woman. N Engl J Med 312:1364–1370.

40. Turkalj I, Braun P, Krupp P. 1982. Surveillance of bromocriptine in pregnancy. JAMA 247:1589–1591.

4. Gonadotroph and other clinically nonfunctioning pituitary adenomas

Peter J. Snyder

Gonadotroph adenomas are the most common pituitary macroadenomas but are the hardest to recognize because they secrete inefficiently and their secretory products usually do not cause a recognizable clinical syndrome. Consequently, they are the pituitary adenomas most likely to be clinically nonfunctioning, although occasionally other pituitary adenomas may also be clinically nonfunctioning.

Etiology

Pituitary adenomas are true neoplasms

For many years it was thought that pituitary adenomas could represent a hyperplastic change a resulting from excessive production of a trophic factor or deficient production of an inhibitory factor. Recently, however, most pituitary adenomas have been shown to be clonal [1,2]. Restriction fragment-length polymorphism analysis has shown that in women who have pituitary adenomas and whose peripheral leukocytes have both alleles of the genes encoding the enzymes hypoxanthine phosphoribosyltransferase (HPRT) or phosphoglycerate Kinase (PGK), the adenomas have only one allele or the other (Fig. 1). This result suggests that each of the adenomas arise from a single somatic mutation, which then expands clonally. These results have been found in all pituitary adenomas, including gonadotroph adenomas. Other recent studies have shown that about 40% of somatotroph adenomas harbor an activating mutation of the gene that encodes Gs-α, called the *gsp* oncogene, resulting in constitutively activated adenyl cyclase [3]. Because increased adenyl cyclase activity can cause cellular proliferation as well as increased hormonal secretion, the gene for Gs-α can be considered a protooncogene and the mutations can be considered oncogenes. Although the oncogenes and the proteins they encode have not yet been identified for the other 60% of somatotroph adenomas, or for any other kind of pituitary adenoma, including gonadotroph adenomas, it seems likely that they do exist.

Andrew Arnold (ed.) ENDOCRINE NEOPLASMS. 1997. Kluwer Academic Publishers. ISBN 0-7923-4354-9.
All rights reserved.

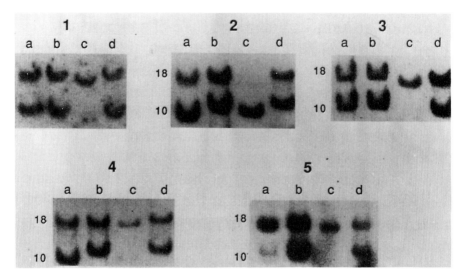

Figure 1. Demonstration of the apparent monoclonality of five pituitary adenomas. The bands represent DNA fragments of the HPRT gene from the peripheral leukocytes (lanes a and b) and pituitary adenoma cells (lanes c and d) of five women known to be heterozygous for the HPRT gene and to have gonadotroph adenomas. The leukocytes of each patient show both alleles (lane a), but the adenoma cells show only one allele (lane c), supporting the hypothesis that these adenomas arose from clonal expansion of a single cell. (From Alexander et al. [1], with permission.)

The search for a specific etiology

Finding a mutation that could be the cause of 40% of somatotroph adenomas has led to a search for mutations that could cause gonadotroph and other pituitary adenomas. The investigation has included known oncogenes, tumor suppressor genes, and hormones and growth factors known to act on the gonadotroph cell. In one study of 19 patients with pituitary adenomas, none of the seven adenomas that appeared to be gonadotroph adenomas by immunostaining exhibited any of three mutations of the *ras* gene known to be oncogenic, although a mutation was found in a highly invasive lactotroph adenoma [4]. Another study showed no mutations of the *ras* gene in five primary pituitary carcinomas or in six invasive adenomas of unspecified type, but point mutations of H-*ras* were found in the distant metastases of three of the carcinomas [5]. In the same study, no mutations were found in exons five through eight of the *p53* tumor suppressor gene.

A study of 18 pituitary adenomas, including 12 that stained for glycoprotein subunits, showed no allelic loss of the retinoblastoma gene [6]. Another study of 34 pituitary adenomas, of which 17 stained immunospecifically for gonadotropin subunits, confirmed those results [7]. An examination of 21 clinically nonfunctioning adenomas showed two that had mutations of the *gsp* oncogene, similar to those found in somatotroph adenomas; none of 27 had mutations of the *gip* gene [8]. What role the *gsp* mutation might play in the pathogenesis of these adenomas is as yet uncertain. In summary, there is little evidence to date for a role of well-known oncogenes in the pathogenesis of gonadotroph adenomas.

Several known growth factors have been found to be expressed by gonadotroph and other pituitary adenomas. Interleukin-6 immunoactivity was found in the media in which 2 of 2 gonadotroph adenomas and 23 of 49 clinically nonfunctioning adenomas were cultured [9]. One of two gonadotroph adenomas was found to express basic fibroblast growth factor mRNA [10]. Two (of two) gonadotroph adenomas expressed transforming growth factor α mRNA [11]. Invasive pituitary adenomas expressed a point mutation on the α isoform of protein kinase C, whereas noninvasive adenomas expressed only the native sequence [12]. Gonadotroph adenomas also express the activin/inhibin β_B subunit, and can therefore presumably synthesize activin B, which is a homodimer of this subunit. In one study, the activin/inhibin β_B subunit was expressed in all 10 gonadotroph adenomas studied [13]. In another study, gonadotroph adenomas were also found to express the activin/inhibin β_B subunit [14]. Whether or not the expression of any of these growth factors by gonadotroph adenomas is pathogenetically related to the development of the adenomas has not yet been established.

Clinical presentation (Table 1)

Gonadotroph adenomas usually come to clinical attention when they become so large as to cause neurologic symptoms but may also be recognized when imaging of the head is performed for an unrelated reason. The large size may also cause deficient hormonal secretion from the nonadenomatous pituitary, and these deficiencies may even be recognizable at the time of presentation, but they are usually not the impetus for the patient to seek medical attention.

Table 1. Clinical presentations of gonadotroph adenomas

Neurologic symptoms (most common)
Visual impairment
Headache
Other (diplopia, seizures, CSF rhinorrhea, etc.)
Incidental finding
When an imaging procedure is performed because of an unrelated symptom
Hormonal symptoms (least common)
Oligorrhea or amenorrhea in a premenopausal woman
Ovarian hyperstimulation when FSH is secreted excessively in a premenopausal woman
Premature puberty when intact LH is secreted in a prepubertal boy
Symptoms of hormonal deficiencies (commonly occur but uncommonly are the presenting symptoms)

CSF = cerebrospinal fluid; FSH = follicle-stimulating hormone; LH = luteinizing hormone.

Gonadotroph adenomas are rarely, if ever, recognized when they are microadenomas because excessive gonadotropin secretion usually does not cause a clinically recognizable syndrome, and also because these adenomas are usually so inefficient hormonally that when they are of 'micro' size (<1 cm) they probably do not produce elevated serum concentrations of gonadotropins or their subunits. Gonadotroph adenomas rarely cause a recognizable clinical syndrome.

Neurologic symptoms

Impaired vision is the symptom that most commonly leads a patient with a gonadotroph adenoma to seek medical attention [15], although other neurologic symptoms may also do so. Visual impairment is caused by suprasellar extension of the adenoma that compresses the optic chiasm. When compression becomes more severe, central visual acuity is also affected. The onset of the deficit is usually so gradual that patients often do not seek ophthalmological consultation for months or even years. Even then the reason for the deficit may not be recognized, unless a visual-field examination is performed and the diagnosis is delayed further. Other neurologic symptoms that may cause a patient with a gonadotroph adenoma to seek medical attention are headaches, caused presumably by expansion of the sella; diplopia, caused by oculomotor nerve compression due to lateral extension of the adenoma; cerebrospinal fluid (CSF) rhinorrhea, caused by inferior extension of the adenoma; and the excruciating headache and diplopia caused by pituitary apoplexy, sudden hemorrhage into the adenoma.

Incidental finding

The common use of magnetic resonance imaging (MRI) to evaluate symptoms in the head or neck, such as head trauma, sinusitis, etc., has resulted in the discovery of many intrasellar lesions unrelated to the symptom that led to the imaging procedure. Although many of these incidentally discovered lesions are small and not clinically functioning, some are >1 cm in diameter and can be recognized as gonadotroph adenomas by the procedures described later.

Hormonal presentations

At the time of the initial presentation due to a neurologic symptom, many patients with gonadotroph adenomas, when questioned, admit to symptoms of pituitary hormonal deficiencies. Ironically, the most common pituitary hormonal deficiency is in luteinizing hormone (LH), the result of compression of the normal gonadotroph cells by the adenoma and the lack of secretion of a substantial amount of intact LH by the adenomatous gonadotroph cells. The result in men is a subnormal serum testosterone concentration, which produces symptoms of decreased energy and libido. The result in premenopausal women is amenorrhea. Any other pituitary hormone might be secreted subnormally as well.

Gonadotroph adenomas rarely present because of excessive hormonal secretion. Excessive and relatively constant secretion of follicle-stimulating hormone (FSH) in a premenopausal woman would be expected theoretically to disrupt cyclical ovarian function and to cause ovarian hyperstimulation and amenorrhea. In fact, one such patient has been reported [16]. Excessive secretion of FSH would not be expected to cause symptoms in men and postmenopausal women. Excessive secretion of LH in men would be expected to cause hypersecretion of testosterone, and in the rare cases of gonadotroph adenomas that do hypersecrete LH, that is what happens. LH hypersecretion in men causes supranormal serum testosterone concentrations [17], but typically no symptoms result. LH hypersecretion in boys causes premature puberty [18,19].

Diagnosis

The process of making the diagnosis of a gonadotroph adenoma usually proceeds first from recognizing that a patient's visual abnormality or other symptom could represent an intrasellar lesion, to confirming the presence of an intrasellar lesion by an imaging procedure, to, finally, finding secretory abnormalities of gonadotropins and their subunits characteristic of a gonadotroph adenoma.

Visual and other abnormalities

The visual abnormality most characteristic of an intrasellar lesion is diminished vision in the temporal fields. Either or both eyes may be affected, and if both, to variable degrees. Diminished visual acuity occurs when the optic chiasm is more severely compressed. Other patterns of visual loss may also occur, so an intrasellar lesion should be suspected when any pattern of visual loss is unexplained. Other neurologic abnormalities that should raise the suspicion of an intrasellar lesion are headaches, oculomotor nerve palsies, and cerebrospinal fluid (CSF) rhinorrhea. The quality of the headaches is not specific.

Imaging of the pituitary

Current imaging techniques are more than sensitive enough to demonstrate any pituitary adenoma that has become so large as to impair vision or to cause any other neurologic symptom. Because gonadotroph adenomas are generally hormonally inefficient, by the time a gonadotroph adenoma produces supranormal serum concentrations of intact gonadotropins or their subunits, it

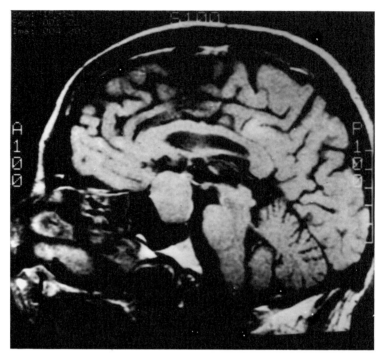

Figure 2. Magnetic resonance imaging showing in a sagittal view of the head a large gonadotroph adenoma extending superior to elevate the optic chiasm. Gonadotroph adenomas are often not recognized until they become large.

is sufficiently large to be seen by imaging (Fig. 2). MRI is currently the best technique for imaging the pituitary gland because of its superior resolution and its ability to demonstrate the optic chiasm. In addition, MRI is able to demonstrate blood, so one is able to recognize hemorrhage into the pituitary and to distinguish an aneurysm from other intrasellar lesions. Computed tomographic (CT) scanning has the advantage of the ability to demonstrate calcium, which is helpful in making the diagnosis of a craniopharyngioma.

If the visual or other symptoms that led to imaging are caused by a gonadotroph adenoma, the imaging will demonstrate the presence of a large intrasellar mass that is likely to extend outside of the sella. MRI will demonstrate if the adenoma is elevating the optic chiasm or extending into the cavernous sinuses or sphenoid sinus. MRI will not distinguish, however, adenomatous tissue from normal pituitary tissue; consequently, a clear distinction between an intrasellar mass lesion and the normal pituitary is evidence that the lesion is not a pituitary adenoma. MRI will also not distinguish a gonadotroph adenoma from other pituitary macroadenomas and often not even from nonpituitary lesions.

Hormonal abnormalities

Intrasellar mass lesions detected by MRI should be evaluated further by measurement of serum concentrations of pituitary hormones to determine if the lesion is of pituitary or nonpituitary origin, and if pituitary, the cell of origin. A pituitary adenoma of gonadotroph or thyrotroph cell origin should be suspected if the serum prolactin concentration is <100 ng/ml, the patient does not appear acromegalic and the serum insulin-like growth factor (IGF)-I concentration is not supranormal, and the patient does not have Cushing's syndrome and does not have supranormal urine cortisol excretion. A 'silent' somatotroph or corticotroph adenoma or a lesion of nonpituitary origin could also account for these findings. Preoperative recognition that an intrasellar mass lesion is of gonadotroph origin depends on finding specific combinations of the serum concentrations of gonadotropins and their subunits (Table 2). The combinations differ somewhat in men and women.

Men. A supranormal basal serum FSH concentration in a man who has an intrasellar mass lesion usually indicates that the lesion is a gonadotroph adenoma [20] (Fig. 3). The diagnosis is strengthened if he also has other characteristic features of a gonadotroph adenoma, such as a supranormal basal serum concentration of the glycoprotein α subunit or responses of intact FSH and LH, or of LHβ, to thyrotropin-releasing hormone (TRH) [20]. A supranormal serum LH accompanied by a supranormal serum testosterone, whether or not accompanied by a supranormal FSH, is strong evidence that the lesion is one of the unusual gonadotroph adenomas that secrete intact LH. A supranormal serum LH accompanied by a serum testosterone that is not elevated suggests that an elevated α subunit is crossreacting in the polyclonal LH immunoassay. This possibility can be confirmed by measuring LH in a highly specific, double monoclonal assay and by measuring the α subunit. A supranormal serum α subunit as the sole basal serum abnormality indicates

Table 2. Hormonal criteria for the diagnosis of gonadotroph adenomas[a] (any one or any combination of the following)

Men	Women
Supranormal basal serum concentrations	
FSH[b]	FSH but not LH
α, LHβ, or FSHβ subunits	Any subunit relative to intact FSH and LH
LH and testosterone	
Supranormal response to TRH	
FSH	FSH
LH	LH
LHβ (most common)	LHβ (most common)

[a] Assuming the patient has a pituitary macroadenoma.
[b] Assuming the patient does not have a history of primary hypogonadism.
FSH = follicle-stimulating hormone; LH = luteinizing hormone.

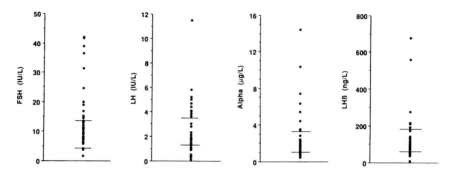

Figure 3. Basal serum concentrations of intact FSH and LH and α and LHβ subunits in 38 men with pituitary macroadenomas that were clinically nonfunctioning. Eleven had elevations of FSH, 10 of LH, 8 of α subunit, and 6 of LHβ subunit. Of the 38 adenomas, 36 were studied in cell culture and 29 could be identified as gonadotroph adenomas by their secretion in culture. (From Daneshdoost et al. [20], with permission.)

that the intrasellar lesion is of gonadotroph or thyrotroph origin. TRH stimulation of intact FSH or LH, or of the LHβ subunit, would confirm a gonadotroph origin.

Women. Recognizing the gonadotroph origin of an intrasellar mass on the basis of basal serum hormone concentrations of intact FSH and LH is more difficult in women that in men. In a woman over 50 years old who has an intrasellar mass and elevated gonadotropins, distinguishing between the adenoma and normal postmenopausal gonadotroph cells as the source is usually not possible on the basis of the basal gonadotropins alone. Similarly, in a woman under 50 years old who has an intrasellar mass and elevated serum gonadotropins, distinguishing between the adenoma and premature ovarian failure as the source of the gonadotropins is also not usually possible on the basis of the FSH and LH values alone. A few combinations of basal FSH, LH, and α subunit values, however, do strongly suggest that an intrasellar mass is a gonadotroph adenoma. A markedly supranormal FSH associated with a subnormal LH, for example, most likely indicates a gonadotroph adenoma, rather than the postmenopausal state or premature ovarian failure [21]. A serum α subunit concentration that is supranormal when intact FSH and LH are not, or is supranormal out of proportion to the FSH and LH, also suggests a gonadotroph adenoma [21]. More commonly, an intrasellar mass in a woman may be recognized as a gonadotroph adenoma by an increase in FSH or LH, or even more frequently, in the LHβ subunit, in response to TRH (Fig. 4) [21].

Distinguishing gonadotroph adenomas from primary hypogonadism. The question of how to distinguish a gonadotroph adenoma from primary hypogonadism is often raised because in both conditions serum concentrations of intact gonadotropins and their subunits may be supranormal and gonadal steroids may be subnormal. Furthermore, longstanding primary hypogonadism may cause some enlargement of the pituitary as a consequence of gonadotroph hyperplasia [22]. In practice, however, making this distinction is usually quite easy because each exhibits a different clinical presentation and each a different set of hormonal secretory characteristics. The major clinical distinction results from the observation that pituitary enlargement due to primary hypogonadism usually does not occur unless the hypogonadism is severe, untreated, and of many years duration. Consequently, such patients, both men and women, often appear hypogonadal clinically. In contrast, men and women who have gonadotroph adenomas may be hypogonadal, but the hypogonadism is usually not severe or of long duration. Consequently, they usually do not appear hypogonadal clinically. The major difference in basal hormonal concentrations is the elevation of both FSH and LH in patients who have primary hypogonadism and the elevation of FSH, but usually not LH, and sometimes by greater elevation of the α subunit, in patients who have gonadotroph adenomas. The major difference in hormonal responses to TRH is that patients who have gonadotroph adenomas often exhibit responses of FSH, LH, and, more commonly, the LHβ subunit, but patients who have

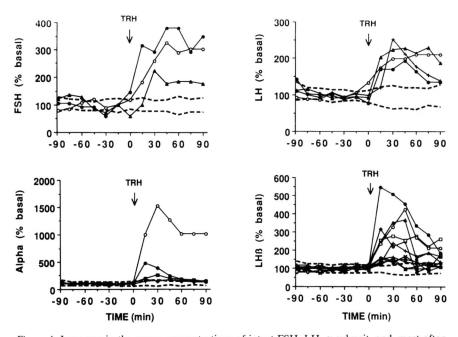

Figure 4. Increases in the serum concentrations of intact FSH, LH, α subunit, and, most often, LHβ subunit to TRH in 16 women with adenomas that were clinically nonfunctioning. The dashed lines show the ranges of serum concentrations in 16 age-matched healthy women. Eleven women with adenomas exhibited significant responses to TRH of the LHβ subunit, four of intact LH and α subunit, and three of FSH. (From Daneshdoost et al. [21], with permission.)

primary hypogonadism do not [23]. Another clear difference is that men who have a subnormal serum testosterone on the basis of a gonadotroph adenoma exhibit an increase to well within the normal range when treated with human chorionic gonadotropin (hCG) for 4 days [24], but men with primary hypogonadism do not.

Abnormal secretion of other pituitary hormones. Pituitary adenomas that secrete intact gonadotropins and/or their subunits usually do not also secrete other pituitary hormones as well, but concomitant secretion of thyroid-stimulating hormone (TSH) and prolactin have been reported rarely. A serum prolactin concentration that is elevated but <100 ng/ml, however, suggests not concomitant secretion by the adenoma but increased secretion by normal lactotroph cells that are less than normally inhibited because of stalk compression by the adenoma. Deficient secretion of other pituitary hormones often occurs due to the mass effect of the typically large gonadotroph adenomas and should always be investigated.

Treatment (Table 3)

Because gonadotroph adenomas usually do not present until they are so large as to cause neurologic symptoms, treatment to relieve those symptoms must be initiated promptly. Currently, trans-sphenoidal surgery is the only treatment that is usually effective in doing so. Surgery is usually not successful in removing all pituitary adenoma tissue, however, so radiation is often necessary to prevent the residual from regrowing. To date no pharmacologic treatment has been shown to be reliably effective.

Table 3. Comparison of standard treatments for gonadotroph adenomas

Treatment	Use	Advantages	Side effects
Trans-sphenoidal surgery	Primary treatment when adenoma causes neurologic symptoms	Rapid decrease of adenoma size	Transient diabetes insipidus and/or SIADH; hormonal deficiencies; decreased vision, hemorrhage, CSF rhinorrhea, meningitis (all uncommon)
Conventional radiation	Adjuvant therapy for residual adenoma after surgery; primary therapy in absence of neurologic symptoms	Prevents regrowth of residual adenoma	Short term: nausea, lethargy, loss of taste and smell; loss of hair at radiation portals. Long term: hypopituitarism
Observation only	Asymptomatic adenomas	No immediate risk	None immediately; risk of future growth

CSF = cerebrospinal fluid.

Surgery

Surgery is performed most successfully and safely by the trans-sphenoidal route. Trans-sphenoidal surgery reduces the size of gonadotroph adenomas and their hormonal hypersecretion in more than 90% of cases, and in about 70% it improves vision [25]. Serious risks of trans-sphenoidal surgery in the immediate postoperative period include worsening vision, hemorrhage, and CSF rhinorrhea, sometimes leading to meningitis, but together these occur in <5% of cases [26,27]. A less serious, but more common, immediate postoperative risk is instability of vasopressin secretion, which can include diabetes insipidus, syndrome of inappropriate secretion of antidiuretic hormone (SIADH), and fluctuations between the two. These fluctuations usually do not last more than 4–5 days after surgery, but diabetes insipidus infrequently is permanent. Surgery may improve hormonal secretion by the nonadenomatous pituitary, worsen it, or leave it unchanged.

The most important preoperative preparations for surgery are identifying the sellar lesion as a gonadotroph adenoma, identifying an experienced pituitary surgeon, and ensuring that the patient is hormonally stable. One reason to identify the mass as a gonadotroph adenoma is to distinguish it from a nonpituitary lesion near the sella, which might best be approached transcranially. Another reason is to find a marker, such as an elevated serum FSH or α subunit concentration, which can be used to monitor the response to surgery and subsequent treatment. Hypothyroidism increases the risk of respiratory arrest due to postoperative administration of narcotics or barbiturates, so hypothyroidism should be corrected preoperatively, or those agents should be used in lower than usual doses.

Postoperative management can be considered in terms of immediate, short term, and long term. In the few days after surgery, the patient may develop diabetes insipidus, SIADH, or both. In this period diabetes insipidus should be treated with aqueous vasopressin, either as subcutaneous bolus doses or as a continuous intravenous infusion. Desmopressin acetate (DDAVP), which is longer acting, should be avoided at this time because it might cause hyponatremia if the diabetes insipidus suddenly remits and especially if it is followed by SIADH. If diabetes insipidus lasts for more than 4–5 days or is present at the time of discharge from the hospital, DDAVP should be used. Maintenance hydrocortisone should be prescribed on discharge from the hospital.

Four to 6 weeks after discharge from the hospital, the patient should be evaluated for the amount of residual adenoma, visual function, and hormonal function of the nonadenomatous pituitary. A crude estimation of the amount of residual adenoma can be determined by MRI, but artifacts of surgery may obscure the actual amount of residual adenoma tissue for several months. The serum concentration of any gonadotroph adenoma product, such as FSH or the α subunit, that had been elevated before surgery will give a more accurate estimate of the amount of residual adenoma. Visual function should be evaluated by acuity and fields. Hormonal function of the nonadenomatous pituitary should be evaluated regardless of whether it was normal or abnormal prior surgery because it can be better, worse, or the same afterwards. This evaluation should include measurement of serum concentrations of thyroxine, early morning cortisol (48 hours after discontinuation of hydrocortisone), and testosterone in a man or estradiol in a premenopausal woman. If the plasma cortisol is $\leq 3\,\mu g/dl$, the patient is hypoadrenal; if it is $\geq 18\,\mu g/dl$, the patient has normal adrenal function. If the plasma cortisol is 4–$17\,\mu g/dl$, a test of adrenocorticotrophic hormone (ACTH) reserve, such as a metyrapone test, should be performed. Measurement of cortisol 1 hour after the administration of $250\,\mu g$ of cosyntropin should not be used because in this situation it may give a falsely normal result [28]. If the patient has significant nocturia at this time, 24-hour urine volume should be determined, and if it is 3–6 liters, a water deprivation test should be performed to assess the possibility of diabetes insipidus. Greater volumes almost certainly indicate diabetes insipidus. Any hormonal deficiencies should be treated.

Long-term evaluation should include testing every 6–12 months initially to detect recurrence of the adenoma and the adequacy of hormonal replacement medications. Evaluation for recurrence should include measurement of whatever serum marker was elevated before surgery and an MRI. If vision was affected by the adenoma, it should be evaluated periodically as well.

Radiation

Radiation therapy is used most commonly after trans-sphenoidal surgery to prevent residual gonadotroph adenoma tissue from regrowing, but occasionally it can be used appropriately as primary therapy. As adjuvant therapy, radiation is administered 6–12 months after surgery if MRI shows significant residual adenoma tissue; if radiation is not administered, the chances are high that the residual adenoma will increase in size within the next few years and require surgery again. If little pituitary tissue remains after surgery, MRI, once a year initially and then less frequently, should detect regrowth soon enough to treat by radiation. As primary therapy, radiation is appropriate if the adenoma is sufficiently large to be threatening the optic chiasm but not actually causing visual impairment or other neurologic symptoms.

Conventional radiation therapy is supervoltage radiation, administered in 23 daily doses of 2 Gy each. Side effects of radiation that occur during treatment include nausea, lethargy, loss of taste and smell, and loss of hair at the radiation portals. The first two remit within 1–2 months, and the latter two usually remit within 6 months. The long-term side effect of radiation is loss of function of the nonadenomatous pituitary. The chances are approximately 50% that at least one pituitary hormone that had been normal prior to radiation will be subnormal within 5 years afterwards.

Two newer methods of radiation treatment, both involving stereotactic delivery, are being tried. A theoretical advantage of these methods is that the number of portals of entry of the radiation is increased infinitely, so the radiation exposure of any one part of the brain is decreased. One method is stereotactic administration of conventional radiation administered in fractionated doses. The other method is administration of gamma radiation from a ⁶⁰Co source that is stereotactically delivered to the adenoma in a single, large dose. This technique is called *radiosurgery* or *gamma knife*. A theoretical disadvantage of this method is that the dose of radiation is so large that it is considered unsafe to treat an adenoma that extends outside the sella because of the risk of damaging nonpituitary tissue, such as the optic chiasm. To date, limited information has been published about the effects of either of these treatments on pituitary adenomas, so it is best to restrict their use to a few centers on an experimental basis until their actual advantages and disadvantages become more clear.

Medications

The extraordinary success of dopamine agonists in reducing the size of, as well as secretion by, lactotroph adenomas has prompted attempts to find a pharmacologic treatment for gonadotroph adenomas. So far, however, no drug has been found that will reduce adenoma size consistently and substantially. Although dopamine does not decrease gonadotropin secretion to an appreciable degree in normal subjects, bromocriptine has been reported to reduce the secretion of intact gonadotropins and the α subunit in a few patients, and even to improve vision in one, but not to reduce adenoma size [29,30].

Based on data showing the presence of somatostatin receptors on the cell membranes of clinically nonfunctioning pituitary adenomas [31,32], two groups administered octreotide to such patients. One group found improvement in visual fields in three of four patients, but no decrease in adenoma size [33]. Another group found among six patients decreases in α-subunit values in three and in size and visual impairment in two each, but no correlation among the three parameters [34].

Agonist analogs of gonadotropin-releasing hormone (GnRH) have been administered to patients with gonadotroph adenomas, based on the rationale that chronic administration of these agonists causes downregulation of GnRH receptors on, and decreased secretion of FSH and LH from, normal gonadotroph cells. Administration of GnRH agonist analogs to patients with gonadotroph adenomas, however, generally produces either an agonist effect or no effect on secretion and no effect on adenoma size [35–37].

The pure GnRH antagonist, Nal-Glu GnRH, is the most effective agent tested so far in suppressing FSH secretion by gonadotroph adenomas, but it does not appear to decrease their size. Administration for 1 week of Nal-Glu GnRH to men with gonadotroph adenomas reduced their elevated FSH concentrations to normal [38]. When Nal-Glu was administered for 6 months,

FSH remained suppressed for the entire period but adenoma size did not decrease [39]. These results suggest that FSH secretion by gonadotroph adenomas is dependent on endogenous GnRH but that adenoma size is not. As a practical matter, no medical treatment tried thus far can be recommended.

No treatment

Gonadotroph adenomas that are asymptomatic and not an immediate threat to vision may not require treatment, especially if the patient is elderly or infirm. This situation is increasingly common as more and more gonadotroph adenomas are detected as incidental findings when MRI is performed to evaluate head trauma, etc. Hormonal deficiencies should still be replaced. Re-evaluation of adenoma size and the function of the nonadenomatous pituitary should be performed at yearly intervals.

References

1. Alexander JM, Biller BMK, Bikkal H, Zervas NT, Arnold A, Klibanski A. 1990. Clinically nonfunctioning pituitary tumors are monoclonal in origin. J Clin Invest 86:336–340.
2. Herman V, Fagin J, Gonsky R, Kovacs K, Melmed S. 1990. Clonal origin of pituitary adenomas. J Clin Endocrinol Metab 71:1427–1433.
3. Landis CA, Masters SB, Spada A, Pace AM, Bourne HR, Vallar L. 1989. GTPase inhibiting mutations activate the chain of Gs to stimulate adenyl cyclase in human pituitary tumors. Nature (Lond) 340:692–696.
4. Karga HJ, Alexander JM, Hedley-Whyte ET, Klibanski A, Jameson JL. 1992. Ras mutations in human pituitary tumors. J Clin Endocrinol Metab 74:914–919.
5. Pei L, Melmed S, Scheithauer B. 1994. H-ras mutations in human pituitary carcinoma metastases. J Clin Endocrinol Metab 78:842–846.
6. Cryns VL, Alexander JM, Klibanski A, Arnold A. 1993. The retinoblastoma gene in human pituitary tumors. J Clin Endocrinol Metab 77:644–646.
7. Zhu J, Leon SP, Beggs AH, Busque L, Gilliland G, Black PM. 1994. Human pituitary adenomas show no loss of heterozygosity at the retinoblastoma gene locus. J Clin Endocrinol Metab 78:922–927.
8. Tordjman K, Stern N, Ouaknine G, Yossiphov Y, Razon N, Nordenskjold M, Friedman E. 1993. Activating mutations of the Gs α-gene in nonfunctioning pituitary tumors. J Clin Endocrinol Metab 77:765–769.
9. Jones TH, Daniels M, James RA, Justice SK, Corkle RM, Price A, Kendall-Taylor P, Weetman AP. 1994. Production of bioactive and immunoreactive interleukin-6 (IL-6) and expression of IL-6 messenger ribonucleic acid by human pituitary adenomas. J Clin Endocrinol Metab 78:180–186.
10. Ezzat S, Smyth HS, Ramyar K, Asa SL. 1995. Heterogenous in vivo and in vitro expression of basic fibroblast growth factor by human pituitary adenomas. J Clin Endocrinol Metab 80:878–884.
11. Ezzat S, Walpola IA, Ramyar L, Smyth MS, Asa SL. 1995. Membrane-anchored expression of transforming growth factor-α in human pituitary adenoma cells. J Clin Endocrinol Metab 80:534–539.
12. Alvaro V, Levy L, Dubray C, Roche A, Peillon F, Querat B, Joubert D. 1993. Invasive human pituitary tumors express a point-mutated α-protein kinase-C. J Clin Endocrinol Metab 77:1125–1129.

13. Haddad G, Penabad JL, Bashey HM, Asa SL, Gennarelli TA, Cirullo R, Snyder PJ. 1994. Expression of activin/inhibin subunit messenger ribonucleic acids by gonadotroph adenomas. J Clin Endocrinol Metab 79:1399–1403.
14. Alexander JM, Swearingen B, Tindall GT, Klibanski A. 1995. Human pituitary adenomas express endogenous inhibin subunits and follistatin messenger ribonucleic acids. J Clin Endocrinol Metab 80:146–152.
15. Snyder PJ. 1985. Gonadotroph cell adenomas of the pituitary. Endocr Rev 6:552–563.
16. Djerassi A, Coutifaris C, West VA, Asa SL, Kapoor SC, Pavlou SN, Snyder PJ. 1995. Gonadotroph adenoma in a premenopausal woman secreting follicle-stimulating hormone and causing ovarian hyperstimulation. J Clin Endocrinol Metab 80:591–594.
17. Snyder PJ, Sterling FH. 1976. Hypersecretion of LH and FSH by a pituitary adenoma. J Clin Endocrinol Metab 42:544–550.
18. Faggiano M, Criscuolo T, Perrone I, Quarto C, Sinisi AA. 1983. Sexual precocity in a boy due to hypersecretion of LH and prolactin by a pituitary adenoma. Acta Endocrinol 102:167–172.
19. Ambrosi B, Basstti M, Ferrario R, Medri G, Giannattosic G, Faglia G. 1990. Precocious puberty in a boy with a PRL-LH-and FSH-secreting pituitary tumor: Hormonal and immuno-cytochemical studies. Acta Endocrinol (Copenh) 122:569–576.
20. Daneshdoost L, Gennarelli TA, Bashey HM, Savino PJ, Sergott RC, Bosley TM, Snyder PJ. 1993. Identification of gonadotroph adenomas in men with clinically nonfunctioning adenomas by the luteinizing hormone β-subunit response to thyrotrophin-releasing hormone. J Clin Endocrinol Metab 77:1352–1355.
21. Daneshdoost L, Gennarelli TA, Bashey HM, Savino PJ, Sergott RC, Bosley TM, Snyder PJ. 1991. Recognition of gonadotroph adenomas in women. N Engl J Med 324:589–594.
22. Samaan NA, Stephans AV, Danziger J, Trujillo J. 1979. Reactive pituitary abnormalities in patients with Klinefelter's and Turner's syndromes. Arch Intern Med 139:198–201.
23. Snyder PJ, Bashey HM, Kim SU, Chappel SC. 1984. Secretion of uncombined subunits of luteinizing hormone by gonadotroph cell adenomas. J Clin Endocrinol Metab 59:1169–1175.
24. Snyder PJ, Bigdeli H, Gardner DF, Mihailovic V, Rudenstein RS, Sterling FH, Utiger RD. 1979. Gonadal function in fifty men with untreated pituitary adenomas. J Clin Endocrinol Metab 48:309–314.
25. Harris RI, Shatz NJ, Gennarelli T, Savino PJ, Cobbs WH, Snyder PJ. 1983. Follicle-stimulating hormone-secreting pituitary adenomas: Correlation of reduction of adenoma size with reduction of hormonal hypersecretion after transsphenoidal surgery. J Clin Endocrinol Metab 56:1288–1293.
26. Trautmann JC, Laws ER. 1983. Visual status after transsphenoidal surgery at the Mayo Clinic, 1971–1982. Am J Ophthalmol 96:200–208.
27. Black PM, Zervas NT, Candia G. 1988. Management of large pituitary adenomas by transsphenoidal surgery. Surg Neurol 29:443–447.
28. Streeten DHP, Anderson GH Jr, Bonaventura MM. 1996. The potential for serious consequences from misinterpreting normal responses to the rapid adrenocorticotropin test. J Clin Endocrinol Metab 81:285–290.
29. Berezin M, Olchovsky D, Pines A, Tadmor R, Lunenfeld B. 1984. Reduction of follicle-stimulating hormone (FSH) secretion in FSH-producing pituitary adenoma by bromocriptine. J Clin Endocrinol Metab 59:1220–1222.
30. Vance ML, Ridgway EC, Thorner MO. 1985. Follicle-stimulating hormone and α-subunit-secreting pituitary tumor treated with bromocriptine. J Clin Endocrinol Metab 61:580–584.
31. Ikuyama S, Nawata H, Kato K, Karashima T, Ibayashi H, Nakagaki M. 1985. Specific somatostatin receptors on human pituitary adenoma cell membranes. J Clin Endocrinol Metab 61:666–671.
32. Reubi JC, Heitz PU, Landolt AM. 1987. Visualization of somatostatin receptors and correlation with immunoreactive growth hormone and prolactin in human pituitary adenomas: Evidence for different tumor subclasses. J Clin Endocrinol Metab 65:65–73.

33. DeBruin TW, Kwekkeboom DJ, Verlaat JWV, Reubi JC, Krenning EP, Lamberts SWJ, Craughs RJM. 1992. Clinically nonfunctioning pituitary adenoma and octreotide response to long term high dose treatment, and studies in vitro. J Clin Endocrinol Metab 75:1310–131.
34. Katznelson L, Oppenheim DS, Coughlin JF. 1992. Chronic somatostatin analog administration in patients with α-subunit-secreting pituitary tumors. J Clin Endocrinol Metab 75:1318–1324.
35. Roman SH, Goldstein M, Kourides IA, Comile F, Bardin CW, Krieger DT. 1964. The luteinizing hormone-releasing hormone (LHRH) agonist [D-Trp^6-Pro-Net] LHRH increased rather than lowered LH and α-subunit levels in a patient with an LH-secreting pituitary tumor. J Clin Endocrinol Metab 58:313–319.
36. Sassolas G, Lejeune H, Trouillas J, Forest MG, Claustrat B, Lahlou N, Loras B. 1988. Gonadotropin-releasing hormone agonists are unsuccessful in reducing tumoral gonadotropin secretion in two patients with gonadotropin-secreting pituitary adenomas. J Clin Endocrinol Metab 67:180–185.
37. Klibanski A, Jameson JL, Biller BMK, Crowley Jr WF, Zervas NT, Rivier J, Vale WW, Bikkal H. 1989. Gonadotropin and α-subunit responses to chorionic gonadotropin-releasing hormone analog administration in patients with glycoprotein hormone-secreting pituitary tumors. J Clin Endocrinol Metab 68:81–86.
38. Daneshdoost L, Pavlou S, Molitch ME. 1993. Inhibition of follicle-stimulating hormone secretion from gonadotroph adenomas by repetitive administration of a gonadotropin-releasing hormone antagonist. J Clin Endocrinol Metab 71:92–97.
39. McGrath GA, Goncalvez R, Udupa J, Grossman RI, Pavlou SN, Molitch ME, Rivier J, Vale WW, Snyder PJ. 1993. New technique for quantitation of pituitary adenoma size: Use in evaluating treatment of gonadotroph adenomas with a GnRH antagonist. J Clin Endocrinol Metab 76:1363–1368.

5. Approach to the incidentally discovered pituitary mass

Mark E. Molitch

Improvements in diagnostic imaging techniques over the last several years have created the dilemma for the clinician of the radiologist being able to detect asymptomatic masses in several organs [1]. Such incidentally found masses have been referred to as *incidentalomas* [2]. When these imaging techniques have been applied to the pituitary gland, similar incidentalomas have been found in seemingly normal subjects [3–11]. At present, these techniques include high-resolution computed tomographic (CT) scanning with infusion of intravenous contrast, and magnetic resonance imaging (MRI), with or without administration of gadolinium [12,13]. It is the purpose of the present discussion to provide information and guidelines for the evaluation of the patient incidentally found to have a mass lesion of the pituitary on a CT or MRI scan that has been performed for some other reason (Fig. 1).

Types of pituitary mass lesions

A number of lesions may be present within the sella turcica and in parasellar areas [12–14] (Table 1). Certainly the most common lesion is the pituitary adenoma. Pituitary adenomas may be classified in various ways [15]. Virtually all are benign, although there may be localized areas of invasion [15]. Although some adenomas may display histologic evidence suggestive of malignancy, such as mitoses, cellular and nuclear pleomorphism, hyperchromatism of nuclei, and an increased nuclear/cytoplasmic ratio, these findings are not specific and only the presence of distant metastases can be used for the definitive designation of malignancy [15]. True pituitary carcinomas with evidence of metastases are so rare as to be individually reportable.

Adenomas generally are classified as to size, with tumors <10 mm in diameter being designated microadenomas and tumors >10 mm in diameter being designated as macroadenomas (Fig. 2). Additional features to note are localized areas of invasion and extrasellar extension. In particular, lesions extending in a suprasellar direction need to be evaluated with respect to possible compression of the optic chiasm by direct visualization on MRI scan and by visual field examination using Goldmann perimetry [16].

Andrew Arnold (ed.) ENDOCRINE NEOPLASMS. 1997. Kluwer Academic Publishers. ISBN 0-7923-4354-9.
All rights reserved.

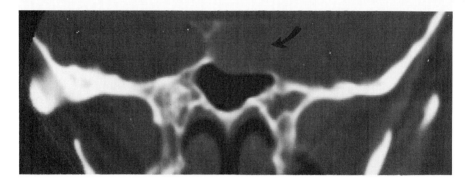

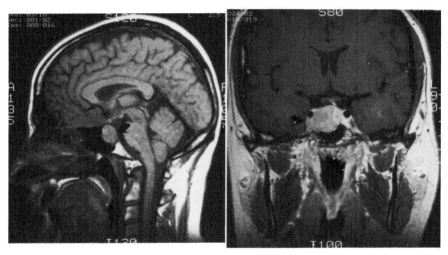

Figure 1. **Top**: CT scan, coronal view, carried out to rule out lesions of internal auditory canals causing deafness. Note the poorly visualized macroadenoma (arrow). **Bottom**: MRI scans, lateral and frontal cuts, showing large macroadenoma (arrows) with suprasellar and lateral parasellar extension. This 30-year-old man was eventually found to have panhypopituitarism and a prolactin of 2200 ng/ml. His deafness was subsequently found to be caused by Wegener's granulomatosis.

In addition to their size, pituitary adenomas are also characterized by their hormonal secretion. The most common tumor is a prolactin (PRL)-secreting tumor (prolactinoma) and the next most common is a clinically non-functioning tumor. The latter frequently secrete intact gonadotropins or their glycoprotein subunits (alpha and/or beta) in vivo or in vitro; technically, therefore, most are really gonadotroph adenomas [17,18]. Rarely, clinically nonfunctioning tumors will be found to stain positively for adrenocorticotrophic hormone (ACTH) or growth hormone (GH) but do not secrete these hormones in excess, and such patients do not have Cushing's disease [19] or acromegaly [20,21]. In various surgical series, prolactinomas and

Table 1. Lesions of the sella turcica and parasellar areas

Pituitary adenomas 　PRL secreting 　GH secreting 　ACTH secreting 　Gonadotropin secreting 　TSH secreting 　Nonsecreting	Gliomas 　Chiasmatic-optic glioma 　Oligodendroglioma 　Ependymoma 　Infundibuloma 　Astrocytoma 　Microglioma
Primitive germ-cell tumors 　Germinoma 　Dermoid 　Teratoma 　Atypical teratoma (dysgerminoma)	Granulomatous, infections, inflammatory 　Abscess, bacterial and fungal 　Sarcoidosis 　Tuberculosis 　Giant-cell granuloma
Benign lesions 　Meningioma 　Enchondroma 　Hypothalamic hamartomas 　Gangliocytomas 　Myoblastomas	Metastatic tumors Vascular aneurysms Miscellaneous 　Arachnoid cyst 　Empty sella syndrome 　Suprasellar-chiasmatic arachnoiditis
Cell rest tumors 　Craniopharyngioma 　Rathke's cleft cyst 　Epidermoid (cholesteatoma) 　Chordoma 　Lipoma 　Colloid cyst	Histiocytosis X (eosinophilic 　　granuloma) 　Lymphocytic hypophysitis 　Mucocele (sphenoid) 　Echinococcal cyst

Modified from Post et al. [14], with permission.
PRL = prolactin; GH = growth hormone; ACTH = adrenocorticotrophic hormone; TSH = thyroid-stimulating hormone.

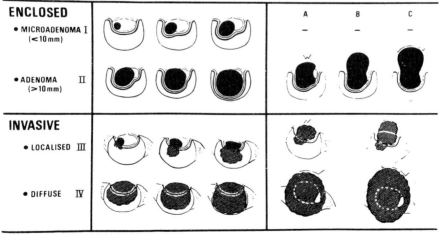

Figure 2. Growth pattern of adenomas. (Reproduced with permission from Hardy J. Transsphenoidal surgery of hypersecreting pituitary tumours. In Kohler PO, Ross GT, eds. Diagnosis and Treatment of Pituitary Tumours. New York: America Elsevier, pp 179–194.)

75

nonsecreting tumors each comprise about 30–40% of all tumors. ACTH-secreting tumors and growth hormone (GH)–secreting tumors comprise 2–10% each and thyrotropin (TSH)–secreting tumors comprise about 1% [15]. Clearly, in the evaluation of patients with pituitary incidentalomas, that is, those without any endocrine symptomatology (see later), these frequencies will be altered towards the clinically nonfunctioning tumors.

A number of other lesions may be found in the sellar area that may mimic a pituitary adenoma. Such lesions include aneurysms of the internal carotid artery, craniopharyngiomas, Rathke's cleft cysts, meningiomas of the tuberculum sellae, gliomas of the hypothalamus and optic nerves, dysgerminomas, cysts, hamartomas, metastases, sarcoidosis, eosinophilic granulomas, sphenoid sinus mucoceles, and focal areas of infarction [12–14]. Lymphocytic infiltration of the pituitary can also masquerade as a pituitary adenoma [22]. Artifacts mimicking pituitary lesions include beam-hardening effects with CT and susceptibility distortions with MRI [13].

Autopsy findings

Pituitary adenomas have been found by sectioning of the gland at autopsy in 1.5–27% of subjects not suspected of having pituitary disease while alive [3,23–40] (Table 2). Except for the study by Muhr et al. [32], which showed only a 1.5% frequency, these studies, comprising 12,300 subjects, found a minimum frequency of adenomas of 5%. In the studies in which PRL immunohistochemistry was performed, 46% of the 298 pituitaries stained positively for PRL [27,28,30,34,36–40]. The tumors were distributed equally throughout the age groups (range 16–86 years) and between the sexes.

In these postmortem studies all but three of the tumors were <10mm in diameter (Table 2), and these three were <15mm in diameter. Thus, microadenomas are present in 10–20% of the adult population. The lack of macroadenomas in these studies suggests that growth from micro- to macro-adenomas must be an exceedingly uncommon event and/or that virtually all macroadenomas come to clinical attention and therefore are not included in these autopsy findings.

Two autopsy studies evaluated other lesions in the sella in addition to pituitary adenomas [3,40]. In specimens removed from 100 random cadavers in whom there had been no clinical suspicion of pituitary disease, Chambers et al. [3] found 24 lesions >3mm in diameter, including 11 microadenomas, 6 pars intermedia cysts, 4 foci of metastatic tumor, and 3 pituitary infarcts. In addition, there were 14 pars intermedia cysts and 3 pituitary microadenomas <3mm in diameter. Teramoto et al. [40] found 61 lesions in 1000 pituitaries that were >2mm in diameter. Of these, 18 were adenomas, 2 were focal hyperplasias, 37 were Rathke's cleft cysts, and 4 were hemorrhages. Generally, only lesions of >3mm diameter will be considered to be significant in this discussion, as this is generally the smallest size lesion that can be distinguished

Table 2. Frequency of pituitary adenomas found at autopsy

Study	No. pituitaries examined	No. adenomas found	Frequency (%)	No. macroadenomas found	Stain for prolactin (%)
Susman [23]	260	23	8.8	—	—
Costello [24]	1,000	225	22.5	0	—
Sommers [25]	400	26	6.5	0	—
McCormick & Halmi [26]	1,600	140	8.8	0	—
Kovacs et al. [27]	152	20	13.2	2	53
Landolt [28]	100	13	13.0	0	—
Mosca et al. [29]	100	24	24.0	0	23
Burrows et al. [30]	120	32	26.7	0	41
Parent et al. [31]	500	42	8.4	1	—
Muhr et al. [32]	205	3	1.5	0	—
Schwezinger & Warzok [33]	5,100	485	9.5	0	—
Coulon et al. [34]	100	10	10.0	0	60
Chambers et al. [3]	100	14	14.0	0	—
Siqueira & Guembarovski [35]	450	39	8.7	0	—
El-Hamid et al. [36]	486	97	20.0	0	48
Scheithauer et al. [37]	251	41	16.3	0	66
Marin et al. [38]	210	35	16.7	0	32
Sano et al. [39]	166	15	9.0	0	47
Teramoto et al. [40]	1,000	51	5.1	0	30
Total	12,300	1395	11.3	3	

reasonably well from background 'image noise' in these types of scanning procedures [3,13].

CT and MRI scans in normal individuals

Three series have evaluated CT scans of the sellar area in normal subjects who were having such scans for reasons unrelated to possible pituitary disease. Chambers et al. [3] found discrete areas of low density >3mm in diameter in 10 of 50 such subjects. In our study of 107 normal women, we found 7 who had focal hypodense areas >3mm in diameter [4]. In one of these seven, a woman with peripheral neurofibromatosis, the serum PRL level was elevated to a value of 36.2 ng/ml (normal <25 ng/ml); the PRL and α subunit values were normal in the other six. Focal high-density regions >3mm in diameter were found in five subjects. One had a PRL level of 48 ng/ml and had a melanotic melanoma metastatic to the brain so that the high-density area may have represented a pituitary metastasis. This patient also had received cranial irradiation, which may increase PRL levels [41]. In a third study, Peyster et al. [6] found focal hypodense areas >3mm in diameter in only 8 of 216 subjects.

77

Two similar studies have been carried out using MRI. Chong et al. [9] found focal pituitary gland hypodensities 2–5 mm (mean 3.9 mm) in 20 of 52 normal subjects with nonenhanced images using a 1.5-T scanner and 3-mm thick sections. With similar scans but with gadolinium-DTPA enhancement, Hall et al. [10] found that in 100 normal volunteers, focal areas of decreased intensity ≥3 mm in diameter compatible with the diagnosis of adenoma were found in 34, 10, and 2 volunteers, depending on whether there was agreement on the diagnosis between one, two, or three independent reviewing neuroradiologists at the National Institutes of Health. This latter study is particularly interesting in that it both confirms prior estimates of incidental adenomas found on scans and points out the degree of uncertainty of diagnosis of adenoma, even among experienced neuroradiologists, at a premier institution.

On the basis of such studies, it can be seen that CT and MRI scans may reveal lesions of ≥3 mm in diameter in 4–20% of normal subjects. However, autopsy studies suggest such a finding is relatively nonspecific, with cysts and old infarcts being almost as common as adenomas. Metastatic foci are also relatively common and need to be considered as well.

Sellar lesions >10 mm in diameter have not been found in such studies, similar to the autopsy experience. However, this author has seen patients with large pituitary tumors found incidentally on skull x-rays, CT scans, and MRI scans done because of head trauma or other reasons (e.g., Fig. 1). In the two series of patients reported with pituitary incidentalomas [8,11], 29 of 52 patients had macroadenomas. In one of these series [8], 5 of the 11 with macroadenomas had tumors ≥2 cm in maximum diameter.

Diagnostic evaluation

Endocrinologic evaluation

Because the most common lesion in the sella is a pituitary adenoma, it is reasonable to evaluate patients endocrinologically, regardless of the size of the lesion seen. Many of the changes occurring with hormone oversecretion syndromes may be quite subtle and only slowly progressive; therefore, it is important to review with the patient changes compatible with the development of a prolactinoma, Cushing's disease, and acromegaly. For Cushing's disease, patients should be questioned and examined for the development of hypertension, hirsutism, hyperpigmentation, centripetal obesity, acne, pigmented striae, weakness, gonadal dysfunction, facial erythema and rounding, and excessive fat deposition in the dorsal and ventral fat pads and supraclavicular fat pads [42]. For acromegaly, a similar evaluation for the development of hypertension, acral enlargement, tongue enlargement, increased spacing between the teeth, and seborrhea may be helpful [43,44].

Women with hyperprolactinemia may experience galactorrhea, amenorrhea, hirsutism, infertility, and loss of libido [45]. Men may similarly have a loss of libido and are usually impotent [45]. Most patients with gonadotroph cell adenomas are male, have very large tumors, and have a history of relatively normal gonadal function [17,18]. Patients with TSH cell adenomas usually display the typical features of hyperthyroidism, although they lack the features specific for Graves' disease, that is, exophthalmos (unless produced by the mass effect of the tumor itself pushing out the eye) and dermopathy [46].

If the clinical evaluation of the patient points to particular hormone oversecretion, then a detailed evaluation of such secretion is warranted to establish the diagnosis. However, because these tumors may also be present with very little in the way of clinical symptomatology, screening for hormonal oversecretion is also warranted, even in patients with no clinical evidence of hormone oversecretion (Table 3). So-called silent somatotroph and corticotroph adenomas have been reported many times, and it is not clear whether these patients with minimal clinical evidence of hormone oversecretion are free from the increased risk for the more subtle cardiovascular, bone, oncological, and possibly other adverse effects we usually associate with such tumors. Screening for hormone oversecretion in such patients has been questioned as to its cost effectiveness [47]. However, evidence from one of the series cited earlier that have screened such patients [8] suggests such screening is worthwhile because 1 of their 18 patients turned out to have a GH-secreting tumor.

Prolactinomas are the most common of the hormone-secreting tumors. In addition, there are a large number of medications and conditions that may cause hyperprolactinemia (Table 4), so that the finding of hyperprolactinemia in a patient with a 'tumor' on scan may be a false-positive finding. The conditions in Table 4 can generally be excluded on the basis of a careful history and physical examination, routine laboratory screening, and checking of

Table 3. Screening tests for pituitary hormone oversecretion

Hormone	Test
GH	Elevated Insulin-like growth factor I (somatomedin C level)
	Failure to suppress GH levels to <2 ng/ml with oral glucose load
ACTH	Elevated 24-hour urinary free cortisol level
	Failure to suppress cortisol levels to <7 ng/ml (193 nmol/l with 1 mg of dexamethasone given orally 2300–2400 h the previous night)
PRL	Elevated basal levels, repeated at least once,
	Exclusion of other causes by history, physical examination, chemistry screening, and thyroid function tests
FSH/LH	Elevated basal levels of FSH, LH, and α subunit
TSH	Elevated basal levels of T4, T3 resin uptake, T3 with nonsuppressed or elevated levels of TSH

Reproduced with permission from Molitch and Russell [7].
GH = growth hormone; ACTH = adrenocorticotrophic hormone; PRL = prolactin; FSH = follicle-stimulating hormone; LH = luteinizing hormone; TSH = thyroid-stimulating hormone.

Table 4. Causes of hyperprolactinemia

Pituitary disease	Neurogenic	Medications
Prolactinomas	Chest wall lesions	Phenothiazines
Acromegaly	Spinal-cord lesions	Butyrophenones
'Empty sella syndrome'	Breast stimulation	Monoamine oxidase inhibitors
Lymphocytic hypophysitis	Other	Tricyclic antidepressants
Cushing's disease	Pregnancy	Reserpine
Pituitary stalk section	Hypothyroidism	Methyldopa
Hypothalamic disease	Renal failure	Metoclopramide
Craniopharyngioma	Cirrhosis	Amoxepin
Meningiomas	Pseudocyesis	Verapamil
Dysgerminomas	Idiopathic	Cocaine
Nonsecreting pituitary tumors		
Other tumors		
Sarcoidosis		
Eosinophilic granulomas		
Neuraxis irradiation		
Vascular		

Reproduced with permission from Molitch ME. 1995. Pituitary, thyroid, adrenal and parathyroid disorders. In Barron WM, Lindheimer MD, eds. Medical Disorders During Pregnancy, 2nd ed. MO: St. Louis, Mosby-Year Book, pp 89–127.

thyroid function. Although all of these conditions may cause modest hyperprolactinemia, PRL levels >200 ng/ml are found exclusively in patients with prolactinomas and patients with renal failure also taking medications known to disrupt hypothalamic dopaminergic regulatory pathways [45]. Because of the episodic secretion of PRL, levels in a normal individual may occasionally be above the upper limit of normal (generally 20–25 ng/ml). Two or three measurements should be obtained at different times to be sure that PRL levels are elevated on a sustained basis before concluding that a patient has hyperprolactinemia.

Various stimulation and suppression tests have been used over the years to aid in the differential diagnosis of hyperprolactinemia. However, there tests yield nonspecific results and have been largely abandoned [45,48]. One important cause of hyperprolactinemia needs to be emphasized. Normally, PRL is under tonic inhibitory control by the hypothalamus via PRL inhibitory factors that are transmitted via the portal system in the hypothalamic-pituitary stalk. Large pituitary lesions (nonsecreting adenomas, craniopharyngiomas, meningiomas, etc.) can cause moderate hyperprolactinemia by interfering with stalk function and the transmission of these inhibitory factors. Rarely do PRL levels get above 200 ng/ml in this fashion, however [49]. Thus, a large lesion (>2 cm in height) that is associated with a PRL level <200 ng/ml should be considered to be something other than a prolactinoma because large prolactinomas generally have PRL levels ranging from several hundred to several thousand nanograms per milliliter.

For GH oversecretion, probably the best single screening test is measuring insulin-like growth factor I (IGF-I, also known as somatomedin C). Although basal GH levels are also usually elevated, such elevations may be only minimal, that is, 2–3 ng/ml [44], and normal individuals commonly have GH levels that may go over 20 ng/ml during one of the secretory surges that occur about every 2 hours [50]. If only GH measurements are available, then GH levels should be obtained after an oral glucose load (100 g of glucose), showing lack of suppression to <2 ng/ml by hyperglycemia [44]. When any of these tests is positive, more detailed evaluation is necessary to establish the diagnosis definitively [44].

Two tests have proven very useful for screening for the presence of Cushing's disease. The measurement of free cortisol in a 24-hour collection of urine has generally been found to be a good screening test for Cushing's disease [51,52]. However, others have noted that some patients may have normal urinary free cortisol measurements on occasion [53]. A second test is the measurement of serum cortisol at 8 a.m. after the patient has received 1 mg of dexamethasone at bedtime the night before. Normally, the cortisol will suppress to ≤7 µg/dl [51,52]. Rarely, patients with Cushing's disease will suppress with this low dose of dexamethasone overnight, and even with the standard 2-day dexamethasone suppression test [51,52]. If there is a clinical suspicion of Cushing's disease in the patient being evaluated and if there is any discrepancy found in one of these two tests, then the second also ought to be done. When these screening tests are positive, more detailed testing will be necessary to establish the diagnosis definitively [42,51,52].

Gonadotroph adenomas can generally be evaluated on a screening basis by measuring basal follicle-stimulating hormone (FSH), luteinizing hormone (LH) and α-subunit levels; isolated FSH and LH β-subunit hypersecretion may be able to be evaluated in the future if radioimmunoassays become commercially available. In the male, testosterone levels are usually normal [18]. In the female, considerable difficulty may be found when trying to differentiate hormone oversecretion by these tumors versus postmenopausal normally elevated gonadotropin levels. When the diagnosis is important to establish, stimulation testing with thyrotropin-releasing hormone (TRH) may demonstrate a gonadotropin response in patients with gonadotroph adenomas [54,55].

Thyrotroph cell adenomas cause biochemical as well as clinical hyperthyroidism, with patients showing elevated thyroxine (T4) and triiodothyronine (T3) levels. The unusual feature in these patients is an inappropriately normal or even elevated, rather than depressed, thyroid-stimulating hormone (TSH) level [46,56].

Microadenomas do not generally cause disruption of normal pituitary function. Of the 22 patients with suspected microadenomas evaluated in the series of Reincke et al. [8] and Donovan and Corenblum [11], all had normal pituitary function. Larger lesions may cause varying degrees of hypopituitarism because of compression of the hypothalamus, the hypothalamic-pituitary stalk that transmits the hypophysiotropic-releasing factors to the pituitary, or the pituitary itself. Of the 27 patients with suspected macroadenomas evaluated in the series of Reincke et al. [8] and Donovan and Corenblum [11], 5 were found to have partial hypopituitarism. Patients with these larger lesions should be evaluated for hypopituitarism.

The most critical hormone axis to be evaluated is the hypothalamic-pituitary-adrenal axis. Morning cortisol and ACTH levels should be obtained. If the cortisol level is <5 ng/ml, then replacement should be started with dexamethasone. If the ACTH level is also low, then the diagnosis is fairly well established, although some would also determine that the adrenal could respond to repetitive doses of ACTH. If the cortisol level is >5 ng/ml, then an overnight metyrapone test could be done. In this test, 30 mg/kg (maximum dose of 2000 mg) is given at bedtime and 11-deoxycortisol (compound S) and cortisol levels are measured at 8 a.m. the next morning. Because metyrapone blocks the 11-hydroxylase step of cortisol synthesis, cortisol levels should be low and, because of decreased feedback causing increased ACTH levels, the precursor 11-deoxycortisol should increase in the blood to >7.5 µg/dl and the cortisol level should decrease [57,58]. This will establish the presence of ACTH reserve deficiency.

Alternatively, the ACTH and cortisol responses to insulin-induced hypoglycemia could be obtained. In this test, hypoglycemia is induced with intravenous insulin given as a bolus (0.1–0.15 U/kg ideal body weight), and cortisol and ACTH are obtained at 0, 30, 60, and 90 minutes. In this test, glucose levels should decline to <50% of baseline, to a level of <50 mg/dl, and the patient should become symptomatic and the plasma cortisol should increase by at least 10 µg/dl to a level of at least 18 µg/dl [17,18].

TSH deficiency can be established by finding low levels of T4, T3, and TSH in the blood. Gonadotropin deficiency is established by finding low levels of gonadotropins, or the absence of cycling in women in conjunction with low target hormone levels, that is, estradiol or testosterone. However, when there is hyperprolactinemia, these assessments of gonadal function are not accurate because the hyperprolactinemia itself will cause a decrease in gonadotropin and gonadal hormone levels [45].

GH deficiency can be determined by finding an inadequate (<7 ng/ml) GH response to hypoglycemic stimulation as described above. Such testing should only be carried out after repletion of thyroid, glurocorthoid and gonadal hormones and when GH repletion therapy is indicated [58].

Radiologic evaluation

The index abnormality being discussed is an abnormality found during a scan. For lesions >1 cm in diameter, the important differential resides between pituitary adenomas and other mass lesions [12–14]. MRI may be done as a secondary procedure if a mass is first detected on CT scan because it can reveal far more anatomic detail of the lesion itself and its relationship to surrounding structures [12,13,59,60]. MRI can demonstrate the decreased signal of flowing blood and therefore can better determine the presence of aneurysms [12].

Aneurysms and adenomas may coexist, however, and occasionally arteriography may be necessary. Meningiomas are associated with (1) hyperostosis of the adjacent bone in 50% of cases [12], (2) a more homogeneous enhancement with gadolinium than macroadenomas, (3) a suprasellar rather than sellar epicenter of tumor, and (4) a tapered extension of an intracranial dural base [61].

Some degree of calcification is present in over 80% of craniopharyngiomas, but calcification has also been demonstrated in pituitary adenomas [12,13]. About 50% of craniopharyngiomas display areas of high intensity on T1-weighted images due to the proteinaceous material present in the cyst fluid. Although cystic components are common to craniopharyngiomas and Rathke's cleft cysts, they may also be seen in pituitary adenomas. Craniopharyngiomas are usually hypointense or hyperintense on MRI T1-weighted images but are usually very hypointense on T2-weighted images [12]. The cyst fluid in Rathke's cleft cysts varies in its protein content, and thus the cyst may be hypointense or hyperintense on T1-weighted images [13]. In Rathke's cleft cysts, contrast enhancement is usually confined to a thin rim along the cyst wall [13]. Gliomas are usually hypointense on T1-weighted images but hyperintense on T2-weighted images. When arising from the optic nerve or chiasm, such gliomas may also cause enlargement of the optic foramen [12]. Metastases may be almost impossible to differentiate from a pituitary adenoma radiologically [12,62] and clinically. The radiologic characteristics of these and other lesions of the sella are obviously complex, and more detailed reviews of this subject are available [12–14]. Because of the lack of specificity of many of the radiologic signs, however, in many cases the only sure way of diagnosing a lesion is by obtaining tissue.

In patients with lesions <10mm, there is a similar lack of specificity and artifacts may contribute to the confusion in establishing a diagnosis [13]. Several studies have compared radiologic studies to operative findings. In three papers from the Montreal General Hospital that analyzed preoperative direct coronal CT scans for ACTH-, PRL-, and GH-secreting adenomas resected by Dr. Jules Hardy, Marcovitz et al. calculated respective sensitivities of 63%, 91.9%, and 81.2%; specificities of 62.5%, 25%, and 100%; and overall accuracies of 62.8%, 87.7%, and 81.2% [63–65]. Similarly, poor sensitivity (30%) and accuracy (39%) of CT for Cushing's syndrome was reported from the National Institutes of Health [66]. Somewhat better data have been reported for MRI using 1.5-T systems by Peck et al. [67], reporting a sensitivity of 71% and specificity of 87% for ACTH-secreting adenomas.

Johnson et al. [68] performed both CT and MRI on patients undergoing surgery and found that correct diagnoses of microadenomas were made in 8 of 14 cases with CT and in 12 of 14 cases with MRI. Thus, specific features, such as focal hypodense or hyperdense areas and deviation of the stalk, are not specific for the presence of a pituitary adenoma or other lesion. In addition, it is important to avoid diagnosing a tumor simply on the basis of a slight increase in the size of the pituitary, because it is increased in size during the normal physiologic states of adolescence [69] and pregnancy [70,71], and is hyperintense during pregnancy [72]. The increase in size during pregnancy continues into the first postpartum week, with some pituitaries increasing to almost 12 mm in height; the pituitaries then rapidly return to normal size despite postpartum breast-feeding [71]. Pituitary volume may also be seen to be homogeneously increased with depression [73].

Recommendations

Microlesions

Clinical judgment must be employed in determining which patients need evaluation, and such things as patient age and other associated illnesses must be considered. Although the diagnostic possibilities are large, there are really only two things to be considered: (1) that this is a functioning pituitary adenoma for which specific treatment might be necessary to correct the hormonal hypersecretion and (2) that this is an adenoma or other lesion that could potentially cause future problems for the patient because of enlargement (Fig. 3). With respect to the first consideration, patients can be evaluated and screened for hormonal oversecretion, as discussed earlier. If hormone oversecretion is found, then further diagnostic evaluation and therapy may be necessary, as indicated for that specific tumor type [74].

If there is no evidence of hormone oversecretion, then the second consideration comes into play. With respect to pituitary microadenomas, it is known that for prolactinomas, at least, the risk of significant tumor enlargement is probably under 5% [75–79]. This low risk of significant enlargement is likely to be true for nonsecreting adenomas as well. The risks of significant enlargement of Rathke's cleft cysts, intrasellar craniopharyngiomas, etc. are unknown, but they also seem to enlarge slowly. There is one case report of a patient whose relatively large, probable craniopharyngioma did not enlarge over a 5-year period of observation [80], but there are no other series in which a substantial number of such patients have been followed without intervention. Therefore, a reasonable approach may be to repeat the scan at yearly intervals for 2 years and, if there is no evidence of growth of the lesion, subsequently lengthen the interval between scans. Because of the radiation exposure with CT [81], consideration should be given to performing the repeat scans with MRI.

Surgery does not seem to be indicated for such nonsecreting lesions unless growth is demonstrated. In the series of patients evaluated by Reincke et al. [8], 1 of 7 patients with suspected microadenomas showed evidence of tumor enlargement (5–9 mm) over an 8-year follow-up period and 1 patient had a regression in tumor size from 8 to 4 mm. In the series of patients evaluated by Donovan and Corenblum [11], none of the 15 patients with suspected microadenomas showed evidence of tumor growth over a mean of 6.7 years of follow-up.

Pituitary Incidentaloma

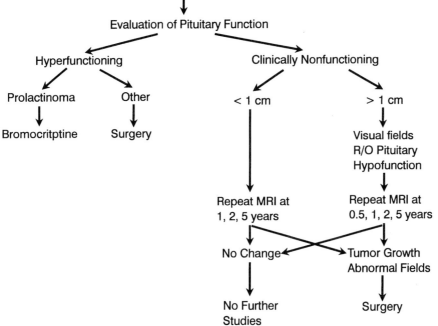

Figure 3. Flow diagram indicating the approach to the patient found to have a pituitary incidentaloma. The first step is to evaluate patients for pituitary hyperfunction and then to treat those found to be hyperfunctioning. Of those patients with tumors that are clinically nonfunctioning, those with macroadenomas are evaluated fruther for evidence of chiasmal compression and hypopituitarism. Scans are then repeated at progressively longer intervals to assess for enlargement of the tumors. (Reproduced from Molitch ME. 1995. Evaluation and treatment of the patient with a pituitary incidentaloma. J Clin Endocrinol Metab 80:3–6. Copyright, The Endocrine Society.)

Macrolesions

Again, two factors should be considered with such lesions: (1) that it is a functioning pituitary adenoma for which specific treatment might be necessary and (2) that because of its size, the lesion may need to be resected. When hormone oversecretion is found, further diagnostic evaluation and therapy may be necessary as indicated for the specific tumor type [74].

Lesions >1 cm in diameter have already indicated a propensity for growth. A careful evaluation of the mass effects of these tumors is indicated, including evaluation of pituitary function and visual-field examination. If a completely asymptomatic lesion is thought to be a pituitary adenoma on the basis of radiologic and clinical findings, then a decision could be made to simply repeat scans (MRI rather than CT to reduce irradiation, as earlier) on a yearly basis, with surgery being deferred until there is evidence of tumor growth. As mentioned, however, the size of these lesions already indicates evidence of tumor growth and early surgery may be of benefit. About 10–15% of nonsecreting adenomas respond to bromocriptine with tumor shrinkage [17], and some may also respond to octreotide [82,83] so that a trial of medical therapy may be worthwhile in the completely asymptomatic patient. If no therapy is chosen initially, repeating scans at 6 and 12 months, and then yearly, to monitor for any increase in tumor size seems warranted. If there is no size change, the interval can subsequently be lengthened. Certainly, with any evidence of significant tumor growth, surgery should be performed.

In the series of Reincke et al. [8], 4 of their 11 patients with incidentally found macroadenomas were operated upon initially because of visual-field abnormalities in 2, chiasmal displacement in 1, and the demonstration of GH excess in 1. The other 7 patients were followed for 17–48 months. Two of these patients had increases in the size of their lesions from 22 to 25 mm and from 14 to 20 mm over about 1.5 years. In the series of Donovan and Corenblum [11], 4 of their 16 patients with suspected macroadenomas experienced tumor enlargement over a mean follow-up period of 6.1 years, with the increase ranging from 2 to 5 mm. In 1 of these 4, the enlargement was associated with visual-field impairment, and he was found to have a craniopharyngioma at surgery. Another developed pituitary apoplexy following heparinization for coronary angiography. The other two patients continue to be followed with no further intervention or complications.

Summary

Incidental pituitary adenomas are being found commonly with our improved neuroradiologic imaging procedures. Screening for hormone oversecretion by these tumors appears to be warranted. For patients with macroadenomas, patients should also be screened for hypopituitarism. In the absence of visual-field abnormalities or hypothalamic/stalk compression, it may be appropriate to observe such patients carefully with repeated MRI scans. A limited amount of data suggest that significant tumor enlargement will occur in <5% of patients with microadenomas [8,11]. However, all macroadenomas must start out as microadenomas, and so periodic follow-up is indicated to assess for this possibility.

Macroadenomas, by their very existence at the time of detection, have already indicated a propensity for growth. Over the limited period of follow-up in the two series reported, significant growth occurred in just over one quarter of the patients with macroadenomas [8,11]. Hemorrhage into such tumors is uncommon, but anticoagulation may predispose to this complication. When there is no evidence of visual-field deficits, an attempt at medical therapy with a dopamine agonist or octreotide is reasonable, realizing that only about 10% of such patients will respond with a decrease in tumor size.

Surgery is indicated if there is evidence of tumor enlargement, especially when such growth is accompanied by compression of the optic chiasm, cavernous sinus invasion, or the development of pituitary hormone deficiencies.

References

1. Copeland PM. 1983. The incidentally discovered adrenal mass. Ann Intern Med 98:940–945.
2. Geelhoed GW, Druy EM. 1982. Management of the adrenal 'incidentaloma.' Surgery 92:866–874.
3. Chambers EF, Turski PA, LaMasters D, Newton TH. 1982. Regions of low density in the contrast-enhanced pituitary gland: Normal and pathologic processes. Radiology 144:109–113.
4. Wolpert SM, Molitch ME, Goldman JA, Wood JB. 1984. Size, shape and appearance of the normal female pituitary gland. Am J Neuroradiol 5:263–267.
5. Mark L, Pech P, Daniels D, Charles C, Williams A, Haughton V. 1984. The pituitary fossa: A correlative anatomic and MR study. Radiology 153:453–457.
6. Peyster RG, Adler LP, Viscarello RR, Hoover ED, Skarzynski J. 1986. CT of the normal pituitary gland. Neuroradiology 28:161–165.
7. Molitch ME, Russell EJ. 1990. The pituitary incidentaloma. Ann Intern Med 112:925–931.
8. Reincke M, Allolio B, Saeger W, Menzel J, Winkelmann W. 1990. The 'incidentaloma' of the pituitary gland. Is neurosurgery required? JAMA 263:2772–2776.
9. Chong BW, Kucharczyk AW, Singer W, George S. 1994. Pituitary gland MR: A comparative study of healthy volunteers and patients with microadenomas. Am J Neuroradiol 15:675–679.
10. Hall WA, Luciano MG, Doppman JL, Patronas NJ, Oldfield EH. 1994. Pituitary magnetic resonance imaging in normal human volunteers: Occult adenomas in the general population. Ann Intern Med 120:817–820.
11. Donovan LE, Corenblum B. 1995. The natural history of the pituitary incidentaloma. Arch Intern Med 153:181–183.
12. Wolpert SM. 1987. The radiology of pituitary adenomas. Endocrinol Metab Clin North Am 16:553–584.
13. Elster AD. 1993. Modern imaging of the pituitary. Radiology 187:1–14.
14. Post KD, McCormick PC, Bello JA. 1987. Differential diagnosis of pituitary tumors. Endocrinol Metab Clin North Am 16:609–645.
15. Kovacs K, Horvath E. 1987. Pathology of pituitary tumors. Endocrinol Metab Clin North Am 16:529–551.
16. Melen O. 1987. Neuro-ophthalmologic features of pituitary tumors. Endocrinol Metab Clin North Am 16:585–608.
17. Klibanski A. 1987. Nonsecreting pituitary tumors. Endocrinol Metab Clin North Am 16:793–804.
18. Snyder PJ. 1995. Gonadotroph adenomas. In Melmed S, ed. The Pituitary. Cambridge, MA: Blackwell Science, pp 559–575.
19. Horvath E, Kovacs K, Killinger DW, Smyth HS, Platts ME, Singer W. 1980. Silent corticotrophic adenomas of the human pituitary gland: A histologic, immunocytologic, and ultrastructural study. Am J Pathol 98:617–638.
20. Klibanski A, Zervas NT, Kovacs K, Ridgway EC. 1987. Clinical silent hypersecretion of growth hormone in patients with pituitary tumors. J Neurosurg 66:806–811.
21. Yamada S, Sano T, Stefaneanu L, Kovacs K, Aiba T, Sawano S, Shishiba Y. 1993. Endocrine and morphological study of a clinical silent somatotroph adenoma of the human pituitary. J Clin Endocrinol Metab 76:352–356.
22. Powrie JK, Powell M, Ayers AB, Lowy C, Sönksen PH. 1995. Lymphocytic adenohypophysitis: Magnetic resonance imaging features of two new cases and a review of the literature. Clin Endocrinol 42:315–322.

23. Susman W. 1933. Pituitary adenoma. Br Med J 2:1215.
24. Costello RT. 1936. Subclinical adenoma of the pituitary gland. Am J Pathol 12:205–215.
25. Sommers SC. 1959. Pituitary cell relations to body states. Lab Invest 8:588–621.
26. McCormick WF, Halmi NS. 1971. Absence of chromophobe adenomas from a large series of pituitary tumors. Arch Pathol 92:231–238.
27. Kovacs K, Ryan N, Horvath E. 1980. Pituitary adenomas in old age. J Gerontol 35:16–22.
28. Landolt AM. 1980. Biology of pituitary microadenomas. In Faglia G, Giovanelli MA, MacLeod RM, eds. Pituitary Microadenomas. New York: Academic Press, pp 107–122.
29. Mosca L, Solcia E, Capella C, Buffa R. 1980. Pituitary adenomas: Surgical versus post-mortem findings today. In Faglia G, Giovanelli MA, MacLeod RM, eds. Pituitary Microadenomas. New York: Academic Press, pp 137–142.
30. Burrows GN, Wortzman G, Rewcastle NB, Holgate RC, Kovacs K. 1981. Microadenomas of the pituitary and abnormal sellar tomograms in an unselected autopsy series. N Engl J Med 304:156–158.
31. Parent AD, Bebin J, Smith RR. 1981. Incidental pituitary adenomas. J Neurosurg 54:228–231.
32. Muhr C, Bergstrom K, Grimelius L, Larsson SG. 1981. A parallel study of the roentgen anatomy of the sella turcica and the histopathology of the pituitary gland in 205 autopsy specimens. Neuroradiology 21:55–65.
33. Schwezinger G, Warzok R. 1982. Hyperplasien und adenome der hypophyse im unselektierten sektionsgut. Zentralbi Allg Pathol 126:495–498.
34. Coulon G, Fellmann D, Arbez-Gindre F, Pageaut G. 1983. Les adenome hypophysaires latents. Etude autopsique. Semin Hop Paris 59:2747–2750.
35. Siqueira MG, Guembarovski AL. 1984. Subclinical pituitary microadenomas. Surg Neurol 22:134–140.
36. El-Hamid MWA, Joplin GF, Lewis PD. 1988. Incidentally found small pituitary adenomas may have no effect on fertility. Acta Endocrinol 117:361–364.
37. Scheithauer BW, Kovacs KT, Randall RV, Ryan N. 1989. Effects of estrogen on the human pituitary: A clinicopathologic study. Mayo Clin Proc 64:1077–1084.
38. Marin F, Kovacs KT, Scheithauer BW, Young WF Jr. 1992. The pituitary gland in patients with breast carcinoma: A histologic and immunocytochemical study of 125 cases. Mayo Clin Proc 67:949–956.
39. Sano T, Kovacs KT, Scheithauer BW, Young WF Jr. 1993. Aging and the human pituitary gland. Mayo Clin Proc 68:971–977.
40. Teramoto A, Hirakawa K, Sanno N, Osamura Y. 1994. Incidental pituitary lesions in 1000 unselected autopsy specimens. Radiology 193:161–164.
41. Huang KE. 1979. Assessment of hypothalamic-pituitary function in women after external head irradiation. J Clin Endocrinol Metab 49:623–627.
42. Aron DC, Findling JW, Tyrrell JB. 1987. Cushing's disease. Endocrinol Metab Clin North Am 16:705–730.
43. Molitch ME. 1992. Clinical manifestations of acromegaly. Endocrinol Metab Clin North Am.
44. Melmed S. 1990. Acromegaly. N Engl J Med 322:966–976.
45. Molitch ME. 1995. Prolactinoma. In Melmed S, ed. The Pituitary. Cambridge, MA: Blackwell Science, pp 443–477.
46. Greenman Y, Melmed S. 1995. Thyrotropin-secreting pituitary tumors. In Melmed S, ed. The Pituitary. Cambridge, MA: Blackwell Science, pp 546–558.
47. Aron DC. 1995. Hormonal screening in the patient with an incidentally discovered pituitary mass: Current practice and factors in clinical decision making. Endocrinologist 5:357–363.
48. Vance ML, Thorner MO. 1987. Prolactinomas. Endocrinol Metab Clin North Am 16:731–753.
49. Molitch ME, Reichlin S. 1985. Hypothalamic hyperprolactinemia: Neuroendocrine regulation of prolactin secretion in patients with lesions of the hypothalamus and pituitary stalk. In MacLeod RM, Thorner MO, Scapagnini U, eds. Prolactin, Basic and Clinical Correlates. Proceedings of the IVth International Congress on Prolactin, Padova, ltaly, Liviana Press, pp 709–719.

50. Winer LM, Shaw MA, Baumann G. 1990. Basal plasma growth hormone levels in man: New evidence for rhythmicity of growth hormone secretion. J Clin Endocrinol Metab 70:1678–1682.
51. Carpenter PC. 1986. Cushing's syndrome: Update of diagnosis and management. Mayo Clin Proc 61:49–58.
52. Kaye TB, Crapo L. 1990. The Cushing's syndrome: An update on diagnostic tests. Ann Intern Med 112:434–444.
53. Streeten DHP, Anderson GH Jr., Dalakow TG, Seeley D, Mallov JS, Eusebio R, Sunderlin FS, Badawy SZA, King RB. 1984. Normal and abnormal function of the hypothalamic-pituitary-adrenocortical system in man. Endocr Rev 5:371–394.
54. Daneshdoost L, Gennarelli TA, Bashey HM, Savino PJ, Sergott RC, Bosley TM, Snyder PJ. 1991. Recognition of gonadotroph adenomas in women. N Engl J Med 324:589–594.
55. Daneshdoost L, Gennarelli TA, Bashey HM, Savino PJ, Sergott RC, Bosley TM, Snyder PJ. 1993. Identification of gonadotroph adenomas in men with clinically nonfunctioning adenomas by the luteinizing hormone beta subunit response to thyrotropin-releasing hormone. J Clin Endocrinol Metab 77:1352–1355.
56. Gesundheit N, Petrick PA, Nissim M, Dahlberg PA, Doppman JL, Emerson CH, Braverman LF, Oldfield EH, Weintraub BD. 1989. Thyrotropin-secreting pituitary adenomas: Clinical and biochemical heterogeneity — case reports and follow-up of nine patients. Ann Intern Med 111:827–835.
57. Abboud CF. 1986. Laboratory diagnosis of hypopituitarism. Mayo Clin Proc 61:35–48.
58. Vance ML. 1994. Hypopituitarism. N Engl J Med 330:1651–1662.
59. Lundin P, Bergstrom K, Thomas KA, Lundberg PO, Muhr C. 1991. Comparison of MR imaging and CT in pituitary macroadenomas. Acta Radiol 32:189–196.
60. Webb SM, Ruscalleda J, Schwarzstein D, Calaf-Alsina J, Rovira A, Matos G, Pulg-Domingo M, de Leiva A. 1992. Computerized tomography versus magnetic resonance imaging: A comparative study in hypothalamic-pituitary and parasellar pathology. Clin Endocrinol 36:459–465.
61. Taylor SL, Barakos JA, Harsh GR, Wilson CB. 1992. Magnetic resonance imaging of tuberculum sellae meningiomas: Preventing preoperative misdiagnosis as pituitary macroadenoma. Neurosurgery 31:621–627.
62. Shubiger O, Haller D. 1992. Metastases to the pituitary-hypothalamic axis. An MR study of 7 symptomatic patients. Neuroradiology 34:131–134.
63. Marcovitz S, Wee R, Chan J, Hardy J. 1987. The diagnostic accuracy of preoperative CT scanning in the evaluation of pituitary ACTH-secreting adenomas. Am J Radiol 149:803–806.
64. Marcovitz S, Wee R, Chan J, Hardy J. 1988. Diagnostic accuracy of preoperative CT scanning of pituitary prolactinomas. Am J Neuroradiol 9:13–17.
65. Marcovitz S, Wee R, Chan J, Hardy J. 1988. Diagnostic accuracy of preoperative CT scanning of pituitary somatotroph adenomas. Am J Neuroradiol 9:19–22.
66. Saris SC, Patronas NJ, Doppman JL, Loriaux DL, Cutler GB Jr., Nieman LK, Chrousos GP, Oldfield EH. 1987. Cushing syndrome: Pituitary CT scanning. Radiology 162:775–777.
67. Peck WW, Dillon WP, Norman D, Newton TH, Wilson CB. 1988. High-resolution MR imaging of microadenomas at 1.5 T: Experience with Cushing disease. Am J Neuroradiol 9:1085–1091.
68. Johnson MR, Hoare RD, Cox T, Dawson JM, Maccabe JJ, Llewelyn DEH, McGregor AM. 1992. The evaluation of patients with a suspected pituitary microadenoma: Computer tomography compared to magnetic resonance imaging. Clin Endocrinol 36:335–338.
69. Elster AD, Chen MYM, Williams DW III, Key LL. 1990. Pituitary gland: MR imaging of physiologic hypertrophy in adolescence. Radiology 174:681–685.
70. Gonzalez JG, Elizondo G, Saldivar D, Nanez H, Todd LE, Villarreal JZ. 1988. Pituitary gland growth during normal pregnancy: An in vivo study using magnetic resonance imaging. Am J Med 85:217–220.
71. Elster AD, Sanders TG, Vines FS, Chen MYM. 1991. Size and shape of the pituitary gland during pregnancy and post partum: Measurement with MR imaging. Radiology 181:531–535.

72. Miki Y, Asato R, Okumura R, Togashi K, Kimura I, Kawakami S, Konishi J. 1993. Anterior pituitary gland in pregnancy: Hyperintensity at MR. Radiology 187:229–231.
73. Krishnan KRR, Doraiswamy PM, Lurie SN, Fiegiel GS, Husain MM, Boyko OB, Ellinwood EH Jr, Nemeroff CB. 1991. Pituitary size in depression. J Clin Endocrinol Metab 72:256–259.
74. Klibanski A, Zervas NT. 1991. Diagnosis and management of hormone-secreting pituitary adenomas. N Engl J Med 324:822–831.
75. March CM, Kletzky OA, Davajan V, Teal J, Weiss M, Apuzzo ML, Marrs RP, Mishell DE Jr. 1981. Longitudinal evaluation of patients with untreated prolactin-secreting pituitary adenomas. Am J Obstet Gynecol 139:835–844.
76. Weiss MH, Teal J, Gott P, Wycoff R, Yadley R, Apuzzo ML, Gianotta SL, Kletzky O, March C. 1983. Natural history of microprolactinomas: Six-year follow-up. Neurosurgery 12:180–183.
77. Koppelman MCS, Jaffe MJ, Rieth KG, Caruso RC, Loriaux DL. 1984. Hyperprolactinemia, amenorrhea, and galactorrhea. Ann Intern Med 100:115–121.
78. Sisam DA, Sheehan JP, Sheeler LR. 1987. the natural history of untreated microprolactinomas. Fertil Steril 48:67–71.
79. Schlechte J, Dolan K, Sherman B, Chapler F, Luciano A. 1989. The natural history of untreated hyperprolactinemia; a prospective analysis. J Clin Endocrinol Metab. 68:412–418.
80. Sharara FI, Chrousos GP, Patronas NJ. 1992. Watchful waiting and craniopharyngioma. Ann Intern Med 117:876–877.
81. Conway BJ, McCrohan JL, Antonsen RG, Rueter GF, Slayton RJ, Suleiman OH. 1992. Average radiation dose in standard CT examinations of the head: Results of the 1990 NEXT survey. Radiology 184:135–140.
82. Katznelson L, Oppenheim DS, Coughlin JF, Kliman B, Schoenfeld DA, Klibanski A. 1992. Chronic somatostatin analog administration in patients with α-subunit-secreting pituitary tumors. J Clin Endocrinol Metab 75:1318–1325.
83. DeBruin TWA, Kwekkeboom DJ, Van't Verlaat JW, Reubi J-C, Krenning EP, Lamberts SWJ, Croughs RJM. 1992. Clinical nonfunctioning pituitary adenoma and octreotide response to long term high dose treatment, and studies in vitro. J Clin Endocrinol Metab 75:1310–1317.

6. Follicular cell–derived thyroid carcinomas

Stefan K.G. Grebe and Ian D. Hay

Cancers derived from the follicular epithelium (papillary, follicular, and poorly differentiated (anaplastic) cancers) comprise about 60–95% of all thyroid carcinomas. The rest are, in decreasing order of frequency, medullary carcinomas, lymphomas, sarcomas, squamous-cell carcinomas, and metastases from tumors elsewhere. Besides being extremely rare, all of the latter, with the exception of medullary thyroid carcinoma, are tumors derived from non-endocrine tissues, and therefore they are not the subject of this review. Medullary thyroid carcinoma is covered in Chapter 20.

Demographics and epidemiology

The annual incidence of thyroid cancer is between 0.5 and 10 per 100,000 population in most countries [1]. Clinical thyroid malignancy is relatively uncommon, comprising less than 1% of clinical human malignancies. Nonetheless, thyroid malignancies are more common and kill more patients than all other endocrine malignancies combined [2]. During 1996 the American Cancer Society estimates there will be 15,600 new cases of thyroid cancer in the U.S. population (90% of endocrine malignancies). An estimated 1210 patients will die of thyroid cancer during this period, accounting for 64% of deaths from endocrine cancers and 0.4% of all deaths from malignancy [3].

The majority of malignant thyroid neoplasms are derived from the follicular epithelium. Amongst those, in most countries rates of papillary thyroid cancer (PTC) are greater than those for follicular cancers (FTC), and either is far more common than anaplastic carcinomas [4,5]. However, the relative proportions of the three cancer types show wide geographic variation. The prevalence rate for anaplastic carcinomas may be as small as 1% or 2%, or as high as 20%, and among the differentiated carcinomas (FTC and PTC) FTC may comprise between 10% and 50%. Anaplastic carcinomas and FTC tend to be relatively more common in endemic goiter areas, and a number of case-control studies have strongly suggested that dietary iodine content is responsible for the increased rates of anaplastic cancer and FTC in these areas [6,7]. This

Andrew Arnold (ed.) ENDOCRINE NEOPLASMS. 1997. Kluwer Academic Publishers. ISBN 0-7923-4354-9.
All rights reserved.

hypothesis is supported by the fact that dietary iodine supplementation has been shown to increase the relative proportion of papillary cancers and to decrease the frequency of FTC [8,9].

Both PTC and FTC are more than twice as common in females as in males and tend to occur more commonly in middle age and later, although PTC patients are somewhat younger than FTC patients [4,5]. The female preponderance of patients with follicular cell–derived thyroid cancer has led to speculation about the role of estrogens as a risk factor. Indeed, other putatively estrogen-dependent tumors, particularly breast cancer, and thyroid cancer occur more frequently in the same individual than expected by chance [10,11]. In addition, case-control studies have suggested a correlation between pregnancy, an extremely high estrogen state, and the onset of thyroid cancer [12]. The biological basis for these epidemiological observations could be that estrogen acts as a growth promoter on thyrocytes, and, indeed, some experimental evidence suggests that thyrocytes express estrogen receptors and estrogen may stimulate thyrocyte growth in cell-culture systems [13,14].

Recently, it has also been shown that the partial estrogen antagonist tamoxifen inhibits growth of PTC cells both in vitro and in vivo [13], although this phenomenon may not be mediated via classical estrogen receptors. On the other hand, risk factors for breast cancer, which lead to increased estrogen exposure (such as low parity and absence of breast feeding) are, with the exception of increased body weight, not associated with an increased risk of thyroid cancer [11,15], and increased parity itself seems to increase thyroid cancer risk. This might suggest that pregnancy per se, rather than the associated estrogen levels, may be associated with increased thyroid cancer risk [16]. On balance, the role of female sex hormones as a risk factor for the development of thyroid cancer in general must still be considered as unresolved.

Genetic factors may play a role in a small group of patients with PTC and FTC. PTC may be associated with other nonthyroid malignancies, as well as premalignant conditions, such as Cowden's syndrome or familial adenomatous polyposis coli (Gardner's syndrome) [17]. Additionally, several cases of familial PTC have now been described [18]. No such distinct associations exist for FTC, but aggregation of FTC cases in families with dyshormonogenesis has been described [19]. Certain HLA types may also predispose to FTC. Depending on ethnic background and environmental iodine content, DR1, Drw6, or DR7 may be associated with FTC.

The most firmly established risk factor for thyroid cancer development is prior exposure to ionizing radiation, particularly to the head and neck region during childhood. This used to be a common problem in some exposed populations in Japan and the Pacific during the 1960s and 1970s, in the aftermath of atomic bomb use at the end of the second world war and atmospheric nuclear bomb tests during the 1950s and 1960s [20,21]. In most other countries, radiation treatment for benign medical conditions, such as acne vulgaris, thymic enlargement, tinea capitis, or inflammatory connective tissue disorders, contributed to rising numbers of thyroid cancer [22–25]. These practices have been long abandoned, and atmospheric nuclear tests have only been (rarely) conducted by France and China during the last two decades. Consequently, radiation exposure as a risk factor has now ceased to be of significant importance in most countries [24]. Exceptions are areas of high natural background radiation, patients who have undergone radiation therapy for malignant conditions [26], and areas of environmental radioactive contamination from military or civilian sources, particularly in a number of countries in the southern part of the former Soviet Union, which were heavily contaminated in the wake of the Chernobyl nuclear reactor accident [27]. The contamination in parts of Byelorussia and the Ukraine was significant and prolonged, and there is mounting epidemiological evidence that this has led to increased rates of thyroid malignancies, often of an unexpectedly aggressive nature [27]. With increasing mobility of eastern European populations, physicians in Western European and North America may well encounter such individuals and should be alert to the increased likelihood of thyroid malignancy in thyroid nodules found in these patients.

Pathology and classification

Main pathological features and classification

Papillary carcinomas of the thyroid are defined as malignant neoplasms of the thyroid gland showing evidence of follicular cell differentiation, typically with papillary and follicular structures, as well as characteristic nuclear changes [28]. The distinct nuclear changes seen in PTC are large, pale-staining nuclei with a 'ground glass' appearance. These typical nuclear changes usually enable unequivocal identification of PTC cells on cytological examination. Papillary structures usually consist of complex branching papillae with a fibrovascular core covered by a single layer of tumor cells. Follicular elements, usually resembling FTC, are often interspersed [28,29].

Follicular carcinomas of the thyroid are defined as malignant neoplasms of the thyroid epithelium that exhibit follicular differentiation and do not fulfill any of the pathological criteria for other types of thyroid malignancies [28,29]. They are characterized by varying degrees of resemblance to normal follicular architecture and function (including colloid formation), capsule formation with capsular invasion, and local tissue and vascular invasiveness. Two major patterns of growth are recognized: a minimally invasive (also referred to as 'encapsulated') type and a widely invasive type. The former is much more common and often closely resembles a benign follicular adenoma in gross and microscopical appearance, occasionally causing significant problems in differential diagnosis. Cytological features can vary considerably, with differing degrees of atypia and no clear distinction from benign follicular tumors [30].

93

Major criteria for malignancy are unequivocal capsular and vascular invasion [28,29,31]. By contrast, the widely invasive type of follicular carcinoma is easily distinguished from a benign adenoma by obvious tissue and vascular invasion on the macroscopic and microscopic level, high mitotic activity, and marked cellular and nuclear atypia.

Anaplastic carcinomas typically are extremely poorly differentiated and often can barely be identified as arising from follicular epithelium. Cytologically, nuclear abnormalities and DNA aneuploidy are almost universal and abundant mitotic figures are present. Cells are uniform and dedifferentiated and seldom form recognizable papillary or follicular structures. Not infrequently, only immunocytochemical staining for epithelial cell surface markers can unequivocally distinguish anaplastic thyroid carcinomas from thyroid lymphomas or sarcomas. However, occasionally more differentiated papillary or follicular elements can be identified within the tumor or coexist separately in nearby areas. This has given rise to speculation that some PTC and FTC may dedifferentiate into anaplastic cancers.

Patterns of spread

Lymph-node involvement at presentation is common in PTC, occurring in 15–60% (mean around 35%) of patients, when only macroscopically suspicious nodes are removed at primary surgery, and in excess of 70% of patients (mean 80%), when more extensive dissection is undertaken [32–39]. By contrast, in FTC lymph-node involvement at presentation is uncommon, usually less than 10% [40].

However, FTC is more likely to spread by hematogenous dissemination. About twice as many patients with FTC (5–40%), as compared with PTC (1–25%), will suffer distant metastatic spread during their illness, and about half of those will have metastases at presentation [41–49]. The favored sites of distant metastasis for PTC and FTC are lung and bone, followed by a variety of other sites, including brain, liver, and skin [41–44]. In PTC about two thirds of metastases are to the lungs [41], whereas in FTC about a third each of metastases are to the lung and bone and the last third to all other organs. Anaplastic cancers typically spread aggressively by local and lymphatic extension, as well as hematogenous dissemination, with the majority of patients either presenting with metastases or developing distant metastatic spread shortly after diagnosis.

Histological subgroups

Most PTC display varying degrees of follicular elements, but this does not seem to impact on biological behavior and the formerly used pathological category of 'mixed' papillary-follicular carcinoma has generally been abandoned. However, in recent years a number of other PTC subtypes, with possibly different prognostic implications, have been recognized, and some authors have made a strong point for separately classifying these particular tumors. Tall cell, columnar cell, and oxyphilic variants of PTC are reputed to have a higher incidence of extrathyroidal invasion and local and distant metastatic spread, and may be associated with increased mortality. The diffuse sclerosing type of PTC may also lead to more frequent regional nodal metastases, but there is no evidence that distant spread or mortality are increased [4,29]. Unfortunately, in all these cases uniform criteria for diagnosing these subtypes are lacking, and the purportedly different implications of the various tumor subtypes are based on very small case series (in each of the above variants the largest case series comprise about 20 tumors). Strict definition of subtypes and systematic review of large, unselected case series will therefore be necessary before such subclassifications can be regarded as useful and recommended for universal use.

Similarly, in FTC a number of morphological subtypes have been recognized, in addition to the distinction between minimally invasive and widely invasive FTC. These include pure (typical) follicular carcinoma, clear-cell carcinoma, oxyphilic (Hürthle-cell, oncocytic) carcinoma, and insular carcinoma. It has been argued that some of these subtypes demonstrate unique biological features and should henceforth be recognized by separate subcategories. This argument has been made particularly for Hürthle-cell (oncocytic) cancers and insular carcinomas, which many publications, including standard pathology atlases [29], now categorize separately. Of these two groups Hürthle-cell carcinoma is the more common subtype; not infrequently a quarter of FTC fall into this category. These tumors both macroscopically and microscopically resemble other follicular cancers, with the exception that they predominantly (>75%) consist of so-called oncocytes (or oxyphilic cells), which are follicular cells with abundant granular acidophilic cytoplasm, caused by extremely large numbers of densely packed mitochondria. They also tend to exhibit a trabecular rather than a follicular growth pattern [29].

Some authors find evidence for a worse clinical outcome in these oncocytic tumors as compared with other follicular cancers [41,50–52], whereas others [53,54], including ourselves, have not observed a significant increase in mortality in this type of thyroid malignancy. However, Hürthle-cell cancers do have a much greater tendency for tumor recurrence, especially in regional nodes. This has implications for cancer therapy and follow-up, and might justify separate pathological classification of these tumors. Insular carcinomas are often extremely poorly differentiated and may be associated with a significantly worse prognosis than typical FTC [55,56]. They consist of well-defined rounded nests of small, poorly differentiated cells, with only occasional microfollicle formation [29]. Abundant mitotic figures and extensive vascular invasion are nearly always present, and hence there is considerable overlap between 'insular carcinomas' and the 'widely invasive' growth pattern of 'ordinary' follicular cancer. These tumors are at the most dedifferentiated end of the spectrum of FTC and may well represent transitional forms towards anaplastic cancers. Indeed, some authors classify insular carcinomas as a 'more benign' subgroup of anaplastic cancer.

Pathogenesis

There is still no widely accepted paradigm for the development of thyroid cancer. Thyroid adenomas and carcinomas are traditionally seen as entirely distinct entities. However, in recent years evidence has mounted suggesting an adenoma to carcinoma multistep pathogenesis, similar to colonic cancer and other adenocarcinomas. This seems to be relatively well supported for FTC, but less well established for PTC.

About half of all hyperplastic nodules, the majority of FA, and probably all FTC are of monoclonal origin, as judged by X-chromosome inactivation analysis [57–62]. Oncogene activation, by mutation or translocation, particularly of the *RAS* oncogene, is also common in both FA and FTC (around 40%), supporting a role in early tumorigenesis [17,63,64]. Finally, there is a spectrum of gradually increasing chromosome abnormalities in all types of benign and malignant thyroid tumors. Numerical chromosome aberrations have been discovered in about 10% of benign hyperplastic thyroid nodules [65], and structural abnormalities involving translocations on chromosome 19 have also been observed [66]. Follicular adenomas display abnormal karyotypes in a larger percentage, about 30% (range, 15–60%) [67–74], with a wide range of chromosomes being involved. Interestingly, translocations involving chromosome band 19q13 have been observed repeatedly [66,70,75,76]. The fact that these translocations involving 19q13 seem identical to those occurring in some benign hyperplastic nodules [66] suggests that the events associated with this translocation could be among the earliest steps in follicular tumorigenesis.

Fluorescent in situ hybridization of cosmid probes from the q arm of chromosome 19 in a transformed thyroid adenoma cell line mapped the breakpoint between the DNA polymerase delta 1 and troponin T1 genes at the boundary between chromosome bands 19q13.3 and 19q13.4. It appears likely that an oncogene, or, less likely, a tumor suppressor gene of pathogenetic importance may be located in this area. Among known genes in this region, potential candidate genes, which may act as oncogenes if mutated or constituitively activated, include two genes encoding zinc finger proteins (*ZNF83* and *ZNF160*), as well as the gene coding for the gamma subunit of protein kinase C. Finally, from FA to FTC one again observes an increase in the frequency of chromosomal abnormalities. Flow cytometry has demonstrated that DNA aneuploidy occurs in 41–64% of typical FTC and in 27–80% of oxyphilic (Hürthle-cell) FTC [77]. Massive chromosomal deletions, often involving 10 or more chromosomes, can be observed in some tumors [68].

Structural chromosomal abnormalities may be even more common and have been observed in a number of euploid tumor cells [70]. Most structural abnormalities represent complex clonal karyotypes [78], although some simple deletions and deletions/rearrangements may also be seen [70]. Among a plethora of reported structural cytogenetic abnormalities, deletions, partial deletions, and deletion/rearrangements involving the p arm of chromosome 3 have been the most commonly observed changes [78,79]. LOH studies have corroborated the cytogenetic studies, with frequently observed LOH on 3p loci [68]. Because LOH at 3p has also been found in both a primary tumor and its metastasis, it appears that loss of genetic material on the p arm of chromosome 3 loss is a nonrandom, inheritable property of certain follicular thyroid cancers and hence of possible etiological and prognostic significance [79].

A number of other neoplasms, including small-cell lung cancer and renal-cell carcinomas [80–82], also exhibit frequent LOH on 3p, giving rise to the concept that one or several tumor suppressor genes may be located on the short arm of chromosome 3. Proof that chromosome 3p contains at least one tumor suppressor comes from the recent positional cloning of the gene responsible for tumorigenesis in von Hippel-Lindau syndrome and clear-cell carcinoma of the kidney (*VHL* gene) [83]. However, in several follicular thyroid cancers exhibiting LOH on chromosome 3p, no mutations in the *VHL* gene were found [83], suggesting that this particular gene is not involved in follicular thyroid carcinogenesis.

Interestingly, LOH on chromosome 3p seems to be limited to follicular thyroid carcinomas. Matsuo et al. [84] were unable to detect LOH using probes from a relatively small region between 3p21.2 and 3p21.3 in 27 follicular adenomas. Also, Hermann et al. [68], using restriction enzyme fragment polymorphism (RFLP) probes mapping to a larger region of chromosome 3p, found no evidence for LOH on chromosome 3p among six papillary and three follicular adenomas, whereas all six follicular carcinomas that were studied exhibited loss at 3p loci. These studies suggest that loss of a tumor suppressor on 3p could be specific for follicular thyroid carcinomas and might be viewed as a key event in the adenoma to carcinoma progression. For FTC tumorigenesis, it therefore appears that a tentative sequence of events, starting with 19q13 rearrangement in hyperplastic nodules, followed by *ras* activation in some adenomas, and finally tumor suppressor loss on 3p, culminating in established FTC, can be proposed.

By contrast, in PTC the concept of gradual, stepwise carcinogenesis is more difficult to support. Histologically, there is no evidence that hyperplastic nodules or follicular adenomas ever undergo gradual change to a malignant papillary tumor. Chromosomes 3 and 19 are infrequently abnormal and *ras* oncogene activation is uncommon. DNA aneuploidy, as determined by flow cytometry, is much less common in PTC than in FTC, and may in fact be even less common than in FA. Most studies show no more than 20% of papillary thyroid carcinomas to be aneuploid [70,77]. However, structural chromosomal abnormalities may occur in about 50% of PTC (but they typically do not involve the same chromosomes as in FA and FTC). In more than half of these cases of structural abnormalities, chromosome 10, particularly 10q, has been involved.

Molecular genetic studies have revealed that the structural chromosomal changes involving chromosome 10 frequently involve the intrachromosomal inversion of the *RET* protooncogene, a member of the receptor tyrosine kinase family. Usually this results in the formation of a chimeric fusion gene with the *H4* (D10S170) gene, leading to the formation of an oncogene, designated *RET/PTC1* [85,86]. The *H4* gene contains no significant homology to known genes, but contains an open reading frame of 585 amino acids with extensive putative alpha-helical domains [87]. The rearranged *RET/PTC1* gene encodes a fusion protein containing the N-terminus of *H4* fused upstream of the *RET* tyrosine kinase domain such that *RET/PTC1* expression is driven by the *H4* gene promoter [88]. Interestingly, the *H4* gene contains a putative oligomerization domain (coiled-coil) and oligomerization of *H4* was observed in vitro [88]. Because oligomerization of receptor tyrosine kinases appears to be an obligate step in their activation, oligomerization of *RET/PTC1* may account in part for its oncogenic properties [88]. In addition, its constitutive expression by the *H4* promoter may well play an important role in its oncogenic activity [88]. In addition to the predominant *RET/PTC1* rearrangement, translocation of the *RET* locus to chromosome 17q23 has been shown to result in formation of the so-called *RET/PTC2* oncogene by fusion with part of the gene coding for the regulatory subunit RIα of protein kinase A [86,89]. Finally, another intrachromosomal rearrangement involving the *RET* locus leads to fusion with the *ele1* gene and formation of the *RET/PTC3* chimeric gene, which functions as an oncogene as a consequence of *RET* overexpression due to the very active *ele1* promoter [86].

Taken together, the three *RET/PTC* chromosomal rearrangements may be observed in about 30% of papillary thyroid cancers [86]. Because RET has not been subjected to extensive sequence analysis in PTC, one may speculate that, in addition to chromosomal rearrangements, activating point mutations, similar to those found in MEN 2, may well occur in some PTC. Overall, the genetic studies suggest that *RET* activation may be a very common feature of papillary thyroid carcinomas. In addition, *RET/PTC* activation has been observed in 11 out of 26 occult thyroid papillary carcinomas, suggesting that *RET/PTC* gene activation represent an early, possibly crucial, event in the process of thyroid oncogenesis [90]. Furthermore, *RET* activation is specific for the papillary subtype of thyroid cancer [91], again suggesting that it represents an early event in the transition of a normal follicular thyroid cell into a papillary cancer cell.

In addition to *RET*, several other oncogenes are occasionally found to be involved in PTC, but the only other oncogene frequently involved is *NTRK1* (also named *TRKA*), which also codes for a receptor tyrosine kinase. *NTRK1* activation may be found in 10–20% of PTC [92]. The ligand of *NTRK1* is believed to be nerve growth factor, and, similar to *RET* activation, recombinant genetic events leading to fusion proteins with other gene products, again often involving genes coding for a coiled-coil motif, or overexpression of NTRK1 due to active promoters in the fusion gene, are the main mechanisms of activation [92,93]. Accordingly, it appears possible that receptor tyrosine kinase activation by *RET* or *NTRK1* rearrangement may often directly lead to papillary cancer formation, without intervening steps.

Theoretically, any event leading to a potential increased frequency of chromosomal breakage and subsequent rearrangement could be responsible for the *RET* and *NTRK1* gene rearrangements. This is consistent with the observation that nonspecific mutagenic stimuli such as radiation exposure result in an increased risk of PTC. Evidence that such radiation-induced lesions can be caused by *RET* gene rearrangements has been shown in vitro using X-irradiation of human undifferentiated thyroid carcinoma and fibrosarcoma cells that lack *RET* oncogene rearrangement [94]. In these studies rearrangements typical of in vivo thyroid cancer and atypical rearrangements not observed in vivo were seen. [94]. Furthermore, 4 of 7 tumors from patients examined after the Chernobyl disaster displayed evidence of *RET* gene rearrangement [95]. Thus increased radiation exposure may be one mechanism for generating activated *RET/PTC* oncogenes. Overall, it therefore appears that PTC may not follow a gradual stepwise course of tumorigenesis as FTC does. Rather, a single event, possibly most often leading to receptor tyrosine kinase activation, such as *RET* or *NTRK1* oncogene activation, may send some follicular thyroid cells down the path of papillary oncogenicity. As a consequence of the putative lack of gradual accumulation of carcinogenic genetic events, PTC tumors generally display less severe cytogenetic and molecular genetic changes than follicular tumors. It may be speculated therefore that they are genomically more stable, thereby resulting in less tendency to dedifferentiation and progression, explaining their somewhat better prognosis as compared with FTC.

Whether either PTC or FTC, if left untreated, ever show a tendency to progress towards anaplastic cancer over time, or whether anaplastic tumors arise de novo remain uncertain. For FTC the presence of extremely poorly differentiated subtypes suggests that such events may occasionally occur. In both PTC and FTC, tumor progression and dedifferentiation are likely to be associated with further oncogene activation and tumor suppressor loss. For example, the tumor suppressor gene p53 is only infrequently mutated in well-differentiated PTC and FTC, but poorly differentiated and anaplastic cancers may show evidence of p53 mutations in around 50% of cases [96,97].

Clinical presentation and diagnosis

Thyroid tumors generally present as anterior neck nodules, which in most cases can be easily localized to the thyroid gland by palpation. Many thyroid nodules will arise in the context of benign hyperplasia, but between 5% and 20% of nodules coming to medical attention will represent true neoplasms, either benign follicular adenomas or malignant carcinomas. Differentiating true neoplasms from hyperplastic nodules, and distinguishing benign from malignant tumors, represent the two major challenges facing the clinician confronted with a patient complaining of a thyroid mass. This can be a formidable task. High-resolution ultrasound studies in large groups of normal volunteers have shown a prevalence of nodular thyroid disease of over 60% in the healthy adult population [98]. Given that clinical thyroid cancer in most populations has a prevalence of much less than 1% [99], the majority of these nodules are obviously benign.

The problem is further compounded by the fact that microscopic foci of thyroid cancer are not uncommon, with reported autopsy prevalence rates ranging between 2% and more than 40% [100–106]. The majority of these minute tumors will never become a clinical problem, but they may still be discovered, and inappropriately treated, if all patients with nodular thyroid disease are submitted to surgical tumor removal and extensive histological examination of the specimen. The main instruments that clinicians may use to identify the minority of patients with thyroid nodules, who should be submitted to surgical exploration/treatment, are history and clinical examination, biochemical testing and imaging, and fine-needle aspiration biopsy (FNAB).

History and examination

Historical features that may suggest possible thyroid malignancy include growth of a nodule over weeks or months rather than a much longer period; changes in speaking, breathing, or swallowing; and systemic symptoms of malignancy, such as weight loss, fatigue, and night sweats. Although uncommon and nonspecific, these symptoms are not rare. Between 5% and 20% of patients with thyroid cancer may have distant metastases at presentation, and, in the absence of disturbances in thyroid function, systemic symptoms can be strong indicators of malignancy [41–43].

On physical examination typical signs of thyroid malignancy should be sought. These include firm consistency of the nodule, irregular shape, and fixation to underlying or overlying tissues. Evidence of suspicious regional lymphadenopathy may be present in up to a third of patients with PTC but will be absent in most patients with hyperplastic nodules, follicular adenomas, and FTC. Although thyroid cancer is more common in older patients and in women, benign nodular thyroid disease is also increased in prevalence in these two groups, and therefore a young, male patient with a thyroid nodule actually has a greater chance of malignancy than an elderly female patient. A history of exposure to ionizing radiation should always be sought and a family history of thyroid and other malignancies can occasionally be helpful.

Overall, a careful history and physical examination performs surprisingly well in identifying cases with a high likelihood of malignancy [107–112]. Sensitivity and specificity rates for history and physical examination in detecting thyroid malignancy have been reported to be around 60% and 80%, respectively. Only about 20% of patients with later confirmed malignancy have, when initially seen, neither suspicious historical feature nor evidence of potential malignancy on physical examination [108]. On the other hand, if the patient is young, has a history of radiation exposure in childhood, and also has a hard nodule, a recently growing nodule, or palpable cervical lymphadenopathy, then the chances of the presenting nodule being neoplastic are around 80%, with more than half being malignant [112].

Biochemical testing and imaging procedures

Thyroid function tests are rarely abnormal in patients with thyroid cancer. Even if biochemical evidence of hypothyroidism- or hyperthyroidism is found, malignancy is not excluded, although it tends to be extremely rare in cases of frank thyrotoxicosis. Both PTC and FTC may produce excessive amounts of thyroglobulin (Tg) or release stored Tg in increased amounts into the circulation. Unfortunately, a considerable degree of overlap in measured values with a number of benign conditions exist, limiting the usefulness of this test in initial diagnosis. However, in the absence of thyrotoxicosis, a serum thyroglobulin level of greater than 10 times the normal value, as established in the measuring laboratory, is highly suspicious for malignancy [113].

Imaging procedures are slightly better suited than biochemical tests in aiding the differential diagnosis of thyroid nodules. The traditional imaging procedure has been thyroid scintigraphy using the isotopes I^{131}, I^{123}, or Tc^{99m}. Thyroid carcinomas tend to be inefficient in trapping and organifying iodine, and will appear on scanning as areas of diminished isotope uptake, so-called 'cool' or 'cold' nodules. However, a significant proportion of benign nodules also fail to concentrate iodine and will appear as cold nodules. Overall, 80% of thyroid nodules scanned for possible cancer may be scintigraphically cold [108]. Furthermore, nodules that exhibit normal or slightly increased uptake are not all benign. A number of investigators have found little difference in cancer rate between cold and warm nodules [114]. Isotopic scanning, therefore, tends to add little or no information to physical examination [107,108,114]. Indeed, most investigators have found that history and physical examination have both higher sensitivity and specificity than radioiodine scanning [107]. Alternative scanning agents such as thallium 201 (TI^{201}) and Tc^{99m}-labeled methoxyisobutylisonitrile (MIBI) may enhance the utility of radioiodine scans. For example, absent TI^{201} uptake in a nodule, which also has decreased uptake on radioiodine or technetium scanning, may have a negative predictive value (i.e., excludes malignancy) as high as 97% [115]. A positive thallium scan under the same circumstances may have a positive predictive value of about 90% [115]. However, when used without prior radioiodine imaging, TI^{201} scanning has limited sensitivity, with a false-negative rate of about 40%; in most centers expertise in the interpretation of such scans is limited.

By contrast, ultrasound scanning is readily available and is capable of identifying even minute, impalpable nodules. Cystic and homogeneously hyperechoic lesions are reputed to carry a low risk of malignancy [116,117], but positive predictive criteria of malignancy are less well defined, with only 64% of malignant nodules displaying patterns typical for malignancy in one study [118]. Nevertheless, in experienced hands ultrasonography may achieve sensitivies of 80% for thyroid malignancies at a specificity of as high as 90% [110]. Unfortunately such excellent results are not achieved in all centers.

Computed tomography (CT) scanning and magnetic resonance imaging (MRI) in most centers are more expensive than sonography, and in our own experience they do not generally provide better quality images of the thyroid and cervical nodes but can be helpful when tracheal invasion is suspected, enabling delineation of intraluminal tumor, a feat impossible for ultrasound because of the acoustic shadowing of the trachea.

Fine-needle aspiration biopsy

FNAB easily eclipses physical examination, biochemical testing, and imaging procedures in the accuracy of diagnosis of malignant thyroid tumors. The technique is easy to learn and has few complications. The diagnosis of PTC by FNAB is particularly reliable and accurate; sensitivity and specificity both approach 100%. However, care must be taken to obtain an adequate specimen, with most authors recommending between three and six aspirations [119,120]. A satisfactory specimen contains at least five or six groups of well-preserved cells, with each group consisting of at least 10–15 cells. In contrast to PTC, FNAB performs much less well for follicular neoplasms. If strict criteria for malignancy are used, sensitivity has been reported to be as low as 8% [110]. On the other hand, if all follicular neoplasms, that are not clearly benign on cytological examination are classified as cancerous, sensitivity rises to around 90% or more, at the cost of markedly reduced specificity, which tends to fall to 50% or less. This seriously limits the usefulness of this technique in geographic regions of high FTC prevalence. Recent attempts at overcoming this problem have focused on thyroid peroxidase (TPO) immunochemistry with a monoclonal antibody (MoAb 47). For a 100% sensitivity, a specificity of almost 70% has been achieved using this technique. Pending independent confirmation of these results, TPO immunocytochemistry may prove to be a valuable adjunct to the standard cytological techniques used in the evaluation of thyroid FNAB.

Apart from the limitations in follicular neoplasms, 'nondiagnostic' specimens, which may occur in up to 20% of cases [120], represent the greatest problem with FNAB. Although repeated aspiration attempts increase both the accuracy and the rate of diagnostic aspirations, sometimes even repeated attempts may fail. A considerable number of persistently nondiagnostic FNABs may be neoplastic, with some authors suggesting around 50% [121]. A trial of thyroxine suppression can sometimes shrink benign nodules [119], but a significant proportion of benign nodules will also fail to shrink and some carcinomas may respond with a decrease in size. Consequently, the value of thyroxine suppression is doubtful, and either close observation or surgical removal of the nodule are probably the best options. Some investigators have also suggested that ultrasound-guided FNAB may ultimately prove helpful in overcoming this problem [122], and in some patients this may be an option to pursue [123].

Primary treatment

There is little question that the primary treatment of almost all follicular cell–derived neoplasms is surgical. However, the extent of surgery continues to be debated. Some advocate local tumor excision or lobectomy only, while others feel that only total thyroidectomy represents adequate treatment. In the past 50 years there has been a tendency towards more extensive primary surgical resection, a trend well illustrated by PTC surgery at Mayo Clinic during 1945–1985 (Fig. 1). Complete removal of the tumor seems important, as testified by the significantly impaired survival of patients with incomplete removal in all studies that have examined this question in PTC and FTC [124–131]. Although some of these studies did not use multivariate analysis, and better survival in completely resected patients may simply reflect less advanced tumor stage in these individuals, with an aggregate patient number of well over 6000, these studies offer quite convincing evidence that complete tumor removal should be attempted whenever possible. This is even true for very extensive tumors invading the aerodigestive tract, which hitherto were often only palliatively treated. Even with such extensive tumors, survival is better for patients who

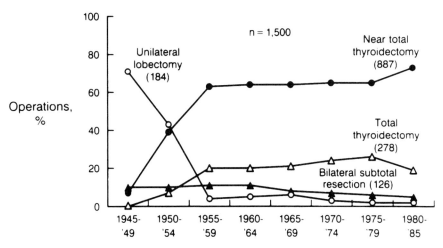

Figure 1. Trends through four decades in the extent of initial surgical resection performed at the Mayo Clinic for the definitive therapy of papillary carcinoma. (From Hay [183], with permission.)

undergo complete tumor removal [132,133]. Without such an intervention about 80% of these patients are dead at 5 years, whereas with complete resection the 5-year survival is generally greater than 50%. These challenging procedures should now probably be considered state of the art in locally extensive thyroid carcinomas.

However, provided the primary tumor was completely removed, there is no evidence that extent of surgery influences survival. The vast majority of studies, that have compared total thyroidectomy to lesser procedures, with combined patient numbers of several thousand, have found no evidence for better survival in those patients who underwent more extensive procedures [33,45,52,130,131,134–155]. We are aware of only five studies that have found evidence that more extensive thyroid resection is followed by improved survival [156–160]. However, there are at least four studies with which we are familiar, in which less invasive surgical procedures were actually associated with better outcomes [161–164], although it appears likely that in most of these studies this represents an artifact of confounding by severity. Overall, there appears to be no survival advantage to total thyroidectomy, as against near-total thyroidectomy, and it may be logical to assume that extending surgery beyond complete local tumor control may rarely be justifiable.

However, there is some evidence that recurrence, particularly in the contralateral lobe, may be reduced by total or near-total thyroidectomy [45,145–147,152–155,165]. This may be a significant problem in PTC, in which about 25% of tumors are reported to be multicentric. On the other hand, later additional surgery, if and when such a problem arises, may be just as satisfactory. Secondary 'completion' thyroidectomies can be performed by skilled surgeons at almost comparable risk to primary interventions [166–168]. Proponents of total thyroidectomy, nevertheless, rightly argue that second operations may carry slightly higher operative morbidity, but total thyroidectomy itself is not a low-risk procedure. It has a good safety record in the hands of some highly trained, dedicated, and experienced surgeons [32,169,170], but almost unacceptable complication rates in the hands of most surgeons, with reported rates of complications being between 10% and 40% for short-term complications and 5–20% for long-term complications (mainly iatrogenic hypoparathyroidism) [145,160,171,172]. In fact, complications related to such radical thyroid surgery represent the single most common cause for malpractice litigation related to the treatment of endocrine neoplasms in the United States, accounting for more than half of the 62 such cases pursed and judged in civil courts in the United States between 1985 and 1991 [173].

One major factor in favor of total thyroidectomy is that postoperative follow-up and some adjuvant treatment modalities, namely, monitoring of serum thyroglobulin levels and radioiodine diagnostic scanning and treatment, may be facilitated. Both serum thyroglobulin monitoring and radioiodine scanning may be ambiguous and difficult to interpret in the presence of a

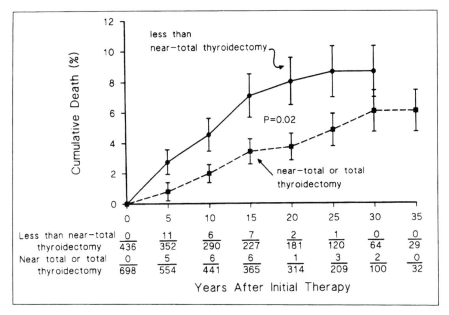

Figure 2. Cancer mortality in 698 patients with Mazzaferri stage 2 or 3 papillary and follicular thyroid cancers treated with near-total or total thyroidectomy, compared with 436 who underwent less extensive surgery. (From Mazzaferri and Jhiang SM. [158], with permission.)

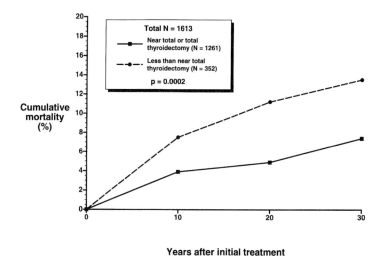

Figure 3. Cause-specific mortality in 1261 patients with Mazzaferri stage 2 or 3 papillary and follicular thyroid cancers treated at Mayo Clinic during 1940–1991 with near-total or total thyroidectomy, compared with 352 who underwent less extensive surgery.

thyroid remnant of significant size, and successful radioiodine treatment may be difficult or impossible in such a setting, with success rates for 'remnant' ablation in such situations being on the order of only 30% [174], and short-term complications of RAI treatment, namely, radiation thyroiditis are significantly increased [175]. In most high-risk patients and some low-risk patients, such a situation might be unacceptable to the clinician and patient, although it remains unclear how much harm beyond patient and physician anxiety this may bring. Nonetheless, a viable compromise may be to perform a near-total thyroidectomy, which will have most of the potential advantages of a total thyroidectomy but is associated with far fewer complications [165,171,172]. Figure 2 illustrates the improved outcome observed after near-total or total thyroidectomy in 698 stage 2 or 3 patients with PTC and FTC when compared with 436 patients undergoing less extensive surgery [158]. Figure 3 shows comparable data for 1613 patients treated at out institution during 1940–1991. At 30 years the mortality rates (cause-specific) were 7.4% after near-total or total thyroidectomy, significantly less than the 12.5% seen after less than near-total thyroidectomy.

In recent times the discussion about the extent of primary thyroid resection has been supplemented with an equally lively argument about the necessity and potential advantages of extensive nodal dissection at primary surgery. For the most part, this discussion is limited to PTC and MTC (the latter is covered in Chapter 20), but some have argued for extensive nodal dissection in all forms of thyroid cancer. Until recently lymphatic tumor spread in PTC was generally not seen as an adverse prognostic sign. Nonetheless, there has been a vocal group of proponents of extensive lymphatic dissection who claim significantly reduced recurrence and improved survival in these operated patients. When we recently reviewed the literature we were unable to find data supporting these claims [40], except in two papers from the 1970s [160,176]. We were neither able to find any published evidence that lymphatic involvement had a significant negative prognostic impact in PTC. However, two recent publications have reopened the question. Noguchi recently reported on the largest single institution series of PTC to date (2192 cases) and found a significant influence of nodal status on survival if the patient suffered from gross nodal involvement [177].

In the same journal, Scheumann et al. reported on their experience with radical lymphatic dissection in PTC, claiming a significant survival benefit in 135 systematically and radically explored patients with PTC when they were compared with 207 patients who had undergone conventional lymphadenectomy [136]. However, maximum follow-up in the systematically lymphadenectomized group was less than 10 years, whereas it approached 25 years in the conventional group, and the authors conceded that their results could at this point only be called preliminary. Whether the evidence presented in these two recent papers weighs heavier than the compound experience of dozens of previous studies on prognostic factors in PTC, with an aggregate number of about 5000 patients, remains to be seen. Clearly, the evidence suggests that if extensive lymphatic dissection plays any role in PTC, it is likely to be small. In FTC the relative rarity of nodal involvement has led to a lesser interest in lymphatic dissection, although the evidence is that those rare FTC patients with lymph-node metastasis at presentation may well have a somewhat worse prognosis [40].

Natural history of treated thyroid cancer, postoperative staging, and assessment of recurrence risk

The natural history of treated thyroid cancer differs with histotype. Undifferentiated thyroid cancer is usually associated with rapid death, with survival beyond 1 year being very uncommon, regardless of treatment. Only a small subgroup, with slightly better differentiated tumors (which may sometimes also be classified as insular carcinomas, that is, a subgroup of FTC) do somewhat better [178,179], with 5–10% surviving for 5 years or longer. The importance of histotype in prognosis of thyroid cancer is underscored by the fact that without any treatment, still more than twice this number of PTC patients will be alive after a similar time interval following initial diagnosis [180]. Indeed, with treatment the great majority of patients with PTC and FTC do exceptionally well. Most studies show a cause-specific mortality of less than 25% at 10 years follow-up for either of these two most common forms of thyroid cancer. Differences between the two tumor types with regard to survival are small, but probably real, with most studies showing slightly worse survival in FTC when compared with PTC [5]. Of 25 studies we recently reviewed, which allowed comparison of survival between PTC and FTC patients, only one showed better survival for FTC patients, five showed similar survival, and the remaining studies all demonstrated poorer survival either in all patients with FTC or at least in some patient subgroups [5].

Despite some methodological problems in a number of these studies, it appears that there is probably about a 10% poorer cause-specific survival at 10 years in FTC as compared with PTC. In Mazzaferri's most recent report [158], FTC mortality rates were more than twice those of PTC. However, when patients with initial distant metastases were excluded, 30-year mortality rates for FTC and PTC were not significantly different, at 10% and 6%, respectively. In both FTC and PTC, recurrence rates are somewhat higher than mortality, but in many instances recurrence has no or little impact on longevity. This is particularly true for regional nodal recurrence in PTC. There is no convincing evidence that such recurrence is associated with increased mortality [40]. In general, nodal metastases in PTC are often curiously indolent. Even massive nodal recurrence or residual nodal disease may have little impact on survival; in one study massive untreated nodal disease was associated with a 79% 5-year survival [181].

Distant metastases are a more ominous sign, but can occasionally still be associated with long survival. Pulmonary metastases in PTC and FTC are associated with 50–70% 5-year survival and a 30–50% 10-year survival. Bone metastases carry a worse prognosis, with survival figures being between 10% and 20% lower at 5 and 10 years than those in patients with only pulmonary metastases. Besides distant metastases, local (soft tissue) recurrence and spread, with eventual upper aerodigestive tract destruction, is the other main cause of death in PTC and FTC. Overall, local tumor extension accounts for slightly less than half on the deaths from PTC and FTC. It is the most common cause of death in patients who have undergone incomplete tumor removal but can also occur in some patients with apparent complete tumor removal, particularly if the tumor was poorly differentiated. Most recurrences and deaths, as recently reviewed for FTC [5], occur within the first 5 years after the initial diagnosis, but, as in most human cancers, later mortality can occur [148].

Given these facts, it would obviously be desirable to identify the subgroup of patients who will do poorly and to concentrate adjuvant treatment efforts and long-term follow-up on these individuals. This could be achieved by accurate disease staging. All staging and risk assessments should be based on the operative findings. Preoperative staging and categorization of patients is imprecise and prone to serious error. Unfortunately, it is nevertheless sometimes inappropriately introduced into discussions about the usefulness of staging, leading to the erroneous conclusion that staging and risk assessment are not useful in thyroid malignancy [146]. We feel that, quite to the contrary, when staging and risk assessment are properly based on the operative findings, extremely useful information can be gained, and comparison of cases and treatment strategies across institutions is facilitated [182]. We therefore feel that it represent an indispensable part of thyroid cancer management.

The international pTNM system of classifying malignant tumors by primary tumor size, lymphatic spread, and distant metastasis is the most widely accepted tool used to assess disease extent for staging [182]. However, in thyroid malignancy the different histotypes are distinctly different in their risk profiles. Moreover, the patient's age is also a strong predictor of survival in thyroid cancer, a fact not reflected in a strictly pathologic-anatomical assessment of tumor spread. Finally, lymphatic spread is a poor predictor of cause-specific mortality in PTC and FTC, the most common types of thyroid cancer. An improved and more refined risk assignment may be achieved by using additional prognostic information for staging. For both PTC and FTC, age at presentation and the extent of disease at diagnosis seem to be the most important risk factors for recurrence and death [5,183]. In addition to age and distant metastases, tumor size, extrathyroidal invasion, and, in the case of FTC, the degree of invasiveness are significant risk factors [5,127,183]. Lymph-node metastases at presentation seem to have little influence on the risk of death from PTC but do increase the risk of locoregional recurrence. When they do occur in FTC, which rarely happens, they may be of significance [40]. Tumor grade is an established risk factor in PTC, but is unfortunately not commonly assessed on routine postoperative histology [183]. In FTC no widely accepted grading scheme has been developed, but poorly differentiated tumors in FTC are also often widely invasive and carry a much worse prognosis than well-differentiated and encapsulated, minimally invasive tumors [5,135,184]. Histological subtypes of PTC, with the possible exceptions of the very rare oxyphilic [185], tall-cell [2], or columnar-cell [29] variants, seem to be of little prognostic importance. In FTC the oxyphilic subtype, as alluded to in the section on pathology, is much more prone to nodal recurrence [5,40], and poorly differentiated 'insular' FTC is associated with a significantly increased risk of death [29,55]. DNA aneuploidy does not appear to be an important prognostic factor in either PTC or typical FTC, but does seem to be of very significant importance in predicting mortality due to oxyphilic FTC [77].

Several staging systems have been developed on the basis of some or all of this prognostic information, and they can be complimentary to pTNM in stratifying patients into low- and high-risk categories, thus helping in the rational planning of postoperative management and follow-up. The AMES system, for example, was based on age of patient, sex of patient, tumor extension (local and distant), and tumor size. This prognostic system has been applied to both PTC and FTC patients [186]. However, in our opinion the most accurate prognostic scoring system for PTC patients is the MACIS system [127]. The MACIS scores take into account the presence of initial distant *M*etastases, *A*ge of patient at diagnosis, *C*ompleteness of primary tumor resection, presence of extrathyroidal *I*nvasion, and primary tumor *S*ize (largest diameter). It is the only system that has been properly crossvalidated, by being first developed on a subset of patients and then independently applied to another set of patients. FTC patients can be assigned to risk categories using a simple, yet quite accurate, staging system developed by Brennan et al. [135]. In addition to age and distant spread at presentation, this scheme takes degree of invasiveness into account. Finally, another recently developed prognostic scheme for follicular thyroid carcinoma found age, primary tumor size, extraglandular invasion, presence of distant metastases at presentation, and oxyphilic histology to be significant risk factors [187]. The Sloan-Kettering group also now considers that in patients with differentiated thyroid cancer, who are 45 years or older, the presence of cervical lymph-node metastases denoted a higher risk status [188].

No staging system is perfect, but it is clear from the recent literature that all succeed fairly well in identifying at least high- and low-risk patients with reasonable accuracy [189,190] despite some opinion to the contrary [146,157]. Adjuvant treatment and intensive follow-up can then be targeted to high-risk patients and a less interventional approach taken for low-risk individuals. As Loree has recently stated. 'prognostic factor and risk group analysis makes a selective approach to differentiated thyroid cancer possible. Such an approach can spare many patients the morbidity and expense of unnecessarily aggressive treatment without compromising outcome' [190].

Further management and follow-up

Based on knowledge of the natural history of thyroid cancer, in addition to accurate postoperative staging and risk assessment, further management and follow-up can be individualized and optimized. The first step in this process is the decision whether to subject the patient to any adjuvant therapy. The main adjuvant treatment modalities in thyroid cancer are thyroid hormone treatment and radiation therapy, with the latter mainly in the form of radioactive iodine (RAI) and occasionally as external-beam radiotherapy. Adjuvant chemotherapy, as established in breast and colon cancer, is only rarely used.

Thyroxine therapy

Thyroxine treatment is based on administration of supraphysiological doses of levothyroxine. The empirical basis of this treatment was laid down in the 1940s and 1950s, when reports of dramatic shrinkage of thyroid cancer metastases after desiccated thyroid therapy began to accumulate. It was quickly assumed that the mechanism of action was analogous to normal physiology, suppression of endogenous thyrotrophin (TSH) production, thereby depriving TSH-dependent differentiated thyroid cancer cells of an important growth-promoting factor. Potential alternative effects of desiccated thyroid extract, namely, other hormones, cytokines, or growth factors possibly contained in the mixture, were not considered at the time. Consequently, with the availability of synthetic thyroid hormone, it was assumed that this would share the beneficial effects of desiccated thyroid, and the treatment was increasingly used as adjuvant therapy after surgery in order to reduce the risk of tumor recurrence. Traditionally, thyroxine therapy aims to suppress pituitary TSH secretion completely, as indicated by undetectable serum TSH levels measured by sensitive immunometric assays, or, in former days, by the absence of a serum TSH rise in response to intravenous or oral thyroid-releasing hormone (TRH) administration. The efficacy of thyroxine therapy is very difficult to assess because the majority of patients operated on in the last 20 years would have undergone sufficiently radical procedures to necessitate thyroxine replacement therapy to avoid hypothyroidism. We are not aware of a single study that has carefully assessed levels of TSH suppression in appropriately treated patients and has correlated these with outcome data. Furthermore, those patients who do not need any thyroid hormone replacement therapy after surgery are likely to have had either unresectable tumors or more limited, potentially incomplete, surgery, both of which could signify a potentially worse prognosis.

Given these limitations, all evidence of potentially beneficial effects of thyroxine treatment has to be viewed very critically. Mazzaferri et al. have repeatedly reported that thyroxine treatment decreased cancer death rates in their patient group, although it was difficult to dissociate this effect from adjuvant radioiodine treatment and it was found only by univariate analysis [153,158]. Simpson et al. also reported that in a group of 568 PTC patients treated by surgery without RAI therapy cause-specific survival was higher in patients who had received postoperative thyroxine, although this advantage became nonsignificant (but still present) when patients were stratified according to other risk factors (pathology, age, and postoperative status) [131]. Staunton confirmed survival benefits for thyroxine-treated patients with differentiated thyroid cancer by multivariate analysis, but his patient series may have been somewhat unusual, as testified by the fact that thyroxine seemed to also convey a survival advantage in patients with anaplastic carcinoma, a malignancy not normally known to respond to thyroxine [137]. Cunningham et al., when they reviewed follow-up data of 2282 patients with differentiated thyroid cancer from the database of the Illinois division of the American Cancer Society, found a significant effect of thyroxine treatment on survival in a multivariate model adjusted for stage, age, race, and sex. This effect on survival was confined to patients older than 50 years and appeared to be independent of postoperative radioiodine treatment, although the use of thyroxine made a 'stronger contribution' [151]. Finally, Szántó et al. showed improved survival with thyroxine therapy by univariate analysis in a series of 169 patients with FTC [154].

In addition to these data on survival, Young et al. have described reduced recurrence in FTC with thyroxine treatment [45], which was also reported in Mazzaferri's PTC papers [153,158]. Because thyroxine treatment is necessary for most patients anyway, and is cheap, easy to monitor, and relatively free of side effects, it would appear prudent, on balance, that almost all patients receive it. Provided that the TSH level is monitored using a sensitive TSH assay and is kept in the 0.1–0.4 mIU/l range for all but very high-risk patients (who should receive full suppressive doses), the risks of such treatment seem to be small. Past concern about the effects of thyroxine on bone metabolism and bone density has been somewhat alleviated by a number of studies published during 1994 that have failed to show a detrimental effect on bone density [191,192], although accelerated bone turnover has been confirmed [193].

Radioactive iodine remnant ablation

Similar to thyroxine treatment, the concept of adjuvant RAI therapy originated from treatment approaches to metastatic thyroid carcinoma and was also based on an equally compelling physiological premise. Because most thyroid carcinoma cells retain some architectural and functional features of normal thyrocytes, iodine trapping, and sometimes organification, may be preserved in these tumors. It would therefore seem appropriate to take advantage of this by trying to eradicate microscopic residual postoperative tumor foci with RAI. Unfortunately, there are a number of biological reasons that partially thwart this approach. Firstly, not all tumors concentrate sufficient amounts of radioiodine to make treatment feasible. Secondly, carcinomas often consist of heterogeneous cell populations, which may vary in their degree of differentiation. In a given tumor, most of an administered dose of radioiodine may therefore be trapped in the most differentiated, least 'malignant' cells, whereas the more dedifferentiated cells may go untreated. Thirdly, the beta-radiation distribution of RAI is such that both very small and very large metastases (<0.5 cm and >5 cm diameter) are unlikely to receive adequate therapeutic doses to all tumor parts. Finally, it may be impossible to deliver sufficient doses without toxicity, when either the residual tumor (or normal remnant thyroid) tissue burden is too large, or when uptake is generally and chronically diminished because of large iodine stores, such as occurs in areas with very high dietary iodine intake, for example, in some parts of Japan. On this background it becomes clear that even on a theoretical basis, adjuvant RAI therapy may often fail. In the context of its clinical application in differentiated thyroid cancer, with its extremely low mortality, it might therefore be expected that it would be difficult to either prove or disprove the putative benefits of adjuvant RAI treatment. Only large, carefully controlled prospective randomized trials will finally confirm or refute the value of this treatment [194]. In the absence of such, a large number of retrospective studies have not surprisingly yielded very conflicting results over the past 35 years.

RAI ablation of thyroid remnants has been defined as 'the destruction of residual macroscopically normal thyroid tissue following surgical thyroidectomy' [195]. The concept of using remnant ablation with RAI to 'complete' a thyroidectomy has existed since at least 1960, when Blahd and his colleagues at UCLA described their first decade's experience with radioisotope therapy [196]. They concluded from a careful analysis of outcome in 26 patients, 11 of whom had only remnant ablation, that 'a realistic appraisal of the I^{131} treatment of thyroid cancer is extremely difficult. The unfortunate muddling of therapeutic modalities and the remarkable longevity of many of these patients for the most part frustrates any forthright analysis.' [196]. Although, by 1970 many groups had further reported on their results of RAI therapy, Beierwaltes and colleagues [197] could not find in the literature 'a comparison of a population treated with surgery followed by ^{131}I, with a population of patients treated surgically without sodium iodide I-131.'

The Ann Arbor group [197] reported in 1970 that 84 patients with 'well differentiated papillary and follicular thyroid carcinoma,' who were aged 40 years and older at the time of postoperative RAI therapy, experienced a 'significantly lower death rate' than 32 'controls' who had surgery alone. These 'control' patients were 'roughly matched' in sex, but not in age, distribution. The extent of the disease was not controlled, with some having remnant tissue, and others metastatic disease. There was, in fact, no description of the disease stage present in the surgery only group. The control patients came from an earlier time period (1933–1947), when less aggressive surgery was performed. Not all patients underwent a standard bilateral surgery, and the presence or absence of postoperative residual disease was not described. Of the 47 deaths from both groups, the cause of death was unknown in 19 (40%), yet mortality as reported included those deaths. All patients who completed RAI therapy were placed on 'full replacement doses of desiccated thyroid,' an advantage not shared by the surgery-only patients. It is sad to reflect that during the following 25 years the majority of retrospective reports describing outcome after postoperative RAI therapy have continued to be plagued with the same flaws of study design that bedeviled the Michigan experience.

Despite severe criticism of their original study design [198,199], Beierwaltes and his colleagues in 1984 confidently stated, based on their cumulative experience of treating 511 patients with RAI, that 'there is no question today that we should ablate normal thyroid tissue as a part of the treatment of well-differentiated thyroid cancer' [200]. It is surprising that only 1 year previously, Sisson, also from Ann Arbor, concluded from his analysis of the literature that 'the aggregate of evidence does not convincingly demonstrate that ablation of small remnants — and especially those remote from the primary tumor — lowers the rate of recurrent cancer' [198]. Indeed, a Mayo clinic group suggested in the same journal issue that ablative therapy with RAI directed to postsurgical remnants represented a 'questionable pursuit of an ill defined goal' [199].

Part of the confusion related to interpreting these retrospective analyses may arise from a period effect, that is, a systematic change in disease behavior over time. Such a possibility was discussed in the late 1970s by Crile [201] and Cady et al. [202], who based their opinions on the outcome analysis of patients with differentiated thyroid cancer treated over many decades at the Cleveland and Lahey Clinics. More recently, such an effect was demonstrable by multivariate analyses performed during the 1980s in both France [203] and Iceland [204]. Coupled with the ever increasing use of RAI remnant ablation [183] over the last two decades (Fig. 4), the question arises as to whether this period effect is the cause or effect of RAI treatment. If, on the one hand, the nature of the disease has changed across all stages, as is evident from declining case numbers of anaplastic cancer and FTC [205] and, on the other hand, the use of RAI has significantly increased in more recent times, any retrospective study would inevitably find ever improving results attributed to RAI treatment, because the majority of patients with 'new', 'milder' disease would be in the RAI-treated cohort.

In this country the cause of RAI remnant ablation, initially championed by Beierwaltes and his University of Michigan group [197,200], has over the past two decades been actively promoted by endocrinology groups from the University of Chicago [146,148,157], the University of Texas [51,152], and the Ohio State University [45,153,158,206], led by DeGroot, Samaan, and Mazzaferri, respectively. The Chicago group has reported separately on 269 patients with PTC [146,157] and 49 patients with FTC [148]. The M.D. Anderson group described outcome results [152] in 1599 patients with differentiated thyroid cancer, which included 1289 PTC, 236 FTC, and 74 Hürthle-cell can-

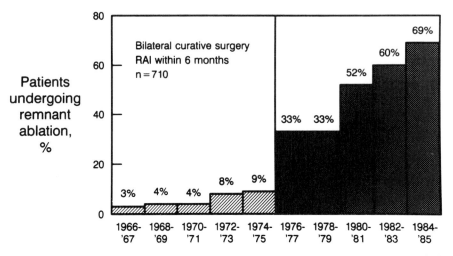

Figure 4. Trend, through 1966 to 1985, in RAI remnant ablation performed at Mayo Clinic within 6 months of bilateral definitive surgery in 710 PTC patients without distant metastases at initial examination. (From Hay [183], with permission.)

cers (HCC). Mazzaferri has now added to his initial study cohort of 907 United States Air Force (USAF) patients [45,153,206], a group of patients treated at Ohio State 'on whom comparable records existed' [158] and has recently reported on the long-term impact of initial therapy on this combined group of 1355 patients, consisting of 1077 PTC and 278 FTC, not excluding HCC.

In a 1994 editorial, DeGroot [207] summarized the present status of RAI remnant ablation as follows: 'Mazzaferri, Young, and coworkers provided, nearly 2 decades ago, the first powerful support for the role of radioactive iodine treatment in reducing recurrences and deaths in differentiated (thyroid) cancer . . . more recent studies by DeGroot and colleagues, and Samaan and coworkers demonstrated, in a careful analysis stratifying patients by extent of diseases, that both more extensive surgery (lobectomy plus subtotal or near-total thyroidectomy) and radioactive iodine treatment reduce the number of recurrences and deaths. Hay and coworkers have thrown their support behind more extensive surgery, but have not yet supported routine radioactive iodide ablation.' It is still our stance that we remain unconvinced by the presently available retrospective data describing the efficacy of RAI remnant ablation in differentiated thyroid carcinoma.

If one were to design a prospective controlled trial to evaluate the role of RAI remnant ablation, one would wish to exclude patients with distant metastases and those who had undergone incomplete resection of primary tumor, that is, restrict entry to patients undergoing potentially curative surgery. One would wish the patients to be matched for age, sex, extent of initial disease, and histology. Ideally, both groups should have a standard primary

114

operation, preferably near-total or total thyroidectomy, performed by specialist surgeons. To qualify as ablative therapy, the RAI would have to be administered for uptake confined to the thyroid bed soon after the operation, typically within 3–6 months. Those patients, who would be randomly allocated to the surgery-only group, should be treated identically with regard to thyroxine (T_4) therapy and followed in a similar manner to the ablated group by the same group of physicians. Follow-up data would require scrupulous evaluation with multivariate analyses.

Obviously, such a prospective trial has not yet been planned. Indeed, Wong and colleagues [194] have suggested that for 45-year old women 'each arm of the trial would require nearly 4000 patients to detect a 10% reduction in mortality after 25 years. . . . If one in every ten patients was enrolled in such a study, enrollment would take 10 years, and results would be available after 35 years.' However, 'even without the benefits of a long term prospective study,' some are convinced that the utility of RAI ablation is now proven [207]. Bearing in mind the importance of appropriate controls, we feel it is relevant to briefly review the most pertinent results from the combined Chicago, Texas, and USAF/Ohio State experience (see Table 1). It should be recognized that in Chicago patients were considered to have received RAI ablation if given >29.9 mCi I-131 with the intent to ablate residual thyroid within 12 months of diagnosis [146,157]. All patients with extrathyroid invasion or distant metastases who were given RAI to ablate as well as to treat metastases were included in the ablated group. By contrast, the M.D. Anderson patients were considered to have RAI as part of their original treatment if it was given within 6 months of surgical intervention [51,152]. In none of the many publications devoted to the USAF/Ohio State cohort have we been able to find details of the timing of RAI administration for postoperative ablative purposes [45,153,158,206].

The studies of Mazzaferri on adjuvant RAI therapy in either FTC or PTC principally concentrated on differences in recurrence rates found between patients treated with thyroid hormone (T4) only and those who in addition received postoperative RAI. When the outcomes in PTC patients with either a primary tumor 1.5 cm or larger, or with multiple primary tumors, local tumor invasion, or cervical metastases were examined, the recurrence rate of 9% in 153 RAI-treated patients was significantly less (p = 0.03) then the 17% rate observed in 311 patients treated with only T4 [206]. No such differences in recurrence rate were found in patients with small primary lesions (<1.5 cm diameter). We ourselves were unable to find any advantage of ablation therapy in node-positive PTC patients with minimal tumors (≤1 cm diameter) [208]. Moreover, we could not demonstrate a significant influence of remnant ablation performed within 6 months of bilateral potentially curative surgery on tumor recurrence or cause-specific mortality in 220 ablated PTC cases, classified by Mazzaferri's scheme as stage 2 (intermediate risk) or stage 3 (high risk) [183]. When similar studies on recurrence rate were performed by Young and Mazzaferri on 51 FTC patients treated by RAI and T4, they were unable to show a significant decrease in recurrence rate (p = 0.28) when compared with 116 patients treated with T4 alone [45]. The findings were similar to those of DeGroot, who could not demonstrate in FTC any decreased risk of death (p = 0.88) or recurrence (p = 0.72) after postsurgical RAI ablation [148].

In their 269 PTC patients DeGroot et al. were also unable to confirm any advantage for RAI ablation by multivariate analysis [157]. Using a Cox model, absence of ablation was not associated with significantly increased risk of death from PTC or tumor recurrence in either the total group or in class I (intrathyroid) or II (node-positive) patients. A nonsignificant trend towards reduced recurrence was found by Cox analysis for class I and II patients with lesions >1 cm in size (p = 0.096). Examination of the recurrence data (Fig. 5) shows that the ablated group was followed for a shorter time, possibly giving rise to a 'period effect.' Clearly, analysis of such data requires the use of a Cox model, which, as DeGroot states, is 'sensitive to duration of follow-up.' However, DeGroot preferred to accept analysis by the 'less rigorous' χ^2 test, which is influenced only by final outcome and not by the duration of observation. By such (perhaps inappropriate) analyses, he concluded that ablation was associated with decreased recurrence in all PTC patients with tumors >1 cm in size and decreased mortality in intrathyroid or node-positive PTC patients with tumors >1 cm diameter [157].

In 1983 Samaan's group, comparing 136 patients with either PTC or FTC who had received ablative therapy with similar patients who had not received RAI found a lower frequency of recurrence after ablation but no difference in survival or disease-free interval (DFI) [51]. The advantage seen with ablation

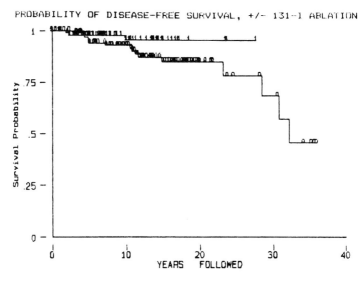

Figure 5. Probability of survival without serious recurrence in relation to postoperative ^{131}I ablation in class I and II patients. (From DeGroot et al. [157], with permission.)

was confined to patients who had total thyroidectomy and those with FTC or mixed papillary-follicular histotypes. A more recent analysis, published in 1992 [152] demonstrated that RAI therapy was the most powerful prognostic indicator for increased DFI and that it ranked third, after age and extent of disease, in the prediction of cause-specific mortality. Samaan also reported that the beneficial effect of RAI extended to AMES [186] low-risk patients, who apparently had significantly fewer recurrences and deaths ($p < 0.001$).

In his most recent multivariate analysis [158] of 1322 stage 1–3 patients with differentiated thyroid cancer (70% PTC), Mazzaferri has found that RAI therapy independently lowered the likelihood of not only tumor recurrence ($p < 0.001$) but also cancer death ($p < 0.05$). Thirty years after initial surgery, recurrence rates in stages 2 and 3 were 16% after RAI and 38% after T4 alone ($p < 0.001$). As noted in Table 1, only 138 (39%) of the 350 patients receiving RAI were given treatment only to ablate remnant tissue. The cumulative recurrence rates in stage 2 or 3 tumors are illustrated by Figure 6. The 30-year rate of 9% seen after ablation was significantly less than the 35% seen in patients who were not ablated ($p = 0.00005$). Even more remarkable are the cumulative mortality data shown in Figure 7. Mazzaferri reports no cancer-related deaths in the 138 stage 2 or 3 tumors treated by RAI remnant ablation, significantly less than the 8% rate seen after 30 years in the 802 patients not so treated.

At our own institution we have treated 2162 patients with differentiated thyroid cancer (1916 PTC, 153 FTC, and 93 HCC) during the period 1940–1991. The mean age at initial therapy of our patients was 46.1 years, more than 10 years, on average, older than the 35.7 years seen in Mazzaferri's series [158]. To date, 142 (7%) of our patients have died of thyroid cancer, comparable with the 5% found in the USAF/Ohio State cohort. Because of the remarkably improved results seen by Mazzaferri in stage 2 and 3 patients, we have chosen to analyze our experience in an identical fashion. Figure 8 illustrates our cumulative recurrence data over 30 years in 1542 stage 2 or 3 patients, divided according to RAI ablative status. The 30-year recurrence rates of 19.1% and

Table 1. Postoperative RAI therapy in 3272 U.S. patients with PTC or FTC treated in three institutions during 1948 through 1993

Study group (time period)	Total No.	Ablation and therapy		Remnant ablation only	
		No.	%	No.	%
Chicago [146,148,157] (1968–1993)	318	167	53	Not stated	Not stated
Texas [51,152] (1948–1989)	1599	736	46	447	28
USAF/Ohio [45,153,158,206] (1950–1993)	1355	350	26	138	13
Total	3272	1253	38	585	20

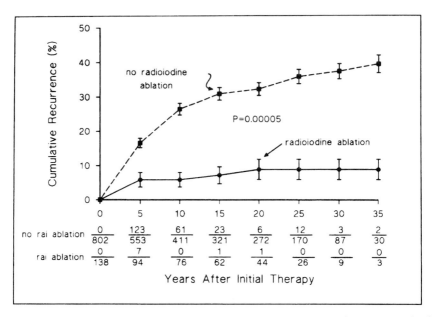

Figure 6. Cancer recurrence in patients with Mazzaferri stage 2 or 3 tumors either treated with (n = 138) or without (n = 802) RAI remnant ablation to destroy presumably normal thyroid gland tissue without tumor. (From Mazzaferri and Jhiang [158], with permission.)

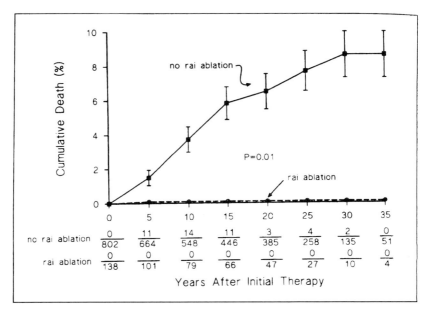

Figure 7. Cancer mortality rates in patients with Mazzaferri stage 2 or 3 tumors either treated with (n = 138) or without (n = 802) RAI remnant ablation to destroy presumably normal thyroid gland tissue without tumor. (From Mazzaferri and Jhiang [158], with permission.)

118

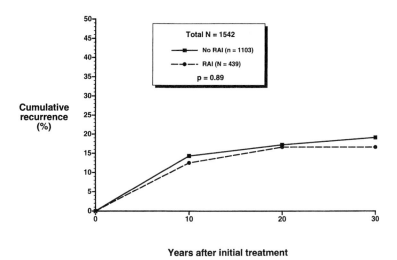

Figure 8. Cumulative recurrence (any site) in 1542 Mazzaferri stage 2 or 3 tumors treated at the Mayo Clinic during 1940–1991, either with (n = 439) or without (n = 1103) RAI ablation. All 1542 patients had complete primary tumor excision, that is, there was no gross postoperative residual disease and 1218 (79%) of the 1542 patients underwent near-total or total thyroidectomy as the primary surgical procedure.

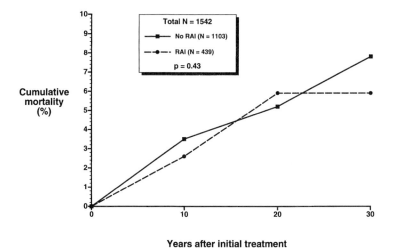

Figure 9. Cumulative cause-specific mortality in 1542 Mazzaferri stage 2 or 3 tumors treated at the Mayo Clinic during 1940–1991, either with (n = 439) or without (n = 1103) RAI ablation. Of the 1542 patients 198 (13%) had FTC.

16.6% seen in the no-RAI and the RAI group are not significantly different (p = 0.89). Both rates seem much lower than the 35% recurrence rate seen at 30 years in Mazzaferri's patients who were not ablated. Our cumulative cause-specific mortality rates are shown in Figure 9. The rates seen in the no-RAI and the RAI group of 7.8% and 5.9%, respectively, at 30 years are not significantly different (p = 0.43). Of our 439 ablated patients, 18 had a less than near-total thyroidectomy as an initial surgical procedure. When those 18 are excluded, the rates for recurrence and mortality seen after ablation were 15.5% and 6.4%, respectively, at 30 years not significantly different from the rates of 16.2% and 5.3% found with near-total or total thyroidectomy alone.

At the present time we do not have a clear explanation for these marked differences in effect of RAI treatment on recurrence and mortality between our data and Mazzaferri's experience. However, they do in part explain why we have, as DeGroot has observed '. . . not yet supported routine radioactive iodide ablation.' Similarly, a number of other North American [47,209], and non-American [130,144,145,147,149,210,211] studies have over the last two decades also failed to confirm a survival benefit for patients treated with adjuvant RAI, despite cumulative patient numbers of over 4500 patients, a third of which were treated with adjuvant RAI. Furthermore, only one of these studies [147] demonstrated reduced recurrence in patients who had received adjuvant RAI, casting additional doubt on the value of routine use of adjuvant RAI therapy.

In contrast to thyroxine therapy, which is essentially nontoxic and most often needed as hormone replacement therapy in any case, RAI remnant ablation has the potential for significant side effects. Short-term side effects include radiation thyroiditis (up to 70%), sialoadenitis (up to 10%; may become chronic), odynophagia, herpes zoster, leukopenia, endocrine and reproductive testicular and ovarian failure (mostly reversible), and radiation cystitis [175,212–218]. Long-term carcinogenic risks may theoretically include leukemia, stomach, breast, and bladder cancer [219]. A recent Swedish study of 834 thyroid cancer patients treated with RAI showed that, although there was a significant increased overall cancer risk, more then 10 years after exposure there was no increased risk of stomach or bladder cancer [220]. In view of these side effects and the present uncertainties about its effectiveness, however, we still feel that, despite all theoretical and philosophical attractions, adjuvant RAI therapy should be used in a selective fashion. We agree with the judgment of Heufelder and Gorman [221] that the current evidence 'does not justify ablation for small, well differentiated, noninvasive and non-metastatic thyroid cancers.' The large group of low-risk PTC and FTC patients, who make up the majority of thyroid cancer victims [188], may not benefit from such treatment and could be exposed to inconvenience and potential harm. Even for high-risk patients, conclusive proof of efficacy would be desirable, but most clinicians would feel that the risk/benefit ratio is probably weighed in favor of adjuvant RAI treatment in such individuals. In our institution we presently recommend RAI remnant ablation routinely in patients with FTC and those high-risk PTC patients who have a postoperative MACIS score of 6.0 or more [127].

Both short-term and long-term side effects are dose related, and it would appear that this mandates usage of the lowest effective dose if remnant ablation is used. Numerous studies have tried to address the problem of RAI remnant ablation dosing. Results have been conflicting, as summarized by Dulgeroff and Hershman [189]. There is no conclusive evidence for the superiority of a particular dose. As little as 30 mCi may be successful, while occasionally doses as high as 200 mCi may fail. Most recently. Mazzaferri and Jhiang were unable to show a difference in recurrence rate (7–9%) between patients who had received 50 mCi or less and those who had received more [158]. Logue et al. found that there was no difference in the likelihood of successful remnant ablation for doses of <100 mCi, as compared with doses of >100 mCi, in 121 patients treated in Toronto between 1977 and 1988 [222]. The amount of residual thyroid tissue and the initial dose rate, rather than the total dose, may be the major determinants of successful ablation [222,223]. The former can be estimated ultrasonogrpahically; the latter can only be estimated from measured uptake over time. The only way to determine uptake prior to treatment is by diagnostic scanning, which in itself can diminish the rate and amount of subsequent therapeutic RAI uptake [224]. Possible ways to overcome this problem may include the use of I-123 rather than I-131 for diagnostic scanning [224], or uptake rate measurements during therapy with additional dosing during the same therapy cycle if necessary [223]. In the interim, for remnant ablation after near-total or total thyroidectomy, empirical initial dosing with 30 mCi as an outpatient, followed by 100 mCi if the initial dose or a second outpatient dose, fails to abolish all uptake, might represent a reasonably practical approach [221]. Patients with very large remnants, who are deemed at high risk of recurrence, may be best advised to undergo additional cytoreductive surgery before ablation is attempted.

External-beam radiation therapy

In addition to thyroxine treatment and RAI remnant ablation, external-beam radiation therapy (XRT) is sometimes used as an adjuvant treatment modality. It has some theoretical advantages over RAI therapy, in that delivered dose and dose rate can be more carefully controlled. However, effects are limited to the irradiated field; micrometastases elsewhere, which putatively may be destroyed by RAI treatment, will not be reached. Furthermore, normal tissues within the radiated field may receive a higher dose than with RAI treatment, and this may lead to increased local side effects compared with RAI. With regards to treatment efficacy, XRT has been less well studied than either thyroxine or RAI therapy [225]. Samaan et al. found XRT by univariate analysis to be effective in reducing both mortality and recurrence rates, but the effect disappeared in a multivariate model [152]. Simpson et al. found postoperative XRT to be as effective as RAI in reducing recurrence and improving survival in patients with residual disease but did not influence those who had undergone complete tumor resection [131]. Tubiana et al. [211] showed XRT to be more effective than RAI treatment in reducing recurrence, but survival was not improved. However, the patients receiving XRT almost invariably had residual disease, and hence fell into a high-risk category. In contrast to these relatively optimistic results, Mazzaferri et al. found in both 1981 and 1994 that XRT was associated with the worst outcomes of all treatment modalities [153,158], but as observed by Brierley and Tsang [225], this may be explained by the higher incidence of initial nodal involvement and the absence of RAI therapy in the XRT patient. Similarly pessimistic observations were made by Staunton [137] and Russell et al. [209].

In addition to these studies comparing different treatment modalities, there have been a few papers from radiation oncology centers reviewing the XRT experience with only limited comparison to other treatments. A recent series from the Royal Marsden Hospital included 113 patients with residual disease after surgery. Survival at 5 years for patients with microscopic residual disease was 85%, but was only 27% for gross residual disease. Those 74 patients who had received RAI had similar survival to those who received only XRT [226].

Overall, it would appear that, similar to adjuvant RAI treatment, the value of postoperative adjuvant XRT remains uncertain, but that it may yield comparable results to RAI, and it is presently unclear whether the effects of RAI treatment and XRT may be additive. We therefore feel that this treatment should be limited to high-risk patients, and probably should be considered as an appropriate alternative to RAI treatment in certain specific circumstances, rather than as additional treatment for those who have already received radioiodine. For example, a patient with oxyphilic FTC, a tumor that rarely exhibits radioiodine uptake, and postoperative residual disease might be regularly a candidate for adjuvant XRT. In contrast to our position, DeGroot has recently recommended that 5000 rads should be prophylactically given to the thyroid bed after RAI treatment in patients with papillary or follicular cancer who are over the age of 45–50 years and have either locally invasive disease or possible residual disease [227]. He also advises similar treatment for recurrent disease in a patient of any age.

An alternative, and perhaps more acceptable, approach to XRT may be that recently proposed by the University of Toronto group [225]. They recommend no XRT in patients with good prognostic features and complete surgical excision. For patients with bulky residual disease they advise XRT to improve 'local control.' A more vexed question relates to the patients with either presumed or definite microscopic residual disease. In the absence of convincing data from prospective randomized controlled trials, the Toronto group now advise 40 Gy over 3 weeks for possible residual disease, and 50 Gy over 4 weeks for definite residual disease. In young patients with minimal residual disease and good RAI uptake, they recommend RAI alone, without XRT.

Other adjuvant treatments

Chemotherapy, or a combination of XRT and chemotherapy, is rarely justified as an adjuvant treatment measure in differentiated thyroid cancer. The results of chemotherapy are generally disappointing, and the prognosis of most patients, even with advanced disease, is fairly reasonable compared with other human cancers, thereby making it difficult to justify use of such toxic treatments in the absence of established progressive disease. However, in anaplastic carcinoma the interest in adjuvant chemotherapy and combination therapy is much greater. Given the lethal nature of the disease and the high mitotic activity of the tumors, basic oncological considerations would suggest the potential usefulness of such an approach. There are no controlled studies assessing the validity of these assumptions, but a large number of case series and retrospective studies suggest that XRT after surgery almost completely abolishes local recurrence, one of the major causes of death in anaplastic carcinoma, whereas the addition of chemotherapy seems to prolong median survival [228–235]. However, whether cure rates are improved remains uncertain, and significant treatment toxicity is the rule. Furthermore, there is at least one study in the literature that suggests impaired survival for patients with anaplastic cancers who received chemotherapy in addition to surgery, presumably as a consequence of treatment toxicity [236]. Despite some initial promise, adjuvant chemotherapy and multimodal treatment for anaplastic thyroid carcinoma continue to be considered experimental, and their use should probably be confined to centers with significant expertise, particularly with chemotherapy.

Follow-up

Similar to adjuvant treatment, follow-up for thyroid cancer patients should be individualized. Given that most recurrences and deaths tend to occur during the first 5 postoperative years, it seems difficult to justify intensive lifelong follow-up for the majority of differentiated thyroid cancer patients. Regardless of the staging system used, over 80% of individuals will fall into low-risk categories, with a lifetime recurrence and cancer death risk of less than 10%, and minimal follow-up after 5 years would seem sufficient for this patient group. High-risk patients will obviously require more intensive follow-up.

For all patients, follow-up strategies should be based on the known biological tumor behavior. Amongst the cancers arising from follicular epithelium, PTC and FTC exhibit distinctly different patterns of recurrence. PTC most often recurs in the neck, especially in regional lymph nodes [40,183]. Between 10% and 30% of PTC patients will eventually have disease recurrence in the neck [40]. Distant metastases also occur, but much less frequently. No more than 10% of PTC patients, who had no evidence of distant spread at presentation, will later develop distant metastases [41,127]. By contrast, typical FTC rarely spreads to regional nodes, but more often spreads hematogenously to distant sites [5]. Between 5% and 40% of patients with FTC will suffer metastatic disease in the course of their illness. Oxyphilic FTC differs from typical FTC in that it exhibits both frequent nodal involvement and distant metastases [5,40].

When distant metastases occur in PTC or FTC (both typical and oxyphilic), the most common sites of involvement are the lungs [237], followed by the bony skeleton [41]. In PTC about two thirds of metastases are to the lungs, whereas in FTC bone metastases are only slightly less frequent than pulmonary spread [41]. Both regional (lymphatic) and distant metastases in PTC and FTC often retain a reasonable degree of differentiation. They may stay responsive to some of the regulatory signals affecting the function of normal thyroid tissue and may also concentrate iodine and secrete thyroglobulin (Tg).

For these reasons it is evident that careful physical examination of the neck is of great importance in the follow-up of patients with PTC and oxyphilic FTC, and is likely to uncover many recurrent lesions in the thyroid remnant or regional nodes. By contrast, in typical FTC the low rate of regional (nodal) recurrence makes neck examination a procedure with a much lesser yield of useful information. Physical examination of the chest and the bony skeleton is too insensitive to discover most metastases, and, particularly in the absence of symptoms, could potentially be omitted.

Measurement of serum thyroid function tests, particularly TSH, is an important part of the follow-up of all patients who are on postoperative thyroxine therapy. The majority of low-risk patients will probably not benefit from extreme TSH suppression and, in order to minimize toxicity whist still reaping some potential benefits of TSH suppression, serum TSH values should be kept just below the reference range. On the other hand, in some high-risk patients one may accept the potential for long-term toxicity and aim for complete TSH suppression.

In FTC and PTC patients, who had a near-total or total thyroidectomy (with or without additional RAI remnant ablation), the small amount of remaining normal thyroid tissue should be dormant, while on thyroxine, and a measurable Tg level may therefore indicate possible recurrence. Measurements are somewhat less reliable, but in most instances still useful, if the patient has residual thyroid tissue [238]. In patients with little or no residual thyroid tissue, sensitivity may be further enhanced if measurements are taken whilst the patient is not receiving thyroxine. However, undetectable serum Tg levels while on thyroxine are seldom observed in patients with recurrent cancer. Hence, thyroid hormone treatment does not usually have to be discontinued in these individuals [238]. Similarly, serum levels <5 ng/ml on thyroxine are also very infrequently, although slightly more often than undetectable levels, seen in patients with recurrent disease. Therefore, repeat Tg measurements off thyroxine may also not be indicated in such patients [238–240]. All other patients should possibly have measurements repeated off thyroxine and may also require additional diagnostic measures. Furthermore, all patients with Tg autoantibodies will need to undergo additional tests because Tg measurements become unreliable in the presence of anti-Tg antibodies. Interestingly, it has been recently suggested that monitoring antibody levels, rather than Tg levels, may be useful in these individuals [241–243]. Antibody production may be dependent on a constant antigen source, and hence declining titers of anti-Tg autoantibodies may signify cure. However, at the moment this is not an established practice and, until these observations are widely confirmed, measurements of anti-Tg antibody titers must not be relied on to exclude persistent or recurrent disease, although they may yield useful complimentary information.

Imaging procedures are not universally required but can be very useful in selected patients. The most commonly used imaging procedures are diagnostic radioiodine scans. However, in unselected patients follow-up radioiodine scans have a low yield. In these patients yearly or biannual diagnostic radioiodine scans are neither cost effective nor totally safe. Over the years patients have had to endure, prior to scanning, multiple episodes of thyroxine withdrawal with resultant morbid hypothyroidism. Furthermore, cumulative radiation dose over many years can be significant and may occasionally result in long-term toxicity [244]. A low-risk PTC or FTC patient who has undergone near-total or total thyroidectomy, with no clinical evidence of recurrence and an undetectable serum Tg level on thyroxine treatment (in the absence of antithyroglobulin autoantibodies), probably does not need to be submitted to any imaging procedures. By contrast, a high-risk patient with clinical or biochemical parameters suggestive of recurrence, but without an obvious site of disease progression, may need extensive imaging procedures.

Diagnostic RAI scanning will not be the most appropriate testing procedure in all of these patients. For patients with PTC or oxyphilic FTC who have suspected recurrence, a high-resolution ultrasound scan of the neck may be highly effective in discovering potential nodal metastases [245,246]. All sonographically suspicious nodules (often clinically impalpable) can be readily biopsied under ultrasound guidance, usually yielding an immediate tissue diagnosis [247]. Many recurrences outside the neck may be diagnosed using diagnostic RAI scanning. Unfortunately, this procedure presently requires patients to discontinue thyroid hormone treatment prior to scanning in order to maximize TSH-driven uptake in metastatic tissue. This is always unpleasant for patients and, in some instances, when TSH levels are completely suppressed, several weeks may go by before the serum TSH level rises to levels adequate for scanning, resulting in significantly symptomatic hypothyroidism in these individuals. Fortunately, recent trials have demonstrated that recombinant human TSH can lead to uptake stimulation similar to that seen after several weeks of thyroxine withdrawal. Therefore, the problem of scanning-related iatrogenic hypothyroidism may soon be historical [248]. Regardless of whether patients are prepared for scanning in the traditional way or by recombinant human TSH administration, serum Tg level measurements should be repeated at the time of scanning in those individuals without autoantibodies. This may provide useful complimentary information to the scan because the serum Tg level off thyroxine may sometimes significantly rise in patients with metastatic disease but negative radioiodine scans.

For those PTC and FTC patients with negative radioiodine scans and neck ultrasonography but elevated serum Tg levels or strong clinical suspicion of recurrence, additional imaging procedures are required. Pulmonary metastases are common in PTC and FTC, and can be clinically completely silent. Mostly they take up radioiodine, but occasionally they are not iodophilic. However, they may still be visible on a chest radiograph, which is a useful and inexpensive additional test in this situation. More often, the metastases are micronodular and may only be visualized by high-resolution CT scanning. Similarly, occult, non-iodophilic osseous metastases can often be localized by isotopic bone scanning. For intra-abdominal metastases sonography, computed tomography (CT), or magnetic resonance imaging (MRI) scanning represent highly sensitive procedures. For intracranial and small intrathoracic metastases, CT or MRI are the procedures of choice. A number of other imaging modalities can occasionally be helpful, particularly if there is a strong local expertise in their application. Such procedures include Tc-99m-sestamibi, Tc-99m pentavalent dimercaptosuccinic acid (DMSA), radiolabeled anti-CEA antibodies, and radioiodinated-131 meta-iodobenzyl guanidine [249]. DMSA seems to perform particularly well in identifying FTC and PTC metastases that do not take up radioiodine, and this procedure may in the future prove to be a viable alternative to conventional imaging.

Management of progressive and recurrent disease

When evidence for progressive or recurrent disease is discovered during follow-up, the available treatment options are essentially the same as for initial treatment, namely, surgery, thyroxine, RAI, XRT, chemotherapy, or a combination of some or all. In addition, a number of potential novel approaches have been tried in recent years, and some of these may eventually find their way into routine management.

Local neck recurrence, whether confined to nodes or not, is probably best treated surgically. There is no evidence that the addition of radiotherapy in any form is superior to successful surgical removal of recurrent tumor. If surgical removal is deemed too difficult or unacceptable to the patient, both RAI and XRT have good success rates for preventing recurrent nodal metastases on the order of an 80% response rate. Similarly, after incomplete surgical removal of recurrent tumor, radiotherapy (with RAI or XRT) may improve outcome, although conclusive proof is lacking.

Management of distant metastases depends on their location and features, including symptoms. Localized, apparently solitary, metastases are best tackled surgically if possible, particularly if they are large. Surgical treatment of solitary metastases may result in 5-year and 10-year survival rates of around

45% and 33%, respectively [250]. RAI treatment almost invariably yields disappointing results in solitary metastases that are larger than 100 g estimated weight [251]. Pulmonary metastases are probably most responsive to RAI treatment. The response rate to RAI treatment for lung metastases in differentiated thyroid cancer is between 25% and 50% [252]. By univariate analysis, survival seems prolonged in patients whose metastases concentrate RAI [252], and to a lesser degree even in young patients without significant uptake in the metastatic tissue [41,237,252]. However, multivariate analysis has cast doubt on the value of RAI treatment in metastatic thyroid cancer, with no evidence of a beneficial effect when data are adjusted for the effects of age and extent of involvement [41,237]. Survival rates at 5 and 10 years for patients with RAI-treated pulmonary metastases in differentiated thyroid cancer are around 50–60% and 30–40%, respectively [44,252,253].

Bone metastases, unless localized and surgically respectable, are also often managed with RAI treatment. Results are rather worse than for lung metastases; more than 70% of patients with bone metastases have died by 7 years after diagnosis [254]. This has led some to question about whether treatment beyond palliative measures is worthwhile for bone metastases. Treatment doses of RAI for both pulmonary and other metastases are generally higher than in remnant ablation and may in some patients occasionally exceed cumulative doses of 1000 mCi. The major dose-limiting factor is bone marrow toxicity. Autologous bone marrow rescue may sometimes be used to overcome this limitation. However, RAI doses of this magnitude are rarely indicated.

XRT can be used on bone lesions. Although large, systematic experience is lacking, fracture risk and pain is likely treated effectively. XRT may also be preferably to RAI treatment with intracranial metastases; the former treatment anecdotally leads to good palliative results [255], whereas the latter (RAI) can be rarely associated with fatal cerebral edema [256]. Chemotherapy, usually including doxorubicin, can be tried in patients who have not responded to other treatment modalities. Long-term cures are rare, but survival times can be significantly prolonged [2,189,236,257].

In addition to these 'conventional' treatment approaches, a number of experimental therapies have emerged, some already in occasional clinical use, others still at the in vitro stage. In an attempt to improve dose distribution and dose rate, alternative isotopes to RAI are being considered for treatment of differentiated thyroid cancer. Astatine 211 (At-211) is chemically related to iodine but is a high-energy alpha-particle emitter, thereby permitting higher and more focused tissue doses within thyroid cancer tissue. Unfortunately, in animal experiments it seems to be associated with a potential for marked toxicity [2,189].

Augmentation of RAI or XRT by the use of 'radiosensitizing' drugs or other drugs aimed at increasing the biological effect of radiotherapy has been occasionally used for some years. Lithium was the first drug in this category to be used. It interfered with iodine transport across membranes, leading to slowed RAI excretion and prolonged RAI storage in thyrocytes. Whilst potentially increasing treatment efficacy, this had also the potential for increased toxicity, both by direct effects of lithium itself as well as indirect effects due to increased RAI dose. Chemotherapeutic drugs in low doses, particularly doxorubicin, (Adriamycin) and cisplatinum, have also been shown to have radiosensitizing effects [2], but at the present time experience with these treatments is extremely limited. Another way to potentially increase the effectiveness of RAI treatment is to decrease the relative proportion of uptake in more differentiated tumor parts and in residual normal thyroid tissue. Retinoids have the ability to induce type I iodothyronine 5'-deiodinase in relatively well-differentiated thyroid-derived cells [258], thereby potentially shortening the half-life of iodine in these cells, and may therefore be useful for this purpose. Hyperthermia leads to improved differentiation of cultured thyroid carcinoma cells in vitro [259]. Because increased differentiation may be associated with increased RAI uptake, this also has the potential to be useful as a therapeutic measure aimed at optimizing RAI therapy.

Hormonal manipulations other than thyroxine therapy include tamoxifen, a partial estrogen antagonist, which has shown encouraging results in cell culture and nude mice models [13]. Somatostatin, and its more commonly used long-acting synthetic analogue octreotide, are known to inhibit the secretion of a large number of hormones and also to diminish the growth rates of a number of endocrine neoplasms. Octreotide has been used in clinical trials to treat metastatic differentiated thyroid cancer. However, in a recent small series of six patients with disseminated differentiated thyroid cancer [260], none of the patients seemed to improve with the treatment. Type I human interferons have been shown to capable of significant growth suppression, inducing redifferentiation and increasing the expression of MHC I in thyroid carcinoma cultures, all of which may aid in the management of advanced thyroid malignancies [261]. Interleukin-1 and TNF-α have also shown promise in vitro, but clinical trials have not yet been conducted [189]. Interleukin-2 plus lymphokine-activated killer (LAK) cells have been used in a patient with thyroid cancer without success [189], on the basis that this treatment, when given for nonthyroid neoplasms, has been shown to lead to a high incidence of hypothyroidism [262,263]. Finally, immunization of patients with tumor extracts has been tried for more than 20 years and has, in concordance with the experience in most other human tumors, proved unsuccessful for follicular cell–derived thyroid malignancies [264].

References

1. Franceschi S, La Vecchia C. 1994. Thyroid cancer. Cancer Surv 19–20:393–422.
2. Robbins J, Merino MJ, Boice JD Jr, et al. 1991. Thyroid cancer: A lethal endocrine neoplasm. Ann Intern Med 115:133–147.
3. Parker SL, Tong T, Bolden S, Wingo PA. 1996. Cancer statistics, 1996. CA Cancer J for Clin 46:5–27.

4. Ain KB. 1995. Papillary thyroid carcinoma. Endocrinol Metab Clin North Am 24:711–760.
5. Grebe SKG, Hay ID. 1995. Follicular thyroid cancer. Endocrinol Metab Clin North Am 24:761–801.
6. Williams ED, Doniach I, Bjarnason O, Michie W. 1977. Thyroid cancer in an iodide rich area: A histopathological study. Cancer 39:215–222.
7. Franceschi S, Levi F, Negri E, Facina A, La Vecchio C. 1991. Diet in thyroid cancer: A pooled analysis of four European case control studies. Int J Cancer 48:395–398.
8. Harach HR, Escalante DA, Onativia A, Lederer Outes J, Saravia Day E. 1985. Thyroid carcinoma and thyroiditis in an endemic goitre region before and after iodine prophylaxis. Acta Endocrinol 108:55–60.
9. Harach HR, Williams ED. 1995. Thyroid cancer and thyroiditis in the goitrous regions of Salta, Argentina, before and after iodine prophylaxis. Clin Endocrinol 43:701–706.
10. Ron E, Curtis R, Hoffman DA, Flannery JT. 1984. Multiple primary breast and thyroid cancer. Br J Cancer 49:87–92.
11. McTiernan A, Weiss NS, Daling JR. 1987. Incidence of thyroid cancer in women in relation to known or suspected risk factors for breast cancer. Cancer Res 47:292–295.
12. Ron E, Kleinerman RA, Boice JD Jr, LiVolsi VA, Flannery JT, Fraumeni JF Jr. 1987. A population-based case-control study of thyroid cancer. J Natl Cancer Inst 79:1–12.
13. Hoelting T, Siperstein AE, Duh QY, Clark OH. 1995. Tamoxifen inhibits growth, migration, and invasion of human follicular and papillary thyroid cancer cells in vitro and in vivo. J Clin Endocrinol Metab 80:308–313.
14. van Hoeven KH, Menendz-Botet CJ, Strong EW, Huvos AG. 1993. Estrogen and progesterone receptor content in human thyroid disease. Am J Clin Pathol 99:175–181.
15. McTiernan AM, Weiss NS, Daling JR. 1984. Incidence of thyroid cancer in women in relation to reproductive and hormonal factors. Am J Epidemiol 120:423–435.
16. Kravdal O, Glattre E, Haldorsen T. 1991. Positive correlation between parity and incidence of thyroid cancer: New evidence based on complete norwegian birth cohorts. Int J Cancer 49:831–836.
17. Farid NR, Shi Y, Zou M. 1994. Molecular basis of thyroid cancer. Endocr Rev 15:202–232.
18. Houlston RS, Stratton MR. 1995. Genetics of non-medullary thyroid cancer. Q J Med 88:685–693.
19. Cooper DS, Axelrod L, De Groot LJ, Vickery AL Jr, Maloof F. 1981. Congenital goitre and the development of metastatic follicular carcinoma with evidence for a leak of non-hormonal iodide: Clinical, pathological, kinetic and biochemical studies and a review of the literature. J Clin Endocrinol Metab 52:294–306.
20. Hamilton TE, van Belle G, LoGerfo JP. 1987. Thyroid neoplasia in Marshall Islanders exposed to nuclear fallout. JAMA 258:629–636.
21. Prentice RL, Kato H, Yoshimoto K, Mason M. 1982. Radiation exposure and thyroid cancer incidence among Hiroshima and Nagasaki residents. Natl Cancer Inst Monogr 62:207–212.
22. Razack MS, Sako K, Shimaoka K, Getaz EP, Rao U, Parthasarathy KL. 1980. Radiation-associated thyroid carcinoma. J Surg Oncol 14:287–291.
23. Paloyan E, Lawrence AM. 1978. Thyroid neoplasms after radiation therapy for adolescent acne vulgaris. Arch Dermatol 114:53–55.
24. Mehta MP, Goetowski PG, Kinsella TJ. 1989. Radiation induced thyroid neoplasms 1920 to 1987: A vanishing problem? Int J Radiat Oncol Biol Phys 16:1471–1475.
25. Schneider AB, Recant W, Pinsky SM, Ryo UY, Bekerman C, Shore-Freedman E. 1986. Radiation-induced thyroid carcinoma. Clinical course and results of therapy in 296 patients. Ann Intern Med 105:405–412.
26. McHenry C, Jarosz H, Calandra D, McCall A, Lawrence AM, Paloyan E. 1987. Thyroid neoplasia following radiation therapy for Hodgkin's lymphoma. Arch Surg 122:684–686.
27. Nikiforov Y, Gnepp DR. 1994. Pediatric thyroid cancer after the Chernobyl disaster. Pathomorphologic study of 84 cases (1991–1992) from the Republic of Belarus. Cancer 74:748–766.

28. Hedinger CE. 1988. Histological typing of thyroid tumours. In Hedinger CE, ed. International Histological Classification of Tumours, Vol. 11. Berlin: Springer-Verlag, pp 22–23.

29. Rosai J, Carcangiu ML, DeLellis RA. 1992. Tumors of the thyroid gland. In Atlas of Tumor Pathology. Washington, DC: Armed Forces Institute of Pathology.

30. Kini SR. 1987. Thyroid. New York: Igaku-Shoin, 57–95.

31. Kahn NF, Perzin KH. 1995. Follicular carcinoma of the thyroid: An evaluation of the histology criteria used for diagnosis. Pathol Annu 18:221–253.

32. Marchegiani C, Lucci S, De Antoni E, et al. 1985. Thyroid cancer: Surgical experience with 322 cases. Int Surg 70:121–124.

33. Høie J, Stenwig AE, Brennhovd IO. 1988. Surgery in papillary thyroid carcinoma: A review of 730 patients. J Surg Oncol 37:147–151.

34. Noguchi M, Kumaki T, Taniya T, Miyazaki I. 1990. Bilateral cervical lymph node metastases in well-differentiated thyroid cancer. Arch Surg 125:804–806.

35. Noguchi M, Kumaki T, Taniya T, et al. 1990. A retrospective study on the efficacy of cervical lymph node dissection in well-differentiated carcinoma of the thyroid. Jpn J Surg 20:143–150.

36. Hamming JF, van de Velde CJ, Goslings BM, Fleuren GJ, Hermans JD, van Slooten EA. 1989. Peroperative diagnosis and treatment of metastases to the regional lymph nodes in papillary carcinoma of the thyroid gland. Surg Gynecol Obstet 169:107–114.

37. Noguchi S, Noguchi A, Murakami N. 1970. Papillary carcinoma of the thyroid. II. Value of prophylactic lymph node excision. Cancer 26:1061–1064.

38. Roka R, Niederle B, Rath T, Wenzl E, Krisch K, Fritsch A. 1982. Die Bedeutung der beidseitigen diagnostischen Lymphadenektomie beim Schilddrusencarcinom. Operationstaktisches Vorgehen beim Ersteingriff. Chirurg 53:499–504.

39. Salvadori B, Del Bo R, Pilotti S, Grassi M, Cusumano F. 1993. 'Occult' papillary carcinoma of the thyroid: A questionable entity. Eur J Cancer 29A:1817–1820.

40. Grebe SKG, Hay ID. 1996. Thyroid cancer nodal metastases: Biological significance and therapeutic considerations. Surg Oncol Clin North Am 5:43–63.

41. Ruegemer JJ, Hay ID, Bergstralh EJ, Ryan JJ, Offord KP, Gorman CA. 1988. Distant metastases in differentiated thyroid carcinoma: A multivariate analysis of prognostic variables. J Clin Endocroinol Metab 67:501–508.

42. Casara D, Rubello D, Saladinin G, Gallo V, Masarotto, G, Busnardo B. 1991. Distant metastases in differentiated thyroid cancer: Long-term results of radioiodine treatment and statistical analysis of prognostic factors in 214 patients. Tumori 77:432–436.

43. Mizukami Y, Michigishi T, Nonomura A, et al. 1990. Distant metastasis in differentiated thyroid carcinomas: A clinical and pathologic study. Hum Pathol 21:283–290.

44. Schlumberger M, Tubiana M, De Vathaire F, et al. 1986. Long-term results of treatment of 283 patients with lung and bone metastases from differentiated thyroid carcinoma. J Clin Endocrinol Metab 63:960–967.

45. Young RL, Mazzaferri EL, Rahe AJ, Dorfman SG. 1980. Pure follicular thyroid carcinoma: Impact of therapy in 214 patients. J Nucl Med 21:733–737.

46. Simpson WJ, McKinney SE, Carruthers JS, Gospodarowicz MK, Sutcliffe SB, Panzarella T. 1987. Papillary and follicular thyroid cancer. Prognostic factors in 1578 patients. Am J Med 83:479–488.

47. Jensen MH, Davis RK, Derrick L. 1990. Thyroid cancer: A computer-assisted review of 5287 cases. Otolaryngol Head Neck Surg 102:51–65.

48. Glanzmann C, Horst W. 1979. Behandlung und Prognose des folliculären and papillären Schilddrüsenkarzinoms. Strahlentherapie 155:515–528.

49. Schröder S, Baisch H, Rehpenning W, et al. 1987. Morphologie und Prognose des folliculären Schilddrüsencarcinoms — Eine klinisch-pathologische und DNS-cytometrische Untersuchung an 95 Tumoren. Langenbecks Arch Chir 370:3–24.

50. Samaan NA, Schultz PN, Haynie TP, Ordonez NG. 1985. Pulmonary metastasis of

differentiated thyroid carcinoma: Treatment results in 101 patients. J Clin Endocrinol Metab 60:376–380.

51. Samaan NA, Maheshwari YK, Nader S, et al. 1983. Impact of therapy for differentiated carcinoma of the thyroid: An analysis of 706 cases. J Clin Endocrinol Metab 56:1131–1138.

52. Crile G Jr, Pontius KI, Hawk WA. 1985. Factors influencing the survival of patients with follicular carcinoma of the thyroid gland. Surg Gynecol Obstet 160:409–413.

53. Har-El G, Hadar T, Segal K, Levy R, Sidi J. 1986. Hurthle cell carcinoma of the thyroid gland. A tumor of moderate malignancy. Cancer 57:1613–1617.

54. Reiners C, Herrmann H, Schaffer R, Borner W. 1983. Incidence and prognosis of thyroid cancer with special regard to oncocytic carcinoma of the thyroid. Acta Endocrinol 252 (suppl.):18.

55. Carcangiu ML, Zampi G, Rosai J. 1984. Poorly differentiated ('insular') thyroid carcinoma. A reinterpretation of Langerhans' 'wuchernde Struma.' Am J Surg Pathol 8:655–668.

56. Flynn SD, Forman BH, Stewart AF, Kinder BK. 1988. Poorly differentiated ('insular') carcinoma of the thyroid gland: An aggressive subset of differentiated thyroid neoplasms. Surgery 104:963–970.

57. Lyon MF. 1988. X-chromosome inactivation and the location and expression of X-linked genes. Am J Hum Genet 42:8–16.

58. Vogelstein B, Fearon ER, Hamilton SR, Fairberg AP. 1985. Use of restriction fragment length polymorphism to determine clonal origine of human tumors. Science 227:642–645.

59. Hicks DG, Li Volsi VA, Neidich JA, Puck JM, Kant JA. 1990. Clonal analysis of solitary follicular nodules in the thyroid. Am J Pathol 137:553–562.

60. Thomas GA, Williams D, Williams ED. 1989. The clonal origin of thyroid nodules and adenomas. Am J Pathol 134:141–147.

61. Namba H, Matsuo K, Fagin JA. 1990. Clonal compostion of benign and malignant human thyroid tumors. J Clin Invest 86:120–125.

62. Aeschimann S, Kopp PA, Kimura ET, Zbaeren J, Tobler A, Fey MF. 1993. Morphological and functional polymorphism within clonal thyroid nodules. J Clin Endocrinol Metab 77:846–851.

63. Namba H, Rubin SA, Fagin JA. 1990. Point mutations of Ras oncogenes are an early event in thyroid tumorigenesis. Mol Endocrinol 4:1471–1479.

64. Suarez HG, Du Villard JA, Caillou M, Schlumberger M, Tubiana C, Parmentier R. 1988. Detection of activated ras oncogenes in human thyroid carcinomas. Oncogene 2:403–406.

65. Roque L, Gomes P, Correia C, Soares P, Soares J, Castedo S. 1993. Thyroid nodular hyperplasia: Chromosomal studies in 14 cases. Cancer Genet Cytogenet 69:31–34.

66. Belge G, Thode B, Bullerdiek J, Bartnitzke S. 1992. Aberrations of chromosome 19. Do they characterize a subtype of benign thyroid adenomas? Cancer Genet Cytogenet 60:23–26.

67. Bondeson L, Bengtsson A, Bondeson AG, Dahlenfors R, Grimelius L, Mark J. 1989. Chromosome studies in thyroid neoplasia. Cancer 64:680–685.

68. Herrmann MA, Hay ID, Bartelt DH Jr, Ritland SR, Dahl RJ, Grant CS, Jenkins RB. 1991. Cytogenetic and molecular genetic studies of follicular and papillary thyroid cancers. J Clin Invest 88:1596–1604.

69. Taruscio D, Carcangiu ML, Ried T, Ward DC. 1994. Numerical chromosomal aberrations in thyroid tumors detected by double fluorescence in situ hybridization. Genes Chromosom Cancer 9:180–185.

70. Teyssier JR, Liautaud-Roger F, Ferre D, Patey M, Dufer J. 1990. Chromosomal changes in thyroid tumors. Relation with DNA content, karyotypic features, and clinical data. Cancer Genet Cytogenet 50:249–263.

71. Bartnitzke S, Herrmann ME, Lobeck H, Zuschneid W, Neuhaus P. 1989. Cytogenetic findings on eight follicular thyroid adenomas including one with a t(10;19). Cancer Genet Cytogenet 39:65–68.

72. Roque L, Castedo S, Gomes P, Soares P, Clode A, Soares J. 1993. Cytogenetic findings in 18 follicular thyroid adenomas. Cancer Genet Cytogenet 67:1–6.

73. Sozzi G, Miozzo M, Cariani TC, Bongarzone I, Pilotti S, Pierotti MA. 1992. A t(2;3) (q12–13; p24–25) in follicular thyroid adenomas. Cancer Genet Cytogenet 64:38–41.

74. Herrmann MA, Hay ID, Bartelt DH Jr, Spurbeck JL, Dahl RJ, Grant CS. 1991. Cytogenetics of six follicular thyroid adenomas including a case report of an oxyphil variant with t(8:14) (q13;q24.1). Cancer Genet Cytogenet 56:231–235.

75. Roque L, Castedo S, Clode A, Soares J. 1992. Translocation t(5;19): A recurrent change in thyroid follicular adenoma. Genes Chromosom Cancer 4:346–347.

76. Dal Cin P, Sneyers W, Aly MS, et al. 1992. Involvement of 19q13 in follicular thyroid adenoma. Cancer Genet Cytogenet 60:99–101.

77. Hay ID. 1991. Cytometric DNA ploidy analysis in thyroid cancer. Diagn Oncol 1:181–185.

78. Jenkins RB, Hay ID, Herath JF, et al. 1990. Frequent occurrence of cytogenetic abnormalities in sporadic nonmedullary thyroid carcinoma. Cancer 66:1213–1220.

79. Roque L, Castedo S, Clode A, Soares J. 1993. Deletion of 3p25→pter in a primary follicular thyroid carcinoma and its metastasis. Genes Chromosom Cancer 8:199–203.

80. Gazdar AF. 1994. The molecular and cellular basis of human lung cancer. Anticancer Res 14:261–267.

81. Kratzke RA, Shimizu E, Kaye FJ. 1992. Oncogenes in human lung cancer. Cancer Treat Res 63:61–85.

82. Kovacs G. 1993. Molecular differential pathology of renal cell tumours. Histopathology 22:1–8.

83. Linehan WM, Lerman MI, Zbar B. 1995. Identification of the von Hippel-Lindau (VHL) gene. Its role in renal cancer. JAMA 273:564–570.

84. Matsuo K, Tang SH, Fagin JA. 1991. Allelotype of human thyroid tumors: Loss of chromosome 11q13 sequences in follicular neoplasms. Mol Endocrinol 5:1873–1879.

85. Pierotti MA, Santoro M, Jenkins RB, et al. 1992. Characterization of an inversion on the long arm of chromosome 10 juxtaposing D10S170 and *ret* and creating the oncogenic sequence *ret/ptc*. Proc Natl Acad Sci USA 89:1616–1620.

86. Bongarzone I, Butti MG, Coronelli S, et al. 1994. Frequent activation of ret protooncogene by fusion with a new activating gene in papillary thyroid carcinomas. Cancer Res 54:2979–2985.

87. Grieco M, Cerrato A, Santoro M, Fusco A, Melillo RM, Vecchio G. 1994. Cloning and characterization of H4 (D10S170), a gene involved in RET rearrangements in vivo. Oncogene 9:2531–2535.

88. Tong Q, Li YS, Smanik PA, et al. 1995. Characterization of the promoter region and oligomerization domain of h4 (d10s170), a gene frequently rearranged with the ret protooncogene. Oncogene 10:1781–1787.

89. Sozzi G, Bongarzone I, Miozzo M, et al. 1994. A t(10;17) translocation creates the RET/PTC2 chimeric transforming sequence in papillary thyroid carcinoma. Genes Chromosom Cancer 9:244–250.

90. Viglietto G, Chiappetta G, Martineztello FJ, et al. 1995. *PET/PTC* oncogene activation is an early event in thyroid carcinogenesis. Oncogene 11:1207–1210.

91. Santoro M, Carlomagno F, Hay ID, et al. 1992. *Ret* oncogene activation in human thyroid neoplasms is restricted to the papillary cancer subtype. J Clin Invest 89:1517–1522.

92. Bongarzone I, Pierotti MA, Monzini N, et al. 1989. Hight frequency of activation of tyrosine kinase oncogenes in human papillary thyroid carcinoma. Oncogene 4:1457–1462.

93. Greco A, Mariani C, Miranda C, et al. 1995. The DNA rearrangement that generates the *TRK-T3* oncogene involves a novel gene on chromosome 3 whose product has a potential coiled-coil domain. Mol Cell Biol 15:6118–6127.

94. Ito T, Seyama T, Iwamoto KS, et al. 1993. In vitro irradiation is able to cause RET oncogene rearrangement. Cancer Res 53:2940–2943.

95. Ito T, Seyama T, Iwamoto KS, et al. 1994. Activated RET oncogene in thyroid cancers of children from areas contaminated by Chernobyl accident. Lancet 344:259.

96. Fagin JA, Matsuo K, Karmakar A, Chen DL, Tang SH, Koeffler HP. 1993. High prevalence of mutations of the p53 gene in poorly differentiated human thyroid carcinomas. J Clin Invest 91:179–184.

97. Ito T, Seyama T, Mizuno T, et al. 1992. Unique association of p53 mutations with undifferentitated but not with differentiated carcinomas of the thyroid gland. Cancer Res 52:1369–1371.

98. Bruneton JN, Balu-Maestro C, Marcy PY. 1994. Very high frequency (13 Mhz) ultrasonographic examination of the normal neck: Detection of normal lymph nodes and thyroid nodules. J Ultrasound Med 13:87–80.

99. Belfiore A, La Rosa GL, Padova G, Sava L, Ippolito O, Vigneri R. 1987. The frequency of cold thyroid nodules and thyroid malignancies in patients from an iodine-deficient area. Cancer 60:3096–3102.

100. Martinez-Tello FJ, Martinez-Cabruja R, Fernandez-Martin J, Lasso-Oria C, Ballestin-Carcavilla C. 1993. Occult carcinoma of the thyroid. A systematic autopsy study from Spain of two series performed with two different methods. Cancer 71:4022–4029.

101. Thorvaldsson SE, Tulinius H, Bjornsson J, Bjarnason O. 1992. Latent thyroid carcinoma in Iceland at autopsy. Pathol Res Pract 188:747–750.

102. Tulinius H. 1991. Latent Malignancies at Autopsy: A Little Used Source of Information on Cancer Biology. Lyon, France: IARC Scientific Publications, pp 253–261.

103. Bisi H, Fernandes VS, de Camargo RY, Koch L, Abdo AH, de Brito T. 1989. The prevalence of unsuspected thyroid pathology in 300 sequential autopsies, with special reference to the incidental carcinoma. Cancer 64:1888–1893.

104. Fukunaga FH, Yatani R. 1975. Geographic pathology of occult thyroid carcinomas. Cancer 36:1095–1099.

105. Sampson RJ, Woolner LB, Bahn RC, Kurland LT. 1974. Occult thyroid carcinoma in Olmsted County, Minnesota: Prevalence at autopsy compared with that in Hiroshima and Nagasaki, Japan. Cancer 34:2074–2076.

106. Harach HR, Franssila KO, Wasenius VM. 1985. Occult papillary carcinoma of the thyroid. A 'normal' finding in Finland. A systematic autopsy study. Cancer 56:531–538.

107. Buraggi GL, Di Pietro S, Doci R, Rodari A. 1976. L'esame clinico e lo studio con radiocesio (131 Cs) nella diagnosi di natura dei noduli freddi tiroidei. Tumori 62:397–405.

108. Hugues FC, Baudet M, Laccourreye H. 1989 Le nodule thyroidien. Une etude retrospective de 200 observations. Ann Otolaryngol Chir Cervicofac 106:77–81.

109. Belanger R, Guillet F, Matte R, Havrankova J, d'Amour P. 1983. The thyroid nodule: Evaluation of fine-needle biopsy. J Otolaryngol 12:109–111.

110. Okamoto T, Yamashita T, Harasawa A, et al. 1994. Test performances of three diagnostic procedures in evaluating thyroid nodules: Physical examination, ultrasonography and fine needle aspiration cytology. Endocr J 41:243–247.

111. Piromalli D, Martelli G, Del Prato I, Collini P, Pilotti S. 1992. The role of fine needle aspiration in the diagnosis of thyroid nodules: Analysis of 795 consecutive cases. J Surg Oncol 50:247–250.

112. Blum M, Rothschild M. 1980. Improved nonoperative diagnosis of the solitary 'cold' thyroid nodule. Surgical selection based on risk factors and three months of suppression. JAMA 243:242–245.

113. Christensen SB, Bondeson L, Ericsson UB, Lindholm K. 1984. Prediction of malignancy in the solitary thyroid nodule by physical examination, thyroid scan, fine-needle biopsy and serum thyroglobulin. A prospective study of 100 surgically treated patients. Acta Chir Scand 150:433–439.

114. Nelson RL, Wahner HW, Gorman CA. 1978. Rectilinear thyroid scanning as a predictor of malignancy. Ann Intern Med 88:41–44.

115. Hermans J, Schmitz A, Merlo P, Bodart F, Beauduin M. 1993. Le thallium 201 permet-il de differencier le nodule thyroidien benin du nodule malin? Ann Endocrinol 54:248–254.

116. Leisner B. 1987. Ultrasound evaluation of thyroid diseases. Horm Res 26:33–41.

117. Solbiati L, Volterrani L, Rizzatto G, et al. 1985. The thyroid gland with low uptake lesions: Evaluation by ultrasound. Radiology 155:187–191.
118. Seya A, Oeda T, Terano T, et al. 1990. Comparative studies on fine-needle aspiration cytology with ultrasound scanning in the assessment of thyroid nodule. Jpn J Med 29:478–480.
119. Hamburger JI. 1994. Diagnosis of thyroid nodules by fine needle biopsy: Use and abuse. J Clin Endocrinol Metab 79:335–339.
120. Gharib H. 1994. Fine-needle aspiration biopsy of thyroid nodules: Advantages, limitations, and effect. Mayo Clin Proc 69:44–49.
121. McHenry CR, Walfish PG, Rosen IB. 1993. Non-diagnostic fine needle aspiration biopsy: A dilemma in management of nodular thyroid disease. Am Surg 59:415–419.
122. Takashima S, Fukuda H, Kobayashi T. 1994. Thyroid nodules: Clinical effect of ultrasound-guided fine-needle aspiration biopsy. J Clin Ultrasound 22:535–542.
123. Yokozawa T, Miyauchi A, Kuma K, Sugawara M. 1995. Accurate and simple method of diagnosing thyroid nodules: The modified technique of ultrasound-guided fine needle aspiration biopsy. Thyroid 5:141–145.
124. Akslen LA, Haldorsen T, Thoresen S, Glattre E. 1991. Survival and causes of death in thyroid cancer: A population based study of 2479 cases from Norway. Cancer Res 51:1234–1241.
125. Akslen LA, Myking AO, Salvesen H, Varhaug JE. 1993. Prognostic importance of various clinicopathological features in papillary thyroid carcinoma. Eur J Cancer 29A:44–51.
126. Ladurner D, Seeber G. 1984. Das follikuläre Schilddrüsenkarzinom. Eine multivariate Analyse. Schweiz Med Wochenschr 114:1087–1092.
127. Hay ID, Bergstralh EJ, Goellner JR, Ebersold JR, Grant CS. 1993. Predicting outcome in papillary thyroid carcinoma: Development of a reliable prognostic scoring system in a cohort of 1779 patients surgically treated at one institution during 1940 through 1989. Surgery 114:1050–1958.
128. Ladurner D, Seeber G, Hofstädter F, Zechmann W. 1985. Das differenzierte Schilddrüsenkarzinom im Endemiegebiet. Dtsch Med Wochenschr 110:333–338.
129. Sethi VK. 1990. Differentiated thyroid cancer: Outcome of treatment in 80 cases. Ann Acad Med 19:433–438.
130. Salvesen H, Njølstad PR, Akslen LA, Albrektsen G, Søereide O, Varhaug JE. 1992. Papillary thyroid carcinoma: A multivariate analysis of prognostic factors including an evaluation of the p-TNM staging system. Eur J Surg 158:583–589.
131. Simpson WJ, Panzarella T, Carruthers JS, Gospodarowicz MK, Sutcliffe SB. 1988. Papillary and follicular thyroid cancer: Impact of treatment in 1578 patients. Int J Radiat Oncol Biol Phys 14:1063–1075.
132. Friedman M, Danielzadeh JA, Caldarelli DD. 1994. Treatment of patients with carcinoma of the thyroid invading the airway. Arch Otolaryngol Head Neck Surg 120:1377–1381.
133. Ballantyne AJ. 1994. Resections of the upper aerodigestive tract for locally invasive thyroid cancer. Am J Surg 168:636–639.
134. Friedman M, Skolnik EM, Baim HM, Becker SP, Katz AH, Montravadi RVD. 1980. Thyroid carcinoma. Laryngoscope 90:1991–2003.
135. Brennan MD, Bergstralh EJ, van Heerden JA, McConahey WM. 1991. Follicular thyroid cancer treated at the Mayo Clinic, 1946 through 1970: Initial manifestations, pathologic findings, therapy, and outcome. Mayo Clin Proc 66:11–22.
136. Scheumann GF, Gimm O, Wegener G, Hundeshagen H, Dralle H. 1994. Prognostic significance and surgical management of locoregional lymph node metastases in papillary thyroid cancer. World J Surg 18:559–67
137. Staunton MD. 1994. Thyroid cancer: A multivariate analysis on influence of treatment on long-term survival. Eur J Surg Oncol 20:613–621.
138. Tourniaire J, Bernard-Auger MH, Adeleine P, Milan JJ, Fleury-Goyon MC, Dutrieux-Berger N. 1989. Les éléments du pronostic des cancers thyroïdiens différenciés. Ann Endocrinol 50:219–224.

134

139. Van Nguyen K, Dilawari RA. 1995. Predictive value of AMES scoring system in selection of extent of surgery in well differentiated carcinoma of thyroid. Am Surg 61:151–155.
140. Böttger T, Klupp J, Sorger K, Junninger T. 1990. Prognostisch relevante Faktoren beim follikulären Schilddrüsenkarzinom. Langenbecks Arch Chir 375:266–271.
141. Ruiz de Almodóvar JM, Ruiz-García J, Olea N, Villalobos M, Pedraza V. 1994. Analysis of risk of death from differentiated thyroid cancer. Radiother Oncol 31:199–206.
142. Böttger T, Klupp J, Gabbert HE, Junginger T. 1991. Prognostisch relevante Faktoren Beim papillären Schilddrüsenkarzinom. Med Klin 86:76–82.
143. Franssila KO. 1975. Prognosis in thyroid carcinoma. Cancer 36:1138–1146.
144. Carcangiu ML, Zampi G, Pupi A, Castagnoli A, Rosai J. 1985. Papillary carcinoma of the thyroid. Cancer 55:805–828.
145. Shaw JH, Dodds P. 1990. Carcinoma of the thyroid gland in Auckland, New Zealand. Surg Gynecol Obstet 171:27–32.
146. DeGroot LJ, Kaplan EL, Straus FH, Shukla MS. 1994. Does the method of management of papillary thyroid carcinoma make a difference in outcome? World J Surg 18:123–130.
147. Rösler H, Birrer A, Lüscher D, Kinser J. 1992. Langzeitverläufe beim differenzierten Schilddrüsenkarzinom. Schweiz Med Wochenschr 122:1843–1857.
148. DeGroot LJ, Kaplan EL, Shukla MS, Salti G, Straus FH. 1995. Morbidity and mortality in follicular thyroid cancer. J Clin Endocrinol Metab 80:2946–2953.
149. Joensuu H, Klemi PJ, Paul R, Tuominen J. 1986. Survival and prognostic factors in thyroid carcinoma. Acta Radiol Oncol 25:243–248.
150. Mizukami Y, Noguchi M, Michigishi T, et al. 1992. Papillary thyroid carcinoma in Kanazawa, Japan: Prognostc significance of histological subtypes. Histopathology 20:243–250.
151. Cunningham MP, Duda RB, Recant W, Chmiel JS, Sylvester J, Fremgen A. 1990. Survival discriminants for differentiated thyroid cancer. Am J Surg 160:344–347.
152. Samaan NA, Schultz PN, Hickey RC, Goepfert H, Haynie TP, Johnston DA. 1992. The results of various modalities of treatment of well differentiated thyroid carcinomas: A retrospective review of 1599 patients. J Clin Endocrinol Metab 75:714–720.
153. Mazzaferri EL. Young RL. 1981. Papillary thyroid carcinoma: A 10 year follow-up report of the impact of therapy in 576 patients. Am J Med 70:511–518.
154. Szántó J, Ringwald G, Karika Z, Liszka G, Péter H, Daubner K. 1991. Follicular cancer of the thyroid gland. Oncology 48:483–489.
155. Guillamondegui OM, Mikhail RA. 1983. The treatment of differentiated carcinoma of the thytoid gland. Arch Otolaryngol Head Neck Surg 109:743–745.
156. Hay ID, Grant CS, Taylor WF, McConahey WM. 1987. Ipsilateral lobectomy versus bilateral lobar resection in papillary thyroid carcinoma: A retrospective analysis of surgical outcome using a novel prognostic scoring system. Surgery 102:1088–1095.
157. DeGroot LJ, Kaplan EL, McCormick M, Straus FH. 1990. Natural history, treatment, and course of papillary thyroid carcinoma. J Clin Endocrinol Metab 71:414–424.
158. Mazzaferri EL, Jhiang SM. 1994. Long-term impact of initial surgical and medical therapy on papillary and follicular thyroid cancer. Am J Med 97:418–428.
159. Andry G, Chantrain G, van Glabbeke M, Dor P. 1988. Papillary and follicular thyroid carcinoma. Individualization of the treatment according to the prognosis of the disease. Eur J Cancer Clin Oncol 24:1641–1646.
160. Wahl R, Nievergelt J, Röher HD, Oellers B. 1977. Radikale Thyroidectomie wegen maligner Schilddrüsentumoren. Dtsch Med Wochenschr 102:13–20.
161. Smith SA, Hay ID, Goellner JR, Ryan JJ, McConahey WM. 1988. Mortality from papillary thyroid carcinoma. Cancer 62:1381–1388.
162. Preda F, Cascinelli N, Pizzocaro G, Zingo L, Stefanoni R, Balzarini GP. 1970. Programmazione terapeutica e prognosi dei tumori maligni della tiroide. Arch Italiano Chir 96:105–135.
163. Blondeau P. 1992. Le cancer thyroïdien est-il un cancer grave? (Étude pronostique de 800 cas opérés dont 143 nodulaires différenciés suivis plus de vingt ans). Bull Acad Natle Med 176:1087–1096.

164. Ito J, Noguchi S, Murakami N, Noguchi A. 1980. Factors affecting the prognosis of patients with carcinoma of the thyroid. Surg Gynecol Obstet 150:539–544.

165. Grant CS, Hay ID, Gough IR, Bergstralh EJ, Goellner JR, McConahey WM. 1988. Local recurrence in papillary thyroid carcinoma: Is extent of surgical resection important? Surgery 104:954–962.

166. Goretzki PE, Simon D, Frilling A, et al. 1993. Surgical reintervention for differentiated thyroid cancer. Br J Surg 80:1009–1012.

167. Calabro S, Auguste LJ, Attie JN. 1988. Morbidity of completion thyroidectomy for initially misdiagnosed thyroid carcinoma. Head Neck Surg 10:235–238.

168. DeGroot LJ, Kaplan EL. 1991. Second operations for 'completion' of thyroidectomy in treatment of differentiated thyroid cancer. Surgery 110:936–993.

169. Clark OH. 1982. Total thyroidectomy: The treatment of choice for patients with differentiated thyroid cancer. Ann Surg 196:361–370.

170. Hamming JF, van de Velde CJH, Goslings BM, et al. 1989. Prognosis and morbidity after total thyroidectomy for papillary, follicular and medullary thyroid cancer. Eur J Clin Oncol 25:1317–1323.

171. McConahey WM, Hay ID, Woolner LB, van Heerden JA, Taylor WF. 1986. Papillary thyroid cancer treated at the Mayo Clinic, 1946 through 1970: Initial manifestations, pathologic findings, therapy, and outcome. Mayo Clin Proc 61:978–996.

172. Staunton MD, Bourne H. 1993. Thyroid cancer in the 1980s a decade of change. Ann Acad Med 22:13–16.

173. Kern KA. 1993. Medicolegal analysis of errors in diagnosis and treatment of surgical endocrine disease. Surgery 114:1167–1173

174. Arad E, O'Mara RE, Wilson GA. 1993. Ablation of remaining functioning thyroid lobe with radioiodine after hemithyroidectomy for carcinoma. Clin Nucl Med 18:662–663.

175. DiRusso G, Kern KA. 1994. Comparative analysis of complications from I-131 radioablation for well-differentiated thyroid cancer. Surgery 116:1024–1030.

176. Block MA, Miller JM, Horn RC Jr. 1971. Thyroid carcinoma with cervical lymph node metastasis. Effectiveness of total thyroidectomy and node dissection. Am J Surg 122:458–463.

177. Noguchi S, Murakami N, Kawamoto H. 1994. Classification of papillary cancer of the thyroid based on prognosis. World J Surg 18:552–557

178. Nel CJ, van Heerden JA, Goellner JR, et al. 1985. Anaplastic carcinoma of the thyroid: A clinicopathologic study of 82 cases. Mayo Clin Proc 60:51–58.

179. Rossi R, Cady B, Meissner WA, Sedwick CE, Werber J. 1978. Prognosis of undifferentiated carcinoma and lymphoma of the thyroid. Am J Surg 135:589–596.

180. Lindahl F. 1975. Papillary thyroid carcinoma in Denmark 1943–68. II. Treatment and survival. Acta Chir Scand 141:504–513.

181. Rossi RL, Cady B, Silverman ML, et al. 1988. Surgically incurable well-differentiated thyroid carcinoma. Arch Surg 123:569–574.

182. Beahrs OH, Henson DE, Hutter RVP. 1992. Manual for Staging Cancer. Philadelphia: J.B. Lippincott.

183. Hay ID. 1990. Papillary thyroid carcinoma. Endocrinol Metab Clin North Am 19:545–576.

184. van Heerden JA, Hay ID, Goellner JR, et al. 1992. Follicular thyroid carcinoma with capsular invasion alone: A nonthreatening malignancy. Surgery 112:1130–1138.

185. Herrera MF, Hay ID, Wu PS-C, et al. 1992. Hürthle cell (oxyphilic) papillary thyroid carcinoma: A variant with more aggressive biological behavior. World J Surg 16:669–675.

186. Cady B, Rossi R. 1988. An expanded view of risk-group definition in differentiated thyroid carcinoma. Surgery 104:947–953.

187. Shaha AR, Loree TR, Shah JP. 1995. Prognostic factors and risk group analysis in follicular carcinoma of the thyroid. Surgery 118:1131–1138.

188. Loree TR. 1995. Therapeutic implications of prognostic factors in differentiated carcinoma of the thyroid gland. Semin Surg Oncol 11:246–255.

189. Dulgeroff AJ, Hershman JM. 1994. Medical therapy for differentiated thyroid carcinoma. Endocr Rev 15:500–515.

190. Davis NL, Bugis SP, McGregor GI, Germann E. 1995. An evaluation of prognostic scoring systems in patients with follicular thyroid cancer. Am J Surg 170:476–480.

191. Giannini S, Nobile M, Sartori L, et al. 1994. Bone density and mineral metabolism in thyroidectomized patients treated with long-term L-thyroxine. Clin Sci 87:593–597.

192. Marcocci C, Golia F, Bruno-Bossio G, Vignali E, Pinchera A. 1994. Carefully monitored levothyroxine suppressive therapy is not associated with bone loss in premenopausal women. J Clin Endocrinol Metab 78:818–823.

193. Taimela E, Taimela S, Nikkanen V, Irjala K. 1994. Accelerated bone degradation in thyroid carcinoma patients during thyroxine treatment, measured by determination of the carboxyterminal telopeptide region of type I collagen in serum. Eur J Clin Chem Clin Biochem 32:827–831.

194. Wong JB, Kaplan MM, Meyer KB, Pauker SG. 1990. Ablative radioactive iodine therapy for apparently localized thyroid carcinoma. A decision analytic perspective. Endocrinol Metab Clin North Am 19:741–760.

195. Maxon HR, III, Smith HS. 1990. Radioiodine-131 in the diagnosis and treatment of metastatic well differentiated thyroid cancer. Endocrinol Metab Clin North Am 19:685–718.

196. Blahd WH, Nordyke RA, Baver FK. 1960. Radioactive iodine (I^{131}) in the postoperative treatment of thyroid cancer. Cancer 13:745–756.

197. Varma VM, Beierwaltes WH, Nofal MM, Nishiyama RH, Copp JE. 1970. Treatment of thyroid cancer. Death rates after surgery and after surgery followed by sodium iodide I-131. JAMA 214:1437–1442.

198. Sisson JC. 1983. Applying the radioactive eraser: I-131 to ablate hormonal thyroid tissue in patients from whom thyroid cancer has been resected. J Nucl Med 24:743–744.

199. Snyder J, Gorman C, Scanlon P. 1983. Thyroid remnant ablation: Questionable pursuit of an ill-defined goal. J Nucl Med 24:659–665.

200. Beierwaltes WH, Rabbani R, Dmuchowski C, Lloyd RV, Eyre P, Mallette S. 1984. An analysis of 'ablation of thyroid remnants' with I-131 in 511 patients from 1947–1984: Experience at University of Michigan. J Nucl Med 25:1287–1293.

201. Crile G, Jr. 1971. Changing end results in patients with papillary carcinoma of the thyroid. Surg Gynecol Obstet 132:460–468.

202. Cady B, Sedgwick CE, Meissner WA, Bookwalter JR, Romagosa V, Werber J. 1976. Changing clinical, pathologic, therapeutic, and survival patterns in differentiated thyroid carcinoma. Ann Surg 184:541–553.

203. Tubiana M, Schlumberger M, Rougier P, et al. 1985. Long-term results and prognostic factors in patients with differentiated thyroid carcinoma. Cancer 55:794–804.

204. Hrafnkelsson J, Jonasson JG, Sigurdson G, Sigvaldson H, Tulinius H. 1988. Thyroid cancer in Iceland 1955–1984. Acta Endocrinol 118:566–572.

205. LiVolsi VA, Asa SL. 1994. The demise of follicular carcinoma of the thyroid gland. Thyroid 4:233–236.

206. Mazzaferri EL. 1987. Papillary thyroid carcinoma: Factors influencing prognosis and current therapy. Semin Oncol 14:315–332.

207. DeGroot LJ. 1994. Long-term impact of initial and surgical therapy on papillary and follicular thyroid cancer. Am J Med 97:499–500.

208. Hay ID, Grant CS, van Heerden JA, Goellner JR, Ebersold JR. 1992. Papillary thyroid microcarcinoma: A study of 535 cases observed in a 50-year period. Surgery 112:1139–1146.

209. Russell MA, Gilbert EF, Jaeschke WF. 1975. Prognostic features of thyroid cancer. Cancer 36:553–559.

210. Schümichen CE, Schmitt E, Scheufele C, Blattmann H, Pauli-Harnasch C. 1983. Einfluß des Therapiekonzepts auf die Prognose des Schilddrüsenkarzinoms. Nucl Med 22:97–105.

211. Tubiana M, Haddad E, Schlumberger M, Hill C, Rougier P, Sarrazin D. 1985. External radiotherapy in thyroid cancers. Cancer 55:2062–2071.

212. Handelsman DJ, Turtle JR. 1983. Testicular damage after radioactive iodine (I-131) therapy for thyroid cancer. Clin Endocrinol 18:465–472.
213. Keldsen N, Mortensen BT, Hansen HS. 1990. Haematological effects from radioiodine treatment of thyroid carcinoma. Acta Oncol 29:1035–1039.
214. Raymond JP, Izembart M, Marliac V, Dagousset F, Merceron RE, Vallee G. 1989. Temporary ovarian failure in thyroid cancer patients after thyroid remnant ablation with radioactive iodine. J Clin Endocrinol Metab 69:186–190.
215. Gunter HH, Schober O, Schwarzrock R, Hundeshagen H. 1987. Hämatologische Langzeitveränderungen nach Radiojodtherapie des Schilddrüsenkarzinoms. II. Knochenmarkveränderungen einschliesslich Leukämien. Strahlenther Onkol 163:475–485.
216. Schober O, Gunter HH, Schwarzrock R, Hundeshagen H. 1987. Hämatologische Langzeitveränderungen nach Radiojodtherapie des Schilddrüsenkarzinoms. I. Periphere Blutbildveränderungen. Strahlenther Onkol 163:464–474.
217. Pacini F, Gasperi M, Fugazzola L, et al. 1994. Testicular function in patients with differentiated thyroid carcinoma treated with radioiodine. J Nucl Med 35:1418–1422.
218. Ahmed SR, Shalet SM. 1985. Gonadal damage due to radioactive iodine (I131) treatment for thyroid carcinoma. Postgrad Med J 61:361–362.
219. Edmonds CJ, Smith T. 1986. The long-term hazards of the treatment of thyroid cancer with radioiodine. Br J Radiol 59:45–51.
220. Hall P, Holm LE. 1995. Cancer in iodine-131 exposed patients. J Endocrinol Invest 18:147–149.
221. Heufelder AE, Gorman CA. 1991. Radioiodine therapy in the treatment of differentiated thyroid cancer: Guidelines and considerations. Endocrinologist 1:273–280.
222. Logue JP, Tsang RW, Brierley JD, Simpson WJ. 1994. Radioiodine ablation of residual tissue in thyroid cancer: Relationship between administered activity, neck uptake and outcome. Br J Radiol 67:1127–1131.
223. Samuel AM, Rajashekharrao B. 1994. Radioiodine therapy for well-differentiated thyroid cancer: A quantitative dosimetric evaluation for remnant thyroid ablation after surgery. J Nucl Med 35:1944–1950.
224. Park HM, Perkins OW, Edmondson JW, Schnute RB, Manatunga A. 1994. Influence of diagnostic radioiodines on the uptake of ablative dose of iodine-131. Thyroid 4:49–54.
225. Brierley JD, Tsang RW. 1996. External radiation therapy in the treatment of thyroid malignancy. Endocrinol Metab Clin North Am 25:141–157.
226. O'Connell ME, A'Hern RP, Harmer CL. 1994. Results of external beam radiotherapy in differentiated thyroid carcinoma: A retrospective study from the Royal Marsden Hospital. Eur J Cancer 30A:733–739.
227. DeGroot LJ. 1995. Thyroid neoplasia. In DeGroot LJ, Besser M, Burger HG, Jameson JL, Loriaux DL, Odell WD, Potts Jr JT, Rubenstein AH, eds. Endocrinology. Philadelphia: W.B. Saunders, pp 834–854.
228. Kim JH, Leeper RD. 1987. Treatment of locally advanced thyroid carcinoma with combination doxorubicin and radiation therapy. Cancer 60:2372–2375.
229. Busnardo B, Girelli ME, Nacamulli D, Pelizzo MR, Daniele O, Rigon A. 1994. Il carcinoma indifferenziato della tiroide. Chir Ital 46:37–41.
230. Tennvall J, Lundell G, Hallquist A, Wahlberg P, Wallin G, Tibblin S. 1994. Combined doxorubicin, hyperfractionated radiotherapy, and surgery in anaplastic thyroid carcinoma. Report on two protocols. The Swedish Anaplastic Thyroid Cancer Group. Cancer 74:1348–1354.
231. Durie BG, Hellman D, Woolfenden JM, O'Mara R, Kartchner M, Salmon SE. 1981. High-risk thyroid cancer. Prolonged survival with early multimodality therapy. Cancer Clin Trial 4:67–73.
232. Tallroth E, Wallin G, Lundell G, Lowhagen T, Einhorn J. 1987. Multimodality treatment in anaplastic giant cell thyroid carcinoma. Cancer 60:1428–1431.
233. Palestini N, Papotti M, Durando R, Fortunato MA. 1993. Il carcinoma scarsamente differenziato 'insulare' della tiroide: Sopravvivenza a distanza. Minerva Chir 48:1301–1305.

234. Cannizzaro MA, De Maria A, Fazzi C, et al. 1993. Il carcinoma anaplastico della tiroide: Sopravvivenza a distanza. Minerva Chir 48:1293–1299.

235. Schlumberger M, Parmentier C, Delisle MJ, Couette JE, Droz JP. 1991. Combination therapy for anaplastic giant cell thyroid carcinoma. Cancer 67:564–566.

236. Benker G, Reinwein D. 1983. Ergebnisse der Chemotherapie des Schilddrusenkarzinoms. Dtsch Med Wochenschr 108:403–406.

237. Dinneen SF, Valimaki MJ, Bergstralh EJ, Goellner JR, Gorman CA, Hay ID. 1995. Distant metastases in papillary thyroid carcinoma: 100 cases observed at one institution during 5 decades. J Clin Endocrinol Metab 80:2041–2045.

238. Ozata M, Suzuki S, Miyamoto T, Liu RT, Fierro-Renoy F, DeGroot LJ. 1994. Serum thyroglobulin in the follow-up of patients with treated differentiated thyroid cancer. J Clin Endocrinol Metab 79:98–105.

239. Berding G, Hufner M, Georgi P. 1992. Thyreoglobulin, 131J-Ganzkorperszintigraphie und Risikofaktoren in der Nachsorge des differenzierten Schilddrusenkarzinomas. Nucl Med 31:32–37.

240. Ericsson UB, Tegler L, Lennquist S, Christensen SB, Stahl E, Thorell JI. 1984. Serum thyroglobulin in differentiated thyroid carcinoma. Acta Chir Scand 150:367–375.

241. Kumar A, Shah DH, Shrihari U, Dandekar SR, Vijayan U, Sharma SM. 1994. Significance of antithyroglobulin autoantibodies in differentiated thyroid carcinoma. Thyroid 4:199–202.

242. Pacini F, Mariotti S, Formica N, Elisei R, Anelli S, Capotorti E. 1988. Thyroid autoantibodies in thyroid cancer: Incidence and relationship with tumour outcome. Acta Endocrinol 119:373–380.

243. Rubello D, Casara D, Girelli ME, Piccolo M, Busnardo B. 1992. Clinical meaning of circulating antithyroglobulin antibodies in differentiated thyroid cancer: A prospective study. J Nucl Med 33:1478–1480.

244. Grebe SKG, Hay ID. 1995. Management of differentiated thyroid cancer. Curr Opin Endocrinol Diab 2:449–454.

245. Delorme S. 1993. Sonographie vergrößerter zervikaler Lymphknoten. Bildgebung 60:267–260.

246. Solbiati L, Cioffi V, Ballarati E. 1992. Ultrasonography of the neck. Radiol Clin North Am 30:941–940.

247. Sutton RT, Reading CC, Charboneau JW, et al. 1988. US-guided biopsy of neck masses in postoperative management of patients with thyroid cancer. Radiology 168:769–760.

248. Meier CA, Braverman LE, Ebner SA, et al. 1994. Diagnostic use of recombinant human thyrotropin in patients with thyroid carcinoma (phase I/II study). J Clin Endocrinol Metab 78:188–196.

249. Mallin WH, Elgazzar AH, Maxon HR. 1994. Imaging modalities in the follow-up of non-iodine avid thyroid carcinoma. Am J Otolaryngol 15:417–422.

250. Niederle B, Roka R, Schemper M, Fritsch A, Weissel M, Ramach W. 1986. Surgical treatment of distant metastases in differentiated thyroid cancer: Indication and results. Surgery 100:1088–1097.

251. Glanzmann C, Horst W. 1979. Therapie des metastasierenden Schilddrüsenadenokarzinoms mit 131-Jod. Erfahrungen bei 103 Patienten aus dem Zeitraum 1963 bis 1977. Strahlentherapie 155:223–229.

252. Maxon HR, Smith HS. 1990. Radioiodine-131 in the diagnosis and treatment of metastatic well differentiated thyroid cancer. Endocrinol Metab Clin North Am 19:685–718.

253. Nemec J, Zamrazil V, Pohunková D, Röhling S. 1979. Radioiodide treatment of pulmonary metastases of differentiated thyroid cancer. Nucl Med 18:86–90.

254. Marcocci C, Pacini F, Elisei R, et al. 1989. Clinical and biologic behavior of bone metastases from differentiated thyroid carcinoma. Surgery 106:960–966.

255. Biswal BM, Bal CS, Sandhu MS, Padhy AK, Rath GK. 1994. Management of intracranial metastases of differentiated carcinoma of thyroid. J Neuro Oncol 22:77–81.

256. Datz FL. 1986. Cerebral edema following iodine-131 therapy for thyroid carcinoma meta-static to the brain. J Nucl Med 27:637–640.
257. Ahuja S, Ernest H. 1987. Chemotherapy for thyroid carcinoma. J Endocrinol Invest 10:303–310.
258. Schreck R, Schnieders F, Schmutzler C, Kohrle J. 1994. Retinoids stimulate type I iodothyronine 5'-deiodinase activity in human follicular thyroid carcinoma cell lines. J Clin Endocrinol Metab 79:791–798.
259. Trieb K, Sztankay A, Amberger A, Lechner H, Grubeck-Loebenstein B. 1994. Hyperthermia inhibits proliferation and stimulates the expression of differentiation markers in cultured thyroid carcinoma cells. Cancer Lett 87:65–71.
260. Zlock DW, Greenspan FS, Clark OH, Higgins CB. 1994. Octreotide therapy in advanced thyroid cancer. Thyroid 4:427–431.
261. Selzer E, Wilfing A, Sexl V, Freissmuth M. 1994. Effects of type I-interferons on human thyroid epithelial cells derived from normal and tumour tissue. Naunyn Schmiedebergs Arch Pharmacol 350:322–328.
262. Atkins MB, Mier JW, Parkinson DR, Gould JA, Berkman EM, Kaplan MM. 1988. Hypothyroidism after treament with interleukin-2 and lymphokine-activated killer cells. N Engl J Med 318:1557–1563.
263. Vialettes B, Guillerand MA, Viens P, et al. 1993. Incidence rate and risk factors for thyroid dysfunction during recombinant interleukin-2 therapy in advanced malignancies. Acta Endocrinol 129:31–38.
264. Amino N, Pysher T, Cohen EP, DeGroot LJ. 1975. Immunologic aspects of human thyroid cancer. Humoral and cell mediated immunity, and a trial of immunotherapy. Cancer 36:963–973.

7. Radiation-induced endocrine tumors

Arthur B. Schneider and Leon Fogelfeld

In 1974 radiation and thyroid cancer were big news in Chicago. The news was not that the two were related, a fact that was relatively well established by that time [1–3], but that thousands of people had received head and neck irradiation during their childhood and were now at risk for developing thyroid cancer. Two years later the concern broadened to the entire United States, when the National Institutes of Health (NIH) initiated a publicity campaign to alert people who may not have been aware that they were exposed to radiation during childhood. Over time more and more people learned that they were exposed to radiation. The U.S. Government belatedly confirmed that many individuals had been exposed to radiation released from the Hanford nuclear reactor and from other nuclear installations.

More recently, the government completed a large effort to identify human experiments involving radioisotopes in which incomplete or no information was provided to the subjects. Similarly, the U.S. military has recently confirmed that aviators and submariners in the 1940s were treated with radiation placed in the nasopharynx to maintain the patency of the eustachian tube in order to permit them to adapt to sudden changes in pressure. Now, one hopes that there will be no more revelations of radiation exposure and no more accidental releases, such as the Chernobyl disaster. In fact, rather than 'big news,' it is more common for the authors to hear comments such as, 'Are you *still* working on radiation and the thyroid?,' or 'Haven't you found everybody yet?' To respond to these question, we will review what has been learned during the last 20 years, where progress is being made, and how long the effects of radiation persist.

This review is divided into three sections. The first considers the evidence establishing a relationship between radiation exposure and tumors of the thyroid, parathyroid, and other tissues in the head and neck area. This section emphasizes dose-response relationships and the evidence that radiation-induced tumors continue to occur. The second section considers the evaluation and treatment of patients who were exposed to childhood radiation. Because this subject has been covered in other reviews [4–7], only the important principles and most recent findings are stressed. Finally, the last section reviews the pathogenesis of radiation-induced endocrine tumors, the potential

Andrew Arnold (ed.) ENDOCRINE NEOPLASMS. 1997. Kluwer Academic Publishers. ISBN 0-7923-4354-9.
All rights reserved.

role of somatic mutations in cancer genes, and the evidence for susceptibility factors.

Evidence for the role of radiation at various sites

Parathyroid glands

Hyperparathyroidism is one of the less common adverse effects of childhood radiation exposure. However, it is useful to consider it first because it illustrates several important points. Among these are the difficulties in establishing the relationship between radiation and hyperparathyroidism in a convincing manner. Case reports and then case-control studies offered the first support for the relationship [8,9]. However, hyperparathyroidism is most often an asymptomatic condition. Therefore, case finding based on clinical presentation or routine clinical care may result in biased ascertainment of cases. Also, the history of childhood radiation may be unreliable, leading to misclassification. Finally, case-control studies cannot establish a dose-response relationship. Cohort (prospective) studies overcome many of these difficulties. By selecting a cohort with known radiation exposure, the following is accomplished: The fact of radiation exposure is established by membership in the cohort, asymptomatic conditions can be detected by screening the cohort, and determination of organ doses is possible. Therefore, the existence of a dose-response relationship in a cohort study is among the most convincing findings supporting a causal role for radiation.

A particular difficulty for studying hyperparathyroidism is the lack of detailed information about the age-dependent frequency of hyperparathyroidism in the general population. Because this is not a malignant condition, registry data are not available. Further, it is rarely, if ever, possible to establish the age of onset. When we found a relatively large number of cases in the cohort we are studying at Michael Reese Hospital, the comparison to the general population was difficult and uncertain. However, we were able to conclude that the cases indicated an effect of radiation [10].

In order to establish a dose-response relationship, it was necessary to determine the organ dose received many years ago; the difficultly of this is obvious. In our study at Michael Reese, the older therapy machines were no longer available, and there was uncertainty about the orientation of rectangular ports. The difficulty of reconstructing the doses received by survivors of the atomic explosions in Japan is well known and is illustrated by the revisions that have occurred. However, dose uncertainty makes it more difficult to show a dose-response relationship, and when one is found, it is even more persuasive.

Three studies establish a dose-response relationship for hyperparathyroidism, one among atomic bomb survivors, one among people treated with x-rays for tuberculous cervical adenitis, and ours among people treated during childhood for benign conditions in the head and neck area. In atomic bomb survivors, Fujiwara et al. [11] found 16 cases in 2365 exposed individuals compared with an expected 4.8 cases. In 444 people treated for cervical adenitis, Tisell et al. [12] found 63 cases of hyperparathyroidism. In the Michael Reese cohort [13], 36 cases were reported in 2555 subjects. The dose-response relationship found in the Michael Reese cohort is shown in Figure 1.

The slope of the dose-response curve is difficult to determine because of the wide confidence interval. This is due, in part, to the relatively small number of cases. Therefore, it is reassuring that the other study that included children, the atomic bomb survivors, had a similar slope (0.11/cGy vs. 0.10/cGy for the excess relative risk). It is important to recognize that one of the factors that may account for the relatively small number of cases is the small size of the parathyroid glands. The effects of radiation on a particular organ are dependent on at least three factors: (1) the dose of radiation, (2) the sensitivity of the tissue, and (3) the volume of the tissue.

The clinical data indicate that the clinical course of hyperparathyroidism in irradiated patients is similar to its course in nonirradiated patients. No cases of parathyroid carcinoma were found in the three cohort studies. Nonfunctioning

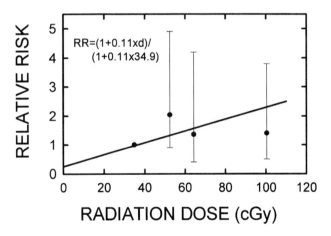

HYPERPARATHYROIDISM

$$RR = \frac{(1 + 0.11 \times d)}{(1 + 0.11 \times 34.9)}$$

Figure 1. Dose-response relationship for hyperparathyroidism for Michael Reese Hospital cohort. There were 36 cases of hyperparathyroidism among 2555 subjects. The doses to the parathyroid glands were divided into four intervals (<50, 50–59, 60–69, ≥70 cGy). The points are placed horizontally at the mean dose for each interval. The line was adjusted to pass through the point for the lowest dose group that was assigned a relative risk of 1. The slope of the relationship was significant, with a 95% confidence interval of 0.0–17.2 around the estimate of 0.11 for excess relative risk per cGy. (From Schneider AB, Gierlowski TC, Shore-Freedman E, et al. Dose-response relationships for radiation-induced hyperparathyroidism. J Clin Endocrinol Metab 80:254–257, 1995. © The Endocrine Society, by permission.)

parathyroid adenomas were found in the Michael Reese cohort and have been reported by others. These are discovered during surgery for radiation-induced thyroid tumors in patients with normal serum calcium levels. It has not been possible to determine whether these occur in excess in irradiated individuals.

One feature may distinguish patients with radiation-induced hyperparathyroidism, that is, they appear to have a higher frequency of radiation-induced thyroid tumors than other individuals exposed to comparable amounts of radiation during childhood [10,14]. As discussed later, this suggests that some patients may be especially sensitive to radiation. Because of the factors mentioned earlier, it is difficult to determine how long the risk of radiation-induced hyperparathyroidism lasts. In the Michael Reese cohort, it is clear that cases of hyperparathyroidism continue to occur, but this may be as much a function of age as of radiation exposure [13]. As long as cases conform to a significant dose-response pattern, it is possible to conclude that there is still an effect of radiation. However, there were too few cases of hyperparathyroidism to determine the time trend for the dose-response curve, as was done for thyroid cancer (see later).

Thyroid gland

One could say, without too much exaggeration, that the thyroid gland has suffered the most and benefitted the most from radiation. It has suffered because it is one of the most sensitive organs to the tumor-producing effects of radiation. This is demonstrated in three ways: (1) the number of radiation-induced thyroid tumors is very high, (2) the slope of the dose-response relationship is high, and (3) nodules and cancer have been demonstrated after very small doses of exposure. The thyroid has benefitted from the use of radioactive iodine and related isotopes for the evaluation of the thyroid and for the treatment of hyperthyroidism and thyroid cancer. This apparently paradoxical situation arises from the incompletely understood differences between external and internal radiation exposure of the thyroid.

Low dose. In Israel, 10,834 immigrant children with tinea capitis had their scalp irradiated to remove their hair to facilitate treatment. Their thyroid glands, being far removed from the site of irradiation, received a mean of 9 cGy. Careful studies of this group showed that even at this low dose, there was a distinct increase in thyroid tumors [15]. Because the thyroid is so sensitive, thyroid nodules or thyroid cancer have been the endpoint of several studies of very low-dose radiation exposure. In China, 27,011 diagnostic x-ray workers developed more thyroid cancer (relative risk = 2.1) than other medical workers [16]. This received partial confirmation in a more recent study that, using thyroid ultrasound to detect nodules, found more nodules in 50 male medical workers with occupational exposure (38%) than in two control groups (19% and 13%) [17]. To determine if exposure to radiation from diagnostic x-ray is associated with thyroid cancer, Inskip et al. [18] ascertained 484 cases of thyroid cancer in Sweden and compared them with controls. The two groups had similar numbers of diagnostic x-rays, at similar ages, and of similar types. Thus, there is no established relationship between diagnostic x-rays and thyroid cancer. Because diagnostic x-rays are delivered over time, dose fractionation, as well as the low dose, may account for this reassuring finding. Whether background radiation is associated with thyroid tumors was studied in China among 1001 older women living in an area of high background radiation (caused by thorium-containing minerals). Compared with controls, there was no increase in thyroid nodularity [19].

For 10 cGy and above, there are many studies that establish a dose-response relationship for radiation and thyroid nodules and thyroid cancer. Figure 2 shows representative data in the form of relative risk versus radiation dose from the Michael Reese Hospital study. In order to take advantage of this surfeit of studies, Ron et al. [20] selected seven studies and performed an analysis of the pooled data. To understand the strength of this analysis, an importance distinction needs to be made. The analysis was made on the pooled individual data points, not just on the summary statistics from the seven studies [15,21–26].

Table 1 lists the conclusions from this analysis and illustrates how much information can be deduced from dose-response analyses when there are

THYROID CANCER

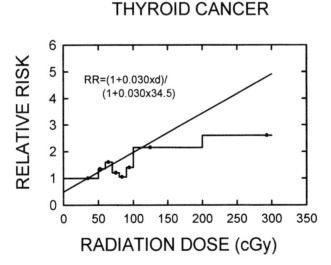

Figure 2. Dose-response relationship for thyroid cancer in the Michael Reese Hospital cohort. The figure includes 309 cases of thyroid cancer. The format is similar to Figure 1. The slope of the relationship was significant with 95% confidence intervals of 0.01–0.40 around the estimate of 0.03 for excess relative risk per cGy. (From Schneider AB, Ron E, Lubin J, et al. Dose-response relationships for radiation-induced thyroid cancer and thyroid nodules: Evidence for prolonged effects of radiation on the thyroid. J Clin Endocrinol Metab 77:362–369, 1993. © The Endocrine Society, by permission.)

Table 1. Conclusions from dose-response analyses of radiation and thyroid cancer

---

1. The probability of developing thyroid cancer is strongly related to the dose of radiation absorbed by the thyroid gland. This is among the strongest indications that radiation is a cause of thyroid cancer.
2. The shortest latency between radiation exposure and the appearance of thyroid cancer is about 5 years.
3. A radiation effect is seen at doses as small as 10 cGy to the thyroid.
4. Over most of the dose range, the data fit best to an excess relative risk (multiplicative) model, although an absolute-risk (additive) model cannot be excluded.
5. The age at radiation exposure is inversely related to the risk of developing thyroid cancer.
6. The relative risk of developing thyroid cancer is about the same for men and women.
7. The introduction of screening increases the number of cases without changing appreciably the excess relative risk.
8. Screening may increases the observed rates by 5- to 10-fold.
9. At the highest doses, the slope of the dose-response relationship decreases and may begin to decline, but the risk remains significant.
10. At the longest times of follow-up, the slope of the dose-response curve may be declining (indicating a waxing of the effects of radiation) but remains significant.

---

sufficient data. Several of the listed conclusions require amplification. The excess risk model means that the effect of radiation is to multiply the background rate, that is, the rate in people not exposed to radiation. Therefore, although the risk is about the same for men and women, most cases of radiation-induced thyroid cancer occur in women because they have a higher background rate.

The dose-response analysis helps understand the effect of screening for thyroid disease. As expected, the rate of thyroid nodules and thyroid cancer is greatly enhanced by screening. If the cases detected by screening are part of the background rate, that is, they are not caused by radiation, the slope of the dose response should decrease or disappear. In the Michael Reese study, even though the rates increased by 5- to 10-fold, the slope of the dose-response relationship did not change. This supports the conclusion that many of the screening-detected nodules and cancers are related to radiation exposure. Similar findings were made among the survivors of the atomic bomb in Japan. Recently, screening sensitivity has been appreciably increased by thyroid ultrasound. The interpretation of the findings with ultrasound remains to be determined (see later).

The shape of the dose-response curve at the highest doses is of interest because it has been hypothesized that cell killing may overtake tumor formation, and the slope would decline and disappear. In fact, with increasing dose the slope (the excess relative risk) stops increasing and probably remains stable. As seen clearly in Figure 2, in which the dose-response relationship is similar to the results of the pooled analysis, the relative risk does not decline to the background at high doses.

From a clinical point of view, the most important finding comes from the analysis of the relative risk over time. It provides the best answer to the question of how long the effects of radiation persist. This question is decep-

146

tively difficult to answer because there is an age-dependent increase in thyroid nodules and cancer, unrelated to radiation. The method to detect a radiation-dependent risk in the background of an age-dependent risk is to determine the slope of the dose-response relationship with time. This shows that radiation has effects on the thyroid that have not disappeared. The relative risk appears to have leveled off, or has begun to decline, but it clearly persists. For irradiated individuals who develop thyroid cancer at later times, this is of concern because thyroid cancer is often more aggressive when it occurs in older patients.

High dose. While radiation therapy for benign childhood conditions has ceased, radiation remains an important modality for the treatment of various malignancies. What are the effects of high-dose radiation exposure on the thyroid? The hypothesis that high-dose exposure causes cell death rather than stimulation to form tumors is no longer tenable. Although cell death may occur, thyroid tumors and cancer also occur after high-dose exposure. At high doses, the dose-response relationship appears to plateau or even begins to decline, but the risk remains distinctly high compared with nonirradiated individuals. The effect of age remains an important factor, with little evidence of an effect when the radiation is administered to adults. Both of these findings are illustrated in the report from the Late Effects Study Group [25]. In 9170 children who were treated for cancer and survived for two or more years, the 23 cases of thyroid cancer that occurred later were distributed in a dose-dependant pattern.

In other instances, radiation may be delivered at a distance from the thyroid and the thyroidal exposure may fall within the range of 'low dose' discussed earlier. A twofold (but not significant) increase in thyroid cancer was found in a large international study of patients treated with radiation for cancer of the cervix [26].

The most regular consequence of high-dose thyroid exposure is impairment of thyroid function, demonstrated by an elevated TSH and sometimes accompanied by clinical hypothyroidism [27]. Because it is likely, although not definitively proven in humans, that TSH promotes thyroid tumors, early intervention with thyroid hormone replacement seems prudent. Whether prophylactic treatment with thyroid hormone reduces the number of thyroid nodules has not been demonstrated.

Radioactive iodine. With so much evidence indicating that radiation causes thyroid cancer, how can we be so confident that radioactive iodine is a safe agent for the diagnosis and treatment of thyroid disorders? The reason is that large, well-designed and persuasive studies have been carried out that confirm the general experience of physicians using radioactive iodine. The cooperative thyrotoxicosis therapy follow-up study included 36,050 patients, 21,714 of whom were treated with radioactive iodine. No increase in thyroid cancer was found in patients treated with radioactive iodine compared with patients treated by other means [28]. Because the effects of radiation are delayed by a latent period of at least 5 years and because the effects last for many years, it is possible that the length of follow-up reported by the cooperative study was not sufficiently long. This concern was diminished by important studies from Sweden, where complete and extensive medical records allow linkage to a national cancer registry. No excess thyroid cancer was found among 10,552 patients with hyperthy-roidism treated with radioactive iodine [29]. The follow-up ranged from 15 years to a maximum of 35 years.

One explanation for these findings is the theory that the thyroid is exposed to such a large dose during the treatment of hyperthyroidism that tumors cannot form. This theory does not fit with the dose-response data cited earlier, nor does it fit with the observations on radioactive iodine used for diagnostic purposes. In 35,074 Swedish patients, no increase in thyroid cancer was observed after the diagnostic use of radioactive iodine [30]. This study was complicated by the fact that some of the diagnostic procedures were performed because of suspected nodular thyroid disease. However, additional analyses showed that this did not affect the conclusion. The average dose absorbed by the thyroid in the study of diagnostic radioactive iodine was 50 cGy, similar to the external doses received by many patients in the studies reviewed earlier, but it was delivered at an older age. The magnitude of the difference in the effects of external and internal thyroid radiation and its explanation remain elusive.

The residents of the Marshall Islands were exposed to radioactive fallout, predominantly I-131, and subsequently developed many thyroid tumors [31]. It is likely that additional isotopes, perhaps combined with radioactive iodine, accounted for the findings. It now appears that thyroid cancer is increasing in children exposed to fallout from the Chernobyl accident. To what extent this is a result of radiation and, if it is, to which isotopes remains to be seen. This important subject has been reviewed [32].

Pituitary

Although two pituitary adenoma were found among the residents of the Marshall Islands exposed to fallout from nuclear tests [33], there are as yet no convincing data indicating that radiation causes the pituitary gland tumors. This may be due to radioresistance and its small size. However, an effect of radiation could easily go unnoticed. Silent pituitary adenomas would not be detectable, except by computed tomography (CT) or magnetic resonance imaging (MRI) screening. Even this might not be conclusive, now that it is recognized how frequently silent pituitary adenomas occur in the general population.

Other tissues in the head and neck area

In patients who develop radiation-induced endocrine tumors, the other radiation-sensitive organs that were exposed require attention. For example,

148

in the Michael Reese Hospital cohort, the parotid glands were in the primary field of radiation therapy.

Salivary gland. For salivary gland cancer, accurate cancer registry data for the general population and dose-response analyses helped establish the relationship to radiation. For benign salivary tumors the information is limited. Because the major salivary glands have a superficial position, few, if any, asymptomatic cases occur. The ratio of benign to malignant salivary gland tumors observed in the Michael Reese cohort is about the same ratio as for benign and malignant thyroid nodules, between two and three benign cases for every cancer [34]. The clinical course of these tumors is usually favorable because early observation leads to prompt treatment. However, some have been aggressive and have led to death.

Neural tumors. The most frequent neural tumors seen in the Michael Reese cohort are schwannomas [34]. These have occurred along peripheral nerves in the field of radiation, along the spinal column, and on cranial nerves, especially the eighth nerve, as vestibular schwannomas (previously called acoustic neuromas). While these are benign tumors, and therefore not included in cancer registries, two factors make it highly likely that these are caused by radiation. First, the frequency is so high that it almost certainly exceeds that of the general population. Second, all but a very few are localized to the area of radiation.

Some individuals have developed multiple schwannomas, without the other findings of neurofibromatosis type 2 (NF2). Therefore, radiation may mimic NF2 and patients with multiple schwannomas should be questioned carefully about radiation exposure. These patients raise the question, discussed later, as to whether susceptibility factors result in their developing multiple tumors. A related concern about radiation for endocrinologists is its use to treat pituitary tumors, usually growth hormone–producing tumors causing acromegaly. After such treatment, patients have an increased risk for the later development of tumors in or near the site of radiation [35].

Approach to the irradiated patient

Natural history of radiation-induced tumors

The clinical evaluation and treatment of an irradiated patient is based on knowledge of which tumors may arise and their natural history. The importance of both is illustrated by thyroid cancer. As reviewed earlier, thyroid cancers of all sizes, from very small ones to quite large ones, are found with increased frequency in irradiated patients. It is necessary to know their natural history (Are they more aggressive than other thyroid cancers? Are the small ones significant at all?) to manage them appropriately.

The available data indicate that radiation-induced thyroid cancers behave in the same way as thyroid cancers occurring in other settings [36,37]. This was analyzed in the Michael Reese cohort by determining which risk factors were associated with recurrences of thyroid cancer. Those factors found to be associated with the risk of recurrence were similar to those reported in nonirradiated thyroid cancer patients. Subsequently, the analysis was extended to members of the cohort who developed thyroid cancer during childhood. Again, the features were similar to the thyroid cancers that developed in children without a history of radiation exposure. We have concluded, therefore, that radiation-induced thyroid cancers should be treated in the same way as other thyroid cancers.

However, there are some features that may distinguish the thyroid cancers in irradiated patients other thyroid cancers. The first is the high frequency of multicentricity and bilateral involvement. The second is that patients with radiation-induced benign nodules are prone to recurrences and some of the recurrences are malignant [38]. In general, malignant recurrences are rare in patients with benign nodular disease. The third distinction is that thyroid hormone treatment reduces the frequency of recurrent benign nodules [38]. Whether this is also true for benign nodular disease not related to radiation remains controversial. The fourth distinction is that the occurrence of a radiation-induced thyroid cancer should increase the concern that other radiation-induced tumors are either present or may develop [39]. Finally, there is some preliminary evidence that the histological type of thyroid cancer occurring in children in the Chernobyl area may be different than thyroid cancers occurring in children living in other areas of the world [40]. This will been hard to confirm because childhood thyroid cancer is rare.

Evaluation

The components of the clinical evaluation follow from knowing which organs are at risk. For some of these, the evaluation is already part of routine health checkups and only require regularity and attentiveness. These regular components include, for example, measurement of serum calcium, examination of the salivary glands, questions about unilateral hearing loss, and a careful physical examination of the thyroid. This subject has been reviewed recently [4]. The main question is in which patients, if any, should the evaluation go beyond routine measures. The factors that would indicate an individual is at higher risk are as follows: (1) large dose, (2) young age at radiation exposure, (3) female, (4) high serum thyroglobulin, (5) rising serum thyroglobulin, (6) other radiation-induced tumors, and (7) radiation-induced tumors in an irradiated sibling.

Almost always the question about additional testing involves imaging of the thyroid. Although the high sensitivity of thyroid scanning in the setting of a high-risk, irradiated patient has been established for many years, its use was limited, in part by concern about additional radiation exposure. Now, how-

150

ever, with the establishment of thyroid ultrasound as an even more sensitive technique, many patients are having this examination, probably more than are indicated by the risk factors mentioned earlier. Abnormalities in the thyroid ultrasound examination may be found in approximately one third of adult, otherwise asymptomatic individuals. We are in the process of evaluating thyroid ultrasound in the high-risk Michael Reese cohort. A representative image is shown in Figure 3. Our preliminary findings indicate that in patients who are unaware of any thyroid disorder and who were screened earlier by conventional means, the frequency of solid and cystic nodules of all sizes is

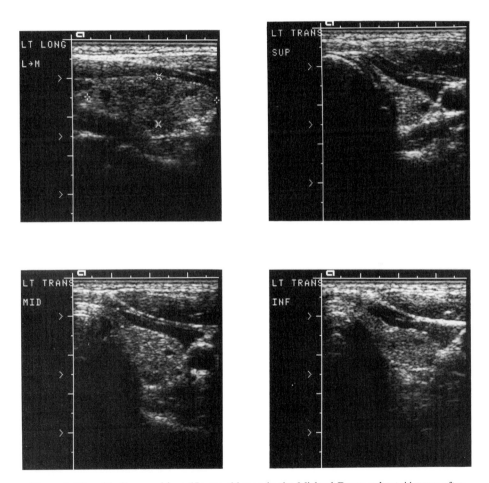

Figure 3. Thyroid ultrasound in a 45-year-old man in the Michael Reese cohort 44 years after childhood radiation exposure for enlarged tonsils. During 21 years of monitoring, starting in 1974, he had normal thyroid scans and normal examinations of his thyroid. The ultrasound shows three predominantly cystic lesions in the left lobe of his thyroid, none larger than 3 mm in any dimension. They are all seen in the anterior portion of the lobe in the longitudinal view (**upper left panel**) and are confirmed by transverse views of the upper (**right upper panel**), middle (**left lower panel**), and lower (**right lower panel**) portions of the thyroid.

very high (>80%) and they are usually multiple. Therefore, thyroid ultrasound should be employed with care and interpreted with even greater care. With our current knowledge, it is difficult to make a recommendation about how to follow high-risk, irradiated patients with one or more ultrasound-

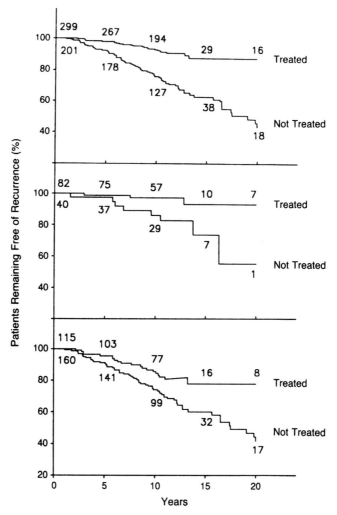

Figure 4. Effect of thyroid hormone treatment on recurrences in patients in the Michael Reese cohort with radiation-induced benign thyroid nodules. Each panel shows follow-up starting from the date of surgery for thyroid nodules that were all benign. The **upper panel** is follow-up for all patients; the **middle panel** for patients with some, but <50%, of their thyroid tissue remaining; and the **bottom panel** for patients with 50% or more of their thyroid tissue remaining. 'Treated' refers to patients receiving thyroid hormone therapy during follow-up. The numbers indicate how many patients were at risk at the beginning of the designated interval. (Reprinted by permission of The New England Journal of Medicine, Fogelfeld L, Wiviott MBT, Shore-Freedman E, et al. 320:835–840, 1989. Copyright 1989. Massachusetts Medical Society. All rights reserved.)

detected small abnormalities in their thyroid gland. It is clear that these small abnormalities are not sufficient to automatically indicate surgery. Their presence does lend support to the use of thyroid hormone and repeat ultrasound imaging.

Treatment of tumors

If one accepts the conclusion that radiation-induced tumors, once they occur, are no more nor less dangerous than similar, non–radiation-related ones, then treatment should follow the guidelines established for the latter. With respect to thyroid tumors, this has been reviewed recently [4–6] and is discussed in Chapter 6. There are, however, some caveats to this simplifying conclusion, related to the effects of radiation. (1) In nonirradiated patients, nontoxic multinodular goiters are usually benign. In irradiated patients they may contain thyroid cancer. (2) Fine-needle aspiration (FNA) appears to be equally useful in individual nodules in irradiated and nonirradiated patients, but the former often have multiple nodules, and some may be difficult to aspirate without ultrasound guidance. We recommend aspirating any nodule ≥10 mm in irradiated patients. (3) In selected, nonirradiated patients undergoing surgery for thyroid nodules, a lobectomy may be adequate. In irradiated patients, the frequency of multiple nodules, multicentric cancers, and the risk of recurrence weigh toward more extensive surgery in almost all cases. (4) The rationale for thyroid hormone treatment, whether thyroid surgery is performed or not, is increased (Fig. 4). (5) Prior to undertaking surgery, the possibility of other radiation-induced conditions, especially hyperparathyroidism, should be evaluated because they could affect the surgical approach.

Pathogenesis of radiation-induced tumors

Radiation elicits a broad range of effects in cells, including induction of point and length mutations, chromosomal aberrations, transient cell-cycle arrest, and eventually cancer. Two types of radiation cause cancer in humans, ionizing and ultraviolet (UV) radiation. UV radiation, with its lower transforming energy, is implicated mainly in skin cancer. Ionizing radiation, with its higher transforming energy, can induce cancers in internal organs. The understanding of the molecular pathogenesis of radiation-induced cancer is evolving rapidly. Radiation-induced cancers are a late consequence of a complex interplay between the type of radiation, the dose and its fractionation, host factors including age at exposure, radiation-sensitive DNA sequences along the genome, the integrity of DNA-repair mechanism, and, in a broader sense, the presence of genetically determined radiosensitivity [41,42].

This section reviews the following concepts important for understanding of the molecular pathogenesis of those endocrine tumors induced by radiation: (1) the effects of radiation on cells, (2) the spectra of genetic mutations induced by radiation in general and in radiation-induced thyroid cancers, and (3) radiation-induced cancer susceptibility and cancer predisposing genes.

Radiation effects on cells

Photons and particles are considered to be ionizing radiation because they have energies greater than 10 eV that exceed the binding energies of electrons in living tissues. Photons with energies of 2–10 eV are in the UV range and are nonionizing. Only UV and ionizing radiation are known to be carcinogenic, and only ionizing radiation affects endocrine glands [43].

Ionizing radiation causes biological damage and cancer that varies according to the average density of energy loss along its path. This is given in units of energy lost per unit of path length (KeV/µm) and is termed the *linear energy transfer* (LET) of the radiation. X-rays give rise to secondary electrons and are considered low LET radiation. The maximally effective radiation has an LET of about 100 KeV, causing ionizations every 20 nm. This corresponds to the diameter of the DNA double helix, and thus might cause the double-strand breaks considered the most important DNA lesion for radiation-induced biological effects [43,44]. The DNA damage caused by ionizing radiation includes base damage, resulting in their alteration or loss, or, more frequently, single-strand and double-strand breaks of the sugar-phosphate backbone [45]. The breaks result in chromosomal aberrations, including deletions, ring formation and acentric fragments, dicentric and acentric fragments, inversions, and translocations.

Radiation-induced genetic damage causes cell killing in a fraction of cells, and in the surviving cells it initiates a complex response involving the activation of several protective mechanisms. One of these is cell cycle arrest [46]. The major function of this is to allow DNA repair mechanisms to function and to prevent the fixing of genetic mutations during subsequent DNA replications. Radiation-induced cell-cycle arrest and DNA repair mechanisms may therefore represent an important safeguard against cancer. Important genes and their products serve as cell-cycle–checkpoint determinants, and mutations in these genes might predispose the irradiated cells to perpetuation of the radiation-induced genetic damage and evolution of cancerous clones.

The p53 tumor suppressor plays a pivotal role in the regulation of cell cycle [47]. Increased expression of p53 in response to radiation arrests the cell in G1 phase. Cells with abnormal p53 function fail to arrest after irradiation and continue to replicate. This may explain the important role of mutated p53 in the common types of human cancer [47]. p53 has an important role in maintaining genetic stability; p53 mutations have been associated with increased gene amplification, chromosomal aneuploidy, and increased recombination [46]. The p53 gene itself might be a direct target to radiation, as is discussed later. In some cells and in some conditions, increased expression of p53 following ionizing irradiation can lead to programmed cell death (apoptosis) [46].

154

Irradiation induces the expression of the ataxia telangiectasia (AT) gene, which in turn induces p53 expression and cell-cycle arrest. Mutations in the AT gene (ATM), recently cloned [48], give rise to ataxia telangiectasia and sensitivity to ionizing radiation. Cells from AT patients do not arrest their cell cycle after irradiation, and their DNA damage repair is defective [49].

Radiation-induced mutations in endocrine tumors

The DNA base mutations and the chromosomal aberrations induced by radiation, described earlier, could lead to structural and functional abnormalities in 'cancer genes' that might initiate and promote carcinogenesis. Radiation could induce base substitutions and gain of function in genes that induce cell proliferation. In the *ras* oncogenes, specific point mutations in codons 12, 13, and 61 decrease their intrinsic GTPase activity, increase their GTP binding, and enhance their growth-promoting effects [50]. In thyroid tumors not related to radiation, *ras* mutations have been found most frequently in follicular carcinomas (53%), but also in follicular adenomas and papillary carcinomas [51,52]. Reports vary about the frequency and pattern of activated *ras* oncogenes in thyroid tumors [53,54].

Activation of the K-*ras* oncogene by radiation has been found in several experimental studies in vivo and in vitro [55,56]. DNA from radiation-induced rat thyroid tumors transfected in NIH3T3 cells showed activation of the K-*ras* oncogene in 8 of the 9 cases [57]. K-*ras* point mutations were found in 3 out of 5 patients with radiation-associated thyroid follicular carcinomas [58]. However, other molecular studies of thyroid cancer in irradiated patients and in children exposed to radiation after the Chernobyl accident failed to show preferential involvement of the K-*ras* oncogene [59–61].

Radiation-induced point mutations can inactivate tumor suppressor genes, such as p53, thereby causing loss of function of genes that inhibit cell proliferation. For p53, point mutations occur in one allele, followed by inactivation of the other allele, usually through allelic loss [62]. Different carcinogens cause characteristic mutations in the p53 gene, presumably related to their different modes of action. Dietary aflatoxin B_1 is associated with G:C to T:A transversions at the third base of condon 249 in hepatocellular carcinoma, and exposure to cigarette smoke is associated with G:C to T:A transversion in lung and head-and-neck carcinomas. UV light is associated with transition mutations at dypirimidine sites, and UV-light–specific p53 mutations are found in skin cancer and in normal skin exposed to UV irradiation involving codons 245 and 247, with transition mutations at dypirimidine sites [63]. Radiation exposure in uranium miners resulted in lung cancer, with preferential G:C to T:A transversion at the second base pair of condon 249 of p53 [64].

In thyroid cancers of patients not exposed to radiation, mutations in the p53 gene are limited, in most reports, to the most advanced and undifferentiated forms [65–69]. One recent study, however, found involvement of p53 in 11 of 44 well-differentiated thyroid carcinomas [70]. In a study of overexpression

155

of mutant p53 protein by immunohistochemistry, 63% of undifferentiated thyroid carcinomas, 14.3% of well-differentiated follicular carcinomas, and 11.1% papillary carcinomas were positive [69]. We found missense p53 point mutations in 4 of 22 radiation-induced thyroid cancer patients. These mutations appeared to be associated with more invasive cancers. Specifically, 3 of the 4 patients with p53 missense mutations had invasion of the cancer beyond the thyroid capsule, compared with 2 of the 17 remaining patients [70a].

In radiation carcinogenesis, length mutations caused by chromosomal aberrations are considered to be most important [45]. Partial chromosomal deletions may result in loss of important tumor suppressor genes. Chromosomal translocations may result in gene rearrangements in which potent translocated promoters from other genes flank oncogenes and increase their expression, or fusion proteins are created that exhibit increased biological activity [71]. An example of this mechanism is the *ret* oncogene rearrangement. *ret* activation by rearrangement is peculiar to thyroid tumors [72]. *ret*, a tyrosine kinase oncogene not expressed in normal thyrocytes, was found expressed in a rearranged form in about 20% of papillary thyroid cancers [72]. The activation occurs by an inversion on the long arm of chromosome 10, resulting in truncation of the transmembrane domain of *ret*, and fusion to the N-terminus of other proteins. Rearranged *ret* localizes to the cytoplasm and becomes constituitively activated by autophosphorylation, either by conformational changes mimicking those produced by the ligand or by substrate availability in the cytoplasm. In two recent reports, *ret*-oncogene rearrangement was found in 4 of 7 and in 4 of 6 children, respectively, exposed to radiation after the Chernobyl nuclear accident [73,74]. Preliminary immunochemistry data show a high frequency of *ret* protein accumulation in these tumors [40].

DNA repair genes and radiation-induced cancer susceptibility

The importance of DNA repair and the integrity of DNA-repair mechanisms after exposure to radiation is illustrated by the existence of human disorders (e.g., ataxia telangiectasia and xeroderma pigmentosum) associated with increased sensitivity to ionizing radiation or UV light. At the molecular level, these disorders are associated with defective processing of radiation-induced DNA damage. These individuals and phenotypically normal family members are predisposed to cancer. Several DNA-repair systems have been identified in mammalian and human cells, including nucleotide excision repair (with mutations in xeroderma pigmentosum, Cockayne syndrome, and trichothiodystrophy), recombinational repair, base-excision repair, postreplication repair, and the repair of DNA double-strand breaks [42]. Hereditary nonpolyposis colorectal cancer (HNPCC), accounting for 10–15% of colon cancers, can be caused by germline mutation of the mismatch repair genes [75]. Four genes (hMSH2, hMLH1, hPMS1, and hPMS2) act in concert to detect and repair any mismatched DNA base pairs occurring during DNA

156

replication. In HNPCC patients, The hMSH2 gene is mutated in 60% and the hMLH1 gene is mutated in 30%.

The existence of individuals prone to develop cancer induced by ionizing radiation has been emphasized by the cloning of the ataxia-telangiectasia (AT) gene [48]. In the rare homozygous form, affected individuals, in addition to telangiectasias and cerebellar degeneration, are extremely sensitive to x-rays and develop malignancies, especially of the lymphoreticular system. More importantly, AT heterozygotes may express two characteristics of the disease, predisposition to cancer and increased sensitivity to radiation. In one study, the higher breast cancer rate in the AT heterozygotes was associated with low-dose radiation exposure in the form of single or multiple fluoroscopic examinations of the chest and abdomen. It is estimated that 0.5–1.4% of the population has an AT gene mutation, and the gene could account for up to 8% of all breast cancers [76].

Radiation-induced thyroid cancer susceptibility in the Michael Reese cohort was addressed by Perkel et al. [77] They studied 286 sibpairs who received childhood radiation and found that there is an independent familial risk factor for developing thyroid neoplasms. Additional analysis of this group (unpublished) shows that in 8 of 322 irradiated sibpairs, both members developed thyroid cancers, about 2.5-fold more than expected. Additional suggestion for radiation-related cancer predisposition in this group comes from analysis of association between thyroid and nonthyroid tumors: In 45 sibpairs in which both members developed thyroid tumors, there were three sibpairs who developed nonthyroid tumors in both siblings, approximately sevenfold higher than expected.

Conclusions

The molecular pathogenesis of radiation-induced thyroid tumors is not understood at present. The emerging data from other radiation-induced cancers suggest that dysfunction of the DNA repair and cell-cycle arrest might predispose certain individuals exposed to radiation to greater risk of thyroid cancer. Therefore, these underlying molecular mechanisms should be investigated in radiation-induced thyroid tumors. Preliminary data suggest a role for *ret* rearrangement in pathogenesis of radiation-induced thyroid tumors. This hypothesis is plausible because *ret* rearrangements represent an expected length mutation after radiation exposure and such lesions are thyroid specific, but more studies are needed to confirm this.

Acknowledgments

The work described from Michael Reese Hospital was supported, in part, by grant CA 21518 (to ABS) from the National Cancer Institute. The authors thank Marge Nickless for her help in preparing the manuscript.

References

1. Duffy BJ, Fitzgerald P. 1950. Thyroid cancer in childhood and adolescence: A report on twenty-eight cases. Cancer 10:1018–1032.
2. Winship T, Rosvoll R. 1970. Thyroid carcinoma in childhood: Final report on a 20-year study. Clin Proc Children's Hospital (Washington, DC) 26:327–348.
3. Degroot LJ, Paloyan E. 1973. Thyroid carcinoma and radiation: A Chicago endemic. JAMA 225:487–491.
4. Sarne DH, Schneider AB. 1995. Evaluation and management of patients exposed to childhood head and neck irradiation. Endocrinologist 5:304–307.
5. Schneider AB. 1990. Radiation-induced thyroid tumors. Endocrinol Metab Clin North Am 19:495–508.
6. Schneider AB, Ron E. 1996. Thyroid diseases: Tumors: Carcinoma of follicular epithelium: Pathogenesis. In Braverman LE, Utiger R, eds. Werner and Ingbar's The Thyroid, 7th ed. Philadelphia: Lippincott-Raven, pp. 902–909.
7. DeGroot L. 1989. Diagnostic approach and management of patients exposed to irradiation to the thyroid. J Clin Endocrinol Metab 69:925–928.
8. Christensson T. 1978. Hyperparathyroidism subsequent to neck irradiation. Cancer 89:216–217.
9. Rao SD, Frame B, Miller MJ, Kleerkorper M, Block MA, Parfitt AM. 1980. Hyperparathyroidism following head and neck irradiation. Arch Intern Med 140:205–207.
10. Cohen J, Gierlowski T, Schneider A. 1990. A prospective study of hyperparathyroidism in individuals exposed to radiation in childhood. JAMA 264:581–584.
11. Fujiwara S, Sposta REH, Akiba S, Neriishi K, Kodama K, Hosoda Y, Shimaoka K. 1992. Hyperparathyroidism among atomic bomb survivors in Hiroshima. Radiat Res 130:372–378.
12. Tisell LE, Carlsson S, Fjalling M, Hansson G, Lindberg S, Lundberg L-M, Oden A. 1985. Hyperparathyroidism subsequent to neck irradiation: Risk factors. Cancer 56:1529–1533.
13. Schneider AB, Gierlowski TC, Shorefreedman E, Stovall M, Ron E, Lubin J. 1995. Dose-response relationships for radiation-induced hyperparathyroidism. J Clin Endocrinol Metab 80:254–257.
14. Tezelman S, Rodriguez JM, Shen W, Siperstein AE, Duh QY, Clark OH. 1995. Primary hyperparathyroidism in patients who have received radiation therapy and in patients who have not received radiation therapy. J Am Coll Surgeons 180:81–87.
15. Ron E, Modan B, Preston D, Alfandary E, Stovall M, Boice JD Jr. 1989. Thyroid neoplasia following low-dose radiation in childhood. Radiat Res 120:516–531.
16. Wang JX, Boice JD Jr, Li BX, Zhang JY, Fraumeni J. 1988. Cancer among medical diagnostic x-ray workers in China. J Natl Cancer Inst 80:344–350.
17. Antonelli A, Silvano G, Bianchi F, Gambuzza C, Tana L, Salvioni G, Baldi V, Gasperini L, Baschieri L. 1995. Risk of thyroid nodules in subjects occupationally exposed to radiation: A cross sectional study. Occup Environ Medicine 52:500–504.
18. Inskip PD, Ekbom A, Galanti MR, Grimelius L, Boice JD Jr. 1995. Medical diagnostic x rays and thyroid cancer. J Nat Cancer Inst 87:1613–1621.
19. Wang Z, Boice JD Jr, Wei L, Beebe G, Zha Y, Kaplan M, Tao Z, Maxon H III, Zhang S, Schneider AB, Tan B, Wesseler T, Chen D, Ershow A, Kleinerman R, Littlefield LG, Preston D. 1990. Thyroid nodularity and chromosome aberrations among women in areas of high background radiation in China. J Natl Cancer Inst 82:478–185.
20. Ron E, Lubin JH, Shore RE, Mabuchi K, Modan B, Pottern LM, Schneider AB, Tucker MA, Boice JD Jr. 1995. Thyroid cancer after exposure to external radiation: A pooled analysis of seven studies. Radiat Res 141:259–277.
21. Thompson DE, Mabuchi K, Ron E, Soda M, Tokunaga M, Ochikubo S, Sugimoto S, Ikeda T, Terasaki M, Izumi S, Preston DL. 1994. Cancer incidence in atomic bomb survivors. Part II: Solid tumors, 1958–1987. Radiat Res 137:S17–S67.
22. Shore R, Hildreth N, Dvoretsky PM, Andresent E, Moseson M, Pasternack B. 1993. Thyroid

158

cancer among persons given x-ray treatment in infancy for an enlarged thymus gland. Am J Epidemiol 137:1068–1080.

23. Schneider A, Ron E, Lubin J, Stoveall M, Gierlowski T. 1993. Dose-response relationships for radiation-induced thyroid cancer and thyroid nodules: Evidence for the prolonged effects of radiation on the thyroid. J Clin Endocrinol Metab 77:362–369.

24. Pottern LM, Kaplan MM, Larsen PR, Silva JE, Koenig RJ, Lubin JH, Stovall M, Boice JD Jr. 1990. Thyroid nodularity after childhood irradiation for lymphoid hyperplasia — A comparison of questionnaire and clinical findings. J Clin Epidemiol 43:449–460.

25. Tucker MA, Jones PH, Boice JD Jr, Robison LL, Stone BJ, Stovall M, Jenkin RD, Lubin JH, Baum ES, Siegel SE, et al. 1991. Therapeutic radiation at a young age is linked to secondary thyroid cancer. The Late Effects Study Group. Cancer Res 51:2885–2888.

26. Boice JD Jr, Engholm G, Kleinerman RA, Blettner M, Stovall M, Lisco H, Moloney WC, Austin DF, Bosch A, Cookfair DL, et al. 1988. Radiation dose and second cancer risk in patients treated for cancer of the cervix. Radiat Res 116:3–55.

27. Schneider A. 1996. Cancer therapy and endocrine disease: Radiation-induced thyroid tumours. In Sheaves P, Jenkins P, Wass J, eds. Clinical Endocrine Oncology. Oxford: Blackwell Scientific Publications, in press.

28. Dobyns BM, Sheline GE, Workman JB, Tompkins EA, McConahey WM, Becker DV. 1974. Malignant and benign neoplasms of the thyroid in patients treated for hyperthyroidism: A report of the Cooperative Thyrotoxicosis Therapy Study. J Clin Endocrinol Metab 38:976–998.

29. Holm LE, Hall P, Wiklund K, Lundell G, Berg G, Bjelkengren G, Cederquist E, Ericsson UB, Hallquist A, Larsson LG, Lidberg M, Lindberg S, Tennvall J, Wicklund H, Boice JD Jr. 1991. Cancer risk after iodine-131 therapy for hyperthyroidism. J Natl Cancer Inst 83:1072–1077.

30. Holm LE, Wilkund KE, Lundell GE, Bergman NA, Bjelkengren G, Cederquist ES, Ericsson UBC, Larsson LG, Lidberg ME, Lindberg RS, Wicklund HV, Boice JD Jr. 1988. Thyroid cancer after diagnostic doses of iodine-131: A retrospective cohort study. J Natl Cancer Inst 80:1132–1138.

31. Robbins J, Adams WH. 1989. Radiation effects in the Marshall Islands. In Nagataki S, ed. Radiation and the Thyroid. Amsterdam: Excerpta Medica, pp 11–24.

32. Becker DV, Robbins J, Beebe G, Bouville AC, Wachholz BW. 1996. Childhood thryoid cancer following the Chernobyl accident: A status report. Endocrinol Metab Clin North Am 25:197–211.

33. Adams WH, Harper JA, Pittmaster RS, Grimson RC. 1984. Pituitary tumors following fallout radiation exposure. JAMA 252:664–666.

34. Schneider A, Shore-Freeman E, Ryo UY, Bekerman C, Favus M, Pinsky S. 1985. Radiation-induced tumors of the head and neck following childhood irradiation: Prospective studies. Medicine 64:1–15.

35. Tsang RW, Laperriere NJ, Simpson WJ, Brierley J, Panzarella T, Smyth HS. 1993. Glioma arising after radiation therapy for pituitary adenoma. A report of four patients and estimation of risk. Cancer 72:2227–2233. [Published erratum appears in Cancer 1994 73:492.]

36. Schneider A, Recant W, Pinsky S, Ryo UY, Bekerman C, Shore-Freeman E. 1986. Radiation-induced thyroid carcinoma: Clinical course and results of therapy in 296 patients. Ann Intern Med 105:405–412.

37. Viswanathan K, Gierlowski TC, Schneider AB. 1994. Childhood thyroid cancer — characteristics and long-term outcome in children irradiated for benign conditions of the head and neck. Arch Pediatr Adolesc Med 148:260–265.

38. Fogelfeld L, Wiviott MBT, Shore-Freeman E, Blend M, Bekerman C, Pinsky S, Schneider AB. 1989. Recurrence of thyroid nodules after surgical removal in patients irradiated in childhood for benign conditions. N Engl J Med 320:835–840.

39. Schneider A, Shore-Freeman E, Weinstein R. 1986. Radiation-induced thyroid and other head and neck tumors: Occurrence of multiple tumors and analysis of risk factos. J Clin Endocrinol Metab 63:107–112.

159

40. Bogdanova T, Bragarnik M, Tronko ND, Harach HR, Thomas GA, Williams ED. 1995. Thryoid cancer in the Ukraine post Chernobyl (abstr). Thyroid 5:S28.
41. Sankaranarayanan K, Chakraborty R. 1995. Cancer predisposition. radiosensitivity and the risk of radiation-induced cancers. 1. Background. Radiat Res 143:121–143.
42. Lohman PH, Cox R, Chadwick KH. 1995. Role of molecular biology in radiation biology. Int J Radiat Biol 68:331–340.
43. Rauth AM. 1992. Radiation carcinogenesis. In Tannock IF, Hill RP, eds. The Basic Science of Oncology. New York: McGraw-Hill, pp 119–135.
44. Hall EJ. 1993. Principles of carcinogenesis: Physical. In DeVita VT, Hellman S, Rosenberg SA, eds. Cancer: Principles and Practice of Oncology. Philadelphia: JB Lippincott, pp 213–227.
45. Ward JF. 1995. Radiation mutagenesis: The initial DNA lesions responsible. Radiat Res 142:362–368.
46. Canman CE, Chen CY, Lee MH, Kastan MB. 1994 DNA damage responses: p53 induction, cell cycle perturbations, and apoptosis. Cold Spring Harb Symp Quant Biol 59:277–286.
47. Kastan MB. 1993 p53: Evolutionarily conserved and constantly evolving. J Natl Inst Health Res 5:53–57.
48. Savitsky K, Bar-Shira A, Gilad S, Rotman G, Ziv Y, Vanagaite L, Tagle D, Smith S, Uziel T, Sfez S, Ashkenazi M, Pecker I, Frydman M, Harnik R, Patanjali S, Simmons A, Clines G, Sartiel A, Gatti R, Chessa L, Sanal O, Lavin M, Jaspers NGJ, Taylor AM, Arlett C, Miki T, Weissman S, Lovett M, Collins F, Shiloh Y. 1995. A single ataxia telangiectasis gene with a product similar to PI-3 kinase. Science 268:1749.
49. Kastan MB, Zhan Q, el-Deiry WS, Carrier F, Jacks T, Walsh WV, Plunkett BS, Vogelstein B, Fornace AJ Jr. 1992. A mammalian cell cycle checkpoint pathway utilizing p53 and GADD45 is defective in ataxia-telangiectasia. Cell 71:587–597.
50. Barbacid M. 1990. ras oncogenes: Their role in neoplasia. Eur J Clin Invest 20:225–235.
51. Lemoine NR, Mayall ES, Wyllie FS, Williams ED, Goyns M, Stringer B, Wynfordthomas. 1989. High frequency of RAS oncogene activation in all stages of human thyroid tumorigenesis. Oncogene 4:159–164.
52. Wright PA, Lemoine NR, Mayall ES, Wyllie FS, Hughes D, Williams ED, Wynfordthomas. 1989. Papillary and follicular thyroid carcinomas show a different pattern of RAS oncogene mutation. Br J Cancer 60:576–577.
53. Namba H, Gutman RA, Matsuo K, Alvarez A, Fagin JA. 1990. H-ras proto-oncogene mutations in human thyroid neoplasms. J Clin Endocrinol Metab 71:223–229.
54. Namba H, Rubin SA, Fagin JA. 1990. Point mutations of RAS oncogenes are an early event in thyroid tumorigenesis. Mol Endocrinol 4:1474–1479.
55. Sawey MJ, Hood AT, Burns FJ, Garte SJ. 1987. Activation of c-myc and c-K-ras oncogenes in primary rat tumors induced by ionizing radiation. Mol Cell Biol 7:932–935.
56. Mizuki K, Nose K, Okamoto H, Tsuchida N, Hayashi K. 1985. Amplification of c-Ki-ras gene and aberrant expression of c-myc in WI-38 cells transformed in vitro by gamma-irradiation. Biochem Biophys Res Commun 128:1037–1043.
57. Lemoine NR, Mayall ES, Williams ED, Thurston V, Wynford-Thomas D. 1988. Agent-specific ras oncogene activation in rat thyroid tumours. Oncogene 3:541–544.
58. Wright PA, Williams ED, Lemoine NR, Wynfordthomas D. 1991. Radiation-associated and spontaneous human thyroid carcinomas show a different pattern of RAS oncogene mutation. Oncogene 6:471–473.
59. Challeton C, Bounacer A, Du Villard JA, Caillou B, De Vathaire F, Monier R, Schlumberger M, Suarez HG. 1995. Pattern of RAS and gsp oncogene mutations in radiation-associatd human thyroid tumors. Oncogene 11:601–603.
60. Nikiforov Y, Nikiforova M, Tang SH, Fagin JA. 1995. Low prevalence of mutations of RAS and p53 in thyroid tumors from children exposed to radiation after Chernobyl (abstr). The Endocrine Society 77th Annual Meeting, Washington DC, p 463.
61. Fugazzola L, Bongarzone I, Pilotti S, Vorontsova TV, Collini P, Degregorio L, Rao S, Astakhova L, Demidchik EP, Prat M, Pacini F, Pinchera A, Pierotti MA. 1995. Papilary

thyroid cancer in children exposed to Chernobyl nuclear accident: Molecular analysis of tumor specimens (abstr). Thyroid 5:S133.

62. Baker SJ, Preisinger AC, Jessup JM, Paraskeva C, Markowitz S, Willson JK, Hamilton S, Vogelstein B. 1990. p53 gene mutations occur in combination with 17p allelic deletions as late events in colorectal tumorigenesis. Cancer Res 50:7717–7722.

63. Harris CC. 1993. p53 — At the crossroads of molecular carcinogenesis and risk assessment. Science 262:1980–1981.

64. Taylor JA, Watson MA, Devereux TR, Michels RY, Saccomanno G, Anderson M. 1994. p53 mutation hotspot in radon-associated lung cancer. Lancet 343:86–87.

65. Wright PA, Lemoine NR, Goretzki PE, Wyllie FS, Bond J, Hughes C, Roher HD, Willi. 1991. Mutation of the p53-gene in a differentiated human thyroid carcinoma cell line, but not in primary thyroid tumours. Oncogene 6:1693–1697.

66. Fagin JA, Matsuo K, Karmakar A, Chen DL, Tang SH, Koeffler HP. 1993. High prevalence of mutations of the p53 gene in poorly differentiated human thyroid carcinomas. J Clin Invest 91:179–184.

67. Ito T, Seyama T, Mizuno T, Tsuyama N, Hayashi T, Hayashi Y, Dohi K, Nakamura N, Aki. 1992. Unique association of p53 mutations with undifferentiated but not with differentiated carcinomas of the thyroid gland. Cancer Res 52:1369–1371.

68. Nakamura T, Yana I, Kobayashi T, Shin E, Karakawa K, Fujita S, Miya A, Mori T, Nish. 1992. p53-gene mutations associated with anaplastic transformation of human thyroid carcinomas. Jpn J Cancer Res 83:1293–1298.

69. Dobashi Y, Sakamoto A, Sugimura H, Mernyei M, Mori M, Oyama T, Machinami R. 1993. Overexpression of p53 as a possible prognostic factor in human thyroid carcinoma. Am J Surg Pathol 17:375–381.

70. Zou MJ, Shi YF, Farid NR, 1993. p53 Mutations in all stages of thyroid carcinomas. J Clin Endocrinol Metab 77:1054–1058.

70a. Fogelfeld L, Bauer TK, Schneider AB, Swartz JE, Zitman R. 1996. p53 gene mutations in radiation-induced thyroid cancer. J Clin Endocrinol Metab 81:3039–3044.

71. Rabbitts TH. 1994. Chromosomal translocations in human cancer. Nature 372:143–149.

72. Viglietto G, Chiappetta G, Martineztello FJ, Fukunaga FH, Tallini G, Rigopoulou D, Visconti R, Mastro A, Santoro M, Fusco A. 1995. RET/PTC oncogene activation is an early event in thyroid carcinogenesis. Oncogene 11:1207–1210.

73. Ito T, Seyama T, Iwamoto KS, Mizuno T, Tronko ND, Komissarenko IV, Cherstovoy ED, Satow Y, Takeichi N, Dohi K, Akiyama M. 1994. Activated RET oncogene in thyroid cancers of children from areas contaminated by Chernobyl accident [letter]. Lancet 344:259.

74. Fugazzola L, Pilotti S, Pinchera A, Vorontsova TV, Mondellini P, Bongarzone I, Greco A, Astakhova L, Butti MG, Demidchik EP, Pacini F, Pierotti MA. 1995. Oncogenic rearrangements of the RET proto-oncogene in papillary thyroid carcinomas from children exposed to the Chernobyl nuclear accident. Cancer Res 55:5617–5620.

75. Fishel R, Lescoe MK, Rao MR, Copeland NG, Jenkins NA, Garber J, Kane M, Kolodner R. 1993. The human mutator gene homolog MSH2 and its association with hereditary nonpolyposis colon cancer. Cell 75:1027–1038. [Published erratum appears in Cell 1994 77:167.]

76. Swift M, Morrell D, Massey R, Chase C. 1991. Incidence of cancer in 161 families affected by ataxia-telangiectasia. N Engl J Med 325:1831–1836.

77. Perkel V, Gail MH, Lubin J, Pee D, Weinstein R, Shore-Freeman E, Schneider AB. 1988. Radiation-induced thyroid neoplasm: Evidence for familial susceptibility factors. J Clin Endocrinol Metab 66:1316–1322.

8. Diagnosis, natural history, and treatment of primary hyperparathyroidism

Shonni J. Silverberg

Primary hyperparathyroidism, one of the most common endocrine disorders, is characterized by hypercalcemia in the presence of elevated parathyroid hormone levels. The disease today bears little resemblance to the severe disorder of 'stones, bones and groans' described by Fuller Albright and others in the 1930s [1–6]. Osteitis fibrosa cystica was the hallmark of classic primary hyperparathyroidism. This skeletal condition was characterized by brown tumors of the long bones, subperiosteal bone resorption, distal tapering of the clavicles and phalanges, and a 'salt and pepper' appearance of the skull on radiograph [7]. Nephrocalcinosis was present in 80% of patients, and neuromuscular dysfunction with muscle weakness was common. With the advent of the automated serum chemistry autoanalyzer in the 1970s, diagnosis of primary hyperparathyroidism became commonplace in the complete absence of symptoms [8–10].

Symptomatic primary hyperparathyroidism is now the exception rather than the rule, with more than three quarters of patients having no signs or symptoms attributable to their primary hyperparathyroidism. Primary hyperparathyroidism is a disease that has 'evolved' from its classic presentation (Table 1). Nephrolithiasis is still seen, although less frequently than in the past. However, radiologically evident bone disease is rare. This chapter presents the clinical picture of primary hyperparathyroidism as it presents today and our current understanding of the etiology of this disease. Issues in the management of this 'new' disorder, many of them as yet unresolved, are also addressed.

Pathology of primary hyperparathyroidism

Parathyroid adenomas

By far the most common lesion found in patients with primary hyperparathyroidism is the solitary parathyroid adenoma [12]. Several risk factors have been identified in the development of primary hyperparathyroidism. These include a history of neck irradiation [13] and prolonged use of lithium therapy for affective disorders [14–17]. However, the vast majority of cases of primary hyperparathyroidism remain idiopathic. Recently much effort has been ex-

Andrew Arnold (ed.) ENDOCRINE NEOPLASMS. 1997. Kluwer Academic Publishers. ISBN 0-7923-4354-9.
All rights reserved.

Table 1. Changing profile of primary hyperparathyroidism

	Cope [2] (1930–1965)	Heath et al. [8] (1965–1974)	Mallette et al. [11] (1965–1972)	Silverberg et al. (1986–1993)
Nephrolithiasis[a]	57	51	37	19.5
Skeletal disease	23	10	14	2
Hypercalciuria	NR[b]	36	40	39
Asymptomatic	0.6	18	22	80

[a] Values are given as percentages.
[b] Not reported.
Reprinted from Bilezikian et al. [12], with permission.

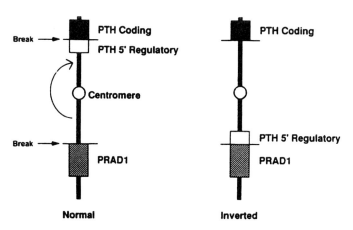

Figure 1. Normal and inverted chromosome showing relative loci of PRAD1 and PTH genes. This molecular rearrangement is responsible for a subset of parathyroid adenomas. (Reprinted from Silverberg et al. [7], with permission.)

pended in the effort to elucidate the pathophysiology of adenoma development in primary hyperparathyroidism. The data suggest an origin in the clonal expansion of cell lines that have undergone a shift in the calcium inhibitory set point [18–21].

The work of Arnold and others has amply demonstrated that most parathyroid adenomas are monoclonal in origin [21–24]. Evidence suggests that the molecular abnormalities leading to clonal emergence are heterogeneous. Among the alterations identified are genetic rearrangement of the PRAD1 (parathyroid adenomatosis 1) oncogene, also known as cyclin D1, which places this important gene in proximity to the 5′ regulatory region of the gene for parathyroid hormone (Fig. 1) [21–23]. In other adenomas, loss of heterozygosity on chromosome 11q13, chromosome 1p, and other loci have been found, implying the existence of parathyroid tumor suppressor genes at these locations [24–26]. In view of the known abnormalities of the calcium set point in patients with parathyroid adenomas, it was postulated that a mutation in the

Ca^{2+}-sensing receptor gene could underlie the development of these tumors [27]. Indeed, such a mechanism has been identified in familial hypocalciuric hypercalcemia and neonatal severe hyperparathyroidism [27,28]. However, studies of primary hyperparathyroidism suggest that mutation or allelic loss in the calcium-sensing receptor gene does not commonly lead to the development of this disease [29,30].

While in most cases, a single adenoma is found, multiple parathyroid adenomas have been reported in 2–4% of cases [31–33]. These may be familial or sporadic. Parathyroid adenomas have been found in a myriad of unexpected anatomic locations. Embryonal migration patterns of parathyroid tissue account for the plethora of possible sites for ectopic parathyroid adenomas. The most common sites for ectopic adenomas are within the thyroid gland, the superior mediastinum, and the thymus [34,35]. Occasionally, the adenoma may ultimately be located in the pharynx, the alimentary submucosa, or the esophagus [36–38]. On histologic examination, most parathyroid adenomas are encapsulated and are composed of parathyroid chief cells. Adenomas containing mainly oxyphilic or oncocytic cells are rare but can give rise to clinical primary hyperparathyroidism.

Parathyroid hyperplasia

In approximately 15% of cases, all four parathyroid glands are involved in the hyperparathyroid process. There are no clinical features that differentiate primary hyperparathyroidism due to adenoma versus hyperplasia. The etiology of parathyroid hyperplasia is multifactorial. In nearly one half of cases, it is associated with a familial hereditary syndrome, such as multiple endocrine neoplasia (MEN) types I and IIa. These syndromes are discussed in detail in chapters 18, 19, and 20. While the pathophysiology of the sporadic cases is unknown, the calcium set point does not seem to be altered [18]. Instead, it seems that the increased number of parathyroid cells in the hyperplastic glands causes the excessive parathyroid hormone secretion. As in the case of parathyroid adenomas, underlying molecular mechanisms are heterogeneous. Some hyperplastic glands are monoclonal, among them certain glands associated with MEN-I [39,40], as well as nonfamilial cases [41]. There are also data suggesting that the loss of tumor suppressor genes at the M27β region of the X-chromosome [41] or on chromosome 11q13 may play a role in some cases of hyperplasia [39,40]. The histology of these glands shows generalized hyperplasia, with chief-cell hyperplasia the most common variety. Water clear-cell hyperplasia, although the first described form of parathyroid hyperplasia, is rarely seen today [42].

Other

Parathyroid carcinoma causes a severe form of primary hyperparathyroidism and is responsible for less than 1% of cases of primary hyperparathyroidism.

This topic is discussed in detail in Chapter 9. Other very rare causes of primary hyperparathyroidism include cystic parathyroid hyperplasia [43,44], and dominant familial parathyroid adenomatosis [45].

Clinical presentation of primary hyperparathyroidism

At the time of diagnosis, 80% of patients with primary hyperparathyroidism have neither symptoms nor signs referable to their disease [7]. History may be obtained of previous neck irradiation or of diseases statistically associated with primary hyperparathyroidism, such as hypertension [8,46–48], peptic ulcer disease (particularly in MEN-I), gout, or pseudogout [49,50]. Constitutional complaints are common, and there is mounting evidence of a neuropsychiatric constellation in some patients [51–56]. Physical examination is generally unremarkable. Band keratopathy, a hallmark of classical primary hyperparathyroidism caused by deposition of calcium-phosphate crystals in the cornea, is now a rare finding that can be seen only on slit-lamp examination.

Biochemical profile of primary hyperparathyroidism

The diagnosis of primary hyperparathyroidism is made by the demonstration of hypercalcemia in the presence of elevated parathyroid hormone levels. Conversely, the other major cause of hypercalcemia, malignancy, is characterized by suppressed parathyroid hormone levels. Improved means of measuring parathyroid hormone, especially immunoradiometric and immunochemiluminometric assays, have far greater sensitivity than previously available assays. They have also eliminated renal insufficiency as a confounding variable in making this diagnosis.

Even using the newer assays, parathyroid hormone is frankly elevated in only 90% of patients at the time of diagnosis [7]. In the rest, levels hover in the high end of the normal range. Many of these individuals will have frankly high values on follow-up. In all such patients, the circulating parathyroid hormone concentration is inappropriately high given the patient's hypercalcemia. Any patient with hypercalcemia should have suppressed levels of parathyroid hormone unless they have primary hyperparathyroidism.

Much less frequently, one sees a patient with 'normocalcemic primary hyperparathyroidism' [7]. These individuals have elevated parathyroid hormone levels but normal serum calcium concentrations. In some, ionized calcium is high and the apparently normal total calcium is caused by a binding protein abnormality. In others, follow-up over time shows the emergence of hypercalcemia.

Other biochemical features of primary hyperparathyroidism include a low normal serum phosphorus, with the frankly low levels seen in classic primary hyperparathyroidism present in less than one quarter of patients. Average

166

total urinary calcium excretion is at the upper end of the normal range, with less than half of all patients having increased excretion levels. Serum 25-hydroxyvitamin D levels tend to be in the lower end of the normal range. While mean values of 1,25-dihydroxyvitamin D3 are in the high normal range, approximately one third of patients have frankly elevated levels of this important hormone [57].

The skeleton in primary hyperparathyroidism

Osteitis fibrosa cystica is rarely seen today. However, using newer, more sensitive techniques, it has become clear that skeletal involvement in the hyperparathyroid process remains ubiquitous. This section reviews the profile of the skeleton in primary hyperparathyroidism as it is reflected in assays for bone markers, bone densitometry studies, and bone histomorphometry. This is not to advocate the performance of these tests as part of the routine evaluation and management of patients with primary hyperparathyroidism (see Evaluation). Indeed, many of the bone turnover markers, and certainly histomorphometric analysis, are appropriate mainly for the research setting.

Bone markers. Both bone resorption and bone formation are increased by parathyroid hormone. Markers of bone turnover, which reflect those increases, provide clues to the extent of skeletal involvement in primary hyperparathyroidism. Bone formation is reflected by osteoblast products, including alkaline phosphatase, bone GLA protein (also known as osteocalcin), and type 1 procollagen [58]. Markers of bone resorption include the osteoclast product tartrate-resistant acid phosphatase (TRAP) and collagen breakdown products, such as hydroxyproline, hydroxypyridinium crosslinks of collagen, and collagen crosslinked N-telopeptide [58].

Despite the emergence of more sensitive measurements of skeletal activity, total alkaline phosphatase is widely assessed in primary hyperparathyroidism [59]. In populations of patients with primary hyperparathyroidism, levels are mildly elevated, yet many individuals have total alkaline phosphatase values within the normal range [60–62]. The bone-specific isoenzyme of alkaline phosphatase is far more sensitive. Unfortunately, the assay is technically difficult, and it is therefore not widely available. Bone-specific alkaline phosphatase is clearly elevated in patients with mild primary hyperparathyroidism. In a small study from our group, bone-specific alkaline phosphatase was correlated with parathyroid hormone levels and bone mineral density at the lumbar spine and femoral neck [63]. Bone GLA protein is also generally increased in patients with primary hyperparathyroidism [64–67]. Bone GLA protein correlates with other indices of bone formation [64–67] and changes within hours after parathyroidenctomy [61]. Assays for procollagen extension peptides reflect bone formation but have little clinical utility in primary hyperparathyroidism [68].

Once the best available marker of bone resorption [69–71], urinary hydroxyproline excretion no longer offers sufficient sensitivity or specificity to make it a useful tool in the assessment of patients with primary hyperparathyroidism. Hydroxypyridinium crosslinks of collagen, on the other hand, are clearly elevated in primary hyperparathyroidism and have been shown to normalize after parathyroidectomy [72]. Studies of the osteoclast product, tartrate-resistant acid phosphatase, in primary hyperparathyroidism are limited, although levels have been shown to be elevated [73]. Assays for collagen crosslinked N-telopeptide levels, a sensitive marker of bone resorption, have yet to be systematically explored in this disease. Thus, sensitive assays reflecting bone formation and bone resorption show both to be increased in mild primary hyperparathyroidism.

Bone densitometry in primary hyperparathyroidism. While markers of bone turnover provide a reflection of the general state of activation of the skeleton, they provide no specific information regarding different skeletal compartments. Bone densitometry at sites containing different amounts of cortical and cancellous bone offers a noninvasive opportunity to gain such information. This is especially well suited to the investigation of states of parathyroid hormone excess, because parathyroid hormone has long been thought of as a hormone with particular proclivity for cortical bone. Consistent with this observation, densitometry studies in primary hyperparathyroidism have shown decreased bone density at the distal radius, which is composed primarily of cortical bone [74,75]. These studies have also shown bone density to be relatively preserved at the lumbar spine, a site containing a preponderance of

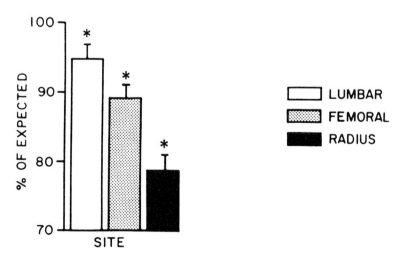

Figure 2. Bone densitometry in primary hyperparathyroidism. Data are shown in comparison with age- and sex-matched normal subjects. Divergence from expected values is different at each site (p = 0.0001). (Reprinted from Silverberg et al. [74], with permission.)

cancellous bone. The femoral neck, intermediate in composition between cortical and cancellous elements, is intermediate in bone density as well (Fig. 2). These data support not only the notion that parathyroid hormone is catabolic in cortical bone, but also the more recently appreciated view that parathyroid hormone is anabolic in cancellous bone [76–78].

It should be noted that the pattern described earlier is also seen on bone densitometry in postmenopausal women with primary hyperparathyroidism [74]. Women with primary hyperparathyroidism, therefore, show a reversal of the pattern usually associated with postmenopausal bone loss. The latter is characterized by preferential loss of cancellous bone. On bone densitometry, this is reflected in reduced bone density at the more cancellous lumbar spine and femoral neck. The reduced bone density at the distal radius (cortical bone) and preserved density at the lumbar spine (cancellous bone) suggest that primary hyperparathyroidism protects these women from postmenopausal bone loss.

Bone histomorphometry. Investigations at a cellular level have supported and extended the data obtained in bone densitometry studies. Cortical thinning has been documented on iliac crest bone biopsy, consistent with the diminution of bone at primarily cortical sites on densitometry [79–81]. Histomorphometric studies, however, have contributed most by elucidating the nature of cancellous bone in this disease. Cancellous bone volume is not only relatively preserved in primary hyperparathyroidism, as was suggested by bone densitometry studies, it is actually increased as compared with normal subjects [79,82,83]. In primary hyperparathyroidism, there is an increase in trabecular number and a decrease in trabecular separation [79]. Using a histomorphometric technique called *strut analysis*, it has been determined that cancellous bone is preserved in primary hyperparathyroidism through the maintenance of well-connected trabecular plates [79,84].

In summary, despite the absence of radiologically evident bone disease, modern-day primary hyperparathyroidism has a clearly defined pattern of skeletal involvement. Bone turnover is increased, and the disease is associated with diminution of cortical bone and preservation of cancellous bone. Unfortunately, no definitive comment can be made on the clinical sequelae of these observations because large-scale fracture data are unavailable. The available data are contradictory [85–89], making this a major area in need of investigation.

Stone disease in primary hyperparathyroidism

Although the incidence of nephrolithiasis is reduced from that seen in classical primary hyperparathyroidism, kidney stones remain the most common manifestation of symptomatic primary hyperparathyroidism (see Table 1). Estimates in recent studies place the incidence of kidney stones at 15–20% of all patients [90]. Other renal manifestations of primary hyperparathyroidism include hypercalciuria, which is seen in approximately 40% of patients, and nephrocalcinosis, the frequency of which is unknown [91]. There was a precept in classical primary hyperparathyroidism that bone and stone disease did not coexist in a given patient [1,92,93]. Today, there is no clear evidence for two distinct subtypes of primary hyperparathyroidism. Cortical bone demineralization is as common and as extensive in those with and without nephrolithiasis [91,93].

Other organs in primary hyperparathyroidism

Classical primary hyperparathyroidism was associated with a distinct neuromuscular syndrome, characterized by type II muscle cell atrophy [94,95]. This is no longer common [96]. As mentioned earlier the neurobehavioral abnormalities seen in primary hyperparathyroidism have yet to be thoroughly characterized, although it remains an area of interest [51–56].

Approach to the patient with primary hyperparathyroidism

Evaluation

The diagnosis of primary hyperparathyroidism is confirmed by demonstrating an elevated parathyroid hormone level in the face of hypercalcemia. Immunoradiometric and immunochemiluminescent assays for parathyroid hormone offer the greatest sensitivity. Further biochemical assessment should include serum phosphate, albumin, creatinine, alkaline phosphatase, and vitamin D studies. Urine should be collected for calcium, creatinine, and, if there are questions, for hydroxypyridinium crosslinks or N-telopeptide levels. We no longer perform skeletal surveys routinely because it is rare to see radiologically evident bone disease. Bone densitometry, on the other hand, is performed in all patients. The only exceptions are those patients who have made an absolute decision to undergo surgery regardless of the extent of skeletal involvement. Densitometry is done at three sites, the lumbar spine, femoral neck, and radius. The three sites together offer a picture of the total effect of the hyperparathyroid process on the skeleton. Bone biopsy is not part of the routine evaluation of primary hyperparathyroidism.

Treatment

Parathyroidectomy remains the only option for cure of primary hyperparathyroidism. As the disease profile has changed, questions have been raised concerning the advisability of surgery in asymptomatic patients. There are data over 5–10 years of follow-up that biochemical and bone densitometric parameters do not worsen in asymptomatic patients, suggesting that in this group at least, primary hyperparathyroidism may not be a progressive disease

[97–99]. At the National Institutes of Health Consensus Development Conference on the Management of Asymptomatic Primary Hyperparathyroidism in 1991, guidelines regarding which patients should be considered for parathyroidectomy emerged [100]. Surgery is advised in patients meeting any of the following criteria:

1. Serum calcium >12 mg/dl
2. Marked hypercalciuria (>400 mg/day)
3. Any overt manifestation of primary hyperparathyroidism (nephrolithiasis, *osteitis fibrosa cystica*, classic neuromuscular disease)
4. Markedly reduced cortical bone density (Z score <-2)
5. Reduced creatinine clearance in the absence of other cause
6. Age <50 years

Surgery. Approximately 50% of patients presenting with primary hyperparathyroidism today will meet one or more of the surgical guidelines listed earlier. It must be noted that these are only guidelines, and data to support mandatory surgery for some (i.e., age <50 years) are lacking. Physician and patient input remain very important in this decision.

Parathyroid surgery requires considerable expertise. Despite a plethora of preoperative localization techniques (see next section), in a neck not previously operated on diligent identification of all four glands at neck exploration remains mandatory. In the immediate postoperative period, patients must be closely observed for signs and symptoms of hypocalcemia. This can be caused by relative hypoparathyroidism, which is generally transient. Another cause of postoperative hypocalcemia is seen in patients with evidence of significant preoperative bone involvement. In patients with significantly increased bone turnover, parathyroidectomy removes the stimulus to bone resorption, leaving a period in which there is only bone formation. Calcium pours into the skeleton. Known as the *hungry bone syndrome*, it can be associated with marked hypocalcemia. Intravenous calcium may be necessary to correct the deficiency.

After parathyroidectomy, recovery is generally rapid. Vague or constitutional symptoms may or may not improve after surgery, while associated disorders (i.e., hypertension, peptic ulcer disease) are unlikely to remit. Parathyroidectomy does lead to the resolution of the biochemical abnormalities of primary hyperparathyroidism [101]. Surgery is also of clear benefit in reducing the incidence of recurrent nephrolithiasis [90,102]. The 5–10% of patients who continue to form kidney stones after parathyroidectomy are thought to have a second cause for their hypercalciuria, which persists despite cure of their hyperparathyroidism [103,104].

Surgery also leads to an improvement in bone mineral density in patients with primary hyperparathyroidism [101]. Our group has shown that in patients meeting surgical criteria, parathyroidectomy leads to a 12% rise in bone density at the mainly cancellous lumbar spine and femoral neck (Fig. 3). This increase is sustained over a 4-year period after surgery. Once again, postmeno-

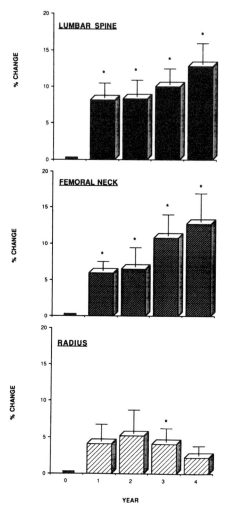

Figure 3. Bone density by site following parathyroidectomy. Data are presented as percentage change from preoperative baseline bone density measurement. Asterisk denotes the change is significant at p < 0.05. (Reprinted from Silverberg et al. [101] with permission.)

pausal women showed a similar pattern of increased bone density. Removing the protection of the hyperparathyroid state did not make them immediately subject to postmenopausal cancellous bone loss. Smaller increases in bone density have been documented at cortical sites. Again, there are no studies of fracture incidence following parathyroidectomy.

Preoperative localization. This topic has generated sufficient controversy to mandate separate consideration. It is well known that the greatest chance for successful parathyroidectomy exists at the time of initial surgery [105].

Preoperative localization techniques have been documented to increase the success of reoperative parathyroid surgery, and there is general enthusiasm for their use in these cases [106]. No such agreement exists regarding the usefulness of preoperative localization techniques for first-time surgery. This is due, in part, to the fact that the ideal localization technique has yet to be developed.

The noninvasive techniques available today are beset with limitations. Ultrasound, thallium/technetium scanning, computed tomography, and magnetic resonance imaging all have significant false-positive rates (15–18%), leading some to require two positive studies before the result is deemed believable [107]. Furthermore, hyperplastic glands often cannot be diagnosed by any of the above-mentioned techniques. Instead, they identify only the dominant hyperplastic gland. Should the surgeon remove only this dominant gland, the patient would remain hyperparathyroid. In addition, only ultrasound can discern lesions of less than 1 cm. Early data on the latest technique to be introduced, radionuclide subtraction scanning with technetium-99m (Tc-99m) sestamibi, has shown improved sensitivity compared with earlier modalities [108–112]. Sestamibi scanning has also been reported to accurately detect hyperplastic glands [112]. At this juncture, however, comparison of the limited sensitivity and high false-positive rate of the noninvasive techniques, with the 90–95% success rate for first-time surgery in experienced hands, has led experts to recommend that localization techniques not be routinely performed prior to initial surgery [105,107].

In the case of the patient who has had previous unsuccessful parathyroid surgery, attempts at preoperative localization are useful. When the noninvasive localization techniques listed earlier are unrevealing, there are invasive techniques that may direct the surgeon. These include parathyroid arteriography and selective venous sampling for parathyroid hormone concentration.

Medical management. Surgical intervention is not warranted in all cases of mild primary hyperparathyroidism. Many of those (approximately one half in our patient population) presenting with asymptomatic hypercalcemia do not meet any of the National Institutes of Health Consensus Conference Guidelines for surgery and often choose to be followed without parathyroidectomy. Data from our group and others have shown remarkable stability in patients with mild primary hyperparathyroidism followed over time [97–99]. We recently reported that in 66 patients, 7 annual measurements showed no change in serum calcium, phosphorus, parathyroid hormone, vitamin D, and alkaline phosphatase, and no change in urinary calcium, hydroxyproline, or hydroxypyridinium crosslink excretion [99]. In sharp contrast to the change in bone mineral density seen in patients after parathyroidectomy, lumbar spine, femoral neck, and radius bone mineral density also showed stability in this group. No change in biochemical indices or bone density at any of the three sites was seen in the subset of postmenopausal women.

In patients followed without surgery, serum and urinary indices should be repeated every 4–6 months, and bone densitometry should be repeated annually. Patients should be instructed to remain well hydrated and to avoid thiazide diuretics [113, 114]. Prolonged immobilization, which can increase hypercalcemia and hypercalciuria, should also be avoided [115]. Dietary calcium intake should be neither very high nor very low. In the latter case, one wishes to avoid the possibility of worsening their underlying disease by causing secondary hyperparathyroidism in response to the low calcium intake.

Fully efficacious medical therapy is not yet available for this disease. Oral phosphate lowers the serum calcium by up to 1 mg/dl [116–118]. While this agent can be used if needed over the short terms, the resulting further increase in parathyroid hormone levels, as well as the possibility of metastatic calcification, limits its utility [119]. Although the most recent bisphosphonates have not been systematically assessed in primary hyperparathyroidism, use of this class of drug in this disorder should probably be limited to therapy of severe hypercalcemia (mainly cases of hyperparathyroid crisis or parathyroid cancer). Estrogen replacement therapy for postmenopausal women with mild primary hyperparathyroidism has wider applicability. It has been associated with a modest (up to 1 mg/dl) decrease in serum calcium, although parathyroid hormone levels are unchanged [120–122].

Agents that inhibit the release of parathyroid hormone hold promise for the future. There was early excitement regarding the organic thiophosphate agent, WR-2721, which successfully inhibits parathyroid hormone release *in vitro* and has been used for malignancy-associated hypercalcemia [123–125]. Unfortunately, dangerous side effects have halted investigation of this agent. More recently, interest has focused on compounds that act on the parathyroid-cell calcium receptor. One such compound, NPS R-568, which is an agonist at the calcium receptor, has been shown to lower serum calcium levels by suppressing parathyroid hormone secretion [126]. A calcimimetic agent of this kind could offer a possible medical alternative to parathyroidectomy for some patients [127].

Acute primary hyperparathyroidism

Known variously as parathyroid crisis, parathyroid poisoning, and parathyroid intoxication, acute primary hyperparathyroidism describes an episode of acute, life-threatening hypercalcemia in a patient with primary hyperparathyroidism [128]. Clinical manifestations of acute primary hyperparathyroidism are mainly those associated with severe hypercalcemia. Many patients have nephrocalcinosis or nephrolithiasis. Radiologic evidence of subperiosteal bone resorption is commonly present. Laboratory evaluation is remarkable not only for very high serum calcium levels but also for extreme elevations in parathyroid hormone to approximately 20 times normal [129]. In this way, acute primary hyperparathyroidism resembles parathyroid carci-

174

noma. A history of persistent mild hypercalcemia has been reported in 25% of patients [129]. However, given the rarity of this condition, the risk of developing acute primary hyperparathyroidism in a patient with mild asymptomatic primary hyperparathyroidism is very low. Possible precipitating conditions include intercurrent medical illness with immobilization. Early diagnosis, with aggressive medical management followed by surgical cure, are essential for a successful outcome in this condition.

Future directions for research

Although our knowledge of primary hyperparathyroidism as it presents today has increased tremendously, there remain many unanswered questions. Active and exciting work on the molecular mechanisms of this disease are ongoing, as are efforts to find a medical 'cure.' Other areas of interest emerge from recent clinical studies. What is the fracture incidence after parathyroidectomy? What is the fracture incidence in primary hyperparathyroidism if left untreated? Can the neurobehavioral component of the disorder be systematically elucidated? Is there an association between primary hyperparathyroidism and cancer [130–132] or heart disease [133–135] as has been suggested? Is the disease truly stable over a longer (more than 7–10 year) period? And if so, should youthfulness no longer be considered an indication for surgery? Multicenter clinical studies will be necessary in order to answer some of these outstanding questions.

References

1. Albright F, Reifenstein EC. 1948. The Parathyroid Glands and Metabolic Bone Disease. Baltimore, MD: Williams & Wilkins.
2. Cope O. 1966. The story of hyperparathyroidism at the Massachusetts General Hospital. N Engl J Med 21:1174–1182.
3. Bauer W. 1933. Hyperparathyroidism: Distinct disease entity. J Bone Joint Surg 15:135–141.
4. Bauer W, Federman DD. 1962. Hyperparathyroidism epitomized: Case of Captain Charles E. Martell. Metabolism 11:21–22.
5. Mandl F. 1925. Therapeutiscle Versuch bei Ostitis fibrosa generalisata mittels Extirpation lines Epithelkoperchentumon. Wein Klin Wochenschr 50:1343–1344.
6. Albright F, Aub JC, Bauer W. 1934. Hyperparathyroidism common and polymorphic condition as illustrated by seventeen proved cases from one clinic. J JAMA 102:1276–1287.
7. Silverberg SJ, Fitzpatrick LA, Bilezikian JP. 1995. Primary hyperathyroidism. In Becker KL, ed. Principles and Practice of Endocrinology and Metabolism. Philadelphia: JB Lippincott, pp 512–519.
8. Heath H, Hodgson SF, Kennedy MA. 1980. Primary hyperparathyroidism: Incidence, morbidity, and economic impact in a community. N Engl J Med 302:189–193.
9. Mundy GR, Cove DH, Fisken R. 1980. Primary hyperparathyroidism: Changes in the pattern of clinical presentation. Lancet 1:1317–1320.
10. Scholz DA, Purnell DC. 1981. Asymptomatic primary hyperparathyroidism. Mayo Clin Proc 56:473–478.

11. Mallette LE, Bilezikian JP, Heath DA, Aurbach GD. 1974. Hyperparathyroidism: A review of 52 cases. Medicine 53:127–147.
12. Bilezikian JP, Silverberg SJ, Gartenberg F, et al. 1994. Clinical presentation of primary hyperparathyroidism. In Bilezikian JP, ed. The Parathyroids: Basic and Clinical Concepts. New York: Raven Press, pp 457–470.
13. Rao SD, Frame B, Miller MJ, Kleerekoper M, Block MA, Parfitt AM. 1980. Hyperparathyroidism following head and neck irradiation. Arch Intern Med 140:205–207.
14. Seely EW, Moore TJ, LeBoff MS, Brown EM. 1989. A single dose of lithium carbonate acutely elevates intact parathyroid hormone levels in humans. Acta Endocrinol 121:174–176.
15. Nordenstrom J, Strigard K, Perbeck L, Willems J, Bagedahl-Strindlund M, Linder J. 1992. Hyperparathyroidism associated with treatment of manic-depressive disorders by lithium. Eur J Surg 158:207–211.
16. McHenry CR, Rosen IB, Rotstein LE, Forbath N, Walfish PG. Lithiumogenic disorders of the thyroid and parathyroid glands as surgical disease. Surgery 108:1001–1005.
17. Krivitzky A, Bentata-Pessayre M, Sarfati E, Gardin JP, Callard P, Delzant G. 1986. Multiple hypersecreting lesions of the parathyroid glands during treatment with lithium. Ann Med Intern 137:118–122.
18. Brown EM, Gardner DG, Brennan MF, Marx SJ, Spiegel AM, Attie MF, Downs RW Jr, Doppman JL, Aurbach GD. 1979. Calcium-regulated parathyroid hormone release in primary hyperparathyroidism. Studies in vitro with dispersed parathyroid cells. Am J Med 66:923–931.
19. Lloyd HM, Parfitt AM, Jacobi JM, Wilgoss DA, Craswell DW, Petrie JJ, Boyle PD. 1989. The parathyroid glands in chronic renal failure: A study of their growth and other properties made on the basis of findings in patients with hypercalcemia. J Lab Clin Med 114:358–367.
20. Parfitt AM, Willgoss D, Jacob J, Lloyd HM. 1991. Cell kinetics in parathyroid adenomas: Evidence for decline in rates of cell birth and tumor growth, assuming clonal origin. Clin Endocrinol 35:151–157.
21. Arnold A, Staunton CE, Kim HG, Gaz RD, Kronenberg HM. 1988. Monoclonality and abnormal parathyroid hormone genes in parathyroid adenomas. N Engl J Med 318:658–662.
22. Arnold A, Kim HG, Gaz RD, Eddy RL, Fukushima Y, Byers MG, Shows TB, Kronenberg HM. 1989. Molecular cloning and chromosomal mapping of DNA rearranged with the parathyroid hormone gene in a parathyroid adenoma. J Clin Invest 83:2034–2040.
23. Friedman E, Bale AE, Marx SJ, Norton JA, Arnold A, Tu T, Aurbach GD, Spiegel AM. 1990. Genetic abnormalities in sporadic parathyroid adenoma. J Clin Endocrinol Metab 71:293–297.
24. Arnold A, Kim HG. 1989. Clonal loss of one chromosome 11 in a parathyroid adenoma. J Clin Endocrinol Metab 69:496–499.
25. Cryns VL, Yi SM, Tahara H, Gaz RD, Arnold A. 1995. Frequent loss of chromosome arm 1p in parathyroid adenomas. Genes Chromosom Cancer 13:9–17.
26. Tahara H, Smith AP, Gaz RD, Cryns VL, Arnold A. 1996. Genomic localization of novel candidate tumor suppressor gene loci in human parathyroid adenomas. Cancer Res 56:599–605.
27. Parfitt AM. 1994. Parathyroid growth, normal and abnormal. In Bilezikian JP, Marcus R, Levine MA, eds. The Parathyroids. New York: Raven Press, pp 373–405.
28. Pollak MR, Brown EM, Chou Y-HW, Herbert SC, Marx SJ, Steinmann B, Levi T, Seidman CE, Seidman JG. 1993. Mutations in the human Ca^{2+}-sensing receptor gene cause familial hypocalciuric hypercalcemia and neonatal severe hyperparathyroidism. Cell 75:1297–1303.
29. Hosokawa Y, Pollak MR, Brown EM, Arnold A. 1995. The extracellular calcium-sensing receptor gene in human parathyroid tumors. J Clin Endocrinol Metab 80:3107–3110.
30. Thompson DB, Samowitz WS, Odelberg S, Davis RK, Szabo J, Heath III H. 1995. Genetic abnormalities in sporadic parathyroid adenomas: Loss of heterozygosity for chromosome 3q markers flanking the calcium receptor locus. J Clin Endocrinol Metab 80:3377–3380.

31. Verdonk CA, Edis AJ. 1981. Parathyroid 'double adenomas': Fact or fiction? Surgery 90:523–526.
32. Harness JK, Ramsburg Sr, Nishiyama RH, Thompson NW. 1979. Multiple adenomas of the parathyroids: Do they exist? Arch Surg 114:468–474.
33. Attie JN, Bock G, Auguste L. 1990. Multiple parathyroid adenomas: Report of thirty-three cases. Surgery 108:1014–1102.
34. Nudelman IL, Deutsch AA, Reiss R. 1987. Primary hyperparathyroidism due to mediastinal parathyroid adenoma. Int Surg 72:104–108.
35. Wheeler MH, Williams ED, Wade JSH. 1987. The hyperfunctioning intrathyroidal parathyroid gland: A potential pitfall in parathyroid surgery. World J Surg 11:110–114.
36. Sloane JA. 1978. Parathyroid adenoma in submucosa of esophagus. Arch Pathol Lab Med 102:242–243.
37. Joseph MP, Nadol JB, Pilch BZ, Goodman ML. 1982. Ectopic parathyroid tissue in the hypopharyngeal mucosa (pyriform sinus). Head Neck Surg 5:70–74.
38. Gilmour JR. 1941. Some developmental abnormalities of the thymus and parathyroids. J Pathol Bacteriol 52:213–218.
39. Thakker RV, Bouloux P, Wooding C, Chotai K, Broad PM, Spurr NK, Besser GM, O'Riordan JL. 1989. Association of parathyroid tumors in multiple endocrine neoplasia type I with loss of alleles on chromosome 11. N Engl J Med 32:218–224.
40. Friedman E, Sakaguchi K, Bale AE, Falchetti A, Streeten E, Zimering MB, Weinstein LS, McBride WO, Nakamura Y, Brandi ML. 1989. Clonality of parathyroid tumors in familial multiple endocrine neoplasia type 1. N Engl J Med 321:213–218.
41. Arnold A, Brown MF, Urena P, Gaz RD, Sarfati E, Drueke TB. 1995. Monoclonality of parathyroid tumors in chronic renal failure and in primary parathyroid hyperplasia. J Clin Invest 95:2047–2053.
42. Albright F, Bloomberg E, Castleman B, Churchill ED. 1934. Hyperparathyroidism due to a diffuse hyperplasia of all parathyroid glands rather than to a parathyroid adenoma of one gland. Clinical studies on three such cases. Arch Intern Med 54:315–329.
43. Clark OH. 1978. Hyperparathyroidim due to primary cystic parathyroid hyperplasia. Arch Surg 113:748–750.
44. Fallon MD, Haines JW, Teitelbaum SL. 1982. Cystic parathyroid hyperplasia. Am J Clin Pathol 77:104–107.
45. Mallette LE, Malini S, Rappaport MP, Kirkland JL. 1987. Familial cystic parathyroid adenomatosis. Ann Intern Med 107:54–60.
46. Ringe JD. 1984. Reversible hypertension in primary hyperparathyroidism: Pre- and postoperative blood pressure in 75 cases. Klin Wochenschr 62:465–469.
47. Broulik PD, Horky K, Pacovsky V. 1985. Blood pressure in patients with primary hyperparathyroidism before and after parathyroidectomy. Exp Clin Endocrinol 86:346–352.
48. Rapado A. 1986. Arterial hypertension and primary hyperparathyroidism. Am J Nephrol 6(Suppl 1):49–50.
49. Bilezikian JP, Aurbach GD, Connor TB, Aplekar R, Freijanes J, Pachas WN, Wells SA, Decker JL. 1973. Pseudogout following parathyroidectomy. Lancet 1:445–447.
50. Geelhoed GW, Kelly TR. 1989. Pseudogout as a clue and complication in primary hyperparathyroidism. Surgery 106:1036–1041.
51. Joborn C, Hetta J, Johansson H, et al. 1988. Psychiatric morbidity in primary hyperparathyroidism. World J Surg 12:476–481.
52. Joborn C, Hetta J, Frisk P, Palmer M, Akerstrom G, Ljunghall S. 1986. Primary hyperparathyroidism in patients with organic brain syndrome. Acta Med Scand 219:91–98.
53. Alarcon RD, Franceschini JA. 1984. Hyperparathyroidism and paranoid psychosis case report and review of the literature. Br J Psychiatr 145:477–486.
54. Ljunghall S, Jakobsson S, Joborn C, Palmer M, Rastad J, Akerstrom G. 1991. Longitudinal studies of mild primary hyperparathyroidism. J Bone Miner Res 6(Suppl 2):S111–S116.
55. Brown GG, Preisman RC, Kleerekoper MD. 1987. Neurobehavioral symptoms in mild

primary hyperparathyroidism: Related to hypercalcemia but not improved by parathyroidectomy. Henry Ford Med J 35:211–215.

56. Kleerekoper M. 1994. Clinical course of primary hyperparathyroidism. In Bilezikian JP, ed. The Parathyroids: Basic and Clinical Concepts. New York: Raven Press, pp 471–484.

57. Vieth R, Bayley TA, Walfish PG, Rosen IB, Pollard A. 1991. Relevance of vitamin D metabolite concentrations in supporting the diagnosis of primary hyperparathyroidism. Surgery 110:1043–1046.

58. Deftos LJ. 1994. Markers of bone turnover in primary hyperparathyroidism. In Bilezikian JP, ed. The Parathyroids: Basic and Clinical Concepts. New York: Raven Press, pp 485–492.

59. Moss DW. 1992. Perspectives in alkaline phosphatase research. Clin Chem 38:2486–2492.

60. Pfeilschifter J, Siegrist E, Wuster C, Blind E, Ziegler R. 1992. Serum levels of intact parathyroid hormone and alkaline phosphatase correlate with cortical and trabecular bone loss in primary hyperparathyroidism. Acta Endocrinol 127:319–323.

61. Minisola S, Scarnecchia L, Carnevale V, Bigi F, Romagnoli E, Pacitti MT, Rosso R, Mazzuoli GF. 1989. Clinical value of the measurement of bone remodeling markers in primary hyperparathyroidism. J Endocrinol Invest 12:537–543.

62. Torres R, De La Pirera C, Papado A. 1989. Osteocalcin and bone remodeling in Paget's disease of bone, primary hyperparathyroidism, hypercalcemia of malignancy and involutional osteoporosis. Scand J Clin Invest 49:279–285.

63. Silverberg SJ, Deftos LJ, Kim T, Hill CS. 1991. Bone alkaline phosphatase in primary hyperparathyroidism. J Bone Miner Res 6:A624.

64. Duda RJ, O'Brien JF, Katzman JA, Paterson JM, Mann KG, Riggs BL. 1988. Concurrent assays of circulating bone Gla-protein and bone alkaline phosphatase: Effects of sex, age, and metabolic bone disease. J Clin Endocrinol Metab 5:1–7.

65. Price PA, Parthemore JG, Deftos LJ. 1980. New biochemical marker for bone metabolism. Measurement by radioimmunoassay of bone Gla-protein in the plasma of normal subjects and patients with bone disease. J Clin Invest 66:878–883.

66. Deftos LJ, Parthemore JG, Price PA. 1982. Changes in plasma bone Gla-protein during treatment of bone disease. Calcif Tissue Int 34:121–124.

67. Eastell R, Delmas PD, Hodgson S, Eriksen EF, Mann KM, Riggs BL. 1988. Bone formation rate in older normal women: Concurrent assessment with bone histomorphometry, clacium kinetics, and biochemical markers. J Clin Endocrinol Metab 67:741–748.

68. Eberlin PR, Peterson JM, Riggs BL. 1992. Utility of type 1 procollagen propeptide assays for assessing abnormalities in metabolic bone diseases. J Bone Mineral Res 7:1243–1250.

69. Deftos LJ. 1991. Bone protein and peptide assays in the diagnosis and management of skeletal disease. Clin Chem 37:1143–1148.

70. Delmas PH. 1991. Biochemical markers of bone turnover: Methodology and clinical use in osteoporosis. Am J Med 91:169–174.

71. Parfitt AM. 1991. Serum markers of bone formation in parenteral nutrition patients. Calcif Tissue Int 49:143–145.

72. Seibel MJ, Gartenberg F, Silverberg SJ, Ratcliffe A, Robins SP, Bilezikian JP. 1992. Urinary hydroxypyridinium cross-links of collagen in primary hyperparathyroidism. J Clin Endocrinol Metab 74:481–486.

73. Kraenzlin ME, Lau KHW, Liang L, Freeman TK, Singer FR, Baylink DJ. 1990. Development of an immunoassay for human serum osteoclastic tartrate-resistant acid phosphatase. J Clin Endocrinol Metab 71:442.

74. Silverberg SJ, Shane E, DeLaCruz L, Dempster DW, Feldman F, Seldin D, Jacobs TD, Siris ES, Cafferty M, Parisien MV, Bilezikian JP. 1989. Skeletal disease in primary hyperparathyroidism. J Bone Miner Res 4:283–291.

75. Bilezikian JP, Silverberg SJ, Shane E, Parisien M, Dempster DW. 1991. Characterization and evaluation of asymptomatic primary hyperparathyroidism. J Bone Miner Res 6(Suppl 1):585–589.

76. Dempster DW, Cosman F, Parisien M, Shen V, Lindsay R. 1993. Anabolic actions of parathyroid hormone on bone. Endocr Rev 14:690–709.

178

77. Canalis E, Hock JM, Raisz LG. 1994. Anabolic and catabolic effects of PTH on bone and interactions with growth factors. In Bilezikian JP ed. The Parathyroids: Basic and Clinical Concepts. New York: Raven Press, pp 65–82.

78. Slovik DM, Rosenthal DI, Doppelt SH, Potts JT, Daly MA, Neer RM. 1986. Restoration of spinal bone in osteoporotic men by treatment with human PTH (1–34) and vitamin D. J Bone Miner Res 1:377–381.

79. Parisien M, Silverberg SJ, Shane E, de la Cruz L, Lindsay R, Bilezikian JP, Dempster DW. 1990. The histormorphometry of bone in primary hyperparathyroidism: Preservation of cancellous bone structure. J Clin Endocrinol Metab 70:930–938.

80. Parfitt AM. 1986. Accelerated cortical bone loss: Primary and secondary hyperparathyroidism. In Uhthoff H, Stahl E, eds. Current Concepts of Bone Fragility. Berlin: Springer-Verlag, pp 279–285.

81. Parfitt AM. 1989. Surface specific bone remodeling in health and disease. In Kleerekoper M, ed. Clinical Disorders of Bone and Mineral Metabolism. New York: Mary Ann Liebert, pp 7–14.

82. van Doorn L, Lips P, Netelenbos JC, Hackengt WHL. 1989. Bone histomorphometry and serum intact PTH (I-84) in hyperparathyroid patients. Calcif Tissue Int 44S:N36.

83. Parisien M, Dempster DW, Shane E, Silverberg S, Lindsay R, Bilezikian JP. 1988. Structural parameters of bone biopsies in primary hyperparathyroidism. In Takahashi HE, ed. Bone Morphometry. Proceedings of the Fifth International Congress on Bone Morphometry, Niigata, Japan. New York: Smith-Gordon, pp 228–231.

84. Christiansen P, Steiniche T, Vesterby A, Mosekilde L, Hessov I, Melsen F. 1992. Primary hyperparathyroidism: Iliac crest trabecular bone volume, structure, remodeling, and balance evaluated by histomorphometric methods. Bone 13:41–49.

85. Wilson RJ, Rao DS, Ellis B, Kleerekoper M, Parfitt AM. 1988. Mild asymptomatic primary hyperparathyroidism is not a risk factor for vertebral fractures. Ann Intern Med 109:959–962.

86. Dauphine RT, Riggs BL, Scholz DA. 1975. Back pain and vertebral crush fractures: An unrecognized mode of presentation for primary hyperparathyroidism. Ann Intern Med 83:365–367.

87. Larsson K, Lindh E, Lind L, Persson I, Ljunghall S. 1989. Increased fracture risk in hypercalcemia. Bone mineral content measured in hyperparathyroidism. Acta Orthop Scand 60:268–270.

88. Lafferty FW, Halsay CA. 1986. Primary hyperparathyroidism: A review of the long-term surgical and non-surgical morbidities as a basis for a rational approach to treatment. Arch Intern Med 149:789–796.

89. Melton LJ 3rd, Atkinson EJ, O'Fallon WM, Heath H. 1992. Risk of age-related fractures in patients with primary hyperparathyroidism. Arch Intern Med 152:2269–2273.

90. Klugman VA, Favus M, Pak CYC. 1994. Nephrolithiasis in primary hyperparathyroidism. In Bilezikian JP, ed. The Parathyroids: Basic and Clinical Concepts. New York: Raven Press, pp 505–518.

91. Silverberg SJ, Shane E, Jacobs TP, Siris ES, Garterbey F, Seldin D, Clemens TL, Bilezikian JP. 1990. Nephrolithiasis and bone involvement in primary hyperparathyroidism. Am J Med 89:327–334.

92. Broadus AE, Horst RL, Lang R, Littledike ET, Rasmussen H. 1990. The importance of circulating 1,25(OH)$_2$D in the pathogenesis of hypercalciuria and renal stone formation in primary hyperparathyroidism. N Engl J Med 302:421–426.

93. Pak CYC, Nicar MJ. Peterson R, Zerwekh JE, Snyder W. 1981. Lack of unique pathophysiologic background for nephrolithiasis in primary hyperparathyroidism. J Clin Endocrinol Metab 53:536–542.

94. Aurbach GD, Mallette LE, Patten BM, Heath DA, Doppman JP, Bilezikian JP. 1973. Hyperparathyroidism: Recent studies. Ann Intern Med 79:566–581.

95. Patten BM, Bilezikian JP, Mallette LE, Prince A, Engel WK, Aurbach GD. 1989. The neuromuscular disease of hyperparathyroidism. Ann Intern Med 80:182–194.

179

96. Turken SA, Cafferty M, Silverberg SJ, de la Cruz L, Cimino C, Lange DJ, Lovelace RE, Bilezikian JP. 1989. Neuromuscular involvement in mild, asymptomatic primary hyperparathyroidism. Am J Med 87:553–557.

97. Rao DS, Wilson RJ, Kleerekoper M, Parfitt AM. 1988. Lack of biochemical progression or continuation of accelerated bone loss in mild asymptomatic primary hyperparathyroidism. J Clin Endocrinol Metab 67:1294–1298.

98. Parfitt AM, Rao DS, Kleerekoper M. 1991. Asymptomatic primary hyperparathyroidism discovered by multichannel biochemical screening: Clinical course and considerations bearing on the need for surgical intervention. J Bone Miner Res 6(Suppl 2):s97–s101.

99. Silverberg SJ, Gartenberg F, Jacobs TP, Shane E, Siris E, Staron RB, Bilezikian JP. 1995. Longitudinal measurements of bone density and biochemical indices in untreated primary hyperparathyroidism. J Clin Endocrinol Metab 80:723–728.

100. National Institutes of Health. 1991. Consensus development conference statement on primary hyperparathyroidism. J Bone Miner Res 6:s9–s13.

101. Silverberg SJ, Gartenberg F, Jacobs TP, Shane E, Siris E, Staron RB, McMahon DJ, Bilezikian JP. 1995. Increased bone mineral density following parathyroidectomy in primary hyperparathyroidism. J Clin Endocrinol Metab 80:729–734.

102. Deaconson TF, Wilson SD, Lemann J. 1987. The effect of parathyroidectomy on the recurrence of nephrolithiasis. Surgery 215:241–251.

103. Kaplan RA, Snyder WH. Stewart A. 1976. Metabolic effects of parathyroidectomy in asymptomatic primary hyperparathyroidism. J Clin Endocrinol Metab 42:415–426.

104. Siminovich JMP, James RE, Esselsytne CBJ, Straffon RA, Banowsky LH. 1980. The effect of parathyroidectomy in patients with normocalcemic calcium stones. J Urol 123:335–337.

105. Savata RM, Jr, Beahrs OH, Scholz DA. 1975. Success rate of cervical exploration for hyperparathyroidism. Arch Surg 110:625–628.

106. Carty SE, Norton J. 1991. Management of patients with persistent or recurrent primary hyperparathyroidism. World J Surg 15:716–723.

107. Doppman JL. 1994. Preoperative localization of parathyroid tissue in primary hyperparathyroidism. In Bilezikian JP, ed. The Parathyroids: Basic and Clinical Concepts. New York: Raven Press, pp 553–566.

108. Halvorson DJ, Burke GJ, Mansberger AR. 1994. Use of technetium Tc 99m sestamibi and iodine 123 radionuclide scan for preoperative localization of abnormal parathyroid glands in primary hyperparathyroidism. South Med J 87:336–339.

109. Wei JP, Burke GJ, Mansberger AR. 1994. Preoperative imaging of abnormal parathyroid glands in patients with hyperparathyroid disease using combination Tc-99 m-pertechnate and Tc-99 m-sestamibi radionuclide scans. Ann Surg 219:568–573.

110. Casas AT, Burke GJ, Sathyanarayana, Mansberger AR, Wei JP. 1993. Prospective comparison of technetium-99 m-sestamibi/iodine-123 radionuclide scan versus high resolution ultrasonography for the preoperative localization of abnormal parathyroid glands in patients with previously unoperated primary hyperparathyroidism. Am J Surg 166:369–373.

111. Thule P, Thakore K, Vansant J, McGarity W, Weber C, Phillips LS. 1994. Preoperative localization of parathyroid tissue with technetium-99 m sestamibi 123-I subtraction scanning. J Clin Endocrinol Metab 78:77–82.

112. Johnston LB, Carroll MJ, Brittan KE, Shand W, Besser GM, Grossman AB. 1996. The accuracy of parathyroid gland localization in primary hyperparathyroidism using sestamibi radionuclide imagery. J Clin Endocrinol Metab 81:346–352.

113. Stier CT, Itskovitz HD. 1986. Renal calcium metablism and diuretics. Ann Rev Pharmacol Toxicol 26:101–116.

114. Sutton RAL. 1985. Diuretics and calcium metabolism. Am J Kidney Dis 5:4–9.

115. Stewart AF, Adler M, Byers CM, Segre GV, Broadus AE. 1982. Calcium homeostatis in immobilization: An example of resorptive hypercalciuria. N Engl J Med 306:1136–1140.

116. Stock JL, Marcus R. 1994. Medical management of primary hyperparathyroidism. In Bilezikian JP, ed. The Parathyroids: Basic and Clinical Concepts. New York: Raven Press, pp 519–530.

117. Purnell DC, Scholz DA, Smith LM, Sizemore GW, Black MB, Goldsmith RS, Arnand CD. 1974. Treatment of primary hyperparathyroidism. Am J Med 56:800–809.
118. Broadus AE, Magee JS, Mallette LE, Horst RL, Lang R, Jensen PS, Gertner JM, Baron R. 1983. A detailed evaluation of oral phosphate thereapy in selected patients with primary hyperparathyroidism. J Clin Endocrinol Metab 56:953–961.
119. Vernava AM III, O'Neal LW, Palermo V. 1987. Lethal hyperparathyroid crisis: Hazards of phosphate administration. Surgery 102:941:948.
120. Marcus R, Madvig P, Crim M, Pont A, Kosek J. 1984. Conjugated estrogens in the treatment of postmenopausal women with hyperparathyroidism. Ann Intern Med 100:633–640.
121. Marcus R. 1991. Estrogens and progestins in the management of primary hyperparathyroidism. J Bone Miner Res 6(Suppl 1):S125–S129.
122. Selby PL, Peacock M. 1986. Ethinyl estradiol and norethinedrone in the treatment of primary hyperparathyroidism in postmenopausal women. N Engl J Med 314:1481–1485.
123. Glover D, Riley L, Carmichael K, Spar B, Glick J, Kligerman MM, Agus ZS, Slatopolsky E, Attie M, Goldfarb S. 1983. Hypocalcemia and inhibition of parathyroid hormone secretion after administration of WR-2721 (a radioprotective and chemoprotective agent). N Engl J Med 309:1137–1141.
124. Glover DJ, Shaw L, Glick JH, Slatopolsky E, Weiler C, Attie M, Goldfarb S. 1985. Treatment of hypercalcemia or parathyroid cancer with WR-2721, S-2-(3-aminopropylamino) ethyl-phosphorothioic acid. Ann Intern Med 103:55–57.
125. Hirschel-Scholz S, Jung A, Fischer A, Trechsel U, Bonjour J-P. 1985. Suppression of parathyroid secretion after administration of WR-2721 in a patient with parathyroid carcinoma. Clin Endocrinol 23:313–318.
126. Fox J, Hadfield S, Petty BA, Nemeth EF. 1993. A first generation calcimimetic compound (NPS R-568) that acts on the parathyroid cell calcium receptor: A novel therapeutic approach for hyperparathyroidism. J Bone Min Res 8, S181.
127. Fox J, Hadfield S, Petty BA, Conklin RL, Nemeth EF. 1993. NPS R-568 acts on calcium receptors to inhibit parathyroid hormone and stimulate calcitonin secretion: A novel therapeutic approach for hyperparathyroidism. J Am Nephrol:4–719.
128. Fitzpatrick LA, Bilezikian JP. 1987. Acute primary hyperparathyroidism. Am J Med 82:275–282.
129. Fitzpatrick LA. 1994. Acute primary hyperparathyroidism. In Bilezikian JP, ed. The Parathyroids: Basic and Clinical Concepts. New York: Raven Press, pp 583–590.
130. Wajngot A, Werner S, Granberg PO, Lindvall N. 1980. Occurrence of pituitary adenomas and other neoplastic diseases in primary hyperparathyroidisms. Surg Gynecol Obstet 151:401–403.
131. Farr HW, Fahey TJ Jr, Nash Ag, Farr CM. 1973. Primary hyperparathyroidism and cancer. Am J Surg 126:539–543.
132. Attie JN, Vardhan R. 1993. Association of hyperparathyroidism with nonmedullary thyroid carcinoma: Review of 31 cases. Head Neck 15:20–23.
133. Ronni-Sivula H. 1985. The state of health of patients previously operated on for primary hyperparathyroidism compared with randomized controls. Ann Chir Gynaecol 74:60–65.
134. Palmer M, Adami H-O, Bergstrom R, Akerstroom G, Ljunghall S. 1987. Mortality after surgery for primary hyperparathyroidism: A follow-up of 441 patients operated on from 1956 to 1979. Surgery 102:1–7.
135. Stefenelli T, Mayr H, Bergler-Klein J, Globits S, Woloszczuk W, Niederle B. 1993. Primary hyperparathyroidism: Incidence of cardiac abnormalities and partial reversibility after successful parathyroidectomy. Am J Medicine 95:197–202.

9. Parathyroid carcinoma

Kerstin Sandelin

Parathyroid carcinoma is the rarest type of endocrine malignant tumor. Consequently, clinicians and pathologists not dealing with endocrine tumors will have a limited experience, which may affect the diagnosis and treatment of this tumor. Its natural growth pattern is that of a slowly growing neoplasm, and when recurrences eventually occur they are predominantly located cervically. This fact may initially lead the surgeon to assume that the tumor is not malignant. The term *atypical adenoma* was coined for borderline lesions with a clinically benign course [1].

Certain clinical characteristics and morphologic features, however, in the histologic architecture, in tumor cytology, and in the DNA pattern of the tumor cells have been found to be consistent with malignancy. Recent advances using molecular techniques have shown chromosomal abnormalities in different types of benign and malignant parathyroid tumors that may to some extent explain the pathogenesis behind the various forms of primary hyperparathyroidism (pHPT). This chapter focuses on the collected experience in diagnosis and management and also covers the more recent attempts to characterize these unusual tumors by means of immunohistochemical and molecular methodology.

Historical background

Some 25 years after the anatomical description of the parathyroid glands made by the Swedish anatomist Sandström [2], the Austrian pathologist Erdheim described the connection between enlarged glands, osteolytic bone deficiency, and the symptoms of hypoparathyroidism on parathyroidectomized rats [3,4]. Simultaneously in the United States, MacCallum at Johns Hopkins Hospital started to publish work on tetany and the use of parathyroid extract to relieve symptoms [5]. During the same time period, Halstead performed thyroidectomies and made similar conclusions about the incidence and treatment of tetany postoperatively.

The clinical and operative description by Mandl in 1925 of a young man with severe osteoporosis (osteitis fibrosa cystica), together with the operative

Andrew Arnold (ed.) ENDOCRINE NEOPLASMS. 1997. Kluwer Academic Publishers. ISBN 0-7923-4354-9.

findings of a large cervical tumor adherent to the recurrent laryngeal nerve, with 4 years of remission and subsequent recurrence of symptoms that eventually had a fatal outcome, is well in accordance with a malignant parathyroid tumor. In the late 1920s, the histopathologic description of parathyroid carcinoma was discussed in two papers in which capsular invasion, polymorphic nuclei, and mitotic figures were findings [6–8].

Incidence

As mentioned initially, this rare tumor represents less than 1% of cases with pHPT. In series from institutions where the number of cases with benign and malignant cases are given, the incidence figures for parathyroid carcinoma vary between 0.3% and 5.6% [9–14]. Possible explanations for these variations are (1) epidemiological differences, which would explain the 5% incidence of carcinoma in the Japanese population [15], (2) a local referral pattern that increases the figures from reporting centers, and (3) overdiagnosis [12,16,17]. In a retrospective international series, 95 cases of patients with the diagnosis of parathyroid carcinoma were thoroughly evaluated [16]. A morphologic study unbiased by clinical data was made in order to assess the histopathologic findings. Two types of tumors were found, namely, one showing clear signs of an invasive growth pattern (n = 41) and one showing various degrees of atypia (n = 54). Fifteen of the equivocal cases, however, had clinical evidence of recurrence, thus establishing the cancer diagnosis with certainty in 56 of 95 patients. Whether the remaining 39 cases, with a median follow-up period of 84 months (4–264), represent overdiagnosis of malignancy or just illustrate indolent clinical behavior of parathyroid carcinoma is not known.

Etiology

There are six publications of associated parathyroid carcinoma in families with concurrent pHPT [18–22]. The number of affected members are small and only few have had local recurrences. Chromosomal analysis of tumor tissue in a study by Streeten et al. showed no tumor-specific gene abnormality nor any chromosomal aberration that has been identified in any other subgroup of tumors from patients with other forms of HPT [23]. To date there have been no reports of malignant parathyroid tumors in either of the multiple endocrine neoplasia syndromes (MEN-I and MEN-II). Based on the studies of other types of tumors in HPT, several defective genes have been identified or localized as being responsible for tumor development [24]. Radiation-induced tumorigenesis is described for head and neck tumors, including benign HPT and thyroid neoplasia, but is not clearly associated with parathyroid carcinoma [25,26].

184

Symptoms and diagnosis

For the most part, patients with parathyroid carcinoma have typical signs and symptoms of severe pHPT. The female/male ratio is equal and the age of onset is often around the fifth decade. The organs mostly affected by complications are the skeleton (40–70%), kidneys (30–60%), gastrointestinal tract (15%), and neuromuscular system. Osteolytic bone changes or osteitis fibrosa cystica presents as bone pain and sometimes fractures. Kidney stones, nephrocalcinosis, polyuria, and polydipsia are common renal features. A severe muscular weakness is also frequent among these patients. Gastrointestinal symptoms, such as pancreatitis and ulcers, occur less frequently, in contrast to the common loss of appetite and vomiting. Neuropsychiatric manifestations often include anxiety and depression but can also be nonspecific. A palpable cervical mass is present in approximately 30%. The majority of symptoms can be related to the metabolic consequences of high serum calcium levels on the target organs.

Current intact parathormone (PTH) assays will accurately exclude other causes of hypercalcemia. Benign pHPT with an acute onset will present with similar symptoms and thus cannot be distinguished from the malignant form. Nevertheless, the clinical and biochemical profile of pHPT has changed over the last 15 years so that the severe symptoms already described should always alert the clinician to the possibility of parathyroid carcinoma. Regardless of etiology, the condition needs urgent treatment and restoration of fluid and electrolyte balance is mandatory. Intravenous saline solution followed later by loop diuretics will restore glomerular function and increase urine calcium secretion. Since the introduction of the bisphosphonates, which are potent osteoclast inhibitors, the need for other drugs has been largely eliminated. Pamidronate, the most potent bisphosphonate when administered intravenously, will often restore calcium balance within 48 hours. Management of hypercalcemic crisis is addressed in more detail in Chapter 10. Some authors suggest that in a patient with hypercalcemic crisis, once the fluid balance is restored, exploration and removal of the tumor is indicated without further delay [27]. On the other hand, bisphosphonates have proven useful in controlling the serum calcium levels while the patient undergoes an appropriate workup [28].

Operative strategy at initial exploration

'There is no time like the initial operation' to find and to possibly cure the patient, according to Albright in his statement of the operative strategy of pHPT in 1934 [29]. This still holds true and particularly applies to parathyroid carcinoma, for which recognition of the disease and appropriate surgical treatment are critical in decreasing the incidence subsequent local relapse. The gross pathology of a parathyroid carcinoma is a grey, whitish hard tumor, often adherent to neighboring structures, such as the ipsilateral thyroid lobe, the recurrent laryngeal nerve, the thyroid vessels, and/or the esophagus. Nevertheless, in a series of 40 patients with proven locally and/or metastatic parathyroid carcinoma, 19 had a benign HPT diagnosis at initial exploration, emphasizing the diagnostic difficulties that might be encountered [30]. The experience of 14 patients treated surgically at Memorial Sloan–Kettering Cancer Center was reported by Vetto et al. [31]. The authors stressed diagnostic difficulties because the majority of their patients were initially thought to have a benign primary tumor.

When different types of initial surgical procedures have been compared (i.e., en-bloc resection vs. additional thyroidectomy and neck dissection), no real advantage in more extensive procedures has been found [1]. The type of procedure did not affect the overall survival in the series of 40 patients. It should be noted that lymph-node metastases are uncommon in parathyroid carcinoma, and therefore a routine neck dissection does not seem justified [16]. The time to recurrence in this series ranged from 1 to 222 months, illustrating the variable growth potential of this tumor [30].

In conclusion, in a symptomatic patient great care should be taken at initial exploration to remove the tumor en–bloc if densely adherent to adjacent structures and to avoid rupture of the capsule, which may cause local implantation, even in benign cases [32,33]. For technical reasons, a lobectomy can be the appropriate maneuver if the tumor is grossly adherent to the thyroid gland. There is no place for open-biopsy frozen sections in the intraoperative assessment.

Morphologic features

A marked *fibrosis*, often surrounding the tumor but also extending within the tumor-forming hyaline bands, separating the tumor into different parts or forming nodules, was a common finding when an extensive morphologic and cytologic study was performed on 56 carcinomas [34]. These cases were verified either histologically by local invasion or by the presence of local or distant metastases during a median follow-up time of 6 years [34]. Three additional features were also more common among these cases. These were areas of focal *necrosis*, a severe *nuclear atypia* with macronucleoli, and the presence of *mitotic figures* seen in high-power fields (HPF) of the parenchyma. When metastasizing tumors (n = 21) were compared with nonrecurrent tumors (n = 12), macronucleoli and >5 mitoses/50 HPF were significantly more common findings in the aggressive tumors.

According to Vetto et al. the most sensitive criterion of malignancy was that of capsular invasion, based on a review of the slides of 10 patients. They were also helped by immunohistochemical methods in differentiating parathyroid carcinoma from medullary thyroid carcinoma [31]. For suspicious primary cases, it is beneficial to obtain a substantial number of blocks from different sections of the tumor. For reoperative cases, it is important to re-evaluate the original slides and to study the operative report. Because most histopathologic criteria described here can be seen occasionally in what seem to be benign tumors, many pathologists refrain from definitively diagnosing parathyroid carcinoma unless distant metastases or major local invasion are present [17].

Ploidy studies

Assessment of tumor ploidy is a crude evaluation of the growth potential of a tumor. This method is used for prognostic evaluation in a number of adenocarcinomas and other endocrine tumors. The DNA distribution pattern, including cell-cycle analysis, can be assessed by using either flow cytometry or with the image technique [35,36]. The former uses tumor cells in suspension in which a fluorochrome dye that binds to the DNA is added. Each cell nucleus emits light signals that result in a DNA histogram. Image cytometry uses structurally identified tumor cell nuclei that are stained with the Feulgen technique. This reaction specifically stains the nuclear chromatin. Both methods can be used on paraffin blocks or on fresh tissue samples. The results from studies on parathyroid carcinoma in both small and larger series all show accordance with an aberrant ploidy pattern or high S-phase reaction and poor prognosis [16,27,30,37–40]. S-phase status as a marker of proliferation may become useful in conjunction with other tumor criteria as a prognostic marker and for choosing therapy regimens in the future.

Proliferative markers and 'tumor-specific genetic defects'

pHPT is a part of several hereditary endocrinopathies. The predisposing genetic defect for MEN-I has been localized to a region on chromosome 11q [41,42]. Tumors from several other forms of familial and sporadic pHPT, including malignant parathyroid tumors, have since been investigated for molecular genetic aberrations with the hope of gaining a better understanding of the mechanisms for tumor development. Parathyroid tumors were analyzed for clonality using X-linked gene inactivation, which showed evidence of monoclonality in both single and multiple abnormal glands [43,44]. These findings are in agreement with histopathologic data that do not discriminate between uniglandular and multiglandular disease [34,45].

To date, genetic abnormalities located on different chromosomes have been identified, suggesting that the etiologic mechanism for parathyroid tumor development involves several genetic rearrangements rather than a single predisposing genetic defect [24,46]. For example, in parathyroid tumors from patients with MEN-I and in approximately 20% of sporadic cases, the molecular mechanism involves a tumor suppressor gene on chromosome 11q13, the so-called *MEN-I* gene, as mentioned previously. In addition, rearrangements of the PTH gene and the PRAD1/cyclin D1 gene were found in a group of benign parathyroid tumors [24]. The gene for familial pHPT associated with jaw tumors was recently mapped to chromosome 1q. There seems to be an increased risk of parathyroid carcinoma among affected members [47].

Recently, two independent research groups further investigated the extra-cellular Ca^{2+}-sensing receptor gene on chromosome 3q as a putative informative gene for tumorigenesis of different parathyroid abnormalities, including carcinomas. Patients with familial hypocalciuric hypercalcemia or infants with neonatal severe hyperparathyroidism have germline mutations in this gene. However, neither study could confirm somatic mutations in those 60 tumors that were informative [48,49].

The Boston group has studied other possible cell-cycle regulators and has found that the retinoblastoma gene (RB gene) and other markers on 13q were allelically deleted in many parathyroid carcinomas, whereas benign parathy-roid tumors rarely showed alleleic losses at the RB locus [50]. That RB itself may be the functional target of such deletions was supported by the fact that the RB protein was not expressed by immunohistochemical staining in the carcinomas [50]. In a family with isolated pHPT with 19 affected members, including one with parathyroid carcinoma, linkage to both the MEN-I and the MEN-II region was excluded [51].

Proliferative activity in benign and malignant parathyroid glands was mea-sured with immunocytochemical staining of the Ki-67–MIB1 antigen–antibody complex. Carcinomas had a significantly increased mean tumor pro-liferative fraction compared with single and multiple enlarged glands [52]. In conclusion, despite the substantial work on different forms of HPT tumors, the only evidence of a specific genetic mechanism as a frequent cause for malig-nant transformation of the parathyroid glands has been the 13q allelic loss studies. These results have recently been confirmed [52a]. It is hoped that additional knowledge of the molecular basis of malignant hyper-parathyroidism will ultimately lead to improved diagnostic and prognostic capability, especially in the setting of 'atypical' tumors.

Operative strategy in reoperative parathyroid surgery

Metastatic parathyroid carcinoma is located most frequently in the lungs, liver, skeleton, and kidneys. Generally, there is an indication to perform localization studies for all reoperative parathyroid operations. The noninvasive studies may include ultrasonography, computed tomography (CT), magnetic reso-nance imaging (MRI), and scintigraphy using thallium/technetium or techne-tium-sestamibi [53]. Bone scans and chest radiographs may also identify lung and bone metastases. Invasive methods are selective venous samplings for parathormone or arteriography [54]. A CT scan of the chest and abdomen will identify distant metastases in these regions. Ultrasonography is user dependent in its sensitivity and specificity.

Scintigraphy with sestamibi is highly sensitive for finding ectopically located parathyroid glands and may image metastatic lesions [55]. As mentioned previously, tumor implants located cervically are usually small and scattered, which may hamper the evaluation of scintigraphy of the neck region. At re-exploration, dissection lateral to the strap muscles can be easier if the dissection plane is previously untouched. For pulmonary metastases, wedge resection of can render the patient eucalcemic. Solitary liver and bone metastases can be approached similarly. There is unanimous consensus that repeated surgical attempts to excise metastases are of benefit if the general condition of the patient permits [1,12,27,31,37,56,57].

Adjuvant treatment

Current medical treatment is directed towards the tumor, kidneys, and osteo-clasts. Single-agent chemotherapy or various combinations directly or indi-rectly affecting DNA synthesis have thus not proven efficacious for any length of time. Plicamycin and calcitonin are both osteoclast inhibitors but are of limited value due to their nephrotoxicity and short duration of action. Other agents used for parathyroid carcinoma are WR 2771 and gallium nitrate, but the experience with these agents thus far is limited [58,59]. The bisphosphonates are well tolerated and have few side effects, and should therefore be considered as primary medical remedy for unremitting hypercalcemia. Pamidronate has demonstrated efficacy but must be given intravenously, and still has a variable duration of action, ranging from a few days to weeks (see Chapter 10). Finally, calcimimetic agents now being devel-oped might prove useful in the future (see Chapter 8).

Prognosis

Parathyroid carcinoma is a tumor with a high potential for recurring locally, and less often at distant sites, even after a long symptom-free period. Lifelong follow-up of these patients is therefore recommended. The median time to recurrence was 7 years in two studies [27,30]. When metastases are found, a surgical approach should always be considered. This will offer the best chance of palliation. Bisphosphonates are useful agents to control hypercalcemia medically.

Acknowledgments

This work was supported by grants from the Swedish Medical Association and the Cancer Society in Stockholm (project no. 96:113). Dr A. Arnold is ac-knowledged for valuable input on the molecular aspects of parathyroid tumorigenesis.

189

References

1. Levin KE, Galante M, Clark OH. 1987. Parathyroid carcinoma versus parathyroid adenoma in patients with profound hypercalcemia. Surgery 101:649–660.
2. Sandström IV. 1880. Om en ny körtel hos meniskan och åtskilliga däggdjur. Uppsala läkareförenings förhandlingar 15:441–471.
3. Erdheim J. 1906. Tetania parathyreopriva. Mitt Grenzgeb Med Chir 16:632–744.
4. Erdheim J. 1907. Über Epithelkörperchenbefunde bei Osteomalacie. SB Akad Wiss Math naturw C1 116:311.
5. MacCallum WC. 1924. On the pathogenesis of tetany. Medecine 3:137–163.
6. Thompson NW. 1990. The history of hyperparathyroidism. Acta Chir Scand 156:5–21.
7. Wellbrock WLA. 1929. Malignant adenoma of the parathyroid glands. Endocrinology 13:285–294.
8. Wilder RM. 1929. Hyperparathyroidism: Tumor of the parathyroid glands association with osteitis fibrosa. Endocrinology 13:231–244.
9. Fujimoto Y, Obara T, Ito Y, Kanazava K, Aiyoshi Y, Nobori M. 1984. Surgical treatment of ten cases of parathyroid carcinoma: Importance of an initial bloc resection. World J Surg 8:392–400.
10. Cohn K, Silverman M, Corrado J, Sedgewick C. 1985. Parathyroid Carcinoma: The Lahey Clinic Experience. Surgery 98:1095–1100.
11. Mattei JF, Audiffret J, Henri JF, Roux H. 1988. Cancer des parathyroides. Revue Rhum Mal Osteoartic 55:519–523.
12. Sandelin K, Thompson NW, Bondeson L. 1991. Dilemmas in management of parathyroid carcinoma. Surgery 110:978–988.
13. Shortell CK, Andrus CH, Phillips CE, Schwartz SI. 1991. Carcinoma of the parathyroid gland: A 30 year experience. Surgery 110:704–708.
14. van Heerden JA, Weiland LH, Re Mine WH, Walls JT, Purnell DC. 1979. Cancer of the parathyroid glands. Arch Surg 114:475–480.
15. Obara T, Fujimoto Y. 1991. Diagnosis and treatment of patients with parathyroid carcinoma: An update and review. World J Surg 15:738–744.
16. Sandelin K, Auer G, Bondeson L, Grimelius L, Farnebo LO. 1992. Prognostic factors in parathyroid cancer. A review of 95 cases. World J Surg 16:724–731.
17. Mc Keown PP, Mc Garity WC, Sewell CW. 1984. Carcinoma of the parathyroid gland: Is it overdiagnosed? Am J Surg 147:292–298.
18. Dinnen JS, Greenwood RH, Jones JH, Walker DA, Williams ED. 1977. Parathyroid carcinoma in familiar hyperparathyroidism. J Clin Pathol 30:966–975.
19. Frayah RA, Nasar VH, Dagher F, Salti IS. 1972. Familial parathyroid carcinoma. Leb Med J 25:299–309.
20. Malette LE, Bilezikian JP, Ketcham AS, Aurbach GD. 1974. Parathyroid carcinoma in familial hyperparathyroidism. Am J Med 57:642–648.
21. Leborgne J, Neel J-C, Buzelin F, Malvy P. 1975. Cancer familial des parathyroïdes. Intérêt de l'angiographie dans le diagnostic des récidives locorégionales. J Chir (Paris) 109:315–326.
22. Visset J, Letissier E, Perchenet AS, Fiche M, Hamy A, Paineau J. 1992. Forme familiale de cancer primitif des glandes parathyroïdes. Chirurgie 118:223–228.
23. Streeten E, Weinstein LS, Norton JA, Mullvihill JJ, While BJ, Friedman E, Jaffe G, Brandi ML, Stewart K, Zimering MB, Spiegel AM, Aurbach GD, Marx SJ. 1992. Studies in a kindred with parathyroid carcinoma. J Clin Endocrinol Metab 75:362–366.
24. Hendy GN, Arnold A. Molecular basis of PTH overexpression. In Bilezikian JP, Raisz LG, Rodan GA, eds. Principles of Bone Biology, San Diego, CA: Academic Press, in press.
25. Fujiwara S, Sposto R, Ezaki H, et al. 1992. Hyperparathyroidsim among atomic bomb survivors in Hiroshima. Radiat Res 130:372–378.
26. Katz A, Braunstein GD. 1983. Clinical, biochemical, and pathologic features of radiation associated hyperparathyroidism. Arch Intern Med 143:79–82.

27. Obara T, Okamoto T, Yamashita T, Kawano M, Nishy T, Tani M, Sato K, Demura H, Fuijimoto Y. 1993. Surgical and medical management of patients with pulmonary metastases from parathyroid carcinoma. Surgery 114:1040–1049.

28. Jansson S, Tisell L, Lindstedt G, Lundberg P-A. 1991. Preoperative treatment with disodium pamidronate (APD) of hyperparathyroid patients with critically raised serum calcium levels. Surgery 110:480–486.

29. Albright F. 1934. Hyperparathyroidism. JAMA 102:1276.

30. Sandelin K, Tullgren O, Farnebo L. 1994. Clinical course of metastatic parathyroid cancer. World J Surg 18:594–599.

31. Vetto JT, Brennan MF, Woodruf J, Burt M. 1993. Parathyroid carcinoma: Diagnosis and clinical history. Surgery 114:5882–5892.

32. Fraker DL, Travis WD, Merendino JJ Jr, Zimering MB, Streeten EA, Weinstein LS, Marx SJ, Spiegel AM, Aurbach GD, Doppman JL, Norton JA. 1991. Locally recurrent parathyroid neoplasms as a cause for recurrent and persistent primary hyperparathyroidism. Ann Surg 213:58–65.

33. Rattner DW, Marrone GC, Kadson E, Silen W. 1985. Recurrent hyperparathyroidism due to implantation of parathyroid tissue. Am J Surg 149:745–748.

34. Sandelin K, Larsson C, Falkmer UG, Farnebo L, Grimelius L, Nordensjköld M. 1992. Morphology, DNA ploidy, and allele losses on chromosome 11 in sporadic hyperparathyroidism and that associated with multiple endocrine neoplasia type 1. Eur J Surg 158:199–206.

35. Harlow S, Roth SI, Bauer K, Marshall RB. 1991. Flow cytometric DNA analysis of normal and pathologic parathyroid glands. Mod Pathol 4:310–315.

36. Howard S, Anderson C, Diels W, Gerres K, Garcia B. 1992. Nuclear DNA density of parathyroid lesions. Pathol Res Pract 188:497–499.

37. August DA, Flynn SD, Jones MA, Bagwell BC, Kinder BK, 1993. Parathyroid carcinoma: The relationship of nuclear DNA content to clinical outcome. Surgery 113:290–296.

38. Bondeson L, Sandelin K, Grimelius L. 1993. Histopathological variables and DNA cytometry in parathyroid carcinoma. Am J Surg Pathol 17:820–829.

39. Obara T, Fujimoto Y, Kanaji Y, et al. 1990. Flow cytometric DNA analysis of parathyroid tumors. Cancer 66:1556–1562.

40. Levin KE, Chew KL, Ljung B-M, Mayhall BH, Siperstein AE, Clark OH. 1988. Deoxyribonucleic acid cytometry helps identify parathyroid carcinomas. J Clin Endocrinol Metab 67:779–84.

41. Byström C, Larsson C, Blomberg C, et al. 1990. Localization of the MEN1 gene to a small region within chromosome 11q13 by deletion mapping in tumors. Proc Natl Acad Sci USA 87:1968–1972.

42. Friedman E, Sakaguchi K, Bale AE, Falchetti A, Streeten E, Zimering M, Weinstein LS, Mc Bride WO, Nakamura Y, Brandi ML, Norton JA, Aurbach GD, Spiegel AM, Marx SJ. 1989. Clonality of parathyroid tumors in familial multiple endocrine neoplasia type 1. N Engl J Med 321:213–218.

43. Arnold A, Staunton CE, Kim HG, Gaz RD, Kronenberg HM. 1988. Monoclonality and abnormal parathyroid hormone genes in parathyroid adenomas. N Engl J Med 318:658–622.

44. Arnold A, Brown M, Urena P, et al. 1995. Monoclonality of parathyroid tumors in chronic renal failure and in primary parathyroid hyperplasia. J Clin Invest 95:2047–2053.

45. Bonjer HJ, Bruining HA, Birkenhäger JC, Nishiyama RH, Jones MA, Bagwell CB. 1992. Single and multiglandular disease in primary hyperparathyroidism: Long term follow up studies, histological studies and flow cytometric DNA analysis. World J Surg 16:734.

46. Cryns VL, Yi SM, Tahara H, Gaz RD, Arnold A. 1995. Frequent loss of chromosome arm 1p DNA in parathyroid tumors. Genes Chromosom Cancer 13:9–17.

47. Szabo J, Heath B, Hill VM, Jackson CE, Zabo RJ, Mallette LE, Chew SL, Besser JM, Thaker RV, Huff V, Leppert MS, Heath H III. 1995. Hereditary hyperparathyroidism-jaw tumor syndrome: The endocrine tumor gene HRPT2 maps to chromosome 1q21–q31. Am J Hum Genet 56:944–950.

191

48. Hosokawa Y, Pollak MR, Brown EM, Arnold A. 1995. Mutational analysis of the extracellular Ca^{2+}-sensing receptor gene in human parathyroid tumors. J Clin Endocrinol Metab 80:3107–3110.

49. Thompson DB, Samowitz WS, Odelberg S, Davies RK, Szabo J, Heath III H. 1995. Genetic abnormalities in sporadic parathyroid adenomas: Loss of heterozygosity for chromosome 3q markers flanking the calcium receptor locus. J Clin Endocrinol Metabol 80:3377–3380.

50. Cryns VL, Thor A, Xu H-J, Wierman ME, Vickery AL, Benedict WF, Arnold A. 1994. Loss of the retinoblastoma tumor suppressor gene in parathyroid carcinoma. N Engl J Med 330:757–761.

51. Wassif WS, Moniz CF, Friedman E, Wong S, Weber G, Nordenskjöld M, Peters TJ, Larsson C. 1993. Familial isolated hyperparathyroidism: A distinct genetic entity with increased risk of parathyroid cancer. J Clin Endocrinol Metab 77:1485–1489.

52. Abbona GC, Papotti M, Gasparri G, Bussolati G. 1995. Proliferative activity in parathyroid tumors as detected by Ki-67 immunostaining. Hum Pathol 26:135–138.

52a. Dotzenrath C, Teh BT, Farnebo F, Cupistik, Svensson A, Toll A, Goretzki P, Larsson C. 1996. Allelic loss of the retinoblastoma tumor suppressor gene: a marker for aggressive parathyroid tumors? J Clin Endocrinol Metab 81:3194–3196.

53. Krubsack AJ, Wilson SD, Lawson T, Kneeland JB, Thorsen K, Collier BD, Hellman RS, Isitman AT. 1989. Prospective comparison of radionucleotide, computed tomographic, sonographic, and magnetic resonance localization of parathyroid tumors. Surgery 106:639–646.

54. Doppman JL. 1994. Preoperative localization of parathyroid tissue in primary hyperparathyroidism. In Bilezikian JP, ed. The Parathyroids. New York: Raven Press, pp 553–565.

55. Hindié E, Mellière D, Simon D, Perlemuter L, Galle P. 1995. Primary hyperparathyroidism: Is technetium 99m-sestamibi/iodine-123 subtraction scanning the best procedure to locate enlarged glands before surgery? J Clin Endocrinol Metab 80:302–307.

56. Fugimoto Y. 1989. Parathyroid malignancy. In van Heerden J, ed. Current Problems in Endocrine Surgery. Chicago: Year Book Medical Publishers, pp 191–193.

57. Dubost C, Jehanno C, Lavergne A, Le Charpentier Y. 1984. Successful resection of intrathoracic metastases from two patients with parathyroid carcinoma. World J Surg 8:574–551.

58. Glover DJ, Shaw L, Glick JH, Slatopolsky E, Weiler C, Attie M, Goldfarb S. 1985. Treatment of hypercalcemia in parathyroid cancer with WR-2721,S-2-(3 aminopropylamino) ethylphosphorotic acid. Ann Intern Med 103:55–57.

59. Warrel RPJ, Israel R, Frisone M, Snyder T, Gaynor JJ, Bockman RS. 1988. Gallium nitrate for acute treatment of cancer related hypercalcemia. Ann Intern Med 108:669–674.

10. Parathyroid hormone-related peptide and hypercalcemia of malignancy

David Goltzman and Janet E. Henderson

Historical background

An association between cancer and hypercalcemia was first noted in the 1920s and was thought to arise exclusively from osteolysis caused by malignant cells in bone [1]. However, in 1936 Gutman et al. documented the occurrence of hypercalcemia and hypophosphatemia in a patient with bronchogenic carcinoma who had no osseous metastases and no obvious parathyroid dysfunction [2]. An interesting conceptual breakthrough was later provided by Fuller Albright in 1941 in the *New England Journal of Medicine* during a review of a case of renal carcinoma metastatic to bone [3]. The patient was found to be hypophosphatemic in addition to being hypercalcemic. Albright reasoned that bone dissolution alone would cause hyperphosphatemia in association with hypercalcemia. He therefore postulated that the tumor released a parathyroid hormone (PTH)–like factor that could not only stimulate bone resorption but could also induce phosphaturia, leading to hypophosphatemia. The concept of *ectopic hyperparathyroidism* or *pseudohyperparathyroidism* as a cause of hypercalcemia in malignancy (HM) was thus born.

Subsequent studies further defined the clinical and biochemical attributes of this disorder and noted its high prevalence amongst patients with squamous-cell carcinoma and hypernephroma. In 1966 Lafferty pointed out apparent differences between HM and primary hyperparathyroidism (PHPT). These included higher blood calcium concentrations in HM and the occasional occurrence of alkalosis, rather than the mild metabolic acidosis frequently associated with PHPT [4].

Two general mechanisms had therefore been invoked to explain the pathogenesis of HM, the first requiring the presence of lytic tumor cells within bone and the second involving a tumor-derived PTH-like humoral factor in the absence of skeletal lesions. In view of the observed similarities between HM and PHPT, attempts were made to identify PTH per se as the humoral factor. Despite reports of elevated circulating levels of PTH [5] in hypercalcemic cancer patients, PTH mRNA was not generally identified in tumors associated with HM [6]. Notwithstanding, at least two interesting reports of verified ectopic PTH production have subsequently been documented, one in associa-

Andrew Arnold (ed.) ENDOCRINE NEOPLASMS. 1997. Kluwer Academic Publishers. ISBN 0-7923-4354-9.
All rights reserved.

tion with an ovarian carcinoma [7] and one with a small-cell carcinoma of the lung [8]. Other agents associated with HM were prostaglandins [9] and 1,25(OH)$_2$D [10]. However, these factors are now thought to play a relatively minor role in the pathogenesis of HM and are associated with a limited number of tumors.

The elusive endocrine factor capable of eliciting hypercalcemia in association with the majority of tumors was finally identified in the late 1980s by virtue of its PTH-like bioactivity. A number of bioassays that had been developed for PTH were used throughout the 1980s to identify PTH-like bioactivity in both the tumors and body fluids of hypercalcemic cancer patients [11–13]. Chromatographic profiles suggested that the circulating material was both larger and more heterogenous than PTH [14]. A unique peptide, sharing limited NH$_2$-terminal sequence homology with PTH, was eventually purified from tumors associated with HM using stimulation of cyclic adenosine monophosphate (cAMP) in PTH target cells to detect bioactivity [15]. The sequence data were subsequently used to generate olignucleotide probes for screening cDNA libraries from which positive clones were identified. The cDNA sequence of human PTHrP predicted a secretory protein with mature isoforms of 139 amino acids, 141 amino acids, and 173 amino acids. Initially referred to as PTH-like peptide (PLP), this entity is now commonly called *PTH-related peptide* (PTHrP).

PTHrP and the pathogenesis of hypercalcemia of malignancy

Genetic characteristics of PTHrP

The human gene encoding PTHrP is assigned to the short arm of chromosome 12, while that for PTH is located on the short arm of chromosome 11. These two chromosomes carry other functionally related genes and are thought to share a common ancestral origin. Furthermore, similarities in the structural organization of the PTH and PTHrP genes exist in that corresponding exons encode similar functional domains. Finally, the two peptides share limited but biologically important amino acid sequence homology in their NH$_2$-terminal domains, where most of the known bioactivity is believed to reside. Consequently, PTH and PTHrP are thought to be members of a single gene family.

The human PTHrP gene spans more than 15 kilobases of DNA and contains a minimum of 7 exons and 3 promoters [16–19]. While alternative promoter usage and/or different splicing patterns account for the heterogeneity of PTHrP mRNA species seen in various tissues on Northern analysis, the significance of the heterogeneity remains unclear because neither tissue-specific nor developmental splicing patterns have been reported. Tumor-specific promoter utilization [20] has been suggested as a possible explanation for the observation that, while many malignant neoplasms express PTHrP mRNA and protein, it is only a subset of cancer patients that produce the peptide in sufficient quantity to develop hypercalcemia.

The evidence to support this hypothesis is, however, far from conclusive. More recent studies have reported the use of multiple promoters in human tumor samples compared with single-promoter usage in normal tissue harvested from the same individual [21] and have suggested that a general increase in transcription, rather than alternative splicing, leads to overexpression of PTHrP and subsequent hypercalcemia in neoplasia. Other mechanisms that have been invoked to explain increased production of PTHrP in malignant relative to normal tissue include region-specific methylation in the promoter region [22] and the occasional occurrence of gene amplification [23].

PTHrP interactions with its receptor

Sequence homology between PTH and PTHrP is restricted to 8 of the first 13 amino acids at the NH_2 terminus, including those at positions +1 and +2, which are critical for activation of adenylyl cyclase (Fig. 1). This limited homology, as well as conformational similarities in the nonhomologous 14–34 sequence permits the 1–34 domain of these two peptides to bind to a common receptor with equal affinity [24]. Thus, amino-terminal fragments of PTH and PTHrP have been shown to bind to a single, 7-transmembrane spanning receptor termed the PTH/PTHrP receptor that is linked by G-proteins to both the adenylate cyclase and phospholipase-C signaling pathways. Consequently, both PTH and PTHrP are equally effective in eliciting PTH-like bioactivity in animals in vivo [25]. A similar spectrum of bioactivity is also elicited by infusing either PTH-(1–34) or PTHrP-(1–34) into normal human subjects [26], indicating that PTHrP possesses the requisite bioactivity to play a significant role in HM.

Although PTHrP has major PTH-like effects on calcium and phosphate ion homeostasis when overproduced by malignant tissue, its primary role under physiological conditions in normal cells appears to be that of a local regulator of cell growth and differentiation [27,28]. These functions may well be mediated through mechanisms distinct from those required for its role in calcium mobilization [29,30].

Cellular mechanism of PTHrP action

Renal. PTHrP, like PTH, activates PTH/PTHrP receptors in renal tubule cells, resulting in stimulation of adenylyl cyclase and an elevation in intracellular cAMP. A fraction of this intracellular cAMP enters the tubule lumen and is subsequently excreted as a nephrogenous portion of urinary cAMP. Consequently, in PTHrP-associated HM, nephrogenous cAMP (NcAMP) in the

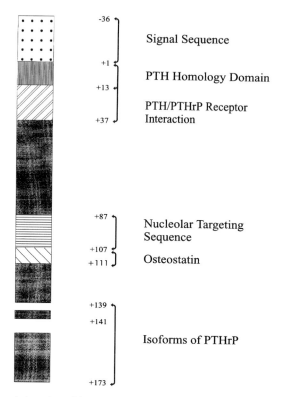

Figure 1. Functional domains of human PTHrP. The translation products of PTHrP mRNA include three related isoforms of a secretory peptide that have distinct COOH termini ending at 139, 141, and 173 amino acids. Although homology to PTH is restricted to 8 of the first 13 amino acids at the NH$_2$ terminus, residues 1–36 are involved in the interaction with the PTH/PTHrP receptor. A basic region between residues 87 and 107 has been identified as a functional nucleolar targeting sequence, and the 107–111 pentapeptide named *osteostatin* is reported to inhibit osteoclast function in vitro.

urine is elevated. Also in a manner similar to PTH, PTHrP inhibits phosphate transport (primarily in the proximal tubule) and stimulates calcium reabsorption (predominantly in the ascending limb of the loop of Henle and in the distal tubule). Numerous experiments have shown that these renal actions of PTHrP are important to both the development and maintenance of several of the biochemical abnormalities associated with HM.

For example, progressive impairment in sodium-phosphate cotransport was observed in renal cortical membranes harvested from rats implanted with the H-500 Leydig cell tumor, ultimately leading to hypophosphatemia [31]. Inhibition of transport was noted as early as 5 days postimplantation, however, well in advance of development of overt hypophosphatemia. In this same animal model, early retention of calcium by the kidney was associated with an increase in NcAMP and a reduction in the fractional excretion of calcium [32].

It was suggested that calcium retention by the kidney accounted for the initial rise in plasma calcium, prior to the onset of osteolysis [33]. Similarly, it has been proposed that this represents the primary mechanism underlying the initial rise in serum calcium in cancer patients with PTHrP-associated HM, whereas increased bone resorption is responsible for the episodes of severe hypercalcemia in advanced stages of the disease [34].

While the effects on renal handling of calcium and phosphorus appear to be elicited in a similar manner by both PTH and PTHrP, bicarbonate ion excretion appears to be handled differently by PTH and PTHrP. Thus, infusion of full-length PTHrP-(1–141) into an isolated perfused rat kidney was shown to have a biphasic effect on bicarbonate excretion [35]. An early increase in urinary bicarbonate concentration was followed at a later time point by a sharp decline in renal bicarbonate excretion. The early increase could be mimicked by treatment with amino-terminal fragments of PTH or PTHrP, whereas the later inhibitory activity was believed to be dependent on a region of PTHrP beyond amino acids 1–34. It was suggested that PTHrP-mediated retention of bicarbonate ion by the kidney might explain the mild metabolic alkalosis sometimes associated with HM (compared with the mild metabolic acidosis seen in PHPT).

PTHrP may also have a distinct mechanism of action with respect to regulation of the renal lα-hydroxylase enzyme in HM. Intravenous administration of amino-terminal fragments of PTH or PTHrP into animals [36] and humans [26] results in an elevation in serum $1,25(OH)_2D$. Likewise, it has been suggested that a positive correlation may also exist between circulating $1,25(OH)_2D$ and PTHrP in the early stage of HM [37]. However, serum $1,25(OH)_2D$ levels are often suppressed in the terminal stages of HM, when plasma PTHrP is elevated and the patient is severely hypercalcemic. One explanation that has been forwarded to explain this inappropriate decrease in circulating $1,25(OH)_2D$ in the presence of excess PTHrP is a direct inhibitory effect of non–NH_2-terminal domains of the PTHrP molecule on the renal lα-hydroxylase enzyme. Alternatively, severe hypercalcemia per se may inhibit the enzyme or a specific inhibitor may be cosecreted with PTHrP by the tumor. These possibilities, however, remain to be substantiated.

The actions of PTHrP in the kidney, therefore, play an essential role in the development and maintenance of biochemical abnormalities associated with HM. Many of these effects are similar for PTH and PTHrP, and are most likely mediated through the same signal transduction pathways. On the other hand, the differential effects of PTH and PTHrP could reflect preferential use of signal transduction pathways and/or the use of alternate receptors [38].

Bone. Cyclical remodeling, which replaces old or damaged bone, occurs at discrete intervals along the bone surface throughout life [39]. A typical cycle involves recruitment and activation of osteoclasts to resorb bone followed by activation of osteoblasts to synthesize, and deposit, an equivalent amount of matrix in the lacuna that was excavated by the osteoclast. Although little is known about the molecular crosstalk involved in the coordination of remodeling, it is clear that osteoclast recruitment and activation are initiated indirectly through signals emanating from osteoblastic cells [40] and that numerous cytokines and systemic hormones, including PTH, are involved [41]. Both PTH and PTHrP interact directly with the common PTH/PTHrP receptor located on osteoblasts and pre-osteoblastic cells [30,42]. Ligand activation of this receptor results in signaling (most probably via cell-bound or soluble cytokines) to osteoclast precursors, ultimately leading to increased osteoclast numbers and activity, and hence to increased bone resorption.

Unlike the highly regulated process of remodeling, pathologic bone resorption associated with cancer is uncontrolled and appears to be mediated through several different mechanisms. All neoplastic cells may produce cytokines and growth factors (such as transforming growth factor alpha), which might directly stimulate osteoclastic bone resorption. Most may also produce enzymes (e.g., collagenase or urokinase), which contribute to bone matrix degradation. However, three patterns seem to occur with respect to osteolysis associated with PTHrP production by tumor cells. The traditional pattern of tumor-induced osteolysis is exemplified by patients with multiple myeloma. Myeloma cells in the bone marrow space release cytokines such as interleukin-1 and interleukin-6, which have been shown to augment osteoclast recruitment and to stimulate their activity in vitro [40,41]. PTHrP is rarely produced by myeloma cells and therefore, most probably makes little or no significant contribution to the pathogenesis of hypercalcemia associated with this disease.

A second paradigm involves the presence of metastatic lesions in bone, for example, in patients with breast cancer. The disseminated, neoplastic cells most likely release locally active cytokines in a manner similar to that seen in myeloma. However, unlike patients with myeloma, who rarely have detectable PTHrP, >90% of breast cancer cells metastatic to bone demonstrate immunopositivity for PTHrP [43]. This observation raises the possibility that the peptide may act at the local level to stimulate the differentiation, and perhaps proliferation, of hematopoietic precursors that give rise to osteoclasts, as has been demonstrated in vitro [44]. In addition, over 50% of patients with breast cancer have increased circulating levels of PTHrP [45]. Therefore, while PTHrP is not thought to generally play a significant role in hypercalcemia associated with multiple myeloma, it most probably makes a significant contribution to hypercalcemia, through both systemic and local mechanisms of action, in patients with breast cancer as well as patients with other cancers metastatic to bone.

The third scenario entails elevated levels of tumor-derived PTHrP in the circulation of patients with HM, in the absence of skeletal metastases. Circulating PTHrP interacts with its receptors in bone to promote the proliferation and differentiation of osteoclast precursors, resulting in enhanced osteoclastic bone resorption. Thus, in these patients with malignancy, bone resorption will increase concomitant with rising levels of circulating PTHrP during progression of the disease to produce the classical manifestations of *pseudohyperparathyroidism, ectopic hyperparathyroidism,* or *humoral hypercalcemia of malignancy* (HHM).

Animal models of hypercalcemia of malignancy

Hypercalcemia occurs in association with a variety of tumors in mammalian species other than humans, and some of these tumor-bearing animal models have been employed in elucidating the pathogensis of PTHrP-associated HM. Additionally, human tumors implanted in immunocompromised mice or rats have also been studied. In several investigations [33,46,47] neutralizing antibodies were administered intravenously to hypercalcemic rodents that had been implanted with PTHrP-producing tumors. Following treatment there was a rapid and sustained reversal of the biochemical abnormalities associated with HM and prolonged survival of the tumor-bearing animals compared with the untreated controls. The initial reduction in plasma calcium and increase in plasma phosphate was accompanied by acute reciprocal urinary changes at an early time point, that is, a rise in urinary calcium excretion and a reduction in urinary phosphate [33]. This most probably reflected an early neutralizing effect of the antibody on the action of PTHrP in the kidney and emphasizes the contribution of renal calcium retention to PTHrP-induced hypercalcemia in neoplasia. Susequently, however, normocalcemia was accompanied by hypocalciuria, which appeared to result from immunoneutralization of the effect of PTHrP in bone. The resultant decrease in the filtered load of calcium, therefore, led to a reduction in urinary calcium excretion.

The role played by circulating PTHrP in bone turnover during the progression of HM has also been examined in nude rats implanted with a PTHrP-producing human squamous carcinoma [48]. This work was undertaken in an attempt to understand the observation in the clinical situation that bone turnover appears to be uncoupled (increased resorption in the absence of increased formation) in HM. During progression of the disease in the animal model, histomorphometric analysis of trabecular bone revealed a coupled increase in turnover in the early stage of disease, prior to detection of circulating PTHrP and hypercalcemia. In contrast, at a later time point, marked inhibition of formation and accelerated bone resorption was seen when the animals had elevated circulating levels of PTHrP and hypercalcemia. A similar impaired osteoblastic response has been noted in patients with advanced myeloma [49] as well as in patients with well-established PTHrP-producing tumors and HM [50]. Taken together, these observations suggest osteoblast activity may be inhibited by severe hypercalcemia, although the mechanism remains unknown. These animal studies have confirmed a central role for PTHrP as an endocrine mediator of HM and have also elucidated some of the characteristics of its action in kidney and bone.

Table 1. Severe, acute hypercalcemia of malignancy

A. Clinical presentation	
Gastrointestinal	Anorexia, nausea, vomiting
Renal	Polyuria, azotemia
Neuromuscular	Weakness, myopathy
Central nervous system	Psychosis, altered conciousness
B. Management	
Rehydration	Expands intravascular volume
	Increases glomerular filtration rate
Loop diuretic	Reduces Na-linked calcium reabsorption
	Effects calciuresis
Calcitonin	Rapidly inhibits osteolysis
Bisphosphonate	Sustained inhibition of osteolysis

Clinical manifestations of hypercalcemia of malignancy

Hypercalcemia is usually a manifestation of advanced rather than early malignancy. Its onset is usually acute and the elevation most often profound (frequently >12 mg/dl or 3 mmol/l). The major symptoms and signs relate to the gastrointestinal, renal, neuromuscular, and central nervous systems, and are most often those associated with acute rather than chronic hypercalcemia (Table 1). Thus, anorexia, nausea, and vomiting are common, whereas constipation, gastritis, and pancreatitis, which generally constitute gastrointestinal evidence of more chronic hypercalcemia, are less frequent. Similarly, polyuria and evidence of dehydration and azotemia are frequent, whereas renal calculi and nephrocalcinosis, which are associated with chronic hypercalcemia, are more unusual. Depression, weakness, and myopathy may occur and the patient's condition may progress toward psychosis, stupor, and coma. The acuteness of onset and severity of the hypercalcemia may, therefore, lead to life-threatening manifestations if left untreated.

Diagnosis of PTHrP-associated hypercalcemia of malignancy

Biochemical abnormalities

The biochemical abnormalities that occur with PTHrP-associated HM are similar, in many respects, to those seen in patients with PHPT (Table 2). These include hypercalcemia (which, however, tends to be more severe in HM than in PHPT), hypophosphatemia, phosphaturia, and calciuria, frequently accompanied by increased NcAMP. In addition, there is an increase in biochemical indices of bone resorption in both disease states as manifested, for instance, by an increase in the level of type I collagen crosslinked N-telopeptides (NTX) or pyridinium crosslinks excreted in urine [51]. These degradation products of osteolysis are replacing the more conventional measurement of hydroxyproline, which lacks sensitivity and specificity.

200

Despite the similarities between PTHrP-associated HM and PHPT, a number of important differences are also evident (see Table 2). Most apparent is the reduction in circulating PTH in patients with HM, which reflects the homeostatic response of the parathyroid gland to an elevation in serum calcium. Serum $1,25(OH)_2D$ levels also tend to be inappropriately low in some patients with PTHrP-associated HM compared with the elevated concentrations often seen in PHPT [52]. Indices of bone formation, such as bone-specific alkaline phosphatase and osteocalcin, are also elevated in patients with PHPT, in whom bone formation is coupled to resorption. In contrast, bone formation and bone resorption appear to be uncoupled, with suppressed formation, in patients with PTHrP-associated HM [50]. Finally, whereas PHPT is often associated with a mild metabolic acidosis, patients with malignancy-associated hypercalcemia may exhibit mild metabolic alkalosis.

PTHrP immunoassays

The rational development of specific and sensitive immunoassays to measure PTHrP has been hampered, to some extent, by the lack of sufficient knowledge regarding regulation of its production, intracellular processing, and metabolic clearance [15,45]. As mentioned previously, the human PTHrP gene encodes three isoforms of the protein, each of which has the potential to undergo complicated post-translational processing within the cell of origin [15,53,54] as well as differential metabolic clearance in the periphery. In view of the complexity of this scheme, it is not surprising that multiple forms of bioactive PTHrP have been identified in the plasma of hypercalcemic cancer patients [14,55]. Characterization of the precise nature of circulating forms of PTHrP, as well as their presence in HM, is essential to the development of

Table 2. PTHrP-associated hypercalcemia of malignancy

Biochemical abnormality	Pathophysiological basis
↑Serum calcium	Volume depletion
	Decreased glomerular filtration rate
	Increased sodium-linked calcium reabsorption
	PTHrP-stimulated calcium reabsorption
	PTHrP-stimulated osteolysis
↑Urine phosphate	PTHrP-inhibited sodium/phosphate transport
↓Serum phosphorous	
↑NcAMP	PTHrP activation of renal PTH/PTHRP receptors
↑Plasma PTHrP	PTHrP released from tumor tissue
↓Plasma PTH	Homeostatic response to hypercalcemia
↑Urine calcium	Increase in PTHrP-stimulated osteolysis
↑Urine NTX	
↓Serum $1,25(OH)_2D$	? Tumor-derived inhibitor of 1α-hydroxylase
Metabolic alkalosis	? PTHrP-inhibited bicarbonate excretion

more sensitive and specific assays for the measurement of PTHrP and remains the subject of intense investigation.

Given the knowledge that HM is characterized by the presence of circulating bioactive forms of PTHrP and that bioactivity resides within the NH_2-terminal region, initial efforts were aimed at the development of immunoassays using antisera raised against synthetic NH_2-terminal fragments of PTHrP. Without exception, all NH_2-terminal radioimmunoassays measured elevated levels of PTHrP in the peripheral circulation of the majority of patients with HM [45]. In some cases, normocalcemic cancer patients also had detectable circulating PTHrP, although the mean values tended to be much lower than those seen in the patients with HM, perhaps reflecting a smaller tumor volume producing insufficient PTHrP to cause hypercalcemia. Alternatively, it is possible that these antisera could recognize both bioactive and bioinert species of the protein.

Two-site, immunoradiometric assays (IRMA) have also been developed to measure larger circulating moieties of PTHrP. This method makes use of two antisera that recognize different epitopes of a protein, the first being used as a *capture antibody* and the second a *signal antibody*. The theoretical advantages of this type of assay are improved specificity, due to the requirement for two epitopes, as well as increased sensitivity. In the case of PTH, which circulates as a single bioactive entity, this approach has greatly improved the clinical utility of PTH measurements. The capacity of PTH IRMAs to distinguish between normal and subnormal concentrations with a high degree of sensitivity is especially useful to the clinician in the differential diagnosis of PHPT and HM, in view of the fact that PTH is generally elevated in the former and suppressed in the latter. However, overlapping situations do occur. Thus, in a recent study using IRMAs for the measurement of PTH and PTHrP in hypercalcemic individuals, 10% of patients whose primary diagnosis was HPT also had elevated circulating PTHrP [56]. Conversely, of those whose primary diagnosis was HM, 13% had coexistent HPT. The PTHrP IRMA used in this study [57] appears to be the most sensitive (detection limit of $<0.5\,pmol/l$) and specific that has been developed. It uses an antibody to PTHrP-(1–34) to capture the protein and a polyclonal antiserum to PTHrP-(37–67) as a signal.

RIAs that identify either midregion or carboxy-terminal fragments of PTHrP have proved to be of less clinical use in the differential diagnosis of HM. A midregion species of PTHrP that was shown to be a secretory product of cultured cells [58] has recently been identified as the predominant circulating form of PTHrP in patients with HM [59]. However, unlike the IRMAs, which have been reported to distinguish between normal controls and patients with HM, the midregion RIAs show considerable overlap between these groups. On the other hand, RIAs that recognize carboxy-terminal fragments of PTHrP show elevated levels in most patients with renal insufficiency as well as in those individuals with malignancy-associated hypercalcemia.

Spectrum of tumors associated with hypercalcemia of malignancy

When the clinical syndrome of ectopic hyperparathyroidism, pseudo-hyperparathyroidism, or HHM was first defined, it was believed to be associated mainly with squamous cell carcinomas from a variety of primary sites and with renal-cell carcinoma. Although breast cancer, for example, was frequently associated with hypercalcemia, the elevation in blood calcium was believed to emanate largely from local osteolysis rather than from a humoral mechanism. With the identification of PTHrP as a causal mechanism of HM, and with the development of molecular biological and immunological methods for its detection, it became clear that PTHrP was produced by many tumors. This led to the realization that elevated circulating levels of PTHrP were associated with a much broader spectrum of histological types of tumors than was previously appreciated. Thus breast cancers produce PTHrP [43], as do endometrial [60] and colon cancers [23], and even mesotheliomas [61]. A variety of endocrine tumors have also been shown to produce PTHrP [62], including pheochromocytomas [63] insulinomas [64], parathyroid adenomas [65], pituitary tumors [66], and thyroid cancers [67]. Furthermore, elevated circulating levels of PTHrP have been detected in some patients with hematological malignancies, notably those with advanced stage lymphomas [68] (Fig. 2), and have been shown to contribute to HM in patients whose hypercalcemia has, in the past, been attributed solely to excess $1,25(OH)_2D$ [10]. It is clear, therefore, that the histological spectrum of tumors elaborating PTHrP, and in which PTHrP is of pathogenetic significance, is much broader than originally thought. Unlike PTH, whose expression is virtually restricted

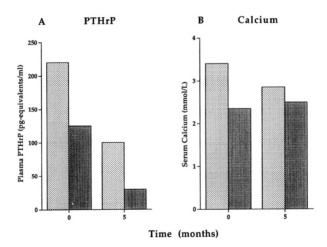

Figure 2. Circulating PTHrP and calcium in patients with B-immunoblastic lymphoma. Decreased levels of plasma PTHrP (**A**) were noted concomitant with reductions in tumor bulk following chemotherapy in both hypercalcemic (light hatching) and normocalcemic (dark hatching) patients with B-immunoblastic lymphoma. However, a significant reduction in serum calcium was seen only in the hypercalcemic patient (**B**). (Modified from Kremer et al. [68], with permission.)

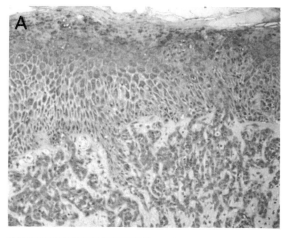

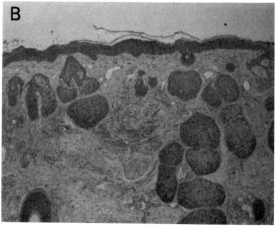

Figure 3. PTHrP immunoreactivity in human skin. In normal skin (**A**) epidermal cells demonstrate strong immunostaining for PTHrP, as do neoplastic regions in squamous carcinoma of skin (**B**).

to cells of the parathyroid gland, PTHrP is broadly expressed by a wide variety of normal fetal and postnatal cells. Consequently, elaboration of PTHrP in neoplasia most likely represents eutopic overproduction by cells that normally synthesize it rather than ectopic synthesis (Figs. 3 and 4).

Treatment

Management of severe, acute hypercalcemia of malignancy

The most important initial step in the treatment of HM is rehydration, followed by therapy aimed at enhancing renal calcium excretion and inhibiting bone resorption (see Table 1). Inhibition of calcium absorption by the gut is usually not necessary in view of the low to normal circulating $1,25(OH)_2D$ levels associated with elevated PTHrP. Hyperabsorption of calcium would not, therefore, be an important mechanism contributing to PTHrP-associated HM. Increased renal calcium clearance is generally initiated by saline infusion to expand the intravascular volume, thereby improving the glomerular filtration rate (GFR), which in turn results in reduced proximal tubular sodium-linked calcium reabsorption. Once the patient is adequately hydrated, a loop diuretic, such as furosemide, can be used in moderation to inhibit renal calcium reabsorption and to produce calciuresis. However, in addition to

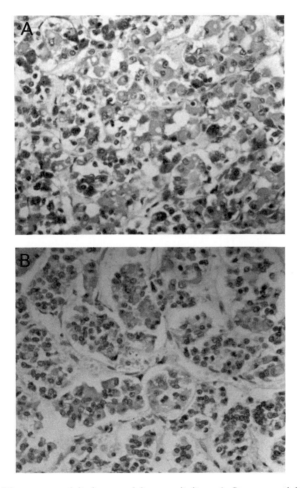

Figure 4. PTHrP immunoreactivity in normal, human pituitary. **A**: Strong reactivity for PTHrP is evident in numerous cells of the adenohypophysis. **B**: Preadsorption of the PTHrP antiserum with synthetic PTHrP-(1–34) abolishes the immunoreactivity in a serial section from the same tissue. (Modified from Asa et al. [62], with permission.)

205

kidney, bone is also a major target tissue of systemically active PTHrP. Thus, the ideal therapeutic modality would inhibit both osteoclastic osteolysis and renal calcium reabsorption. The 32 amino-acid peptide hormone, calcitonin, binds directly to osteoclasts and inhibits their lytic activity as well as stimulating an acute increase in renal calcium excretion. Although it is generally effective in reducing blood calcium within 2–4 hours of administration, its efficacy as an antihypercalcemic agent is limited due to its short-lived effect, most likely due to receptor downregulation, which causes tachyphylaxis.

To date the development of bisphosphonates represents the most significant advance in the management of hypercalcemia associated with malignancy. Bisphosphonates are nonhydrolyzable analogues of pyrophosphate, a naturally occurring inhibitor of bone turnover, in which the O in the pyrophosphate bond is replaced by a C. This P-C-P structure accounts for the metabolic stability of bisphosphonates, as well as their rapid uptake by bone, where they are thought to inhibit resorption by binding to and stabilizing hydroxyapatite crystals, as well as by directly inhibiting the lytic action of osteoclasts. Different side-chain substitutions have generated analogues of increasing potency to the point that the efficacy of the newest analogues is estimated to be 10,000-fold that of the first generation of bisphosphonates.

In view of the low rate of intestinal absorption of bisphosphonates and the frequently associated nausea and altered mental status of the severely hypercalcemic patient, intravenous (IV) infusion is the preferred method of administration to these individuals. Unlike treatment with calcitonin, which elicits a relatively mild hypocalcemic response (seldom >2 mg/dl) of rapid onset and limited duration, a single IV dose of 40–60 mg of pamidronate or 1500 mg of clodronate, for example, results in a steady decline in serum calcium over several days (Fig. 5). A nadir is usually reached within the normal range by 5 days, and this may be sustained for several days thereafter. After an initial IV course of therapy, further intermittent IV therapy or treatment with oral bisphosphonates appears to be effective in maintaining serum calcium within the normal range. Because relapses depend on the type of tumor, the stage of malignancy, and the use of antitumor therapy, long-term maintenance should be adjusted to the individual case [69].

A number of recent studies have examined the relationship between circulating PTHrP concentrations and the overall response to bisphosphonate therapy in hypercalcemic cancer patients [70–73]. Overall, these studies identify a subset of patients with high circulating levels of PTHrP who are considered to be 'poor responders' to IV bisphosphonate therapy due to the presence of a substantial renal component to their hypercalcemia. Pretreatment levels of circulating PTHrP may, therefore, prove useful in predicting the acute response to bisphosphonate therapy and thus allow appropriate adjustments to be made in dosage and/or the frequency of administration.

The efficacy of treatment with bisphosphonates can be conveniently monitored using commercially available assays for the detection of matrix crosslinking compounds, such as NTX, pyridinoline, or deoxypyridinoline,

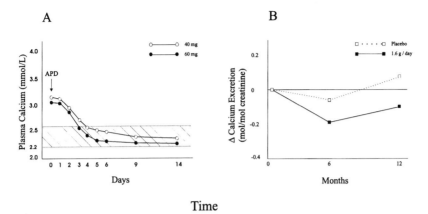

Figure 5. Management of HM with bisphosphonates. **A**: Time-dependent decrease in plasma calcium in patients with severe, acute hypercalcemia in response to intravenous doses of either 40 mg/day (O—O) or 60 mg/day (•—•) pamidronate (APD). Hatched lines depict the normal range. **B**: Changes in urinary calcium excretion over time in patients with breast cancer metastatic to bone treated with either placebo control (□—□) or 1.6 g/day of oral clodronate (■—■). (Modified from Paterson et al. [76], with permission.)

released into the urine as a result of osteolysis [51,74]. The use of fasting urinary calcium excretion, another index of osteolysis, would be less helpful in individuals with detectable PTHrP levels in view of the known effects of the peptide on promoting renal calcium reabsorption.

Other antiosteolytic agents that have been assessed in the treatment of HM are plicamycin (mithramycin) and gallium nitrate. Use of the cytotoxic antibiotic plicamycin as a mechanism to inhibit osteoclastic activity has been limited largely due to its hematopoietic, hepatic, and renal toxicity when administered frequently and in high concentration. Gallium nitrate binds to the mineral phase of bone, thus inhibiting its dissolution in much the same manner as the bisphosphonates. However, unlike the bisphosphonates, which appear to have minimal side effects, gallium nitrate is nephrotoxic and should therefore be used with extreme caution in hypercalcemic cancer patients whose renal function may already be compromised. In general, glucocorticoids have a minimal role to play in the treatment of PTHrP-associated HM because these patients most often do not exhibit enhanced gastrointestinal absorption of calcium. Nevertheless, they may be essential chemotherapeutic agents in patients with susceptible tumors.

In summary, a treatment modality involving initial rehydration followed by simultaneous administration of calcitonin and/or furosemide (for rapidity) and intravenous bisphosphonate (for potency) would be most efficacious in correcting serum calcium. Intermittent intravenous or oral bisphosphonate could then maintain serum calcium within normal limits. It must be emphasized, however, that ultimately the treatment of HM involves antineoplastic therapy, and the initiation of aggressive antihypercalcemic therapy may be questionable when the underlying malignancy is well established and the prognosis is known to be poor.

Antiosteolytic therapy

In addition to their use in the treatment of episodes of acute hypercalcemia, bisphosphonates have been used in the long-term management of osteolysis. They have been used, with some success, both in patients with myeloma, in whom PTHrP is not generally believed to play a role in osteolysis, and in patients with extensive skeletal metastases resulting from breast cancer, in whom PTHrP is thought to play a significant role in osteolysis. Development of pathological fractures and intractable bone pain as well as hypercalcemia are common features in both patient groups, compromising their quality of life and representing a notable health care cost. Preliminary results from several carefully controlled studies using large patient cohorts suggest that the use of oral bisphosphonates reduced the number and degree of hypercalcemic episodes, delayed the onset of osteolytic bone lesions, and decreased bone pain [76–78]. Health care costs, notably hospital admissions for the treatment of fractures and hypercalcemia, and radiotherapy for pain control, were significantly reduced in patients receiving bisphosphonate treatment for disseminated breast cancer [78]. On the other hand, a subsequent careful cost-benefit analysis of the use of a bisphosphonate in the management of multiple myeloma showed no such saving [79]. Patient compliance and lack of drug bioavailability persist as major drawbacks in the use of oral bisphosphonates. However, the advent of analogues having vastly improved potency will hopefully diminish the impact of these problems and allow the widespread use of bisphosphonates as adjuvant therapy in the palliative management of cancer patients with osseous involvement.

Potential new directions for treatment

The most effective therapy for hypercalcemia associated with neoplasia lies in reducing the tumor mass by surgical, radiologic, or chemical means, particularly in cases in which PTHrP has been identified as the major pathogenetic agent. Indeed, a reduction in tumor bulk following chemotherapy has been shown to correlate with a decrease in both serum calcium and circulating PTHrP [55,68]. Alternative modalities that are currently under investigation include the use of receptor antagonists to interfere with the peripheral action of PTHrP [24] and the use of vitamin D analogues to reduce the production of bioactive peptide [80,81]. In addition, antisense technology has been used to interfere with the production and intracellular processing of PTHrP [82].

The potential for the therapeutic use of receptor antagonists was first recognized in studies examining clinical disorders associated with excessive secretion of PTH [24]. With the revelation that PTHrP and PTH bind to and activate the same cell-surface receptor in kidney and bone [83,84], the potential for therapeutic applications for these antagonists increased substantially. Although peptide analogues have been developed that are highly sensitive and specific as antagonists for the PTH/PTHrP receptor in vitro, their efficacy in vivo appears to be hampered, at least in part, as a result of nonspecific binding to plasma proteins [85].

In addition to its role as a calcitropic hormone, $1,25(OH)_2D$ inhibits proliferation and induces differentiation in numerous target tissues [86]. It has also been shown to inhibit the production of PTHrP by normal and transformed cells in vitro through both transcriptional [87,88] and post-translational mechanisms [89–92]. However, although its administration in vivo is associated with a reduction in tumor volume [93] as well as inhibition of PTHrP production, undesirable side effects, such as hypercalcemia and hypercalciuria, ensue from the intrinsic action of the sterol. Several vitamin D analogues have, however, been developed that retain their antiproliferative capacity but that have minimal calcitropic activity. In the laboratory setting these agents have proven to be useful for inhibiting both tumor growth and PTHrP production in animal models of malignancy-associated hypercalcemia [80,94] (Fig. 6).

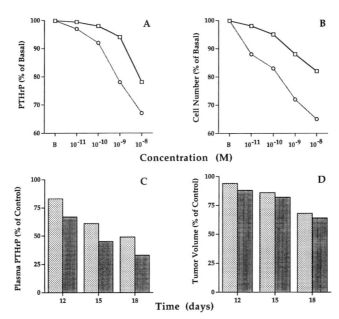

Figure 6. Vitamin D analogs in the treatment of HM. In vitro both $1,25(OH)_2D$ (□—□) and a low calcemic analog (○—○) produced dose-dependent decreases in PTHrP secreted into the medium (**A**), and dose-dependent reductions in cell numbers (**B**) when added to cultures of human HPK1A keratinocytes. In a similar manner, continuous infusion in vivo of 50 pmol/24 hr $1,25(OH)_2D$ (light hatching) or 200 pmol/24 hr of the low calcemic analog (dark hatching) produced time-dependent reductions in plasma PTHrP (**C**) and in tumor volume (**D**) in rats implanted with a hypercalcemic (H-500 Leydig cell) tumor. (Modified from Haq et al. [80] and Yu et al. [81], with permission.)

An alternative approach has used antisense technology to block PTHrP expression in neoplastic tissue. This has also been observed to retard tumor growth and progression in vivo [82,95,96]. Antisense inhibition of the prohormone convertase furin appeared to have an even greater suppressive effect on tumor growth in vivo than that seen when the PTHrP gene product per se was targeted [82]. This observation suggests that, in addition to processing prepropTHrP to its biologically active form, furin may also be involved in the cleavage of other agents required for neoplastic growth. Inhibition of furin action could therefore impede the formation of both PTHrP and other growth factors. Consequently, in the future, gene transfer techniques may be employed to inhibit production of the etiological agent responsible for PTHrP-associated HM rather than directing therapy at the target tissues upon which PTHrP acts.

Acknowledgments

The authors thank George Chan for artwork. Support was provided in part by grants to D.G. from the National Cancer Institute of Canada and the Medical Research Council of Canada.

References

1. Zondek H, Petrow H, Siebert W. 1923. Die bedeutung der calcium-bestimmung in blute fur die diagnose der nierrenin-siffizientz. Z Clin Med 99:129–132.
2. Gutman AB, Tyson TL, Gutman EB. 1936. Serum calcium, inorganic phosphorus and phosphatase activity in hyperparathyroidism, Paget's disease, multiple myeloma and neoplastic disease of the bones. Arch Intern Med 57:379–413.
3. Albright F. 1941. Case records of the Massachusetts General Hospital (case 27461). N Engl J Med 225:789–791.
4. Lafferty FW. 1966. Pseudohyperparathyroidism. Medicine 45:247–260.
5. Sherwood LM, O'Riordan JLH, Aurbach GD, Potts JT. 1967. Production of parathyroid hormone by nonparathyroid tumors. J Clin Endocrinol Metab 27:140–144.
6. Simpson EL, Mundy GR, D'Souza SM, Ibbotson KJ, Bockman MD, Jacobs JW. 1983. Absence of parathyroid hormone messenger RNA in non-parathyroid tumors associated with hypercalcemia. 309:325–330.
7. Nussbaum SR, Gaz RD, Arnold A. 1990. Hypercalcemia and ectopic secretion of parathyroid hormone by an ovarian carcinoma with rearrangement of the gene for parathyroid hormone. N Engl J Med 323:1324–1328.
8. Yoshimoto K, Yamasaki R, Sakai H, Tezuka U, Takahashi M, Iizuka M, Sekiya T, Saito S. 1989. Ectopic production of parathyroid hormone by a small cell lung cancer in a patient with hypercalcemia. J Clin Endocrinol Metab 68:976–981.
9. Robertson RP, Baylink DJ, Marini JJ, Adkison HW. 1975. Elevated prostaglandins and suppressed parathyroid hormone associated with hypercalcemia and renal cell carcinoma. J Clin Endocrinol Metab 41:164–167.
10. Breslau NA, McGuire JL, Zerwech JE, Frenkel EP, Pak CYC. 1984. Hypercalcemia associated with increased calcitriol levels in three patients with lymphoma. Ann Intern Med 100:1–7.

11. Goltzman D, Stewart AF, Broadus AE. 1981. Malignancy associated hypercalcemia: Evaluation with cytochemical bioassay for parathyroid hormone. J Clin Endocrinol Metab 53:899–904.

12. Rodan SB, Insogna KL, Vignery AMC, Stewart AF, Broadus AE, D'Souza SM, Bertolini DR, Mundy GR, Rodan GA. 1983. Factors associated with humoral hypercalcemia of malignancy stimulate adenylate cyclase in osteoblastic cells. J Clin Invest 72:1511–1515.

13. Nissenson RA, Abbott SR, Teitelbaum AP, Clark OH, Arnaud CD. 1981. Endogenous biologically active human parathyroid hormone measurement by a guanyl nucleotide-amplified renal adenylate cyclase assay. J Clin Endocrinol Metab 52:840–844.

14. Goltzman D, Bennet HPJ, Koutsilieris M, Mitchell J, Rabbani SA, Rouleau M. 1986. Studies of the multiple molecular forms of bioactive parathyroid hormone and parathyroid hormone-like substances. Recent Prog Horm Res 48:665–703.

15. Broadus AE, Stewart AF. 1994. Parathyroid hormone-related protein: Structure, processing and physiological actions. In Bilezekian JP, Marcus R, Levine MA, eds. The Parathyroids: Basic and Clinical Concepts. New York: Raven Press, pp 259–294.

16. Yasuda T, Banville D, Hendy GN, Goltzman D. 1989. Characterization of the human parathyroid hormone-like peptide gene. J Biol Chem 264:7720–7725.

17. Mangin M, Ikeda K, Dreyer BE, Broadus AE. 1989. Isolation and characterization of the human parathyroid hormone-like peptide gene. Proc Natl Acad Sci USA 86:2408–2412.

18. Suva LJ, Mather KA, Gillespie MT, Webb GC, Ng KW, Winslow GA, Wood WI, Martin TJ, Hudson PJ. 1989. Structure of the 5' flanking region of the gene encoding human parathyroid hormone-related protein (PTHrP). Gene 77:95–105.

19. Vasavada RC, Wysolmerski JJ, Broadus AE, Philbrick WM. 1993. Identification and characterization of a GC-rich promoter of the human parathyroid hormone-related peptide gene. Mol Endocrinol 7:273–282.

20. Campos RV, Wang C, Drucker DJ. 1992. Regulation of parathyroid hormone-related peptide (PTHRP) gene transcription: Cell and tissue-specific promoter utilization mediated by multiple positive and negative cis-acting DNA elements. Mol Endocrinol 6:1642–1652.

21. Southby J, O'Keefe LM, Martin TJ, Gillespie MT. 1995. Alternative promoter usage and mRNA splicing pathways for parathyroid hormone-related protein in normal tissues and tumours. Br J Cancer 72:702–707.

22. Holt EH, Vasavada RC, Bander NH, Broadus AE, Philbrick WM. 1993. Region-specific methylation of the parathyroid hormone-related peptide gene determines its expression in human renal carcinoma cell lines. J Biol Chem 268:20639–20645.

23. Sidler B, Alpert L, Henderson JE, Deckelbaum R, Amizuka N, Silva JE, Goltzman D, Karaplis AC. 1996. Amplification of the parathyroid hormone-related peptide (PTHrP) gene in a colonic carcinoma. J Clin Endocrinol Metab 81:2841–2847.

24. Chorev M, Rosenblatt M. 1994. Structure-function analysis of parathyroid hormone and parathyroid hormone-related protein. In Bilezekian JP, Marcus R, Levine MA, eds. The Parathyroids: Basic and Clinical Concepts. New York: Raven Press, pp 139–156.

25. Murray TM, Rao LG, Rizzoli RE. 1994. Interactions of parathyroid hormone, parathyroid hormone-related protein, and their fragments with conventional and nonconventional sites. In Bilezekian JP, Marcus R, Levine MA, eds. The Parathyroids: Basic and Clinical Concepts. New York: Raven Press, pp 185–211.

26. Fraher LJ, Hodsman AB, Jonas K, Saunders D, Rose CI, Henderson JE, Hendy GN, Goltzman D. 1992. A comparison of the in vivo biochemical responses to exogenous parathyroid hormone (1–34) and parathyroid hormone-related peptide (1–34) in man. J Clin Endocrinol Metab 75:417–423.

27. Goltzman D, Hendy GN, Banville D. 1989. Parathyroid hormone-like peptide: Molecular characterization and biological properties. Trends Endocrinol Metab 1:39–44.

28. Philbrick WM, Wysolmerski JJ, Galbraith S, Holt E, Orloff JJ, Yang KH, Vasavada RC, Weir EC, Broadus AE, Stewart AF. 1996. Defining the roles of parathyroid hormone-related protein in normal physiology. Physiol Rev 76:127–173.

29. Henderson JE, Amizuka N, Warshawsky H, Biasotto D, Lanske BMK, Goltzman D, Karaplis

211

AC. 1995. Nucleolar targeting of PTHrP enhances survival of chondrocytes under conditions that promote cell death by apoptosis. Mol Cell Biol 15:4064–4075.

30. Amizuka N, Karaplis AC, Henderson JE, Warshawsky H, Lipman ML, Matsuki Y, Ejiri S, Tanaka M, Izumi N, Ozawa H, Goltzman D. 1996. Haploinsufficiency of parathyroid hormone-related peptide (PTHrP) results in abnormal post-natal bone development. Dev Biol 175:166–176.

31. Sartori L, Insogna KL, Barrett PQ. 1988. Renal phosphate transport in humoral hypercalcemia of malignancy. Am J Physiol F1078–1084.

32. Sica DA, Martodam RR, Aronow J, Mundy GR, 1983. The hypercalcemic rat Leydig cell tumor: A model of the humoral hypercalcemia of malignancy. Calcif Tiss Int 35:287–293.

33. Henderson JE, Bernier S, D'Amour P, Goltzman D, 1990. Effects of passive immunization against parathyroid hormone (PTH)-like peptide and PTH in hypercalcemic tumor-bearing rats and normocalcemic controls. Endocrinology 127:1310–1318.

34. Ralston SH, Boyce BF, Cowan RA, Gardner MD, Fraser WD, Boyle IT. 1989. Contrasting mechanisms of hypercalcemia in patients with early and advanced humoral hypercalcemia of malignancy. J Bone Miner Res 4:103–111.

35. Ellis AG, Adam WR, Martin TJ. 1990. Comparison of the effects of parathyroid hormone (PTH) and recombinant PTH-related protein on bicarbonate excretion by the isolated, perfused rat kidney. J Endocrinol 126:403–408.

36. Horiuchi N, Caulfield MP, Fisher JE, Goldman ME, McKee RL, Reagan JE, Levy JJ, Nutt RF, Rodan SB, Schofield TI, Clemens TI, Rosenblatt M. 1987. Similarity of synthetic peptide from human tumor to parathyroid hormone in vivo and in vitro. Science 238:1566–1568.

37. Schweitzer DH, Hamdy NA, Frolich M, Zwinderman AH, Papapoulos SE. 1994. Malignancy-associated hypercalcemia: Resolution of controversies over vitamin D metabolism by a pathophysiological approach to the problem. Clin Endocrinol 41:251–256.

38. Orloff JJ, Stewart AF. 1995. Editorial: The carboxy-terminus of parathyroid hormone: Inert or invaluable. Endocrinology 136:4729–4731.

39. Parfitt AM. 1995. Bone remodeling, normal and abnormal: A biological basis for the understanding of cancer-related bone disease and its treatment. Can J Oncol 5(S1):1–10.

40. Suda T, Udagawa N, Nakamura I, Miyaura C, Takahashi N. 1995. Modulation of osteoclast differentiation by local factors. Bone 17(S2):S87–S91.

41. Mundy GR. 1993. Bone resorbing cells. In Favus MJ, ed. Primer on the Metabolic Bone Diseases and Disorders of Mineral Metabolism. New York: Raven Press, pp 25–32.

42. Rouleau MF, Mitchell J, Goltzman D. 1990. Characterization of the major parathyroid hormone target cell in the endosteal metaphysis of rat long bones. J Bone Miner Res 5:1043–1053.

43. Powell GJ, Southby J, Danks JA, Stilwell RG, Haymen JA, Henderson MA, Bennett RC, Martin TJ. 1991. Localization of parathyroid hormone-related protein in breast cancer metastases: Increased incidence in bone compared with other sites. Cancer Res 51:3059–3061.

44. Sugimoto T, Kanatani M, Kaji H, Yamaguchi T, Fukase M, Chihara K. 1993. Second messenger signaling of PTH and PTHrP-stimulated osteoclast-like cell formation from hemopoietic blast cells. Am J Physiol 265:E367–373.

45. Kremer R, Goltzman D. 1994. Assays for parathyroid hormone-related protein. In Bilezekian JP, Marcus R, Levine MA, eds. The Parathyroids: Basic and Clinical Aspects. New York: Raven Press, pp 321–339.

46. Kukreja SC, Shevrin DH, Wimbiscus SA, Ebeling PR, Danks JA, Rodda CP, Wood WI, Martin TJ. 1988. Antibodies to parathyroid hormone-related protein lower serum calcium in athymic mouse models of malignancy-associated hypercalcemia due to human tumors. J Clin Invest 82:1798–1802.

47. Sato K, Yamakawa Y, Shizume K, Satoh T, Nohtomi K, Demura H, Akatsu T, Nagata N, Kasahara T, Ohkawa HK, Ohsumi. 1993. Passive immunization with anti-parathyroid hormone-related protein monoclonal antibody markedly prolongs survival time of hypercalcemic nude mice bearing transplanted human PTHrP-producing tumors. J Bone Miner Res 8:849–860.

48. Yamamoto H, Nagai Y, Inoue D, Ohnishi Y, Ueyama Y, Ohno H, Matsumoto T, Ogata E,

Ikeda K. 1995. In vivo evidence for progressive activation of parathyroid hormone-related peptide gene transcription with tumor growth and stimulation of osteoblastic bone formation at an early stage of humoral hypercalcemia of cancer. J Bone Miner Res 10:36–44.

49. Mundy GR, Yoneda T. 1995. Facilitation and suppression of bone metastases. Clin Orthop Rel Res 312:34–44.

50. Stewart AF, Vignery A, Silvergate A, Ravin ND, LiVolsi V, Broadus AE, Baron R. 1982. Quantitative bone histomorphometry in humoral hypercalcemia of malignancy: Uncoupling of bone cell activity. J Clin Endocrinol Metab 55:219–227.

51. Body JJ, Delmas PD. 1992. Urinary pyridinium cross-links as markers of bone resorption in tumor-associated hypercalcemia. J Clin Endocrinol Metab 74:471–475.

52. Stewart AF, Horst R, Deftos LJ, Cadman EC, Lang R, Broadus AE. 1980. Biochemical evaluation of patients with cancer-associated hypercalcemia: Evidence for humoral and non-humoral groups. N Engl J Med 303:1377–1383.

53. Rabbani SA, Haq M, Goltzman D. 1993. Biosynthesis and processing of endogenous parathyroid hormone-related peptide (PTHrP) by the rat Leydig cell tumor H-500. Biochemistry 32:4931–4937.

54. Yang KH, dePapp AE, Soifer NE, Dreyer BE, Wu TL, Porter SE, Bellantoni M, Burtis WJ, Insogna KL, Broadus AE, Philbrick WP, Stewart AF. 1994. Parathyroid hormone-related protein: Evidence for isoform and tissue-specific post-translational processing. Biochemistry 33:7460–7469.

55. Henderson JE, Shustik C, Kremer R, Rabbani SA, Hendy GN, Goltzman D. 1990. Circulating concentrations of parathyroid hormone-like peptide in malignancy and hyperparathyroidism. J Bone Miner Res 5:105–113.

56. Walls J, Ratcliffe WA, Howell A, Bundred NJ. 1994. Parathyroid hormone and parathyroid hormone-related protein in the investigation of hypercalcemia in two hospital populations. Clin Endocrinol 41:407–413.

57. Ratcliffe WA, Norbury S, Stott RA, Heath DA, Ratcliffe JG. 1991. Immunoreactivity of plasma parathyrin-related peptide: Three region-specific radioimmunoassays and a two-site immunoradiometric assay compared. Clin Chem 37:1781–1787.

58. Soifer NE, Dee KE, Insogna KL, Burtis WJ, Matvicik LM, Wu TL, Milstone LM, Broadus AE, Philbrick WM, Stewart AF. 1992. Parathyroid hormone-related protein: Evidence for secretion of a novel mid-region fragment by three different cell lines in culture. J Biol Chem 267:18236–18243.

59. Burtis WJ, Dann P, Gaich GA, Soifer NE. 1994. A high abundance midregion species of parathyroid hormone-related protein: Immunological and chromatographic characterization in plasma. J Clin Endocrinol Metab 78:317–322.

60. Sachmechi I, Kalra J, Molho L, Chawla K. 1995. Paraneoplastic hypercalcemia associated with uterine papillary serous carcinoma. Gynecol Oncol 58:378–382.

61. McAuley P, Asa SL, Chiu B, Henderson JE, Goltzman D, Drucker DJ. 1990. Parathyroid hormone-like peptide in normal and neoplastic mesothelial cells. Cancer 66:1975–1979.

62. Asa SL, Henderson JE, Goltzman D, Drucker DJ. 1990. Parathyroid hormone-like peptide in normal and neoplastic human endocrine tissues. J Clin Endocrinol Metab 71:1112–1118.

63. Kimura S, Nishimura Y, Yamaguchi K, Nagasaki K, Shimada K, Uchida H. 1990. A case of pheochromocytoma producing parathyroid hormone-related protein and presenting with hypercalcemia. J Clin Endocrinol Metab 70:1559–1563.

64. Drucker DJ, Asa SL, Henderson JE, Golzman D. 1988. The parathyroid hormone-like peptide gene is expressed in the normal and neoplastic human endocrine pancreas. Mol Endocrinol 3:1589–1595.

65. Ikeda K, Arnold A, Magin M, Kinder B, Vydelingum NA, Brennan MF, Broadus AE. 1989. Expression of transcripts encoding a parathyroid hormone-related peptide in abnormal human parathyroid tissues. J Clin Endocrinol Metab 69:1240–1248.

66. Ito M, Enomoto H, Usa T, Villadolid MC, Ohtsuru A, Namba H, Sekine I, Yamashita S. 1993. Expression of parathyroid hormone-related peptide in human pituitary tumors. J Clin Pathol 46:682–683.

67. Nakashima M, Ohtsuru A, Luo WT, Nakayama T, Enomoto H, Usa T, Kiriyama T, Ito M, Nagataki S, Yamashita S. 1995. Expression of parathyroid hormone-related peptide in human thyroid tumors. J Pathol 175:227–236.
68. Kremer R, Shustik C, Tabak T, Papavasiliou V, Goltzman D. 1996. Parathyroid hormone-related peptide (PTHrP) in hematological malignancies. Am J Med 100:406–411.
69. Bonjour JP, Rizzoli R. 1991. Treatment of hypercalcemia of malignancy with clodronate. Bone 12(S1):S19–S23.
70. Walls J, Ratcliffe WA, Howell A, Bundred NJ. 1994. Response to intravenous bisphosphonate therapy in hypercalcemic patients with and without bone metastases: The role of parathyroid hormone-related protein. Br J Cancer 70:169–172.
71. Wimalawansa SJ. 1993. Significance of plasma PTHrP in patients with hypercalcemia of malignancy treated with bisphosphonate. Cancer 73:2223–2230.
72. Body JJ, Dumon JC, Thirion M, Cleeren A. 1993. PTHrP concentrations in tumor-induced hypercalcemia: Influence on the response to bisphosphonate and changes after therapy. J Bone Miner Res 8:701–706.
73. Gallacher SJ, Fraser WD, Logue FC, Dryburgh FJ, Cowan RA, Boyle IT, Ralston SH. 1992. Factors predicting the acute effect of pamidronate on serum calcium in hypercalcemia of malignancy. Calcif Tiss Int 51:419–423.
74. Garnero P, Shih WJ, Gineyts E, Karpf DB, Delmas PD. 1994. Comparison of new biochemical markers of bone turnover in late postmenopausal osteoporotic women in response to alendronate treatment. J Clin Endocrinol Metab 79:1693–1700.
75. Lahtinen R, Laakso M, Palva I, Virkkunen P, Elomaa L. 1992. Randomised, placebo-controlled multicentre trial of clodronate in mutiple myeloma. Lancet 340:1049–1052.
76. Paterson AHG, Powles TJ, Kanis JA, McCloskey E, Hanson J, Ashley S. 1993. Double-blind controlled trial of oral clodronate in patients with bone metastases from breast cancer. J Clin Oncol 11:59–65.
77. Berenson JR, Lichtenstein A, Porter L, Dimopoulos MA, Bordoni R, George S, Lipton A, Keller A, Ballester O, Kovacs MJ, Blacklock HA, Bell R, Simeone J, Reitsma DJ, Heffernan M, Seaman J, Knight RD. 1996. Efficacy of pamidronate in reducing skeletal events in patients with advanced multiple myeloma. N Engl J Med 334:488–493.
78. Biermann WA, Cantor RI, Fellin FM, Jakobowski J, Hopkins L, Newbold RC III. 1991. An evaluation of the potential cost reductions resulting from the use of clodronate in the treatment of metastatic carcinoma of the breast. Bone 12(S1):537–542.
79. Laakso M, Lahtinen R, Virkkunen P, Elomaa I. 1994. Subgroup and cost-benefit analysis of the Finnish multicentre trial of clodronate in multiple myeloma. Br J Hematol 87:725–729.
80. Haq M, Kremer R, Goltzman D, Rabbani SA. 1993. A vitamin D analogue (EB1089) inhibits parathyroid hormone-related peptide production and prevents the development of maignancy-associated hypercalcemia in vivo. J Clin Invest 91:2416–2422.
81. Yu J, Papavasiliou V, Rhim J, Goltzman D, Kremer R. 1995. Vitamin D analogs: New therapeutic agents for the treatment of squamous cancer and its associated hypercalcemia. Anti Cancer Drugs 6:101–108.
82. Liu B, Amizuka N, Goltzman D, Rabbani SA. 1995. Inhibition of processing of parathyroid hormone-related peptide by antisense furin: Effect in vitro and in vivo on rat Leydig (H-500) tumor cells. Int J Cancer 63:1–6.
83. Jüppner H, Abou-Samra A-B, Freeman M, Kong XF, Schipani E, Richards J, Kolakowski LF, Hock J, Potts JT, Kronenberg HM, Segre GV. 1991. A G protein-linked receptor for parathyroid hormone and parathyroid hormone-related peptide. Science 254:1024–1026.
84. Abou-Samra AB, Jüppner H, Force T, Freeman MW, Kong XF, Schipani E, Urena P, Richards J, Bonventre JV, Potts JT Jr, Kronenberg HM, Segre GV. 1992. Expression cloning of a common receptor for parathyroid hormone and parathyroid hormone-related peptide from rat osteoblast-like cells: A single receptor stimulates intracellular accumulation of both cAMP and inositol trisphosphates and increases intracellular free calcium. Proc Natll Acad Sci USA 89:2732–2736.
85. Kukreja SC, D'Anza JJ, Wimbiscus SA, Fisher JE, McKee RL, Caulfield MP, Rosenblatt M.

214

1994. Inactivation by plasma may be responsible for lack of efficacy of parathyroid hormone antagonists in hypercalcemia of malignancy. Endocrinology 134:2184–2188.

86. Walters MR. 1995. Newly identified actions of the vitamin D endocrine system. In Negro-Vilar A, ed. Hormonal Regulation of Bone Mineral Metabolism, Vol. 4. Bethesda, MD: The Endocrine Society, pp 1–46.

87. Kremer R, Karaplis AC, Henderson JE, Gulliver W, Banville D, Hendy GN, Goltzman D. 1991. Regulation of parathyroid hormone-like peptide in cultured normal human keratinocytes. J Clin Invest 87:884–893.

88. Inoue D, Matsumoto T, Ogata E, Ikeda K. 1993. 22-Oxacalcitriol, a noncalcemic analogue of calcitriol, suppresses both cell proliferation and parathyroid hormone-related peptide gene expression in human T cell lymphotropic virus type 1-infected T cells. J Biol Chem 268:16730–16736.

89. Henderson JE, Sebag M, Rhim J, Goltzman D, Kremer R. 1991. Dysregulation of parathyroid hormone-like peptide expression and secretion in a keratinocyte model of tumor-progression. Cancer Res 51:6521–6528.

90. Liu B, Goltzman D, Rabbani SA. 1993. Regulation of parathyroid hormone-related peptide production in vitro by the rat hypercalcemic Leydig cell tumor H-500. Endocrinology 132:1658–1664.

91. Sebag M, Henderson JE, Rhim J, Kremer R, 1992. Relative resistance to 1,25-dihydroxyvitamin D_3 in a keratinocyte model of tumor progression. J Biol Chem 267:12162–12167.

92. Sebag M, Henderson JE, Goltzman D, Kremer R. 1994. Regulation of parathyroid hormone-related peptide production in normal human mammary epithelial cells in vitro. Am J Physiol 267:C723–C730.

93. Eisman JA, Barkla DH, Tutton PJM. 1987. Suppression of in vivo growth of human solid cancer tumor xenografts by 1,25-dihydroxyvitamin D3. Cancer Res 47:21–27.

94. Abe J, Nakano AT, Nishii Y, Matsumoto T, Ogata E, Ikeda K. 1991. A novel D3 analog, 22-oxa-1,25-dihydroxyvitamin D3, inhibits the growth of human breast cancer in vitro and in vivo without causing hypercalcemia. Endocrinology 129:832–837.

95. Akino K, Ohtsuru A, Yano H, Ozeki S, Namba H, Nakashima M, Ito M, Matsumoto T, Yamashita S. 1996. Antisense inhibition of parathyroid hormone-related peptide gene expression reduces malignant pituitary tumor progression and metastases in the rat. Cancer Res 56:77–86.

96. Rabbani SA, Gladu J, Liu B, Goltzman D. 1995. Regulation in vivo of the growth of Leydig cell tumors by antisense RNA for parathyroid hormone-related peptide. Endocrinology 136:5416–5422.

11. Neoplasms of the adrenal cortex
Clinical and basic aspects

Ana C. Latronico and George P. Chrousos

Cushing's syndrome due to adrenocortical tumors was reported at the turn of the century, almost a decade before the description of the syndrome and homonymous disease by Harvey Cushing [1]. At the time, the adrenal cortices were known to secrete an active principle necessary for life, the absence of which led to Addison's disease. However, the crucial role of the pituitary gland in the control of adrenal secretion was not suspected. Since then, we have learned a great deal about adrenocortical tumors, their incidence, clinical presentation, diagnosis, therapy, and prognosis. Some research on the cell biology of these tumors has also been done, mostly in the last decade. Rapidly advancing knowledge in the biology of other more frequent nonendocrine or endocrine tumors promises that better understanding of adrenal tumorigenesis is also forthcoming.

Treating adrenocortical malignancies has been utterly frustrating for both endocrinologists and oncologists. The desperate situation of the usually young patients with these vicious neoplasms makes the discovery of effective therapeutic modalities as urgent as ever. The purpose of this brief review is to present the state of the art in this field and to suggest new avenues of research.

Classification

Adrenocortical tumors are divided into benign and malignant. Either can be hormonally silent or hormone secreting. The vast majority of adrenocortical tumors are benign and hormonally silent [2,3]. The hormone-secreting tumors can produce glucocorticoids, androgens, mineralocorticoids, estrogens, and combinations thereof [4–12]. Adrenocortical tumors can be sporadic or hereditary, with the former representing the overwhelming majority.

Diffuse or nodular adrenocortical hyperplasia resulting from adrenocorticotropin hormone (ACTH) hyperstimulation in ACTH-dependent Cushing's syndrome, and in congenital adrenal hyperplasia due to defects of cortisol biosynthetic enzymes, and nodular hyperplasia associated with isolated primary micronodular or massive macronodular adrenal disease or Carney's

Andrew Arnold (ed.) ENDOCRINE NEOPLASMS. 1997. Kluwer Academic Publishers. ISBN 0-7923-4354-9.
All rights reserved.

Table 1. Clinical and molecular features of syndromes associated with benign and/or malignant adrenocortical neoplasms

	Clinical features	Chromosomal and molecular defects
Carney's complex	PPNAD, atrial, and other myxomas, schwannomas, lentigines, and blue nevi of the skin and mucosae	2p16 (Carney locus)
Congenital adrenal hyperplasia	Female and male pseudohermarphroditism, cortisol deficiency, mineralocorticoid deficiency or excess	Inborn errors of cortisol biosynthesis enzymes resulting in chronic hypersecretion of ACTH
Li-Fraumeni syndrome	Familiar susceptibility to a variety of cancers	Germline mutations of p53 tumor suppressor gene
McCune-Albright syndrome	Precocious puberty, café-au-lait spots, polyostotic fibrous dysplasia	Overactivity of the Gs protein signaling pathway
Multiple endocrine neoplasia type I (MEN-I)	Hyperparathyroidism, pancreatic-duodenal and pituitary tumors	11q13 (MEN-I locus)
Wiedemann-Beckwith syndrome	Neonatal macrosomia, macroglossia, and omphalocele	Allelic loss of 11p15

PPNAD = primary pigmented nodular adrenocortical disease; ACTH = adrenocorticotrophic hormone.

complex, are considered low-grade premalignant states [13–16]. Table 1 summarizes the clinical and molecular features of genetic syndromes associated with benign and malignant adrenocortical neoplasms.

Incidence and epidemiology

Small benign adrenocortical tumors are present in up to 2% of adults over age 50. Usually they are discovered incidentally, in the context of abdominal computed tomography (CT) or magnetic resonance imaging (MRI) scans performed for various unrelated purposes [2]. Hormone-secreting benign adrenal adenomas are rare, and equally rare are hormonally silent or hormone-secreting adrenocortical carcinomas. Malignant neoplasias of the adrenal cortex account for 0.05–0.2% of all cancers, with an approximate prevalence of two new cases per million of population per year [17,18]. Adrenal cancer occurs at all ages, from early infancy to the seventh and eighth decades of life [4–12]. A bimodal age distribution has been reported, with the first peak occurring before age 5, and the second in the fourth to fifth decade [7]. In all published series, females clearly predominate, accounting for 65–90% of the reported cases [5,9,10,12]. Whereas some investigators report a left-sided prevalence, others note a right-sided preponderance [10,12,19,20]. Bilaterality has been reported in 2–10% of the cases [5,10,12].

218

Clinical presentation

Patients with hormone-secreting adrenocortical neoplasms have associated endocrine syndromes that result from secretion of cortisol and its precursors, adrenal androgens and their precursors, or, rarely, estrogen or mineralocorticoids. The most common syndrome associated with adrenal tumors in adults is Cushing's syndrome [4,7,12]. It is present in 30–40% of patients with adrenocortical carcinoma.

Virilization occurs in 20–30% of adults with functional adrenal neoplasms, while it is the most common hormonal syndrome in children with adrenocortical tumors [4,7,8,10–12]. Virilization is secondary to hypersecretion of adrenal androgens, including dehydroepiandrosterone (DHEA) and its sulfate derivative (DHEA-S), Δ5-androstenediol and Δ4-androstenedione, all of which may be converted finally to testosterone and 5α-dihydrotestosterone. The signs and symptoms in adult females include oligoamenorrhea, hirsutism, cystic acne, excessive muscle mass, temporal balding, increased of libido, and clitoromegaly. In young girls heterosexual precocious puberty occurs. A combination of Cushing's syndrome and virilization is seen in 10–30% of patients [4,7,10]. This combined syndrome is usually associated with secretion of multiple steroid precursors.

Feminization and hyperaldosteronism, as pure hormonal syndromes, are quite rare manifestations of adrenocortical neoplasms. Even more unusual presentations of adrenal cancers include hypoglycemia, non–glucocorticoid-related insulin resistance, and polycythemia [4,7,8,10].

Slightly over half of the adult patients with adrenocortical carcinoma have no recognizable endocrine syndrome. These patients present either with abdominal pain or fullness, or with the incidental finding of an adrenal mass on imaging studies done for unrelated reasons. A palpable abdominal mass is present in about half of the patients with nonfunctional adrenocortical carcinoma at the time of diagnosis [5,6,8,10]. Finally, metastatic disease may cause symptoms before a primary diagnosis is established in a significant proportion of the patients [7,10]. Local invasion commonly involves the kidneys and inferior vena cava, while metastatic disease may be found in the retroperitoneal lymph nodes, lungs, liver, or bone.

Laboratory studies

Several laboratory studies are useful in the establishment or confirmation of excessive steroid secretion and the monitoring of patients with adrenocortical neoplasms. A single-dose (1 mg) overnight dexamethasone suppression test may be helpful as a screening test [21]. Hypercortisolism is best established by measuring the 24 hour excretion of urine free cortisol (UFC) [7,10,21]. Over 90% of patients with Cushing's syndrome have UFC values $>200 \mu g/24 \, hr$, while 97% of normal individuals have UFC values $<100 \mu g/24 \, hr$ [7,21].

Several plasma and urinary steroids are elevated in patients with Cushing's syndrome due to functioning adrenocortical tumors. These include DHEA, DHEAS, Δ5-androstenediol, Δ4-androstenedione, pregnenolone, 17-hydroxypregnenolone, and 11-deoxycortisol in the plasma, and 17-hydroxysteroids, 17-ketosteroids, and the tetrahydro metabolite of 11-deoxycortisol in the urine. Despite the fact that steroidogenic precursors, such as 17-hydroxyprogesterone and 11-deoxycortisol, are not essential in the evaluation of hypercortisolism, they may occasionally provide clues to the presence of an adrenal malignancy in patients with Cushing's syndrome [11,13]. Generally, many of the steroid biosynthesis enzymes are defective in adrenocortical carcinomas, providing an inefficient machinery for steroid production and associated with plasma level patterns of steroid precursors typical of enzymatic blocks [11,13].

A low plasma adrenocorticotrophic hormone (ACTH) level associated with elevated concurrent plasma cortisol concentrations is indicative of autonomous activity of the adrenal glands [13,21]. There are several dynamic endocrine tests for the differential diagnosis of adrenal Cushing's syndrome from the ACTH-dependent forms of the condition [21]. These include the classic high-dose dexamethasone suppression test and the ovine corticotropin-releasing hormone (CRH) stimulation test. Typically, both tests are associated with lack of responsiveness of cortisol secretion to dexamethasone and CRH.

The clinical diagnosis of adrenally induced virilization may be confirmed by measurement of plasma adrenal androgens and testosterone, and 24-hour urinary excretion of 17-ketosteroids. Feminization or hyperaldosteronism can be confirmed by measurements of elevated plasma estradiol and/or estrone, or aldosterone, 11-deoxycorticorticosterone, and/or corticosterone, respectively. All patients, and particularly those with nonfunctional adrenal masses, should also be screened for pheochromocytoma, even in the absence of sustained hypertension.

Imaging procedures

The diagnosis of adrenal neoplasms depends on the identification of an adrenal mass on CT and/or MRI. Both normal and abnormal adrenal glands are easily visible on CT because of the adipose tissue that surrounds these glands in the retroperitoneum [22]. The presence of a large unilateral adrenal mass with irregular borders is virtually diagnostic of adrenal cancer [7,10,19,22]. CT provides information about size, homogeneity, presence of calcifications, areas of necrosis, and the extent of local invasion, thus also being helpful in making decisions about the resectability of the lesion. Tumors as small as 0.5 cm have been detected by CT, although the relative lack of retroperitoneal fat in children might decrease the sensitivity of the test in this age group [10,24,25].

220

Whether MRI will prove to be superior to CT scanning in diagnosing and differentiating adrenal masses remains to be seen. MRI provides information about the invasion of an adrenocortical carcinoma into blood vessels, particularly the inferior vena cava and the adrenal and renal veins, in which tumor thrombi may be identified occasionally. Studies have reported that MRI can distinguish with a fair degree of accuracy among primary malignant adrenocortical tumors, nonfunctioning adenomas, and pheochromocytomas by comparing the ratio of the signal intensity of each type of adrenal mass with that of liver [10,22,26]. Thus, primary malignant adrenocortical lesions have an intermediate to high signal intensity on T2-weighted images. Nonfunctional adenomas have low signal intensity, whereas pheochromocytomas have an extremely high signal intensity.

Other imaging modalities, such as iodo-cholesterol scanning, venography, and arteriography, are rarely indicated [7,10,22]. The [125]iodo-cholesterol scan is usually negative in malignant adrenocortical neoplasms and positive in steroid-secreting adenomas. [125]Iodo-cholesterol uptake may help define whether there is unilateral or bilateral autonomous steroidosynthetic tissue when adrenal masses are seen bilaterally on CT or MRI imaging. Also, it may help with the localization of adrenal rests or adrenal remnants after adrenalectomy. On occasion, selective arteriography may help distinguish between adrenal masses and upper pole renal tumors. Inferior vena cava venography may be indicated if CT or MRI findings suggest the presence of a tumor thrombus in this vessel. In general, these invasive techniques are reserved for the rare instance in which CT or MRI cannot supply the information needed.

Pathology, staging, and prognosis

Histologically, adrenocortical tumors consist of lipid-depleted cells with granular cytoplasm and large multiple nuclei and nucleoli [13,28]. Tumor cells have varying mitotic activity. The differentiation of benign from malignant adrenocortical neoplasms solely on the basis of histologic findings is difficult, if not impossible [8,11,13,29]. Thus, several reports demonstrated that patients whose operatively excised tumors exhibited histologically benign features subsequently developed local recurrences or distant metastases, whereas others whose tumors had a microscopic appearance typical of malignancy lived tumor-free for many years.

Several macroscopic and microscopic criteria are collectively used to define the malignancy of an adrenocortical tumor and to predict its behavior [28–30]. Macroscopically, wet weight of >500 g, a grossly lobulated cut surface, the presence of necrotic areas and/or calcifications, and intratumor hemorrhages predict malignancy. Microscopically, architectural disarray, frequent mitoses, marked cellular pleomorphism, nuclear atypia, and hyperchromasia, as well as invasion of the capsule, suggest malignancy.

221

Abnormal DNA contents have been detected in adrenocortical carcinomas by flow-cytometric DNA analysis [31,32]. Aneuploidy occurs in neoplastic subpopulations through genetic instability and mitotic irregularities. Bowlby et al. reported that 83% of the carcinomas showed aneuploidy, suggesting that flow-cytometric analysis may prove to be a complement to the conventional histopathologic methods and a valuable tool in predicting the prognosis of patients with adrenocortical tumors [31].

The staging system for adrenocortical carcinomas depends on tumor size, nodal involvement, invasion of adjacent organs, and the presence of distant metastases (Table 2) [6,7,33]. Staging is helpful in defining prognosis and therapy. Only patients with stage I and II disease are curable with surgery. Unfortunately, the great majority of the patients have either stage III or IV disease at the time of diagnosis. Despite complete resection, virtually 100% of patients with stage III disease have recurrent and metastatic disease within 5 years of tumor resection. Moreover, the 5-year survival for stage III adrenal carcinoma is generally less than 30%. The most frequent sites of metastasis are lymph nodes (25–46%), lungs (47–97%), liver (53–68%), abdomen (33–43%), and bones (11–33%). Metastases have been reported in the ovary spleen, pleura, thyroid, pharynx, tonsils, mediastinum, myocardium, brain, spinal cord, skin, and subcutaneous tissue [6–8,10]. Despite aggressive surgical therapy, the mean 5-year survival of patients with stage IV disease is 15–25%.

Therapy

Surgical resection is the only therapy that unquestionably cures or prolongs survival significantly, particularly if the disease is detected at stages I and II [7,9,13,20,33–35]. Radical excision with en-bloc resection of any local invasion offers the best chance for cure. A wide exposure is needed, using an extended

Table 2. Staging of adrenocortical carcinoma

Stage	T,N,M	Description
I	T1, N0, M0	Tumor <5 cm, confined to adrenal gland
II	T2, N0, M0	Tumor >5 cm, confined adrenal gland
III	T1 or T2, N1, M0	Tumor confined to adrenal gland with involvement of local lymph nodes
		or
	T3, N0, M0	Tumor extending beyond the adrenal gland but not invading adjacent organs
IV	T3 or T4, N1, M0 any T, M1	Tumor extending beyond the adrenal, invading adjacent organs, and involving local lymph nodes, or any tumor with metastases

Adapted from Macfarlane [••], with permission.
T = tumor; N = lymph node; M = metastases; 0 = negative.

222

subcostal incision or a thoracoabdominal approach [13,30,34]. Patients apparently cured with surgery require continued surveillance. Mitotane after complete macroscopic resection in stage III and IV disease may be given to increase the duration between recurrences; however, this has not been tested in a controlled study [7,10,13,20,36]. An excellent review on the treatment of adrenal cancer appeared recently [37].

Mitotane has been used extensively in patients with adrenocortical carcinoma; however, this drug has been generally ineffective in prolonging overall survival in the advanced stages of the disease [9,20,12,37]. Mitotane acts as an adrenolytic agent, possibly by causing alterations in mitochondrial function, blocking adrenal steroid 11-β-hydroxylation and altering the extra-adrenal metabolism of cortisol and androgens. Studies demonstrated that high oral doses (up to 12–14 g/day) of mitotane caused remission of hypercortisolism in 50–60% of patients with adrenocortical carcinoma; however, short-lived 6–10 month objective tumor responses occurred in less than 20% of these patients [35]. The side effects of mitotane are largely dose related. Weakness, somnolence, confusion, lethargy, and headache are reported in half of the patients treated [10,12,13,35,36]. More serious neurotoxicity, such as ataxia and dysarthria, may also occur [13]. Gastrointestinal side effects include anorexia, nausea, and diarrhea, which are present in most patients. Skin rash, toxic retinopathy with papilledema, and interstitial cystitis are less commonly seen.

Several alternative chemotherapeutic regimens have been used for the treatment of metastatic adrenocortical carcinoma. They include cisplatin, etoposide, 5-fluorouracil, doxorubicin, vincristine, gossipol, suramin, and melphalan [38–43]. Gossipol, a spermatoxin derived from crude cottonseed oil, inhibits the growth of human adrenocortical tumors in nude mice. Oral gossipol (30–70 mg/day) was used with relative safely in outpatients with metastatic adrenal cancer; however, a partial tumor response rate was observed in only 17% [38]. This is consistent with the generally poor response of adrenal cancer to most medical therapies.

Genetic mechanisms of human adrenocortical tumorigenesis

General mechanisms of tumorigenesis

Except in periods of life characterized by rapid growth, the accrual of a certain type of cells in a tissue is equal to the withdrawal of the same type and number of cells (Fig. 1). New cell accrual is stimulated by genes that activate the cell cycle (protooncogenes) and inhibited by others that suppress it (tumor suppressor genes). Cell withdrawal, on the other hand, takes place by programmed cell death (apoptosis), differentiation to a different type of cell, or natural senescence. Tumorigenesis occurs when the equation between cell accrual and withdrawal is disturbed by defects in one or more of multiple

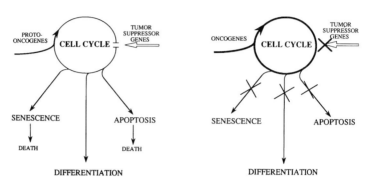

NORMAL CELL　　　　　　　　　　　TUMOR CELL

Figure 1. Except in the periods of life that are characterized by rapid growth, the accrual of a certain type of cells in a tissue is equal to the withdrawal of the same type and number of cells from this tissue. New cell accrual is stimulated by genes that activate the cell cycle (protooncogenes) and is inhibited by genes that suppress it (tumor suppressor genes). Cell withdrawal takes place by apoptosis, differentiation to a different type of cell, or natural senescence. Tumorigenesis occurs when the equation between cell accrual and withdrawal is disturbed by defects in one or more of the multiple checkpoints indicated in the right panel, leading to the accumulation of tumor cells.

checkpoints in the life of a cell that ensures control of the cellular composition of a tissue.

In 1914 Boveri predicted the importance of genetic alterations of somatic cells in the development of cancer [44]. Indeed, in the last 20 years molecular and cell biology studies have revealed that activation of protooncogenes and/or loss of function of tumor suppressor genes represents key mechanisms in the formation of many animal and human cancers [45–47]. At this time, more than 50 oncogenes and 12 tumor suppressor genes have been identified in the human genome; however, only a small proportion of these have been actually implicated in the development of specific human neoplasms.

Protooncogenes are present in all mammalian cells, where they are thought to play key roles in normal cellular growth, proliferation, and differentiation [45]. If these genes are overexpressed or their protein products are inappropriately activated by such mechanisms as gene amplification, point mutation, insertion, or translocation, they may increase cellular growth and proliferation, and inhibit differentiation, leading eventually to tumor formation [45,47]. The tumor suppressor genes are also present in all mammalian cells, coding for proteins that are involved in the control of cellular growth and proliferation. If these negative growth-controlling genes or their protein products are inactivated by such mechanisms as gene deletion, point mutation, insertion, or translocation, they may allow uncontrolled cellular growth and proliferation to take place and, thus, also lead to tumor formation [45–47].

With the exception of germ cells, most other cells in the organism are destined to die after a number of duplications in a process defined as senescence or by induction of programmed cell death (apoptosis). Cancer cells are immortal in the sense that senescence mechanisms are not operational and the apoptosis mechanisms are neutralized. The enzyme telomerase is crucial for providing immortality to germ cells by protecting the chromosomal telomeres after each mitosis. The same enzyme act in immortal cancer cells. On the other hand, proteins that regulate apoptosis are altered in cancer cells to generally prevent apoptosis from occurring.

Genomic instability

Recently, the clonal composition of adrenocortical tumors was determined using X-chromosome inactivation analysis [48,49]. Like most tumors, adrenal adenomas and carcinomas were most often monoclonal, whereas ACTH-induced diffuse and macronodular hyperplasias were polyclonal. These findings support the fundamental contemporary assumption that tumors arise as monoclonal expansions of a single cell, which become tumorous in response to a series of multistep genetic aberrations involving overexpression of protooncogenes and/or inactivation of tumor suppressor genes, as well as alterations of the proteins involved in the normal progression of senescence, induction of apoptosis, and differentiation [50–52]. The rate of DNA defects developed and passed on with each replication, also called the rate of genomic instability, is proportional to the rate of development of clones with survival advantages and, therefore, is proportional to the potential of a tumor to grow and prevail over the host. The ability of the cell to rapidly repair DNA aberrations is then crucial for the prevention of clonal expansion and tumorigenesis. Defects in proteins responsible for DNA repair may also participate in tumorigenesis.

c-Oncogenes

Dysfunctional receptors can inappropriately trigger or amplify signals that result in genes being transcribed out of their normal context. G protein–coupled receptors were recently proposed as candidate protooncogenes [53]. Thus, somatic mutations in the carboxy-terminal portion of the third cytoplasmic loop of the thyrotropin receptor (TSH-R) were recently identified in receptor genes from hyperfunctioning thyroid adenomas [54]. That hyperstimulation of the adrenals by ACTH could result in adrenocortical tumors was directly suggested by isolated case reports of carcinomas arising 3–36 years after the diagnosis of classic congenital adrenal hyperplasia [14,15]. Recently, the adrenocorticotrophic hormone receptor (ACTH-R) gene, a G-protein–coupled receptor, was cloned and its chromosomal localization and sequence were determined [55,56]. The direct sequencing of ACTH-R did not reveal constitutively activating mutations in a series of 25 sporadic adrenal cortical neoplasms and two cancer cell lines, indicating that this mechanism is not frequent in human adrenocortical tumorigenesis [57].

The abnormalities in components of signal-transduction pathways that control the intracellular production of cAMP, such as G-protein–coupled membrane receptors, the stimulatory guanine nucleotide-binding protein (Gs), and the inhibitory G protein (Gi), adenyl cyclase, kinase A, phosphokinases of kinase A, the family of cyclic AMP responsive element-binding protein (CREB), and the phosphokinases, might be implicated in the neoplastic transformation of adrenocortical tissue. Activating mutations of the Gsα gene (*gsp* mutations) were described in affected tissues from patients with McCune-Albright syndrome, and these included hyperfunctioning adrenocortical adenomas (see Table 1) [58]. These findings demonstrated that overactivity of the G-protein–signaling pathway might occasionally lead to the development of adrenocortical tumors. On the other hand, point mutations in Giα2, corresponding to codons 201 and 227 of Gsα, were identified in 3 of 11 sporadic adrenocortical neoplasms [59]. Although defects in the Gs and Giα2 were not confirmed in a large series of sporadic benign and malignant adrenal neoplasms, a small proportion of adrenocortical tumors might be related to mutations in the G-protein genes [60].

Similarly, abnormalities in components of signal-transduction pathways that control the intracellular production of phosphoinositol breakdown products and diacylglycerol, such as G-protein–coupled receptors, phospholipase C, protein kinase C (PKC), and the rest of its cascade, including the transcription factors c-*jun* and c-*fos*, might also be implicated in adrenocortical tumorigenesis [61,62].

PKC activity is a potential marker for human malignant diseases, such as breast tumors, pituitary tumors, and malignant gliomas [63–65]. Calcium-dependent PKC activity was recently described, however, as nonincreased in adrenocortical tumors (benign and malignant), and in diffuse and macronodular adrenal hyperplasia compared with normal adrenal tissue, suggesting that this molecular mechanism is infrequent in adrenocortical tumorigenesis [66].

Tumor suppressor genes

Molecular defects of tumor suppressor genes were recently identified in hereditary and sporadic adrenocortical neoplasms. The Li-Fraumeni syndrome, a rare autosomal dominant susceptibility to a variety of cancers, which include carcinomas of the adrenal cortex and breast, tumors of the brain and muscle, and leukemias, has been associated with germline mutations of the p53 tumor suppressor gene [67–69]. This is the most common known tumorigenesis-related gene mutated in human cancers, found altered in 40–50% of several frequent forms of malignant neoplasms, including those of the breast and colon [70–73]. This gene is composed of 11 exons and has been mapped on human chromosome 17p13.1 [72]. The loss of the normal inhibitory function of the p53 tumor suppressor protein on the cell cycle leads to tumorigenesis. More than 90% of all mutations of p53 discovered in human tumors have been detected in four regions that lie between exons 5 and 8, which are highly conserved among several different species [70–73].

Mutations of the p53 tumor suppressor gene were recently reported in sporadic adrenocortical carcinomas and adenomas [74,75]. Reincke et al. described p53 mutations in exons 5–8 in 27% of adrenocortical carcinomas and the two tumor adrenal cancer cell lines available but in none of the benign cortisol-secreting adrenal adenomas examined [75]. This study demonstrated an excellent correlation between the p53 immunohistochemical findings and the DNA abnormalities. Furthermore, Lin et al. demonstrated a high frequency of p53 gene mutations in 10 of 13 benign aldosteromas. In 75% of the cases, these mutations were clustered in exon 4 [74].

The retinoblastoma susceptibility gene (Rb), a tumor suppressor gene located at chromosome 13q, has been implicated in the pathogenesis of several tumors, including retinoblastoma and osteosarcoma [76]. Overexpression of Rb was identified in the adrenocortical carcinoma of a patient from a family with the Li-Fraumeni syndrome, suggesting that Rb might constitute a secondary event in the adrenal tumorigenesis of this syndrome or might play a role in compensating for the inadequacy of p53, a primary defect in this condition [77].

Recently, intrinsic components of the cell cycle were shown to act as tumor suppressor genes [78]. The p16 gene located on chromosome 9p21 encodes a protein that binds to and inhibits cyclin-dependent kinase 4 (Cdk4), one of several Cdks, whose activity propels cells through the cell cycle and into cell division [78–80]. Deletions or mutations in the p16 gene may affect the relative balance of functional p16, resulting in abnormal cell growth. Consistent with this view, deletions and mutations of this gene in over 70% of cell lines derived from tumors of the lung, breast, brain, bone, skin, bladder, kidney, ovary, and lymphoid tissue were recently found, suggesting that p16 has a pivotal role in inhibiting the development of several human cancers [79]. The high incidence of p16 gene abnormalities in a large variety of tumor cell lines suggests that mutations or deletions of this gene might also be present in adrenocortical carcinomas.

Genes involved in cell senescence/immortality, apoptosis, and genomic instability

Humans share similar telomeric sequences with other vertebrates [81]. Telomere loss or senescence is a major hurdle in the progression of human tumors, and this obstacle is circumvented by activation of the enzyme telomerase, which synthesizes and replaces telomeric DNA in cancer cells [82]. Counter et al. reported that extremely short telomeres are maintained in metastatic cells of epithelial ovarian carcinoma and that tumor cells, but not isogenic nonmalignant cells, express the telomerase enzyme [82]. These findings suggest that telomerase activation is an obligatory step in the immortalization of human cancer cells. The telomerase activity of adrenocortical neoplasms has not been examined as yet.

Apoptosis is genetically encoded and is characterized by specific morphologic and biochemical changes [83–85]. Morphologically, there is rapid condensation and budding of the cell, with the formation of membrane-enclosed 'apoptotic' bodies containing well-preserved organelles, which are phagocytosed and digested by nearby resident macrophages. A characteristic biochemical feature of the process is the double-strand cleavage of nuclear DNA at the linker regions between nucleosomes, leading to the production of oligonucleosomal fragments.

Diverse factors modulate apoptosis, including growth factors, intracellular mediators of signal transduction, and nuclear proteins regulating gene expression [83–85]. Consistent with this view, c-*myc* and c-*fos* expression was shown to be involved in the initiation of apoptosis, the wild-type p53 tumor suppressor gene was found to cause extensive apoptosis, while, in contrast, *bcl-2* inhibited apoptosis [85]. bcl-2, originally identified as an oncogene at the chromosomal breakpoint in follicular B-cell lymphoma, demonstrated a profound capacity to block apoptosis, probably by acting downstream of initiators such as p53 [85].

Apoptosis occurs spontaneously in virtually all untreated malignant tumors and is enhanced in tumors treated by diverse modalities, such as irradiation, cytotoxic chemotherapy, heating, and hormone ablation [83]. Clones in which the mechanisms of apoptosis are disrupted survive, however, and expand, allowing local growth and metastases of the tumor [51]. The study of apoptosis as a complex phenomenon subject to stimulation and inhibition may lead to further knowledge on the mechanisms of oncogenesis, and may provide novel approaches for the prevention, diagnosis, staging, and treatment of neoplastic diseases, including adrenocortical tumors.

There are enzymes in the nucleus whose function is to repair abnormalities of DNA within a given time. Proper functioning of these enzymes and adequate time allow repair to occur and maintain the low rate of genomic instability. Defective DNA repair enzymes or rapid replication of cells is thus associated with increased genomic instability and rates of clonal expansion and tumorigenesis. MSH2 is a recently described DNA repair enzyme that was found to be defective in patients with familial nonpolyposis colon cancer [86]. No studies of DNA-repair enzyme defects in adrenocortical neoplasms have been reported as yet.

Potential mechanisms of transformation associated with adrenocortical tissue-specific factors

Peripheral-type benzodiazepine receptors (PBRs) were found to be related to the regulation of steroid biosynthesis and steroidogenic cell proliferation [87,88]. PBRs are abundant in steroidogenic cells and are implicated in the acute stimulation of steroidogenesis, possibly by promoting the entry, distribution, and/or availability of cholesterol in the mitochondria [87,88]. In addition, differences in PBRs levels in proliferating tumorigenic cells have been reported [88]. High levels of PBRs were found in glioma tumors, colonic adenocarcinoma, and ovarian carcinoma when compared with normal tissues. Initial studies using high concentrations of synthetic ligands of PBRs indicated that these compounds could inhibit DNA synthesis and block mitogenesis in different cell lines [88]. Whether these receptors or their natural ligand(s) play a role in the induction of adrenocortical tumorigenesis remains unknown.

Another interesting adrenocortical protein that needs to be mentioned is the recently described steroidogenic acute regulatory protein [89]. This protein enhances the mitochondrial conversion of cholesterol into pregnenolone, by the cholesterol side-chain cleavage enzyme, suggesting that it is crucial for normal adrenal and gonadal steroidogenesis. Defects of the steroidogenic acute regulatory protein were recently associated with the syndrome of congenital lipoid adrenal hyperplasia [89]. It is not known whether overexpression of this gene could participate in the tumorigenesis of steroid-secreting adrenocortical neoplasms.

A cell-specific orphan nuclear receptor, designated steroidogenic factor I (SF-1), was recently identified as a key regulator of the steroid hydroxylases in adrenocortical cells [90–92]. Consistent with this role, SF-1 in adult mice is expressed all primary steroidogenic tissues, including the adrenal cortex, testicular Leydig cells, and ovarian theca and granulosa cells and corpus luteum [91]. Targetted disruption of the Ftz-F1 gene, which encodes SF-1, produced mice homozygously deficient in both alternative isoforms of this gene. Ftz-F1 null mice had no adrenal glands and/or gonads, suggesting that this nuclear receptor was essential for embryonic gonadal differentiation [92]. Whether abnormalities in the Ftz-F1 gene and SF-1 protein play a role in human adrenocortical tumorigenesis remains unknown.

X-linked adrenal hypoplasia congenita is a developmental disorder of the human adrenal gland that results in profound adrenal insufficiency, which is lethal if untreated [93,94]. Recently, the DAX-1 gene, a new member of the nuclear hormone receptor superfamily, was isolated and was found to be deleted or mutated in several patients with X-linked adrenal hypoplasia [92,93]. The DAX-1 product acts as a dominant negative regulator of transcription mediated by the retinoic acid receptor [93]. Whether abnormalities in DAX-1 gene or its product can be associated with human adrenocortical tumorigenesis remains unknown.

The study of the mechanisms by which cancer cells evade chemotherapy has led to the identification of several distinct genes related to drug resistance. The human multidrug drug resistance (MDR1) gene confers a highly active efflux mechanism for chemotherapeutic drugs, which prevents accumulation of these drugs in the cytoplasm of multidrug-resistant cells [95]. MDR1 encodes a cell surface polypeptide of 170kD and 12 transmembrane regions, known as P-glycoprotein. P-glycoprotein was found in a small number of human specific sites, such as the liver, pancreas, kidney, colon, and jejunum. Most tissues examined revealed very little P-glycoprotein. Interestingly, high levels of P-glycoprotein were diffusely detected on the surface of cells in both the human adrenal cortex and medulla [95]. This suggests that the multidrug transporter P-glycoprotein might play a role as a pump for the secretion of physiological metabolites and certain anticancer drugs in the human adrenal gland and may set adrenocortical neoplasms apart from other cancers by explaining the profound resistance of these neoplasms to chemotherapeutic agents.

Association with chromosomal abnormalities and genetic syndromes

The possibility that there is an inherited predisposition to develop adrenocortical tumors has been previously entertained [67,97,98,100–103]. Adrenocortical carcinoma has been reported in siblings, and a high incidence of diverse malignancies has been noted in families and relatives of patients with adrenocortical carcinomas [67,97,101]. Also, high frequencies of congenital anomalies and secondary tumors have been demonstrated in patients with adrenal cancer [97,98,100,103]. There are several recognized genetic syndromes that have been associated with adrenocortical neoplasms, which are discussed later (see Table 1).

Patients with the Li-Fraumeni syndrome have a high incidence of adrenocortical carcinomas [67]. Germline mutations in p53, located on 17p, were identified in families with this syndrome [67,68]. In addition, Yano et al. described abnormalities of chromosome 17 in adrenocortical carcinomas, which was compatible with loss of heterozygosity and defective tumor suppressor activity of p53, as was later demonstrated in 27% of malignant adrenocortical tumors and two adrenocortical tumor cell lines examined [75,103]. The loss of heterozygosity at 17p was consistently demonstrated in adrenal carcinomas, but not in adrenal adenomas, supporting a malignant transformation-inhibitory role for p53 in adrenocortical tissue [75,104].

The Wiedemann-Beckwith syndrome, a growth disorder associated with allelic loss of 11q15 and characterized by neonatal macrosomia, macroglossia, and omphalocele, has an increased incidence of Wilm's tumors and adrenocortical carcinomas [99,100]. Koufos et al. suggested that a recessive oncogene located on chromosome 11p confers a predisposition to adrenal cortical tumors, hepatoblastoma, and rhabdomyosarcoma [101]. In agreement with this, structural abnormalities at the 11p15 locus were described in 28.5% of sporadic adrenocortical tumors [103]. Particularly, uniparental disomy at the 11p15.5 locus, which includes the H-ras-1, IGF-II, and insulin genes, was observed in human adrenocortical carcinomas [102]. Gicquel et al. also detected very high IGF-II mRNA contents in 83% (5 of the 6 carcinomas) of the adrenocortical carcinomas examined [102]. Four of these five carcinomas showed abnormalities at locus 11p15.5, suggesting that there is a strong relation between IGF-II overexpression and rearrangements at the 11p15 locus in adrenocortical tumors. These findings suggest that structural abnormalities and/or overexpression of the IGF-II gene may play a key role in the multistep process of adrenocortical tumorigenesis.

The Carney complex, an autosomal dominant disorder, is characterized by the association of primary pigmented nodular adrenocortical disease (PPNAD); myxomas, particularly of the heart; and psammomatous melanotic schwannomas involving the peripheral nervous system, spotty pigmentation, and blue nevi of the skin or mucosa and diverse endocrine neoplasms [16,105,106]. Testicular Sertoli cell tumors, growth hormone–producing adenomas, thyroid follicular carcinomas, ovarian cysts, and adrenocortical tumors were associated with this familiar syndrome, whose chromosomal locus was recently mapped on 2p16 but whose pathophysiologic mechanism(s) remains unknown [16,107]. Cytogenetic and microsatellite studies of Carney tumors revealed the presence of genomic instability. But no deletions in the 2p16 area, suggesting that these tumors are caused by activation of a c-oncogene rather than inactivation of a tumor suppressor gene [108].

The familial and genetic nature of multiple endocrine neoplasia type I (MEN-I) syndrome was first pointed out by Wermer in 1954, who suggested that an autosomal dominant gene with high penetrance controls the trait [109]. Recently, the gene for MEN-I was mapped to chromosome 11q13, and several alterations in this region have been described in affected individuals [110–112]. The most frequent endocrinopathies in MEN-I are hyperparathyroidism, pancreatic-duodenal tumors, and pituitary tumors [112]. However, other tumors are also seen more frequently than in the general population, including adrenocortical and thyroid tumors, carcinoids, lipomas, and pinealomas [112]. In MEN-I, benign enlargement of adrenal cortex has been found in about one third of necropsy cases [112]. Diffuse and nodular cortical hyperplasia, adenomas, and a single case of adrenocortical carcinoma were described in patients with MEN-I [110,111]. Loss of constitutional heterozygozity for alleles at 17p, 13q, 11p, and 11q was found in the MEN-I adrenocortical carcinoma, while the benign adrenal lesions retained heterozygosity for the MEN-I locus at 11q13 [111].

Conclusions and future directions

A breakdown in the balanced relation of cells between production (growth and replication) and withdrawal by senescence, apoptosis, or differentiation leads to tumorigenesis (see Fig. 1). The involvement of many control points underscores the complexity of the growth mechanisms that maintain the integrity of the normal cell. Although the sequence of events leading to adrenal tumorigenesis is presently unclear, the process is clearly multistep and is variable from case to case. A multiplicity and variety of genetic abnormalities may account for the phenotypic heterogeneity of adrenocortical tumors.

The studies targeting cellular oncogenes and tumor suppressor genes, as well as genes involved in normal senescence, apoptosis, and differentiation, might provide not only knowledge of the mechanisms of tumorigenesis but also a new generation of cancer markers, which could help identify subjects at high risk for developing specific malignancies, including adrenocortical carcinomas. Also, tests for the early diagnosis and prognosis of cancers might help with the development of better management prevention strategies for these patients.

The advances in our understanding of molecular mechanisms of oncogenesis may also provide a better choice and administration schedule of therapeutic agents. New compounds are likely to be developed that take advantage of the differences between the control of the cell cycle in normal and cancer cells to maximize therapeutic effectiveness. Telomerase inhibitors, apoptosis inducers, genomic instability suppressants, and inducers of adreno-cortical differentiation are among potential future classes of agents that could be administered or directed using gene-therapy methods in adrenocortical cells to produce the long elusive cure for adrenocortical cancer. The use of monoclonal antibodies against adrenocortical antigens or promoters expressed specifically in adrenocortical cells coupled to powerful toxins are probably worthwhile alternatives to pursue.

References

1. Medvei VC. 1982. A History of Endocrinology. Hingham, MA: MTP Press.
2. Ross NS, Aron DC. 1990. Hormonal evaluation of the patient with an incidentally discovered adrenal mass. N Engl J Med 323:1401–1405.
3. Abecassis M, McLoughlin MJ, Langer B, Kudlow JE. 1985. Serendipitous adrenal masses: Prevalence, significance, and management. Am J Surg 149:783–788.
4. Bertagna C, Orth David. 1981. Clinical and laboratory findings and results of therapy in 58 patients with adrenocortical tumors admitted to a single medical center (1951 to 1978). Am J Med 71:855–875.
5. Sullivan M, Boileau M, Hodges CV. 1978. Adrenal cortical carcinoma. J Urol 120:660–665.
6. Nader S, Hickey RC, Sellin RV, Samaan NA. 1983. Adrenal cortical carcinoma. A study of 77 cases. Cancer 52:707–711.
7. Flack MR, Chrousos GP. 1996. Neoplasms of adrenal cortex. In JF Holland, RC Bast Jr, DL Morton, E Frei III, DW Kufe, RR Weichselbaum, Eds. Cancer Medicine, 4th edi., Williams and Wilkins, Baltimore Vol 1, pp 1563–1570.
8. Stewart DR, Jones PHM, Jolleys A. 1974. Carcinoma of the adrenal gland in children. J Pediatr Surg 9:59–67.
9. Henley DJ, van Heerden JA, Grant CS, Carney A, Carpenter PC. 1983. Adrenal cortical carcinoma — A continuing challenge. Surgery 94:926–931.
10. Chudler RM, Kay R. 1989. Adrenocortical carcinoma in children. Urol Clin North Am 163:469–479.
11. Mendonca BB, Lucon AM, Menezes CAV, Saldanha LB, Latronico AC, Zerbini C, Madureira G, Domenice S, Albergaria MA, Camargo MH, Halpern A, Liberman B, Arnhold IJP, Bloise W, Andriolo A, Nicolau W, Silva FAQ, Wroclaski E, Arap S, Wajchenberg BL. 1995. Clinical, hormonal and pathological findings in a comparative study of adrenal cortical neoplasms in childhood and adulthood. J Urol, 154:2004–2009.

12. Luton JP, Cerdas S, Billaud L, Thomas G, Guilhaume B, Bertagna X, Laudat MH, Louvel A, Chapius Y, Blondeau P, Bonnin A, Bricaire H. 1990. Clinical features of adrenocortical carcinoma, prognostic factors and the effect of mitotane therapy. N Engl J Med 322:1195–1201.

13. Barzilay JI, Pazianos AG. 1989. Adrenocortical carcinoma. Urol Clin North Am 16:457–468.

14. Pang S, Becker D, Cotelingham J, et al. 1981. Adrenocortical tumor in a patient with congenital adrenal hyperplasia due to 21-hydroxylase-deficiency. Pediatrics 68:242–246.

15. Bauman A, Bauman CG. 1982. Virilizing adrenocortical carcinoma: Development in a patient with salt-losing congenital adrenal hyperplasia. JAMA 248:3140–3141.

16. Carney JA, Young WF. 1992. Primary pigmented nodular adrenocortical disease and its associated conditions. Endocrinologist 2:6–21.

17. Third National Cancer Survey: Incidence Data National Cancer Institute Monograph 41. March 1975. DHEW Publication No. (NIH) 75–787; US Department of Health. Education and Welfare: Public Health Service, Bethesda, MD: National Institute of Health, National Cancer Institute.

18. Young JL Jr, Miller RW. 1975. Incidence of malignant tumors in U.S. children. J Pediatr 86:254–258.

19. King DR, Lack EE. 1979. Adrenal cortical carcinoma. A clinical and pathologic study of 49 cases. Cancer 44:239–244.

20. Pommier RF, Brennan MF. 1992. An eleven-year experience with adrenocortical carcinoma. Surgery 112:963–971.

21. Crapo L. 1979. Cushing's syndrome a review of diagnostic test. Metabolism 28:955–977.

22. Shapiro B, Fig LM, Gross MD, Khafagi F. 1990. Contributions of nuclear endocrinology to the diagnosis of adrenal tumors. Recent Results Cancer Res 118:113–138.

23. Jones GS, Shan KJ, Mann JR. 1985. Adreno-cortical carcinoma in infancy and childhood: A radiological report of ten cases. Clin Radiol 36:257–262.

24. Daneman A, Chan HSL, Martin J. 1983. Adrenal carcinoma and adenoma in children: A review of 17 patients. Pediatr Radiol 13:11–18.

25. Eghraki M, McLoughlin MJ, Rose IE, St. Louis EL, Wilson SR, Yeung HP. 1980. The role of computed tomography in assessment of tumoral pathology of the adrenal glands. J Comput Assist Tomogr 4:71–77.

26. Glazer GM, Woolsey EJ, Borello J, et al. 1986. Adrenal tissue characterization using MRI imaging. Radiology 158:73–79.

27. Ribeiro RC, Sandrini Neto RS, Schell MJ, Lacerda L, Sampaio GA. 1990. Adrenocortical carcinoma in children: A study of 40 cases. J Clin Oncol 8:67–74.

28. Hogan TF, Gilchrist KW, Westring DW, Citrin DL. 1980. A clinical and pathological study of adrenocortical carcinoma: Therapeutics implications. Cancer 45:2880–2883.

29. Weiss LM. 1984. Comparative histologic study of 43 metastasizing and nonmetastasizing adrenocortical tumors. Am J Surg Pathol 8:163–169.

30. Saeger. 1990. Tumours of the adrenal gland. Recent Results Cancer Res 118:79–96.

31. Bowlby LS, DeBault L, Abraham SR. 1986. Flow cytometric analysis of adrenal cortical tumor DNA. Cancer 58:1499–1505.

32. Taylor S, Roederer M, Murphy R. 1987. Flow cytometric DNA analysis of adrenocortical tumors in children. Cancer 59:2059–2063.

33. Macfarlane DA. 1958. Cancer of the adrenal cortex: The natural history, prognosis and treatment in a study of fifty-five cases. Ann Coll Surg Eng 23:155–186.

34. Brennam MF. 1987. Adrenocortical carcinoma. Cancer 37:348–365.

35. Schwarz RJ, Schimidt N. 1991. Efficient management of adrenal tumors. Am J Surg 161:576–579.

36. Hutter AM, Kayhoe DE. 1966. Adrenal cortical carcinoma: Results of treatment with o′p′ DDD in 138 patients. Am J Med 41:581.

37. Schteingart DE. 1992. Treating adrenal cancer. Endocrinologist 2:149–157.

38. Flack MR, Pyle RG, Mullen NM, Lorenzo B, Wu YW, Knazek. Nisula BC, Reidenberg MM.

1993. Oral gossypol in the treatment of metastatic adrenal cancer. J Clin Endocrinol Metab 76:1019–1024.

39. Haq MM, Legha SS, Samaan NA, Bodey GP, Burgess MA. 1980. Cytotoxic chemotherapy in adrenal cortical carcinoma. Cancer Treat Rep 64:909–913.

40. Hesketh PJ, McCaffrey RP, Finkel HE, Larmon SS, Griffing GT, Melby JC. 1987. Cisplatin-based treatment of adrenocortical carcinoma. Cancer Treat Rep 71:222–224.

41. Johnson DH, Greco FA. 1986. Treatment of metastatic adrenal cortical carcinoma with cisplatin and etoposide (VP-16). Cancer 58:2198–2202.

42. Schlumberger M, Ostronoff M, Bellaiche M, Rougier P, Droz JP, Parmentier C. 1988. 5-Fluorouracil, doxorubicin, and cisplatin regimen in adrenal cortical carcinoma. Cancer 61:1492–1494.

43. van Slooten H, van Oosterom AT. 1983. CAP (cyclophosphamide, doxorubicin, and cisplatin) regimen in adrenal cortical. Cancer Treat Rep 67:377–379.

44. Boveri TH. 1914. Zur Frage der Enstsehung maligner Tumoren. Jena: Verlag von Gustav Fisher.

45. Duffy MJ. 1993. Cellular oncogenes and suppressor genes as prognostic markers in cancer. Clin Biochem 26:439–447.

46. Weinberg RA. 1992. The integration of molecular genetics into cancer management. Cancer 70:1653–1658.

47. Sugimura T, Terada M, Yokota J, Hirohashi S, Wakabayashi K. 1992. Multiple genetic alterations in human carcinogenesis. Environ Health Perspect 98:5–12.

48. Beuschlein F, Reincke M, Karl M, Travis WD, Jaursch-Hancke C, Abdelhamid S, Chronsos GP, Allolio B. 1994. Clonal composition of human adrenocortical neoplasms. Cancer Res 54:4927–4932.

49. Gicquel C, Leblond-Francillard M, Bertagna X, Louvel A, Chapuis Y, Luton JP, Girard F, LeBouc Y. 1994. Clonal analysis of human adrenocortical carcinomas and secreting adenomas. Clin Endocrinol (Oxf) 40:465–477.

50. Weiner T, Cance WG. 1994. Molecular mechanisms involved in tumorigenesis and their surgical implications. Am J Surg 167:428–434.

51. Hartwell LH, Kastan MB. 1994. Cell cycle control cancer. Science 266:1821–1828.

52. Webster K, Cavenee, White RL. 1995. The genetic basis of cancer. Sci Am March: 74–79.

53. Allen LF, Lefkowitz RJ, Caron MG, Cotecchia S. 1991. G-protein-coupled receptors as protooncogenes: Constitutively activating mutations of the α1B-adrenergic receptor enhances mitogenesis and tumorigenesis. Proc Natl Acad Sci USA 88:11354–11358.

54. Parma J, Duprez L, Van Sande J, Cochaux P, Gervy C, Mockel J, Dumont J, Vassart G. 1993. Somatic mutations in the thyrotropin receptor gene cause hyperfunctioning thyroid adenomas. Nature 365:649–651.

55. Mountjoy KG, Robbins LS, Marty TM, Cone RD. 1992. The cloning of a family of genes that encode the melanocortin receptors. Science 257:1248–1251.

56. Vamvakopoulos NC, Rojas K, Overhauser, Durkin S, Nierman WC, Chrousos GP. 1993. Mapping the human melanocortin 2 receptor (adrenocorticotropic hormone receptor; ACTHR) gene (MCR2) to the small arm of chromosome 18 (18p11.21-pter). Genomics 18:454–455.

57. Latronico AC, Reincke M, Mendonça BB, Arai K, Mora P, Allolio B, Wajchenberg BI, Chrousos GP, Tsigos C. 1995. No evidence for oncogenic mutations in the adrenocorticotropin receptor (ACTH-R) gene in human adrenocortical neoplasms. J Clin Endocrinol Metab 80:875–877.

58. Weinstein LS, Shenker A, Gejman PV, Merino MJ, Friedman E, Spiegel A. 1991. Activating mutations of the stimulatory G protein in the McCune-Albright syndrome. N Engl J Med 325:1688–1695.

59. Lyons J, Landid CA, Harsh G, Vallar L, Grunewald K, Feichtinger H, Duh QY, Clark OH, Kawasaki E, Bourne HR. 1990. Two G protein oncogenes in human endocrine tumors. Science 249:655–659.

60. Reincke M, Karl M, Travis W, Chrousos GP. 1993. No evidence for oncogenic mutations in guanine nucleotide-binding proteins of human adrenocortical neoplasms. J Clin Endocrinol Metabol 77:1419–1422.
61. Nishizuka Y. 1984. The role of protein kinase C in cell surface signal transduction and tumour promotion. Nature 308:693–698.
62. Castagna M, Takai Y, Kaibuichi K, Sano K, Kikkawa U, Nishizuka Y. 1982. Direct activation of calcium-activated, phospholipid-dependent protein kinase by tumor-promoting phorbol esters. J Biol Chem 257:7847–7851.
63. O'Brian CA, Vogel VG, Singletary SE, Ward NE. 1989. Elevated protein kinase C expression in human breast tumor biopsies relative to normal breast tissue. Cancer Re 49:3215–3217.
64. Alvaro V, Touraine P, Raisman Vozari R, Bai-Grenier F, Birman P, Joubert (Bression) D. 1992. Protein kinase C activity and expression in normal and adenomatous human pituitaries. Int J Cancer 50:724–730.
65. Coudwell WT, Antel JP, Yong VW. 1992. Protein kinase C activity correlates with the growth rate of malignant gliomas: Part II. Effects of glioma mitogens and modulators of protein Kinase C. Neurosurgery 31:717–724.
66. Latronico AC, Mendonça BB, Bianco AC, Villares SM, Lucon MA, Nicolau W, Wajchenberg BL. 1994. Calcium-dependent protein kinase-C activity in human adrenocortical neoplasms, hyperplastic adrenals, and normal adrenocortical tissue. J Clin Endocrinol Metab 79:736–739.
67. Li FP, Fraumeni JF. 1982. Prospective study of a family cancer syndrome. JAMA 247:2692–2694.
68. Malkin D, Li FP, Strong LC, Fraumeni JF, Nelson CE, Kim DH, Kassel J, Gryka MA, Bischoff FZ, Tainsky MA, Friend SH. 1990. Germ line p53 mutations in a familial syndrome of breast cancer, sarcomas, and other neoplasms. Science 250:1233–1238.
69. Warneford SG, Wilton LJ, Townsend ML, Rowe PB, Reddel RR, Dalla-Pozza L, Symonds G. 1992. Germ-line splicing mutation of the p53 gene in a cancer-prone family. Cell Growth Differ 3:839–846.
70. Levine AJ, Momand J, Finlay CA. 1991. The p53 tumour suppressor gene. Nature 351:453–456.
71. Hollstein M, Sidransky D, Vogestein B, Harris CC. 1991. P53 mutations in human cancer. Science 253:49–53.
72. Roemer K, Friedmann T. 1994. Mechanisms of action of the p53 tumor suppressor and prospects for cancer gene therapy by reconstitution of p53 function. Ann NY Acad Sci 716:265–282.
73. Fromentel CC, Soussi T. 1992. tp53 tumor suppressor gene: A model for investigating human mutagenesis. Genes Chromosom Cancer 4:1–15.
74. Lin SR, Lee YJ, Tsai JH. 1994. Mutations of the p53 gene in human functional adrenal neoplasms. J Clin Endocrinol Metab 78:483–491.
75. Reincke M, Karl M, Travis WH, Mastorakos G, Allolio B, Linehan HM, Chrousos GP. 1994. p53 mutations in human adrenocortical neoplasms: Immunohistochemical and molecular studies. J Clin Endocrinol Metab 78:790–794.
76. Horowitz JM, Park S-H, Bogenmann E, Cheng J-C, Yandell DW, Kaye FJ, Minna JD, Dryja TP, Weinberg RA. 1990. Frequent inactivation of the retinoblastoma anti-oncogene is restricted to a subset of human tumor cells. Proc Natl Acad Sci USA 87:2775–2779.
77. Warneford S, Townsend M, Rowe PB, Dalla-Pozza L, Symonds G. 1991. Overexpression of the retinoblstoma gene in a familial adrenocortical carcinoma. Cell Growth Differ 2:439–445.
78. Marx J. 1994. New tumor suppressor may rival p53. Science 264:344–345.
79. Kamb A, Gruis NA, Weaver-Feldhaus J, Liu Q, Harshman K, Tavtigian SV, Stockert E, Day RS 3rd, Johnson BE, Skolnick MH. 1994. A cell cycle regulator potentially involved in genesis of many tumor types. Science 264:436–440.
80. Marx J. 1994. A challenge to p16 gene as a major tumor suppressor. Science 264:1846.

81. Lange T. 1994. Activation of telomerase in a human tumor. Proc Natl Acad Sci USA 91:2882–2885.
82. Counter CM, Hirte HW, Bacchetti S, Harley CB. 1994. Telomerase activity in human ovarian carcinoma. Proc Natl Acad Sci USA 91:2900–2904.
83. Kerr JFR, Winterford CM, Harmon BV. 1994. Apoptosis. Its significance in cancer and cancer therapy. Cancer 73:2013–2026.
84. Ruoslahti E, Reed J. 1994. Anchorage dependence, integrins, and apoptosis. Cell 77:477–478.
85. Fisher DE. 1994. Apoptosis in cancer therapy: Crossing the threshold. Cell 78:539–542.
86. Fishel R, Lescoe MK, Rao MR, Copeland NG, Jenkins NA, Garber J, Kane M, Kolocher R. 1993. The human mutator gene homolog MSH2 and its association with hereditary nonpolyposis colon cancer. Cell 75:1027–1038.
87. Papadopoulos V, Berkovich A, Krueger KE. 1991. The role of diazepam binding inhibitor and its processing products at mitochondrial benzodiazepine receptors: Regulation of steroid biosynthesis. Neuropharmacology 30:1417–1423.
88. Papadopoulos V. 1993. Peripheral-type benzodiazepine/diazepan binding inhibitor receptor: Biological role in steroidogenic cell function. Endocr Rev 14:222–240.
89. Lin D, Sugawara T, Strauss JF 3rd, Clark BJ, Stocco DM, Saenger P, Rogol A, Miller WL. 1995. Role of steroidogenic acute regulatory protein in adrenal and gonadal steroidogenesis. Science 267:1780–1781.
90. Parker KL, Schimmer BP. 1993. Transcriptional regulation of adrenal steroidogenic enzymes. Trends Endocrinol Metab 4:46–50.
91. Ikeda Y, Shen W-H, Ingraham HA, Parker K. 1994. Developmental expression of mouse steroidogenic factor-1, an essential regulator of steroid hydroxylase. Mol Endocrinol 8:654–662.
92. Luo X, Ikeda Y, Parker K. 1994. A cell-specific nuclear receptor is essential for adrenal and gonadal development and sexual differentiation. Cell 77:481–490.
93. Muscatelli F, Strom TM, Walker AP, Zanaria E, Recan D, Meindl A, Bardoni B, Guioli S, Zehetner G, Rabl W, Schwarz HP, Kaplan J-C, Camerino G, Meitinger T, Monaco AP. 1994. Mutations in the DAX-1 gene give rise to both X-linked hypoplasia congenita and hypogonadotropic hypogonadism. Nature 372:672–676.
94. Zanaria E, Muscatelli F, Bardoni B, Strom TM, Guioli S, Guo W, Lalli E, Moser C, Walker AP, McCabe ERB, Meitinger T, Monaco AP, Sassone-Corsi P, Camerino G. 1994. An unusual member of the nuclear hormone receptor superfamily responsible for X-linked adrenal hypoplasia congenita. Nature 372:635–641.
95. Thiebaut F, Tsuruo T, Hamada, Gotlesman MM, Pastan I, Willingham MC. 1987. Cellular localization of the multidrug-resistance gene product P-glycoprtotein in normal human tissues. Proc Natl Acad Sci USA 84:7735–7738.
96. Miller RW. 1978. Peculiarities in the occurrence of adrenal cortical carcinoma. Am J Dis Child 132:235.
97. Levine GW. 1978. Adrenocortical carcinoma in two children with subsequent primary tumors. Am J Dis Child 132:238–240.
98. Didolkar MS, Bescher A, Elias G, Moore RH. 1981. Natural history of adrenal cortical carcinoma: A clinicopathologic study of 42 patients. Cancer 47:2153–2161.
99. Junien C. 1992. Beckwith-Wiedmann syndrome, tumourigenesis and imprinting. Curr Opin Genet Dev 2:431–438.
100. Ping AP, Reeve AE, Law DJ, Young MR, Boehnke M, Feinberg AP. 1989. Genetic linkage of Beckwith-Wiedmann syndrome to 11p15. Am J Hum Genet 44:720–723.
101. Koufos A, Hansen MF, Copeland NG, Jenkins NA, Lampkin BC, Cavenee WK. 1987. Loss of heterozygosity in three embryonal tumours suggests a common pathogenic mechanism. Nature 316:330–334.
102. Gicquel C, Xavier B, Schneid H, Francillard-LeBlond M, Luton JP, Girard F, LeBouc Y. 1994. Rearrangement at the 11p15 locus and overexpression of insulin-like growth factor-II gene in sporadic adrenocortical tumors. J Clin Endocrinol Metab 78:1444–1453.

103. Yano T, Linehan M, Anglard P, Lerman MI, Daniel LN, Stein CA, Robertson CN, LaRocca R, Zbar B. 1989. Genetic changes in human adrenocortical carcinoma. J Natl Cancer Inst 81:518–523.

104. Rosenberg C, Della-Rosa VA, Latronico AC, Mendonca BB, Vianna-Morgante AM. 1995. Selection of adrenal tumor cells in culture demonstrated by interphase cytogenetics. Cancer Genet Cytogenet 79:36–40.

105. Carney JA, Gordon H, Carpenter PC, Shenoy BV, Go VLW. 1985. The complex of myxomas, spotty pigmentation, and endocrine overactivity. Medicine (Baltimore) 64:270–283.

106. Young WF Jr, Carney JA, Musa BU, Wulffraat NM, Lens JW, Drexhage HA. 1989. Familial Cushing's syndrome due to primary pigmented nodular adrenocortical disease. Reinvestigation 50 years later. N Engl J Med 321:1659–1664.

107. Stratakis CA, Carney A, Ping J, Papanicolaou DA, Karl M, Kastner DL, Pras E, Chrousos GP. 1996. Carney Complex, a Familial Multiple Neoplasia and Lentiginosis Syndrome: Analysis of 11 Kindreds and Linkage to the Short Arm of Chromosome 2. J. Clin Invest 97:699–705.

108. Stratakis CA, Jenkins RB, Pras E, Mitsiadis CS, Raff SB, Stalboerger PG, Tsigos C, Carney A, Chrousos GP. 1996. Cytogenetic and Mircosatellite Alterations in Tumors from Patients with the Syndrome of Myxomas, Spotty Skin Pigmentation, and Endocrine Overactivity (Carney Complex). J Clin Endocrinol Metab 81:3607–3614.

109. Wermer P. 1954. Genetics aspects of adenomatosis of endocrine glands. Am J Med 16:363–371.

110. Larsson C, Friedman E. 1994. Localization and identification of the multiple endocrine neoplasia type 1 disease gene. Endocrinol Metabol Clin North Am 23:67–79.

111. Thakker RV. 1994. The role of molecular genetics in screening for multiple endocrine neoplasia type I. Endocrinol Metab Clin North Am 23:117–135.

112. Skogseid B, Larsson C, Lindgren PG, Kvanta E, Rastad J, Theodorsson E, Wide L, Wilander E, Oberg K. 1992. Clinical and genetic features of adrenocortical lesions in multiple endocrine neoplasia type 1. J Clin Endocrinol Metab 75:76–81.

12. Pheochromocytoma and primary aldosteronism

William F. Young, Jr.

The hormonal hypersecretion associated with adrenal neoplasms can result in unique clinical presentations. The diagnostic and therapeutic approaches to two such adrenal tumors are reviewed in this chapter. Pheochromocytoma is associated with spectacular cardiovascular disturbances and, when correctly diagnosed and properly treated, it is curable; when undiagnosed or improperly treated, it can be fatal. Although primary aldosteronism is not associated with a dramatic clinical presentation or lethal consequences if undiscovered, this form of secondary hypertension and the associated hypokalemia are also amenable to a surgical cure.

Pheochromocytoma

Catecholamine-producing tumors that arise from chromaffin cells of the adrenal medulla and sympathetic ganglia are termed *pheochromocytomas* and *paragangliomas*, respectively. However, the term *pheochromocytoma* has become the generic name for all catecholamine-producing tumors and will be used in this chapter to refer to both adrenal pheochromocytomas and paragangliomas. Since the first successful operations in 1926 [1,2], considerable progress has been made in the diagnosis and treatment of pheochromocytoma.

Prevalence estimates for pheochromocytoma vary from 0.01% to 0.1% of the hypertensive population. Although pheochromocytoma is rare, it is important to suspect, confirm, localize, and resect these tumors (1) because the associated hypertension is curable with surgical removal of the tumor, (2) because of the risk of lethal paroxysm, and (3) because 10% of the tumors are malignant. These tumors occur equally in men and women, primarily in the third through fifth decades. Patients harboring a pheochromocytoma may be asymptomatic. However, symptoms usually are present and are due to the pharmacologic effects of excessive levels of catecholamines in the plasma. Signs and symptoms associated with pheochromocytoma are outlined in Table 1. The hypertension may be sustained or paroxysmal. Paroxysmal hypertension is associated primarily with epinephrine-secreting tumors [3]. Episodic

Andrew Arnold (ed.) ENDOCRINE NEOPLASMS. 1997. Kluwer Academic Publishers. ISBN 0-7923-4354-9.
All rights reserved.

Table 1. Signs and symptoms associated with pheochromocytoma

Spell-related
  Headache
  Palpitation
  Diaphoresis
  Epigastric and chest pain
  Pallor
  Nausea
  Dyspnea
  Anxiety
  Hypertension
  Tremor
  Weakness and exhaustion after the spell
Chronic
  Hypertension
  Orthostatic hypotension
  Grade II to IV retinopathy
  Tremor
  Fever
  Weight loss
  Congestive heart failure
  Hyperglycemia
  Constipation
  Painless hematuria (associated with urinary bladder pheochromocytoma)
  Ectopic hormone secretion-dependent symptoms (e.g., CRH/ACTH, GHRH, PTH-RP,
    VIP)
Not typical of pheochromocytoma
  Flushing

ACTH = corticotropin; CRH = corticotropin-releasing hormone; GHRH = growth hormone–releasing hormone; PTH-RP = parathyroid hormone–related peptide; VIP = vasoactive intestinal polypeptide.

symptoms may occur in spells, or paroxysms, which can be extremely variable in their presentation. They may be spontaneous or precipitated by postural change, anxiety, exercise, or maneuvers that increase intra-abdominal pressure. Although the interindividual variability in the types of spells is high, the spells tend to be stereotypical for each patient. A spell usually lasts from 10 to 60 minutes and may occur anywhere in frequency from daily to only several times per year. Pheochromocytoma is not the most common cause of hypertension-related spells [4]. The differential diagnosis of these spells is outlined in Table 2.

A 'rule of 10' has been quoted for pheochromocytomas: 10% are extra-adrenal, 10% occur in children, 10% are multiple or bilateral, 10% recur after surgical removal, 10% are malignant, and 10% are familial [5]. The familial autosomal neurocristopathic syndromes include familial pheochromocytoma, multiple endocrine neoplasia type IIA (with pheochromocytoma, medullary carcinoma of the thyroid, and hyperparathyroidism), and type IIB (with pheochromocytoma, medullary carcinoma of the thyroid, mucosal neuromas, thickened corneal nerves, intestinal ganglioneuromatosis, and marfanoid body habitus), neurofibromatosis, and von Hippel-Lindau syndrome (retinal hemangiomatosis, cerebellar hemangioblastoma, pheochromocytoma, and renal-cell carcinoma).

Diagnosis

Biochemical documentation of catecholamine hypersecretion should *precede* any form of imaging. Most laboratories now measure catecholamines by high-

Table 2. Spells: Differential diagnosis of pheochromocytoma-type spells

Endocrine
  Pheochromocytoma
  Thyrotoxicosis
  Primary hypogonadism (menopausal syndrome)
  Medullary thyroid carcinoma
  Pancreatic tumors (e.g., insulinoma)
  Hypoglycemia
  Carbohydrate intolerance
  'Hyperadrenergic spells'
Cardiovascular
  Labile essential hypertension
  Cardiovascular deconditioning
  Pulmonary edema
  Syncope
  Orthostatic hypotension
  Baroreflex dysfunction
  Paroxysmal cardiac arrhythmia
  Angina
  Renovascular disease
Psychologic
  Anxiety and panic attacks
  Somatization disorder
  Hyperventilation
Pharmacologic
  Withdrawal of adrenergic inhibitor
  Monoamine oxidase inhibitor treatment and tyramine (in foods) or sympathomimetic drugs
  Sympathomimetic ingestion
  Illegal drug ingestion (e.g., cocaine, PCP, LSD)
  Chlorpropamide-alcohol flush
  Vancomycin ('red man syndrome')
Neurologic
  Postural orthostatic tachycardia syndrome (POTS)
  Autonomic neuropathy
  Migraine headache
  Diencephalic epilepsy (autonomic seizures)
  Stroke
  Cerebrovascular insufficiency
Other
  Mastocytosis — systemic or activation disorder
  Environmental allergies
  Carcinoid syndrome
  Recurrent idiopathic anaphylaxis
  Unexplained flushing spells
  Polycythemia vera
  POEMS syndrome (polyneuropathy, organomegaly, endocrinopathy, M-protein spike, and
    skin changes)

pressure liquid chromatography with electrochemical detection. This has overcome the problems associated with fluorometric analysis (e.g., false-positive results caused by α-methyldopa and other drugs with high native fluorescence). To interpret the measurements of catecholamines and catecholamine metabolites, it is critical to know the methodology a laboratory uses and the accuracy of the measurements for these compounds. In our laboratory, the most reliable screening method is measurement of metanephrines in a 24-hour urine [6]. The measurement of plasma metanephrines, although not widely available, is also an accurate test to diagnose pheochromocytoma [7]. If clinical suspicion is high, then epinephrine, norepinephrine, dopamine, and vanillylmandelic acid measurements are

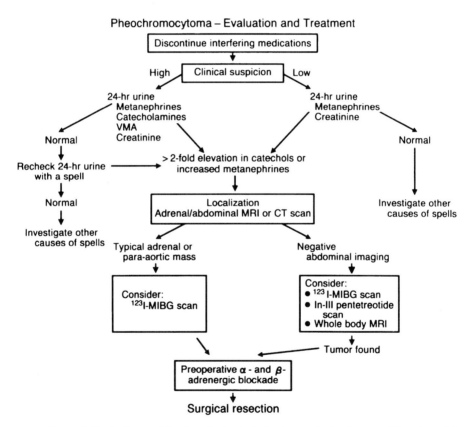

Figure 1. Evaluation and treatment of catecholamine-producing tumors. Clinical suspicion is triggered by the following: paroxysmal symptoms (especially hypertension); hypertension that is intermittent, unusually labile, or resistant to treatment; family history of pheochromocytoma or associated conditions; or incidentally discovered adrenal mass. The details are discussed in the text. CT = computed tomography; MRI = magnetic resonance imaging; ^{123}I-MIBG = ^{123}I-meta-iodobenzylguanidine; VMA = vanillylmandelic acid. (Modified from Young [17]. Reproduced with permission.)

added to the 24-hour urine studies (Fig. 1). For a patient with episodic hypertension, the 24-hour urine collection should start with the onset of a spell. When collected in this manner, patients with pheochromocytoma have more than a twofold increase above the upper limit of normal in one of the three catecholamines measured in the 24-hour urine or increased levels of urinary metanephrines (see Fig. 1).

Although it is best to evaluate patients who are not receiving any medication, most medications may be continued, with some of the exceptions listed in Table 3. Labetalol is the most frequently used antihypertensive agent that interferes with most metanephrine and catecholamine assays. Labetalol must be discontinued for 4–7 days before initiating the diagnostic evaluation for pheochromocytoma. Although plasma catecholamine measurements are convenient, they add little information to that obtained from the 24-hour urinary measurements. Because of the advances in catecholamine measurements, suppression [8] and provocative [9] tests are rarely needed.

Localization studies should not be initiated until biochemical studies have confirmed the diagnosis of pheochromocytoma (see Fig. 1). However, in the 1990s endocrinologists are frequently asked to evaluate patients for pheochromocytoma *after* computerized abdominal imaging (performed for other reasons) discloses an adrenal mass [10]. Computer-assisted adrenal and abdominal imaging [magnetic resonance imaging (MRI) or computed tomography (CT)] is the first localization test (sensitivity >95%, specificity >65%) [11] (Fig. 2). Approximately 90% of these tumors are found in the adrenal glands and 98% in the abdomen [12]. However, tumors may arise at any site where chromaffin tissue is located, from the base of the skull to the scrotum. The most common locations of extra-adrenal pheochromocytoma include superior abdominal para-aortic region, 46%; inferior abdominal para-

Table 3. Medications that may alter measured levels of catecholamines and metabolites

Increase values
    Tricyclic antidepressants
    Labetalol
    Levodopa
    Drugs containing catecholamines
    Amphetamines
    Sotolal hydrochloride
    Methyldopa
    Withdrawal from clonidine hydrochloride and other drugs
    Ethanol
    Benzodiazepines
Decrease values
    Metyrosine
    Methylglucamine[a]

[a] A component of iodinated contrast media that may cause metanephrine values to be falsely normal for as long as 72 hours when measured with Pisano's spectrophotometric method.

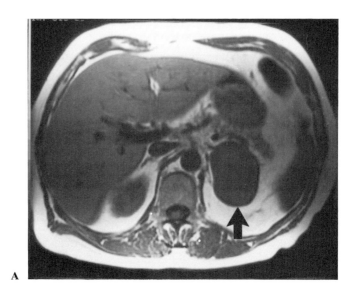

A

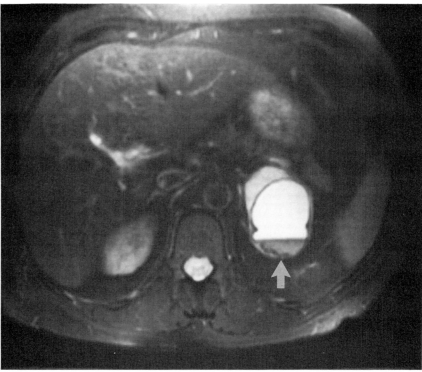

B

Figure 2. Magnetic resonance imaging (MRI) scans from a 61-year-old woman with hypertension and spells. **A:** MRI scan with T_1-weighted partial saturation sequences demonstrates a 6.5 × 4.5 cm cystic left adrenal mass (arrow). **B:** MRI scan with T_2-weighted partial saturation sequences demonstrates the high signal intensity of the solid tissue typical of pheochromocytoma (arrow).

244

aortic region, 29%; urinary bladder, 10%; thorax, 10%; head and neck, 3%; and pelvis, 2% [13]. Tumor size does not correlate with the degree of increase in catecholamine levels [3].

Scintigraphic localization with radiolabeled-MIBG is indicated in the following circumstances: (1) if the results of abdominal imaging are negative, (2) if the patient has a known extra-adrenal pheochromocytoma and it is important to exclude additional paragangliomas, and (3) if metastatic disease is suspected (Fig. 3). This radiopharmaceutical agent accumulates preferentially in catecholamine-producing tumors (sensitivity 88%, specificity 99%) [14]. Computer-assisted chest, neck, and head imaging and central venous sampling are additional localizing procedures that can be used, although they are rarely required. Somatostatin-receptor imaging with In-111–labeled pentetreotide [15,16] may also assist in difficult cases.

Treatment

The treatment of choice for pheochromocytoma is surgical resection. Most pheochromocytomas are benign and can be totally excised. Preoperatively, the chronic and acute effects of excess circulating catecholamines must be corrected. Combined α- and β-adrenergic blockade are required preoperatively to control blood pressure and to prevent intraoperative hypertensive crises. α-Adrenergic blockade should be started at least 10 days preoperatively to

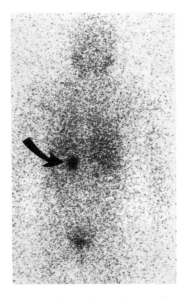

Figure 3. ^{131}I-meta-iodobenzylguanidine (MIBG) scan from a 60-year-old woman with a 4.2-cm left adrenal pheochromocytoma. Adrenal scintigraphic images at 24 hours after administration of ^{131}I-MIBG. Focal increased left suprarenal ^{131}I activity (arrow) was present and was consistent with left adrenal pheochromocytoma.

allow for expansion of the contracted blood volume. A liberal salt diet is advised during the preoperative period. After adequate α-adrenergic blockade is achieved, β-adrenergic blockade may be initiated (e.g., 3 days preoperatively) [17].

Phenoxybenzamine is an irreversible long-acting α-adrenergic blocking agent. The initial dosage is 10 mg given orally one to two times daily; the dosage is increased by 10–20 mg every 2 days as needed to normalize blood pressure and to eliminate spells. The effects of daily administration are cumulative for nearly a week. The average dosage is 20–100 mg daily. Side effects include postural hypotension, tachycardia, miosis, nasal congestion, inhibition of ejaculation, diarrhea, and fatigue. Prazosin, terazosin, and doxazosin are selective α_1-adrenergic blocking agents. The initial dose is 1 mg orally at bedtime to avoid the occasional syncope that follows the first dose. The dosage, up to 20 mg orally (in divided doses for prazosin), is then increased every 2 days as needed to control blood pressure. Phenoxybenzamine is the preferred drug for preoperative preparation because it provides α-adrenergic blockade of long duration. Effective α-adrenergic blockade permits expansion of blood volume, which usually is decreased as a result of excessive adrenergic vasoconstriction.

The β-adrenergic antagonist should be administered only after α-adrenergic blockade is effective because β-adrenergic blockade alone may produce more severe hypertension due to the unopposed α-adrenergic stimulation. Preoperative β-adrenergic blockade is indicated to control the tachycardia associated with both the high concentrations of circulating catecholamines and the α-adrenergic blockade. Caution is indicated if the patient is asthmatic or has congestive heart failure. Chronic catecholamine excess can produce myocardiopathy and may become evident with initiation of β-adrenergic blockade resulting in acute pulmonary edema. Noncardioselective β-adrenergic blockers, such as propranolol and nadolol, or cardioselective β-adrenergic blockers, such as atenolol and metoprolol, may be used. When administration of the β-adrenergic blocker is initiated, the drug should be used cautiously and at a low dose. For example, propranolol is usually initiated at 10 mg every 6 hours at least 1 week after the initiation of α-adrenergic blockade. The dose is then increased and converted to a long-acting β-adrenergic blocker as necessary to control tachycardia. Labetalol should be avoided until all diagnostic studies have been completed because it can interfere with the measurement of catecholamines and metabolites and with ^{123}I-MIBG uptake by pheochromocytomas.

α-Methyl-para-L-tyrosine (metyrosine) inhibits the synthesis of catecholamines by blocking the enzyme tyrosine hydroxylase. Side effects include sedation, diarrhea, anxiety, nightmares, crystalluria and urolithiasis, galactorrhea, and extrapyramidal manifestations. It is used most effectively in those patients who have persistent catecholamine-producing tumors that (for cardiopulmonary reasons) cannot be treated with combined α- and β-adrenergic blockade.

Resection of a pheochromocytoma is a high-risk surgical procedure and requires an experienced surgeon/anesthesiologist team. The last oral doses of α- and β-adrenergic blockers can be administered early in the morning on the day of operation. Continuous measurement of intra-arterial pressure and heart rhythm is required. Hypertensive episodes should be treated with intravenous infusion of phentolamine or nitroprusside. Lidocaine or esmolol are used for cardiac arrhythmia. Because intra-abdominal pheochromocytoma may be multiple and extra-adrenal, an anterior midline abdominal surgical approach is used in most cases. If the tumor is in the adrenal gland, the entire gland should be removed. If the tumor is malignant, as much tumor should be removed as possible. When performed by experienced surgeons, laparoscopic adrenalectomy for sporadic solitary adrenal pheochromocytomas is effective [18]. Paragangliomas of the neck, chest, and urinary bladder require specialized approaches.

Hypotension may occur after surgical resection of the pheochromocytoma and should be treated with fluids and colloids. Postoperative hypotension is less frequent in patients who have had adequate α-adrenergic blockade preoperatively. If both adrenal glands have been manipulated, adrenocortical insufficiency should be considered as a potential cause of postoperative hypotension. Hypoglycemia can occur in the immediate postoperative period; therefore, blood glucose levels should be monitored and the fluid that is given intravenously should contain 5% dextrose.

Blood pressure usually is normal by the time of dismissal from the hospital. Some patients remain hypertensive for up to 4–8 weeks postoperatively. Longstanding persistent hypertension does occur and may be related to accidental ligation of a polar renal artery, resetting of baroreceptors, established hemodynamic changes, structural changes of the blood vessels, altered sensitivity of the vessels to pressor substances, renal functional or structural changes, or coincident essential hypertension. Approximately 2 weeks postoperatively, a 24-hour urine sample should be obtained for measurement of catecholamines and metanephrines. If the levels are normal, the resection of the pheochromocytoma can be considered to have been complete. Increased levels of catecholamines postoperatively indicate the presence of residual tumor, a second primary lesion, or occult metastases. The 24-hour urinary excretion of catecholamines should be checked annually for at least 5 years as surveillance for recurrence in the adrenal bed, metastatic pheochromocytoma, or delayed appearance of multiple primary tumors [19]. A more prolonged follow-up may be indicated if tumor DNA ploidy is abnormal [20,21]. Recurrent tumor in patients with malignant pheochromocytoma may not become evident until an average of 8 years following the initial operation [22].

Malignant pheochromocytoma

The distinction between benign and malignant catecholamine-producing tumors cannot be made on the basis of clinical, biochemical, or histopathologic

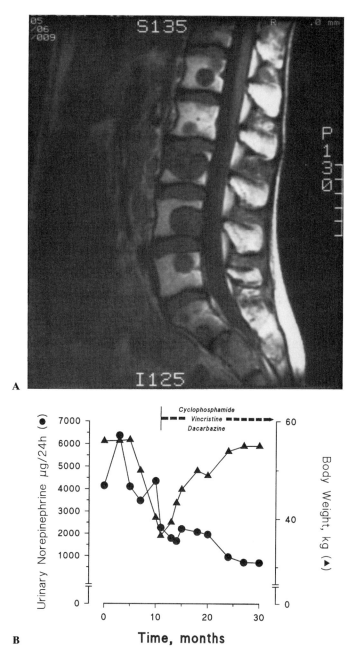

Figure 4. **A:** Magnetic resonance imaging scan of the spine from a 17-year-old woman showing metastatic pheochromocytoma throughout the axial skeleton. **B:** Urinary norepinephrine levels and body weight prior to and during chemotherapy with cyclophosphamide, vincristine, and dacarbazine.

characteristics. Malignancy is based on finding direct local invasion or disease metastatic to sites that do not normally have chromaffin tissue, such as lymph nodes, bone, lung, and liver. Although 5-year survival is less than 50%, the prognosis is variable [22]. Many patients may have an indolent form of the disease, with life expectancy of more than 20 years. Metastatic lesions should be resected if possible. Painful skeletal metastatic lesions can be treated with external radiation therapy. Soft tissue metastases may also respond to external radiation therapy. Local tumor irradiation with therapeutic doses of ^{131}I-MIBG has produced partial and short-term responses in approximately one third of patients [23–25]. If the tumor is clinically aggressive and the quality of life is affected, combination chemotherapy may be considered. A chemo-therapy program consisting of cyclophosphamide, vincristine, and dacarbazine given cyclically every 21–28 days has proven beneficial but not curative in these patients (Fig. 4) [26,27]. Embolization of inoperable tumors may be of benefit in a selected group of patients. However, hypertensive crises may occur following the embolization. Hypertension and spells can be controlled with combined α- and β-adrenergic blockade or inhibition of catecholamine synthesis with metyrosine.

Pheochromocytoma in pregnancy

Pheochromocytoma in pregnancy can cause the death of both the fetus and the mother. The treatment of hypertensive crises is the same as for nonpregnant patients. Although there is some controversy about the most appropriate management [28], pheochromocytomas should be removed immediately if diagnosed during the first two trimesters of pregnancy. Preoperative preparation is the same as for nonpregnant patients. If medical therapy is chosen or if the patient is in the third trimester, cesarean section and removal of the pheochromocytoma in the same operation are indicated. Spontaneous labor and delivery should be avoided.

Primary aldosteronism

Hypertension, hypokalemia, suppressed plasma renin activity (PRA), and increased aldosterone excretion characterize the syndrome of primary aldosteronism first described in 1955 [29,30]. Prevalence estimates for primary aldosteronism vary from 0.05% to 2% of the hypertensive population [31,32]. At least seven subtypes of primary aldosteronism have been identified (Table 4). Aldosterone-producing adenoma (APA) and idiopathic hyper-aldosteronism (IHA) are found in approximately 64% and 32% of the patients with primary aldosteronism, respectively (see Table 4) [33].

Primary adrenal hyperplasia (PAH) and renin-responsive APA are uncommon subtypes. A hyperplastic adrenal that resembles IHA morphologically but mimics the APA response to physiologic maneuvers and unilateral adrenalectomy characterizes PAH [34–36]. The renin-responsive APA

Table 4. Types of primary aldosteronism

Type	Prevalence (%)
Aldosterone-producing adenoma (APA)	64 ± 10 (±SD)
Corticotropin-responsive (common)	
Renin-responsive (rare)	
Idiopathic hyperaldosteronism (IHA)	32 ± 10 (±SD)
Primary adrenal hyperplasia	<2
Aldosterone-producing adrenocortical carcinoma	1
Aldosterone-producing ovarian tumor	<1
Familial hyperaldosteronism (FH)	
Glucocorticoid-remediable aldosteronism (FH type I)	<2
FH type II (APA or IHA)	<2

appears as an APA morphologically and in response to unilateral adrenalectomy, but it responds to physiologic maneuvers, as do the hyperplastic glands of IHA [35–38].

Two forms of familial hyperaldosteronism (FH) have been described. Two isozymes of 11-β-hydroxylase encoded by two genes on chromosome 8 are responsible for aldosterone and cortisol biosynthesis. The isozyme in the zona glomerulosa ($P450_{aldo}$) catalyzes the conversion of deoxycorticosterone to corticosterone to 18-hydroxycorticosterone to aldosterone. The isozyme in the zona fasciculata ($P450_{c11}$) catalyzes the conversion of 11-deoxycortisol to cortisol and does not catalyze aldosterone synthesis. Glucocorticoid-remediable aldosteronism (GRA, FH type I) is autosomal dominant in its inheritance and is associated with variable degrees of hyperaldosteronism, high levels of hybrid steroids (e.g., 18-hydroxycortisol), and suppression with exogenous glucocorticoids. The mutation in patients with GRA is fusion of the promoter region of the gene for $P450_{c11}$ and the coding sequences of $P450_{aldo}$, resulting in ACTH-dependent activation of the aldosterone synthase effect on cortisol, corticosterone, and cortisol precursors [39]. Therefore, these patients are biochemically unique in having markedly increased levels of 18-oxocortisol and 18-hydroxycortisol. The second form of FH, FH type II, was reported by Stowasser et al. [40] and refers to the familial occurrence of APA or IHA or both.

Distinguishing the subtype of primary aldosteronism is critical to appropriate therapy. Unilateral adrenalectomy cures the hypertension and hypokalemia in most patients who have APA and PAH, whereas pharmacologic therapy is more effective for patients with IHA and GRA.

Clinical features

The diagnosis of primary aldosteronism is usually made in patients in the third to sixth decades. Few symptoms are specific to the syndrome. Patients with marked hypokalemia may have muscle weakness, muscle cramping, headaches, palpitations, polydipsia, polyuria, or nocturia. There are no specific physical findings. The degree of hypertension is usually moderate to severe and may be resistant to usual pharmacologic intervention [41].

In addition to the hypokalemia, abnormalities detected on routine clinical laboratory testing should raise suspicion of the presence of primary aldosteronism. For example, mild metabolic alkalosis (serum bicarbonate, >31 mEq/l) and relative hypernatremia (serum sodium, >142 mEq/l) are frequent findings. The relative hypernatremia is most likely associated with decreased vasopressin release due to plasma volume expansion or to a hypokalemia-induced abnormality in vasopressin release and action [42,43]. Chronic potassium depletion can inhibit insulin secretion and action, resulting in increased fasting plasma glucose levels in about 25% of the patients. Electrocardiographic changes of mild left ventricular hypertrophy and hypokalemia, including prolonged ST segment, U waves, and T-wave inversion, may be found.

Diagnosis

The diagnostic approach to primary aldosteronism can be considered in three stages: screening testing, confirmatory testing, and subtype evaluation. Spontaneous or easily provoked hypokalemia in a hypertensive patient should prompt the clinician to screen for primary aldosteronism. Spontaneous hypokalemia is uncommon in patients with uncomplicated hypertension and, when present, strongly suggests associated mineralocorticoid excess. However, *normokalemia does not exclude primary aldosteronism*. Several studies have shown that 7–38% of patients with primary aldosteronism [32,44,45] and most patients with GRA [46] have baseline serum potassium levels in the normal range. Patients with hypertension and hypokalemia (regardless of presumed cause, e.g., diuretic treatment) and most patients with treatment-resistant hypertension should be screened for primary aldosteronism.

Screening of suspected patients can be accomplished by measuring serum potassium, 24-hour urinary potassium, and paired random PAC to PRA ratio (Fig. 5). Because approximately 30% of patients with essential hypertension and almost all patients with primary aldosteronism have subnormal upright PRA levels [47], a low PRA level is not specific for primary aldosteronism. A high ratio of PAC (in ng/dl) to PRA (in ng/ml/hr) is more specific for primary aldosteronism. Although Hiramatsu et al. [48] found the ratio to be <20 in patients with essential hypertension and >40 in patients with primary aldosteronism due to APA, others have found more overlap in the ratio between patients with essential hypertension and those with primary aldosteronism [49]. PAC to PRA ratios exceeding 25 or 33 [49,50] have been recommended to trigger further studies to confirm primary aldosteronism. Weinberger and Fineberg [51] found the combination of PAC/PRA ratio >30 and PAC >20 ng/dl to be 90% sensitive and 91% specific for primary aldosteronism. Patients with at least two of the following findings should be evaluated further for the possibility of primary aldosteronism: (1) spontaneous

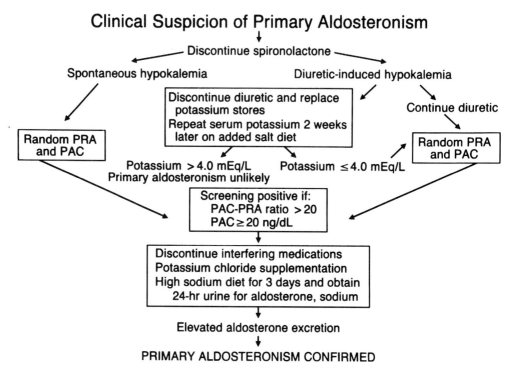

Clinical Suspicion of Primary Aldosteronism

Discontinue spironolactone

Spontaneous hypokalemia   Diuretic-induced hypokalemia

Discontinue diuretic and replace
potassium stores
Repeat serum potassium 2 weeks
later on added salt diet

Continue diuretic

Random PRA
and PAC

Random PRA
and PAC

Potassium > 4.0 mEq/L   Potassium ≤ 4.0 mEq/L
Primary aldosteronism unlikely

Screening positive if:
PAC-PRA ratio > 20
PAC ≥ 20 ng/dL

Discontinue interfering medications
Potassium chloride supplementation
High sodium diet for 3 days and obtain
24-hr urine for aldosterone, sodium

Elevated aldosterone excretion

PRIMARY ALDOSTERONISM CONFIRMED

Figure 5. Screening and confirmatory studies for primary aldosteronism. PRA = plasma renin activity; PAC = plasma aldosterone concentration. (Modified from Young et al. [53]. Reproduced with permission.)

or easily provoked hypokalemia, (2) random PRA <2.0 ng/ml/hr, and (3) random PAC to PRA ratio of >20 (see Fig. 5).

The second stage in the evaluation of the patient with suspected primary aldosteronism is to confirm the disorder by demonstrating increased aldosterone excretion or increased PAC despite volume expansion. The list of drugs and hormones capable of affecting the renin-angiotensin-aldosterone axis is extensive, and frequently, in patients with severe hypertension, a 'medication-contaminated' evaluation is unavoidable. The optimal antihypertensive agents to be used during this evaluation include α_1-adrenergic receptor antagonists and guanadrel; however, calcium-channel blockers and β-adrenergic receptor blockers do not affect the diagnostic accuracy in most cases [33]. It is impossible to interpret data obtained from patients receiving treatment with spironolactone. Therefore, spironolactone treatment *should not be initiated* until the evaluation is completed and the final decisions about treatment are made. If a patient suspected of primary aldosteronism is under treatment with spironolactone, it should be discontinued for at least 6 weeks before initiating diagnostic studies.

Aldosterone suppression testing can be performed with orally administered sodium chloride and measurement of urinary aldosterone [33,45] or with

252

intravenous sodium chloride loading and measurement of PAC [32,44]. Our practice has been oral salt loading over 3 days. Patients should receive a high sodium diet (supplemented with 1-g sodium chloride tablets if needed) for 3 days. The risk of increasing dietary sodium in patients with severe hypertension must be assessed in each case. Because the high-sodium diet can increase kaliuresis, vigorous replacement of potassium chloride should be prescribed. On the third day, a 24-hour urine is collected for measurement of aldosterone, sodium, potassium, cortisol, and creatinine. The 24-hour urinary sodium excretion should exceed 200 mEq to document adequate sodium repletion. Urinary aldosterone excretion >12 µg/24 hr is consistent with hyperaldosteronism. After age 50 the normal excretion rate of aldosterone falls [52]. The age-related 'normal' range for the laboratory should be known. The intravenous saline infusion test is performed after an overnight fast and in a recumbent patient. Two liters of normal saline is infused over 4 hours, and at the end of infusion blood is obtained for measurement of PAC. If the PAC is >10 ng/dl, unsuppressibility of aldosterone secretion is documented. If the PAC is <5 ng/dl following the saline infusion, primary aldosteronism is unlikely [32,44].

The third stage of the evaluation of the patient with primary aldosteronism guides the therapeutic approach by distinguishing APA and PAH from IHA and GRA (Fig. 6). Unilateral adrenalectomy in patients with an APA or PAH results in normalization of hypokalemia in all these patients and of hypertension in approximately 60–70% of them. In IHA and GRA, unilateral or bilateral adrenalectomy seldom corrects the hypertension [33]. The studies outlined in this section should be considered only after the diagnosis of primary aldosteronism is confirmed. This differentiation may require one or more studies, the first of which is imaging the adrenal with computed tomography (CT) or magnetic resonance imaging (MRI) (see Fig. 6). The diagnostic accuracy of adrenal CT scanning is approximately 70–90% [53]. Patients with APAs have more severe hypertension, more profound hypokalemia (<3.0 mEq/l), higher plasma (>25 ng/dl) and urinary (>30 µg/ 24 hr) levels of aldosterone, and younger age (<50 years) than those with IHA [54].

Patients fitting these descriptors are considered to have a 'high probability of APA' (see Fig. 6). Unfortunately, these factors are not absolute predictors of unilateral versus bilateral adrenal disease. The patient with a high probability of APA who has a unilateral adrenal nodule >1 cm should be considered for unilateral adrenalectomy. However, even in this group, there is a risk of operating on a nonfunctioning adrenal nodule. The concern about apparent adrenal microadenomas (≤1 cm) is that they may represent areas of hyperplasia and unilateral adrenalectomy would be inappropriate [55]. The most frequent error may be incorrectly labeling a small APA as IHA on the basis of CT findings of bilateral multinodularity or normal-appearing adrenals [56]. Adrenal venous sampling for aldosterone helps resolve these diagnostic dilemmas (Fig. 7).

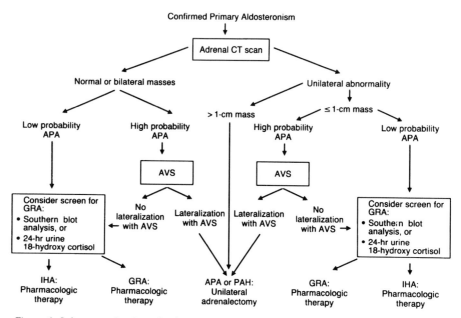

Figure 6. Subtype evaluation of primary aldosteronism. The details are discussed in the text. CT = computed tomography; APA = aldosterone-producing adenoma; IHA = idiopathic hyperaldosteronism; PAH = primary adrenal hyperplasia; GRA = glucocorticoid-remediable aldosteronism; AVS = adrenal venous sampling. (Modified from Young et al. [53]. Reproduced with permission.)

Selective adrenal venous sampling for aldosterone was one of the first tests used to distinguish APA from IHA [56,57]. Although it continues to be the most accurate test when both adrenal veins are sampled, it is an invasive and difficult technique. The failure rate for catheterization of the right adrenal vein in the cases reported in the literature is 26% [33], necessitating the performance of this test in referral centers. Bilateral adrenal/peripheral cortisol gradients validate successful catheterization of both adrenal veins. Normal adrenal vein PACs are in the range of 100–400 ng/dl [58]. After infusion of cosyntropin, patients with APA and PAH have adrenal vein PACs of 1000–20,000 ng/dl: PAC lateralization ratio of >10:1 (APA or PAH adrenal PAC: contralateral adrenal PAC); 'cortisol-corrected' (PAC divided by plasma cortisol concentration) PAC lateralization ratio >5:1 (APA or PAH adrenal PAC/cortisol:contralateral adrenal PAC/cortisol); and PAC:plasma cortisol ratio from unaffected adrenal less than the ratio from the peripheral vein [56,58]. Measuring epinephrine concentrations in the adrenal effluent, although rarely needed, will detect patients suspected of having cortisol cosecretion from an adenoma because this may suppress cortisol secretion from the contralateral gland, resulting in apparent suboptimal sampling of adrenal venous effluent. The effective use of high-resolution adrenal computerized imaging and adrenal venous sampling has made many

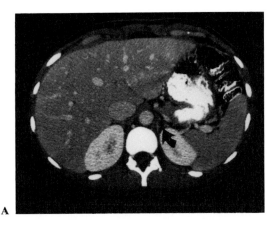

A

Results of Bilateral Adrenal Vein Sampling*

Vein	Adosterone (A) ng/dL	Cortisol (C) mcg/dL	A/C Ratio	Aldosterone Ratio*
RT Adrenal Vein	431	613	0.7	
LT Adrenal Vein	11,341	709	16.0	22.8
IVC	109	30	3.6	

B *Left adrenal vein A/C ratio divided by right adrenal vein A/C ratio

Figure 7. **A:** Computed tomographic (CT) scan from a 26-year-old woman who presented with new-onset hypertension and spontaneous hypokalemia (2.8 mEq/l). The screening plasma aldosterone to plasma renin activity ratio was 56. The 24-hour urinary excretion of aldosterone was 67 μg (with urinary sodium >200 mEq). The CT scan shows a 1-cm nodule in the lateral limb of the left adrenal gland (arrow). **B:** The results of adrenal vein sampling confirmed the left adrenal gland to be the source of excess aldosterone. Following laparoscopic removal of the left adrenal gland with a 0.5-cm cortical adenoma, the hypertension and hypokalemia resolved.

subtype tests obsolete (e.g., posture stimulation test, adrenal scintigraphy with [131]I-19-iodocholesterol, and the plasma 18-hydroxycorticosterone concentration).

Patients with primary aldosteronism who have normal findings with adrenal computerized imaging, or no lateralization of aldosterone on adrenal venous sampling, should be evaluated for the possibility of GRA (see Fig. 6). Typically, the diagnosis in these patients is made in the first to third decades. Also, the patients usually have a positive family history of onset of hypertension at a young age. A 24-hour urine 18-hydroxycortisol excretion in excess of 3000 nmol [46,59] or direct genetic blood testing to detect the chimeric gene [39] confirm the diagnosis.

The treatment goal is to prevent morbidity and mortality associated with hypertension and hypokalemia. The cause of the primary aldosteronism determines the appropriate treatment. Although hypertension is frequently cured with unilateral adrenalectomy in patients with APA and PAH, the average cure rate for IHA is only 19% with unilateral or bilateral adrenalectomy [33]. IHA and GRA should be treated medically.

The treatment of choice for APA and PAH is unilateral total adrenalectomy. The blood pressure response to spironolactone preoperatively often predicts the blood pressure response to unilateral adrenalectomy in patients with APA [60,61]. To decrease the surgical risk, hypokalemia should be corrected with spironolactone before the operation. Accurate preoperative localization permits unilateral posterior surgical approach, which is associated with shorter hospitalization and minimal morbidity and mortality than the abdominal approach [62,63]. Unilateral adrenalectomy obviates the need for corticosteroid coverage. Laparoscopic adrenalectomy appears to be a safe alternative surgical approach with a significantly shorter hospital stay and posthospitalization recovery [64,65].

Typically, the hypertension takes 1–6 months to resolve. Although nearly 100% of patients have improved blood pressure control postoperatively, average long-term cure rates with unilateral adrenalectomy for APA are 60–70% [53]. Persistence of hypertension may be related to change in baroreceptor sensitivity, established hemodynamic changes, structural changes of the blood vessels, altered sensitivity of the vessels to pressor substances, renal functional or structural changes, and coincident primary hypertension.

The nonpharmacologic treatment of IHA includes dietary sodium restriction (<100 mEq sodium/day), maintenance of ideal body weight, and alcohol avoidance. Potassium supplementation in the form of medication or as a diet rich in potassium is ineffective in correcting the hypokalemia of primary aldosteronism. Spironolactone often controls the hypertension and hypokalemia. Unfortunately, spironolactone also blocks both testosterone biosynthesis and peripheral androgen action. Impotence, decreased libido, gynecomastia, menstrual irregularities, and minor gastrointestinal tract symptoms may be found with spironolactone treatment. Amiloride is the drug of choice for men and for women who are intolerant of spironolactone. If hypertension persists despite adequate tolerable doses, a second-step agent [e.g., calcium-channel antagonist, angiotensin-converting enzyme (ACE) inhibitor, angiotensin II receptor blocker, or a thiazide diuretic] should be added. Nifedipine decreases plasma aldosterone levels and normalizes blood pressure in some patients with primary aldosteronism [66]. The ACE inhibitor enalapril returns blood pressure to normal values, decreases aldosterone secretion rates, and improves potassium balance in selected patients with IHA. Lisinopril, benazepril, ramipril, and fosinopril, other long-acting ACE inhibitors, and angiotensin II receptor blockers (e.g., losartin) should be similarly effective. Hypervolemia is a major reason for drug resistance. Low doses (e.g., 12.5–50 mg of hydrochlorothiazide daily) of a thiazide diuretic add to blood-pressure control when used in combination with the potassium-sparing diuretic [41].

Glucocorticoids given in physiologic to suppressive doses correct the hypertension and hypokalemia in patients with GRA. However, spironolactone is just as effective and may be more practical for long-term therapy [67].

Although one of the first instances of primary aldosteronism to be described [68] was due to an aldosterone-producing adrenal carcinoma, it is the rarest form of primary aldosteronism. Distinguishing histologically between benign and malignant adrenal cortical tumors is inherently difficult and remains controversial [69]. The only absolute criterion is the presence of local invasion or metastatic lesions. Adrenal carcinoma should be suspected in patients with aldosterone-producing tumors >3 cm in diameter (Fig. 8). Over 60 cases of aldosterone-producing adrenocortical carcinoma have been reported in the literature [70]. However, more than one half of the reported instances have been associated with excessive excretion of glucocorticoid, androgen, or aldosterone precursors. Isolated excessive aldosterone secretion from an adrenocortical carcinoma is rare. In general, carcinoma of the adrenal cortex carries a poor prognosis, with an overall 5-year survival rate of 16–30% [71].

Because of its low incidence, well-designed prospective therapeutic trials involving large numbers of patients with adrenocortical carcinoma are lacking. Surgical excision is the treatment of choice. Most patients with metastatic

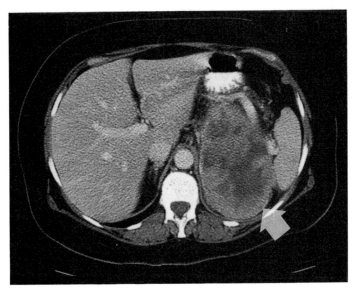

Figure 8. Abdominal computed tomographic (CT) scan from a 54-year-old woman with hypertension and hypokalemia caused by primary aldosteronism. The CT image shows a 13 × 8 cm left adrenal mass, which proved to be a 890 g grade 2 adrenocortical carcinoma at surgery.

257

disease are treated with mitotane (o,p'-DDD). However, the effectiveness of mitotane is controversial [71,72]. One study has shown mitotane to be effective only if high drug blood levels are achieved [73]. Suramin is an adrenal toxic agent that has limited efficacy and serious toxicity [74]. Spironolactone is effective in blocking the effects of excessive aldosterone secretion. If the tumor cosecretes excessive glucocorticoids, the hypercortisolism may be controlled with ketoconazole.

Conclusion

The diagnosis of a pheochromocytoma or an aldosterone-producing adrenal tumor provides the clinician with a unique treatment opportunity, that is, to render a surgical cure or achieve a dramatic response to pharmacologic therapy. Major advances have been made in the diagnosis and treatment of pheochromocytoma and primary aldosteronism since the first surgical cures in 1926 and 1955, respectively. The biochemical diagnoses are now straightforward. Localization of both of these tumor types has advanced with the revolution in computerized imaging. Specialized localization studies, such as MIBG scintigraphy and adrenal venous sampling, are options in specific instances of pheochromocytoma and primary aldosteronism, respectively. The major challenge that remains is the need for physicians to suspect these two disorders on the basis of the clinical presentations.

References

1. Mayo CH. 1927. Paroxysmal hypertension with tumor of retroperitoneal nerve. JAMA 89:1047–1050.
2. Saegesser F. 1984. Cesar Roux (1857–1934) et son epoque. Rev Med Suisse Romande 104:403–454.
3. Ito Y, Fujimoto Y, Obara T. 1992. The role of epinephrine, norepinephrine, and dopamine in blood pressure disturbances in patients with pheochromocytoma. World J Surg 16:759–764.
4. Young WF Jr, Maddox DE. 1995. Spells: In search of a cause. Mayo Clin Proc 70:757–765.
5. Manger WM, Gifford RW Jr. 1977. Pheochromocytoma. New York: Springer-Verlag.
6. Sheps SG, Jiang N-S, Klee GG. 1988. Diagnostic evaluation of pheochromocytoma. Endocrinol Metab Clin North Am 17:397–414.
7. Lenders JWM, Keiser HR, Goldstein DS, Willemsen JJ, Friberg P, Jacobs M-C, Kloppenborg PW, Thien T, Eisenhofer G. 1995. Plasma metanephrines in the diagnosis of pheochromocytoma. Ann Intern Med 123:101–109.
8. Sjoberg RJ, Simcic KJ, Kidd GS. 1992. The clonidine suppression test for pheochromcytoma: A review of its utility and pitfalls. Arch Intern Med 152:1193–1197.
9. Grossman E, Goldstein DS, Hoffman A, Keiser HR. 1991. Glucagon and clonidine testing in the diagnosis of pheochromocytoma. Hypertension 17:733–741.
10. Nadler JL, Radin R. 1991. Evaluation and management of the incidentally discovered adrenal mass. Endocrinologist 1:5–9.
11. Jackson JA, Kleerekoper M, Mendlovic D. 1993. Endocrine grand rounds: A 51-year-old man with accelerated hypertension, hypercalcemia, and right adrenal and paratracheal masses. Endocrinologist 3:5–13.

12. van Gils APG, Falke THM, van Erkel AR, Arndt J-W, Sandler MP, van der Mey AGL, Hoogma RP. 1991. MR imaging and MIBG scintigraphy of pheochromocytomas and extraadrenal functioning paragangliomas. Radiograph 11:37–57.

13. Whalen RK, Althausen AF, Daniels GH. 1992. Extra-adrenal pheochromocytoma. J Urol 147:1–10.

14. Shapiro B, Gross MD, Fig L, Khafagi F. 1990. Localization of functioning sympathoadrenal lesions. In Biglieri EG, Melby JC, eds. Endocrine Hypertension. New York: Raven Press, p 235.

15. Lamberts SWJ, Bakker WH, Reubi J-C, Krenning EP. 1990. Somatostain-receptor imaging in the localization of endocrine tumors. N Engl J Med 323:1246–1249.

16. Tenenbaum F, Lumbroso J, Schlumberger M, Mure A, Plouin PF, Caillou B, Parmentier C. 1995. Comparison of radiolabeled octreotide and meta-iodobenzylguanidine (MIBG) scintigraphy in malignant pheochromocytoma. J Nucl Med 36:1–6.

17. Young WF Jr. 1993. Pheochromocytoma: 1926 to 1993. Trends Endocrinol Metab 4:122–127.

18. Gagner M, Lacroix A, Bolte E. 1992. Laparoscopic adrenalectomy in Cushing's syndrome and pheochromocytoma. N Engl J Med 327:1033.

19. van Heerden JA, Roland CF, Carney A, Sheps SG, Grant CS. 1990. Long-term evaluation following resection of apparently benign pheochromocytoma(S)/paraganglioma(s). World J Surg 14:325–329.

20. Cope C, Delbridge L, Philips J, Friedlander M. 1991. Prognostic significance of nuclear DNA content in phaeochromocytoma. Aust NZ J Surg 61:695–698.

21. Nativ O, Grant CS, Sheps SG, O'Fallon JR, Farrow GM, van Heerden JA, Lieber MM. 1992. The clinical significance of nuclear DNA ploidy pattern in 184 patients with pheochromocytoma. Cancer 69:2683–2687.

22. Mornex R, Badet C, Peyrin L. 1992. Malignant pheochromocytoma: A series of 14 cases observed between 1966 and 1990. J Endocrinol Invest 15:643–649.

23. Krempf M, Lumbroso J, Mornex R, Brendel AJ, Wemeau JL, Delisle MJ, Aubert B, Carpenter P, Fleury-Goyon MC, Gibold C. 1991. Use of m-[[131]-I]iodobenzylguanidine in the treatment of malignant pheochromocytoma. J Clin Endocrinol Metab 72:455–461.

24. Shapiro B, Sisson JC, Wieland DM, Mangner TJ, Zempel SM, Mudgett E, Gross MD, Carey JE, Zasadny KA, Beierwaltes WH. 1991. Radiopharmaceutical therapy of malignant pheochromocytoma with [[131]-I] metaiodobenzylguanidine: Results from ten years of experience. J Nucl Biol Med 35:269–276.

25. Schlumberger M, Gicquel C, Lumbroso J, Tenenbaum F, Comoy E, Bosq J, Fonseca E, Ghillani PP, Aubert B, Travagli JP. 1992. Malignant pheochromocytoma: Clinical, biological, histologic and therapeutic data in a series of 20 patients with distant metastases. J Endocrinol Invest 15:631–642.

26. Averbuch SD, Steakley CS, Young RC, Gelman EP, Goldstein DS, Stull R, Keiser HR. 1988. Malignant pheochromocytoma: Effective treatment with a combination of cyclophosphamide, vincristine, and dacarbazine. Ann Intern Med 109:267–273.

27. Sasaki M, Iwaoka T, Yamauchi J, Tokunaga H, Naomi S, Inoue J, Oishi S, Umeda T, Sato T. 1994. A case of Sipple's syndrome with malignant pheochromocytoma treated with ^{131}I-metaiodobenzyl guanidine and a combined chemotherapy with cyclophosphamide, vincristine, and dacarbazine. Endocr J 41:155–160.

28. Harper MA, Murnaghan GA, Kennedy L, Hadden DR, Atkinson AB. 1989. Phaeochromocytoma in pregnancy: Five cases and a review of the literature. Br J Obstet Gynaecol 96:594–606.

29. Conn JW. 1955. Presidential address: Part I. Painting background, Part II. Primary aldosteronism, a new clinical syndrome. J Lab Clin Med 45:3–17.

30. Mader IJ, Iseri LT. 1955. Spontaneous hypopotassemia, hypomagnesemia, alkalosis and tetany due to hypersecretion of corticosterone-like mineralocorticoid. Am J Med 19:976–988.

31. Berglund G, Andersson O, Wilhelmsen L. 1976. Prevalence of primary and secondary hypertension: Studies in a random population sample. Br Med J 2:554–556.

32. Streeten DHP, Tomycz N, Anderson GH Jr. 1979. Reliability of screening methods for the diagnosis of primary aldosteronism. Am J Med 67:403–413.
33. Young WF Jr, Klee GG. 1988. Primary aldosteronism: Diagnostic evaluation. Endocrinol Metab Clin North Am 17:367–395.
34. Banks WA, Kastin AJ, Biglieri EG, Ruiz AE. 1984. Primary adrenal hyperplasia: A new subset of primary hyperaldosteronism. J Clin Endocrinol Metab 58:783–785.
35. Irony I, Kater CE, Biglieri EG, Shackleton CHL. 1990. Correctable subsets of primary aldosteronism: Primary adrenal hyperplasia and renin responsive adenoma. Am J Hypertens 3:576–582.
36. Melby JC, Azar ST. 1993. Adrenal steroids and hypertension: New aspects. Endocrinologist 3:344–351.
37. Gordon RD, Hamlet SM, Tunny TJ, Klemm SA. 1987. Aldosterone-producing adenomas responsive to angiotensin pose problems in diagnosis. Clin Exp Pharmacol Physiol 14:175–179.
38. Tunny TJ, Gordon RD, Klemm SA, Cohn D. 1991. Histological and biochemical distinctiveness of atypical aldosterone-producing adenomas responsive to upright posture and angiotensin. Clin Endocrinol 34:363–369.
39. Lifton RP, Dluhy RG, Powers M, Rich GM, Cook S, Ulick S, Lalouel JM. 1992. A chimaeric 11β-hydroxylase/aldosterone synthase gene causes glucocorticoid-remediable aldosteronism and human hypertension. Nature 355:262–265.
40. Stowasser M, Gordon RD, Tunny TJ, Klemm SA, Finn WL, Krek AL. 1992. Familial hyperaldosteronism type II; Five families with a new variety of primary aldosteronism. Clin Exp Pharmacol Phys 19:319–322.
41. Bravo EL, Fouad-Tarazi FM, Tarazi RC, Pohl M, Gifford RW, Vidt DG. 1988. Clinical implications of primary aldosteronism with resistent hypertension. Hypertension 11(Suppl I):I207–I211.
42. Ganguly A, Robertson GL. 1980. Elevated threshold for vasopressin release in primary aldosteronism (abs). Clin Res 28:330A.
43. Nakada T, Koike H, Katayama T. 1987. Evidence for a defect in urinary concentrating ability in primary aldosteronism and its reversal by adrenal surgery. Urol Int 42:295–301.
44. Weinberger MH, Grim CE, Hollifield JW, Kem DC, Ganguly A, Kramer NJ, Yune HY, Wellman H, Donohue JP. 1979. Primary aldosteronism: Diagnosis, localization, and treatment. Ann Intern Med 90:386–395.
45. Bravo EL, Tarazi RC, Dustan HP, Fouad FM, Textor SC, Gifford RW, Vidt DG. 1983. The changing clinical spectrum of primary aldosteronism. Am J Med 74:641–651.
46. Rich GM, Ulick S, Cook S, Wang JZ, Lifton RP, Dluhy RG. 1992. Glucocorticoid-remediable aldosteronism in a large kindred: Clinical spectrum and diagnosis using a characteristic biochemical phenotype. Ann Intern Med 116:813–820.
47. Jose A, Kaplan NM. 1969. Plasma renin activity in the diagnosis of primary aldosteronism: Failure to distinguish primary aldosteronism from essential hypertension. Arch Intern Med 123:141–146.
48. Hiramatsu K, Yamada T, Yukimura Y, Komiya I, Ichikawa K, Ishihara M, Nagata H, Izumiyama T. 1981. A screeening test to identify aldosterone-producing adenoma by measuring plasma renin activity: Results in hypertension patients. Arch Inter Med 141:1589–1593.
49. Sigurdsson JA, Bengtsson C, Tibblin E, Wojciechowski J. 1983. Prevalence of secondary hypertension in a population sample of Swedish women. Eur Heart J 4:424–433.
50. McKenna TJ, Sequeira SJ, Heffernan A, Chambers J, Cunningham S. 1991. Diagnosis under random conditions of all disorders of the renin-angiotensin-aldosterone axis, including primary hyperaldosteronism. J Clin Endocrinol Metab 73:952–957.
51. Weinberger MH, Fineberg NS. 1993. The diagnosis of primary aldosteronism and separation of two major subtypes. Arch Int Med 153:2125–2129.
52. Hegstad R, Brown RD, Jiang NS, Kao P, Weinshilboum RM, Strong C, Wisgerhof M. 1983. Aging and aldosterone. Am J Med 74:442–448.

53. Young WF Jr, Hogan MJ, Klee GG, Grant CS, van Heerden JA. 1990. Primary aldosteronism: Diagnosis and treatment. Mayo Clin Proc 65:96–110.
54. Blumenfeld JD, Sealey JE, Schlussel Y, Vaughan ED Jr, Sos TA, Atlas SA, Muller FB, Acevedo R, Ulick S, Laragh JH. 1994. Diagnosis and treatment of primary hyper-aldosteronism. Ann Intern Med 121:877–885.
55. Radin DR, Manoogian C, Nadler JL. 1992. Diagnosis of primary hyperaldosteronism: Importance of correlating CT findings with endocrinologic studies. Am J Roentgenol 158:553–557.
56. Doppman JL, Gill JR Jr, Miller DL, Chang R, Gupta R, Friedman TC, Choyke PL, Feuerstein IM, Dwyer AJ, Jicha DL. 1992. Distinction between hyperaldosteronism due to bilateral hyperplasia and unilateral aldosteronoma: Reliability of CT. Radiology 184:677–682.
57. Melby JC, Spark RF, Dale SL, Egdahl RH, Kahn PC. 1967. Diagnosis and localization of aldosterone-producing adenomas by adrenal-vein catheterization. N Engl J Med 277:1050–1056.
58. Melby JC. 1984. Primary aldosteronism (clinical conference). Kidney Int 26:769–778.
59. Walker BR, Edwards CRW. 1993. Dexamethasone-suppressible hypertension. Endocrinologist 3:87–97.
60. Ferriss JB, Brown JJ, Fraser R, Haywood E, Davies DL, Kay AW, Lever AF, Robertson JIS, Owen K, Peart WS. 1975. Results of adrenal surgery in patients with hypertension, aldosterone excess, and low plasma renin concentration. Br Med J 1:135–138.
61. Saruta T, Suzuki H, Takita T, Saito I, Murai M, Tazaki H. 1987. Pre-operative evaluation of the prognosis of hypertension in primary aldosteronism owing to adenoma. Acta Endocrinol (Copenh) 116:229–234.
62. Grant CS, Carpenter P, van Heerden JA, Hamberger B. 1984. Primary aldosteronism: Clinical management. Arch Surg 119:585–590.
63. Russell CF, Hamberger B, vanHeerden JA, Edis AJ, Ilstrup DM. 1982. Adrenalectomy: Anterior or posterior approach? Am J Surg 144:322–324.
64. Stanley DG. 1994. Laparoscopic adrenalectomy. Int Surg 79:253–258.
65. Schlinkert RT, van Heerden JA, Grant CS, Thompson GB, Segura JW. 1995. Laparoscopic left adrenalectomy for aldosteronoma: Early Mayo Clinic experience. Mayo Clin Proc 70:844–846.
66. Nalder JL, Hsueh W, Horton R. 1985. Therapeutic effect of calcium channel blockade in primary aldosteronism. J Clin Endocrinol Metab 60:896–899.
67. Ganguly A, Grim CE, Bergstein J, Brown RD, Weinberger MH. 1981. Genetic and pathophysiologic studies of a new kindred with glucocorticoid-suppressible hyper-aldosteronism manifest in three generations. J Clin Endocrinol Metab 53:1040–1046.
68. Foye LV Jr, Feightmeir TY. 1955. Adrenal cortical carcinoma producing solely mineralocorticoid effect. Am J Med 19:966–975.
69. Hough AJ, Hollifield JW, Page DL, Hartmann WH. 1979. Prognostic factors in adrenal cortical tumors: A mathematical analysis of clinical and morphologic data. Am J Clin Pathol 72:390–399.
70. Rainwater LM, Young WF Jr, Farrow GM, Grant CS, van Heerden JA, Lieber MM. 1989. Flow cytometric analysis of deoxyribonucleic acid ploidy in benign and malignant aldosterone-producing neoplasms of the adrenal gland. Surg Gynecol Obsertrics 168:491–496.
71. Wooten MD, King DK. 1993. Adrenal cortical carcinoma: Epidemiology and treatment with mitotane and a review of the literature. Cancer 72:3145–3155.
72. Vassilopoulou-Sellin R, Guinee VF, Klein MJ, Taylor SH, Hess KR, Schultz PN, Samaan NA. 1993. Impact of adjuvant mitotane on the clinical course of patients with adrenocortical cancer. Cancer 71:3119–3123.
73. Haak HR, Hermans J, van de Velde CJH, Lentjes EGWM, Goslings BM, Fleuren G-J, Krans HM. 1994. Optimal treatment of adrenocortical carcinoma with mitotane: Results in a consecutive series of 96 patients. Br J Cancer 69:947–951.
74. Arlt W, Reincke M, Siekmann L, Winkelmann W, Allolio B. 1994. Suramin in adrenocortical cancer: Limited efficacy and serious toxicity. Clin Endocrinol 41:299–307.

13. Incidentally discovered adrenal masses

Richard T. Kloos, Melvyn Korobkin, Norman W. Thompson,
Isaac R. Francis, Brahm Shapiro, and Milton D. Gross

Currently, adrenal masses are discovered incidentally in 0.35–5% of patients imaged with computed tomography (CT) and are referred to as adrenal *incidentalomas* [1,2]. As a result, the diagnostic dilemma of separating the small fraction of hypersecretory and/or malignant masses from the majority that are nonhypersecretory adrenal adenomas has become common. Given the fourfold greater autopsy incidence of adrenal adenomas compared with the radiographic incidence, and the oncology data that only 20–41% of adrenal metastases are detected by CT [1,3], it is likely that an increase in prevalence will occur if the spatial resolving capacity of abdominal imaging improves, if abdominal imaging occurs more frequently, and if routine abdominal imaging slice thickness is decreased.

This chapter reviews current approaches to adrenal incidentaloma, including biochemical evaluation, mass size, unenhanced CT attenuation values, chemical-shift magnetic resonance (MR), adrenocortical scintigraphy, percutaneous adrenal biopsy, and surgery. Further, current experimentation regarding the utility of 1-hour post contrast CT attenuation values, positron emission tomography (PET), ethanol injection therapy, surgical resection of adrenal metastases, and subtotal adrenalectomy surgery are also discussed.

Epidemiology

The differential diagnosis of adrenal masses and their relative prevalences as incidentalomas are shown in Tables 1 and 2. The highest values are most likely overestimated due to the small sample sizes of the studies from which they were derived (e.g., adrenocortical carcinoma, cysts, and metastases in non-oncology patients). The majority of adrenal incidentalomas are nonhypersecretory adenomas, likely representing 70–94% of all adrenal masses in non-oncologic and general patient populations [1]. They occur equally in males and females, are uncommon under age 30 years, and their

Partial support for this manuscript was provided by the Cancer Research Training in Nuclear Medicine Grant NCI 2 T32 CA09015-19 and the Department of Veterans Affairs.

Andrew Arnold (ed.) ENDOCRINE NEOPLASMS. 1997. Kluwer Academic Publishers. ISBN 0-7923-4354-9.
All rights reserved.

Table 1. Etiological classification and relative frequency of various adrenal incidentalomas

Mass etiology	Frequency among incidentalomas
Adrenal cortex	
Adenoma	
Non-oncology and non-selected series	36–94%
Oncology patients	7–68%
Pigmented nodules ('black adenomas')	
Nodular hyperplasia	7–17%
Carcinoma	0–25%
Adrenal medulla	
Carcinoma	
Ganglioneuroma	0–6%
Ganglioneuroblastoma	
Pheochromocytoma	0–11%
Neuroblastoma (children)	
Other adrenal masses	
Angioma/hemangioma	
Angiomyolipoma	
Angiosarcoma	
Abscess	
Amyloidosis	
Cysts	4–22%
Parasitic (echinococcal most common): 6% of cysts	
Retention: 2% of cysts	
Endothelial (lymphatic or angiomatous): 44% of cysts	
Degenerative adenomas: 7% of cysts	
Pseudocyst (most likely hemorrhage into normal tissue or adrenal neoplasm): 39% of cysts	
Other (e.g., dermoid): 2% of cysts	
Extramedullary hematopoiesis	
Fibroma	
Granulomatous/infectious-(blastomycosis, coccidiomycosis, cryptococcosis, cytomegalovirus, histoplasmosis, mycobacterium, sarcoidosis)	
Hamartoma	
Hematoma/hemorrhage	0–4%
Leiomyosarcoma	
Leiomyoma	
Lipoma	0–11%
Liposarcoma	
Lymphangioma	
Myelolipoma (0.2% autopsy incidence)	7–15%
Myoma	
Neurofibroma	
Teratoma	
Xanthomatosis	
Metastases	
Non-oncology and nonselected series	0–21%
Oncology patients	32–73%
Breast carcinoma	
Kidney	
Leukemia	
Lung cancer	
Lymphoma	
Melanoma	

Table 1. (cont.)

Mass etiology	Frequency among incidentalomas
Ovarian	
Others	
Pseudo- and peri-adrenal masses	
Paraganglioma; gastric diverticulum; lesions and pseudolesions of the diaphragmatic crura, stomach, gallbladder, kidney, liver, lymphactics (para-aortic, paracaval, retropancreatic, retocrural), omentum, pancreas, retroperitonium (neoplasm, hematoma, cyst), small and large bowel, spleen/accessory spleen, and vasculature (especially aneurysms, varices, tortuosities, dilated inferior vena cava, renal veins)	
Technical artifacts (particularly with prior abdominal surgery)	

Modified with permission from Kloos et al. [1]. © The Endocrine Society.

Table 2. Suggested biochemical screening tests for adrenal incidentalomas

Hypersecretory state	Frequency among incidentalomas	Screening test	Cost[a] (U.S. $)
Pheochromocytoma	0–11%	Serum catecholamines	$139
		or	
		24-hour urinary catecholamines	$102
		or	
		24-hour urinary metanephrines	$79
Cushing's or pre-Cushing's syndrome	0–18%	1-mg oral overnight dexamethasone suppression test for 0800-hour serum cortisol	$70
Mineralocorticoid hypertension	0–7%	Blood pressure	$0
		Serum potassium	$15[b]
		In hypertensive patients.	
		Paired upright plasma renin activity	$90
		Plasma aldosterone concentration	$160
Masculinizing tumor	0–11%	Serum dehydroepiandrosterone sulfate (DHEAS)	$96
		(Serum total and free testosterone and congenital adrenal hyperplasia evaluation in virilized females and boys with precocious sexual development)	
Feminizing tumor	Rare	(Serum estradiol in feminized men)	
		Total cost	$260–570

[a] At the University of Michigan Medical Center (January 1996).
[b] Often obtained previously for other reasons in a biochemical panel ($40).
Modified with permission from Kloos et al. [1]. © The Endocrine Society.

prevalence increases with age [1,4]. Nonhypersecretory adrenal adenomas are associated with hypertension, black versus white race, diabetes mellitus (two-to fivefold), obesity, heterozygote carriers of congenital adrenal hyperplasia (CAH), multiple endocrine neoplasia (MEN), and the McCune-Albright syndrome [1,5]. Adrenocortical adenomas may be monoclonal (43%), polyclonal (28.5%), or of an intermediate form (28.5%); however, the pathogenesis of adrenocortical tumors remains poorly understood [1,5,6].

In patients having no known extra-adrenal primary malignancy, the chance is low that an adrenal incidentaloma is a metastasis or primary adrenal malignancy (see Table 1). Between 8% and 38% of patients with known extra-adrenal malignancies have adrenal metastases at autopsy, most commonly from the breast, lung, kidney, melanoma, and lymphoma [1]. Malignancy rates of adrenal masses with a known extra-adrenal primary malignancy have ranged from 32% to 73%, while benign masses have been reported in 27–68% of such cases [1]. Further, in this setting malignancy rates in adrenal masses ≤3 cm have ranged from 0% to 50%, while in adrenal masses >3 cm, malignancy rates have ranged from 43% to 100% [1]. The distinction between a metastasis and other causes of adrenal masses may be critical in patients who may benefit from curative surgery if their primary malignancy is not disseminated. Further, a small and controversial literature suggests that the resection of isolated adrenal metastases from some extra-adrenal primary malignancies may be beneficial [2,7,8].

Biochemical evaluation

Hypersecretory masses require specific therapy, usually surgical extirpation. However, adrenal surgery is not generally indicated for CAH, primary aldosteronism secondary to bilateral adrenal hyperplasia, or adrenocorticotrophic hormone (ACTH)–dependent Cushing's syndrome with secondary macronodular adrenal hyperplasia. History and physical examinations must consider hypersecretion of cortisol, androgens, estrogen, mineralocorticoids, and catecholamines. However, biochemical screening of all adrenal masses lacking an obvious radiological diagnosis (e.g., simple cyst, myelolipoma; Fig. 1), regardless of the history and physical examinations, cannot be over-emphasized. CT and MR are unable to distinguish hypersecretory from nonhypersecretory lesions, while clinically silent hypersecretory adrenal masses are common (see Table 2) [1]. Fifty to 70% of adrenocortical carcinomas are hypersecretory [1,10–12]. Partially cystic lesions warrant complete evaluations regarding their secretory status and as potential malignancies. Table 2 suggests a minimal, yet adequate, initial screening evaluation of the adrenal incidentaloma.

The prevalence of pheochromocytoma in patients with classic symptoms of episodic headache, palpitations, and diaphoresis is comparable with that of pheochromocytoma amongst adrenal incidentalomas (see Table 2) [1]. Be-

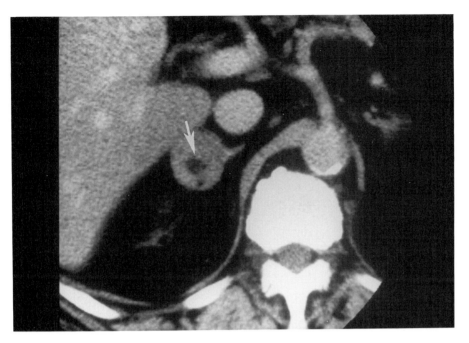

Figure 1. Adrenal myelolipoma. A small amount of fat-attenuation tissue (arrow) is seen within this right adrenal mass. (Reprinted with permission from Korobkin and Francis [9].)

tween 19% and 76% of pheochromocytomas are not diagnosed during life, while up to 80% of unsuspected pheochromocytoma patients who underwent surgery or anesthesia have died [1]. Sixty-five percent of pheochromocytomas have an overlap with adrenal metastases in relative signal intensity on T2-weighted spin-echo MR, and percutaneous adrenal biopsy of pheochromocytoma may precipitate hypertensive crisis, severe retroperitoneal bleeding, and death [1].

Plasma or urinary catecholamines and metanephrines, and urinary vanillylmandelic acid (VMA), are of approximately equal utility; however, the latter may be the least sensitive [1,13]. An understanding of factors that may result in false-negative and false-positive tests is required for proper test selection, performance, and interpretation (Table 3) [14]. Pharmacological stimulation or suppression tests may rarely be helpful [14,15]. Clonidine decreases catecholamines in nonpheochromocytoma subjects but has little effect in pheochromocytoma. Clonidine decreases plasma aldosterone concentration (PAC) and plasma renin activity (PRA) in normal and hypertensive subjects but has little effect in primary aldosteronism (Table 4). Thus, clonidine may be the antihypertensive agent of choice in patients with adrenal incidentalomas in whom antihypertensive therapy must be continued during diagnostic investigations.

We advocate metaiodobenzylguanidine (MIBG) scintigraphy for further

Table 3. Drug interactions with pheochromocytomas and their diagnosis

Drugs	Contraindicated with possible pheochromocytoma	Increase catecholamines and metabolites	Reduce MIBG uptake	Interval of drug withdrawl before MIBG imaging
Acute clonidine or alcohol withdrawl, beta-blockers, minoxidil, hydralazine	Yes	Yes	No	None
Phenoxybenzamine, phentolamine, prazosin, doxazosin, diuretics, spironolactone, amiloride, levodopa, methyldopa	No	Yes	No	None
Cocaine, sympathomimetics	Yes	Yes	Yes	1 week
Dopamine, dopaminergic drugs	Yes	Yes	Possible	1 week
Clonidine, ACE inhibitors	No	No	No	None
Butyrophenones, amphetamines	No	Yes	Possible	1 week
Labetalol	No	Yes	Yes	4 weeks
Guanethidine, guanadrel	Yes	No	Possible	1 week
Phenothiazines	Possible	Variable	Possible	1 week
Tricyclic antidepressants	No	Variable	Yes	4 weeks
Calcium-channel blockers	No	No	Possible	1 week
Methylglucamine (component of iodinated contrast)	No	False normal up to 72 hours	No	None
Reserpine	No	No	Yes	4 weeks

Adapted from Kloos et al. [1] and Bravo [14], with permission.

evaluation of suspected pheochromocytoma when biochemical screening tests are abnormal (Fig. 2). [^{123}I or ^{131}I] MIBG and [^{111}In] pentetreotide (OctreoScan®) detect pheochromocytomas almost equally (sensitivity 88%) and may detect additional paragangliomas or evidence of metastatic disease. MIBG offers advantages of greater sensitivity for neuroblastoma (92% vs. 77%) and ganglioneuroma (100%), with absent or minimal confounding normal renal and hepatic radiotracer accumulation, and the potential for therapy should the neural crest tumor be malignant [21,22]. Normal adrenal glands are visualized in up to 10% and 32% of patients studied with [^{131}I] and [^{123}I] MIBG, respectively (Fig. 2) [23]. [^{123}I] MIBG is an investigational drug with significantly better radiation dosimetry, superior image quality, and better identification of metastatic foci than [^{131}I] MIBG. [^{123}I or ^{131}I] MIBG is administered as a slow intravenous injection. Imaging is performed after 24 and 48 hours with additional imaging after 72 hours for [^{131}I] MIBG [1]. Some data suggest that [^{123}I or ^{131}I] MIBG and [^{111}In] pentertreotide may serve complementary roles [1,24]. The utility of MIBG scintigraphy in patients with normal biochemistry and discordant adrenocortical scintigraphy is uncharacterized [25].

It is likely that a spectrum of cortisol excess exists and that clinically obvious manifestations occur relatively late, while blunting of diurnal variation and loss of cortisol suppressibility occurs before baseline steroid hormone excretion exceeds normal limits [1]. Given the prevalence of Cushing's and pre-Cushing's syndrome (biochemical evidence of Cushing's syndrome without physical stigmata) amongst adrenal incidentalomas (see Table 2) [1,26–28], we suggest that cortisol secretory status be investigated with an overnight 1.0-mg dexamethasone suppression test (DST). One may consider measures of cortisol secretory rhythm with paired 0800-hour and 1600-hour cortisol levels [1],

Table 4. Drug interactions with aldosterone and renin determinations

Renin-angiotensin system drugs	Effect on PRA	Effect on PA	Effect on PA:PRA ratio	Values diagnostic of primary aldosteronism	Values suggesting possible primary aldosteronism	Interval of drug withdrawl before further study
None, prazosin, doxazosin, guanadrel, guanethidine	None (Ø)	Ø	Ø	a	b, c, or d	None
Clonidine	Decrease (D)	D	Ø	a	b, c, or d	None
Minoxidil, hydralazine	Increase (I)	I	Ø or D	a	b, c, d, e, or f	1–2 weeks
Diuretics, spironolactone, amiloride	I	I	Ø or D	a	b, c, d, e, or f	4–6 weeks
ACE inhibitors, calcium-channel blockers	I	D	D	a	b, c, d, g, or h	1–2 weeks
Beta-blockers, antisympathetic agents, NSAIDS	D	Ø or minor D	I	a	b, c, or d	None or 1–2 weeks

[a] Suppressed PRA and elevated PA, either supine or upright.
[b] Upright PRA <1 ng/ml/hr (normal range 1.0–7.0) and PA >10 ng/dl (normal range 4.0–31.0).
[c] Upright PRA <3.0 ng/ml/hr and PA >15 ng/dl.
[d] Supine PRA <2.5 ng/ml/hr (normal range 0.5–3.5) and PA >15 ng/dl (normal range 1.0–16.0).
[e] Upright PA/PRA ratio >30 and PA >20 ng/dl.
[f] Elevated PA, either supine or upright.
[g] Upright PA >15 ng/dl.
[h] Upright PA/PRA ratio >20.
Adapted from Weinberger et al. [16], Weigel et al. [17], Melby and Azar [18], Bravo [19], and Bunnag and Tuck [20].

269

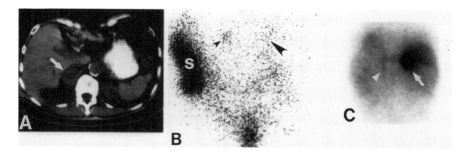

Figure 2. Pheochromocytoma. **A:** Unenhanced abdominal CT obtained for constipation following prostate cancer radiation therapy demonstrates a 5–6 cm right adrenal mass (arrow) containing areas of low density in a normotensive and asymptomatic man with urine catecholamines and metabolites ranging from normal to 4.6 times the upper limits of normal. **B:** Posterior NP59 scan 7 days post–radiotracer administration demonstrates a discordant image pattern with diminished and distorted right adrenal gland uptake (large arrowhead), normal left adrenal gland uptake (small arrowhead), and marked stool (S) radiotracer activity throughout the colon despite laxatives. **C:** Posterior [^{123}I]MIBG scan 24 hours after radiotracer administration reveals intense right adrenal mass uptake (arrow) with normal left adrenal gland (arrowhead) and liver uptake.

or a single 2400-hour cortisol value [29,30]. However, support of surgical intervention for an abnormal serum cortisol rhythm with a normal overnight DST, 24-hour urinary free cortisol (UFC) excretion, and absent physical stigmata of Cushing's syndrome is not available [1]. We recommend NP59 scintigraphy for patients with ACTH-independent Cushing's and pre-Cushing's syndrome, which would demonstrate unilateral radiotracer uptake within the tumor and absent uptake in the contralateral adrenal gland in all Cushing's adenomas and very rarely in cortisol-secreting well-differentiated adrenocortical carcinomas, which usually demonstrate bilateral adrenal nonvisualization (see later). Bilateral adrenal visualization on NP59 scintigraphy should raise the suspicion of bilateral macro-nodular and micronodular hyperplasia (ACTH-dependent or independent).

While some evidence suggests a shift of steroidogenesis from the mineralocorticoid to the glucocorticoid pathway in nonhypersecretory adrenal adenomas [31], blood pressure and serum potassium should be measured to exclude mineralocorticoid excess. In the absence of hypertension, we do not pursue mineralocorticoid excess if the serum potassium is normal (>3.5 mmol/l). Spontaneous or easily provoked hypokalemia (≤3.5 mmol/l) or diuretic-induced hypokalemia (≤3.0 mmol/l) should prompt further investigation [1]. In patients with hypertension, we also obtain a (>2 hours because supine) paired upright PAC and PRA. These determinations are most accurate after interfering medications have been discontinued for an appropriate interval (see Table 4). However, reasonable exclusion of primary aldosteronism may be achieved in the majority of patients in the presence of continued interfering medications. An elevated PAC with a suppressed PRA is always diagnostic of primary aldosteronism. PAC and PRA values suggesting the possibility of primary aldosteronism should be further evaluated following discontinuation of all potentially interfering medications with repetition of baseline values, and/or saline or captopril suppression testing. Suppressed PRA and PAC values with hypokalemia suggest non–aldosterone-mediated mineralocorticoid hypertension [e.g., deoxycorticosterone (DOC)].

The incidentaloma patient found to have primary aldosteronism requires an investigation to distinguish a unilateral process from bilateral adrenal hyperplasia. Further discussion of these techniques may be found in Chapter 12. Briefly, they include the magnitude of the PAC, the PAC/PRA ratio, the 18-hydroxycorticosterone level, postural PAC and PRA studies, dexamethasone-suppressed NP59 scintigraphy, and bilateral adrenal vein hormone sampling.

In the setting of a unilateral process (almost always an adenoma, and rarely unilateral hyperplasia or a well-differentiated hypersecretory adrenocortical carcinoma), a dexamethasone-suppressed NP59 scan demonstrates early radiotracer uptake in the lesion and nonvisualization of the contralateral adrenal gland [32–35]. In the setting of bilateral adrenal hyperplasia, the dexamethasone-suppressed NP59 scan will demonstrate early bilateral adrenal visualization. In the rare setting of a hypersecretory adrenocortical carcinoma or a glucocorticoid-remediable form of primary aldosteronism, the dexamethasone-suppressed NP59 scan will demonstrate absent early adrenal visualization bilaterally. In the former setting, the late images will characteristically demonstrate absent or decreased radiotracer accumulation in the mass relative to the normal contralateral adrenal gland. In the later setting, the blood pressure and biochemical abnormalities will normalize on dexamethasone and the late images will demonstrate a normal (non-lateralizing) NP59 image pattern.

As none of the noninvasive tests are 100% accurate in distinguishing a unilateral from a bilateral etiology of primary aldosteronism, and because bilateral adrenal vein catheterization requires a skilled and experienced angiographer, we recommend that a combination of noninvasive tests be performed. Bilateral adrenal vein catheterization is recommended when the results are discrepant. These functional tests are important because of the relatively high prevalence of coexistant nonhypersecretory adrenal adenomas, and due to the fact the bilateral adrenal hyperplasia may occur asymmetrically.

Some evidence suggests that adrenocortical carcinomas may demonstrate an enzymatic defect (11-beta hydroxylase) in the mineralocorticoid synthetic pathway. A significant, although incomplete, separation of adrenocortical carcinomas from adenomas has been demonstrated by comparison of mineralocorticoid precursor levels to the end product aldosterone by the calculation (aldosterone $\times$ 100)/(DOC + 18-OH-DOC) or (aldosterone $\times$ 100)/DOC. The two patients studied with malignancy metastatic to the adrenal gland demonstrated ratios similar to those of adrenocortical carcinomas; however, neither had an elevated baseline DOC level, in contrast to all the adrenocortical carcinomas studied [36].

Dehydroepiandrosterone sulfate (DHEAS) as a marker of adrenal androgen excess (e.g., virilizing adenomas, adrenocortical carcinomas, and CAH) should always be measured. Low DHEAS values may represent suppressed normal adrenal androgen secretion by autonomous cortisol hypersecretion [26,28,37,38], and thus DHEAS should not be measured concomitantly with the overnight DST. A low DHEAS value may also suggest primary adrenal insufficiency [26]. We do not routinely obtain screening testosterone or estradiol levels in asymptomatic patients [39].

We do not advocate serum 17-OH progesterone or Cortrosyn stimulation testing for CAH in asymptomatic individuals because NP59 scintigraphy in uncomplicated cases will suggest a benign process [1,38]. This approach implies that clinically silent CAH does not require therapy. CAH should be considered in the differential diagnosis of androgen and mineralocorticoid excess. Interestingly, an increased 17-OH-progesterone response to ACTH stimulation has been demonstrated in some patients with incidental nonhypersecretory adrenal adenomas, which returned to normal after unilateral adrenalectomy, suggesting an acquired 21-hydroxylase deficiency intrinsic to the adrenal lesion [38].

Computed tomography

The CT appearance of most adrenal masses does not allow one to differentiate a benign from a malignant lesion. Adrenal hemorrhage (high attenuation) and adrenal myelolipoma (fat attenuation; see Fig. 1), however, have CT features sufficiently characteristic to permit a confident diagnosis in most cases [40–43]. For patients with adrenal lesions typical of myelolipoma, observation can be advised in the asymptomatic patient. Larger myelolipomas (>5 cm) are often associated with pain and are treated by adrenalectomy [44,45]. The diagnosis of an adrenal cyst is sometimes made by CT, but many large cysts have suspicious features that require surgical resection to exclude a malignancy [46]. A simple thin-walled adrenal cyst may be aspirated rather than surgically excised. Thick-walled cysts are more likely to be neoplasms with central necrosis. We have encountered both pheochromocytomas and adrenocortical carcinomas that were originally considered to be benign cysts. Tuberculosis, histoplasmosis, or other granulomatous infections usually involve both glands, but often asymmetrically. The CT findings are nonspecific and include soft-tissue masses, cystic changes, and calcification reflecting the age of the process and degree of necrosis [47]. Percutaneous biopsy is often required to confirm that diagnosis and to identify the organism.

Patients with adrenal hemorrhage and adrenal myelolipoma represent only a small fraction of those with CT-detected, nonhypersecretory adrenal masses.

In the remaining patients, the problem is to differentiate benign from malignant lesions. In patients without a known or suspected extra-adrenal primary neoplasm, the main differential diagnosis is between an adrenocortical adenoma and an adrenocortical carcinoma.

Lesions >5 cm or those with irregular margins have often been surgically removed because they are atypical of benign adenoma. Features typical of carcinoma are size >5 cm; central areas of low attenuation due to tumor necrosis; tumor calcification; and evidence of hepatic, nodal, or venous spread [48,49]. Classical CT features typical of benign adenomas include smooth contour, sharp margination, and size <5 cm. When these features are present and biochemical studies are normal, surveillance with CT at 6 and 12 months has often been recommended to confirm lack of growth. However, size criteria are weak discriminators between adenomas and nonadenomas [50,51]. In our own study of 135 adrenal masses, the mean diameter of the adenomas was significantly lower than the nonadenomas (2.4 cm vs. 4.5 cm), but there was sufficient overlap between the two groups at the smallest sizes that a threshold value for a highly specific diagnosis was not present [52]. Another word of caution regarding the serial CT follow-up of adrenal incidentalomas based on their small size (<3.5–5.0 cm), lack of biochemical hypersecretion, and/or lack of suspicious anatomic imaging is that we have now seen three unfortunate patients with tumors ranging from 3 to 5 cm in diameter when initially found who were advised against operation after an initial evaluation. These patients were followed for 1–2 years elsewhere and then reassured that there was no further risk. Each patients was subsequently referred to our center 3–7 years later with obviously progressed adrenocortical carcinomas.

When an adrenal mass is the only finding suspicious of metastatic disease in an oncologic patient, confirmation of its nature may be crucial in determining whether curative therapy of the primary neoplasm is warranted. Although some CT features are more commonly found in metastases, no single feature or combination of features can reliably distinguish a metastasis from an adenoma. Metastases tend to be larger, less well defined, have inhomogeneous attenuation, and a thick irregular enhancing rim. Adenomas tend to be smaller with a homogeneous density. Because morphologic CT features alone do not usually allow an unequivocal differentiation of adrenal adenoma from metastasis, recent attention has centered on the value of CT densitometry.

Many adrenal adenomas have relatively low unenhanced CT attenuation values. Several studies have compared the attenuation values of adrenal adenomas and nonadenomas, and have reported the sensitivity/specificity ratio for diagnosing an adrenal mass as an adenoma at a given threshold attenuation value. In one series, the mean attenuation value of 38 adenomas was 2.2 HU, compared with 28.9 HU for 28 metastases [51]. In another series, the mean value for adenomas versus nonadenomas was 8.6 HU and 30.7 HU, respectively [53]. In our own recent study, we found a mean unenhanced attenuation value of 2.5 HU in 41 adenomas versus 32 HU in 20 nonadenomas

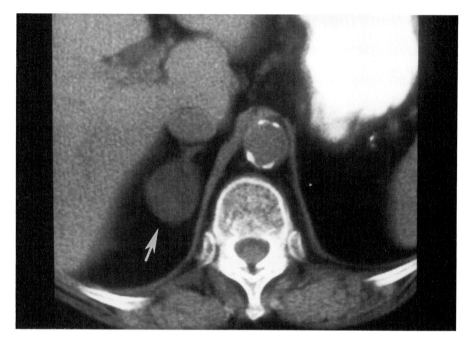

Figure 3. Adrenal adenoma. Unenhanced CT shows a small, sharply marginated right adrenal mass (arrow). The visible low attenuation of the mass measured close to 0 HU is highly suggestive of a benign lesion. (Reprinted with permission from Korobkin and Francis [9].)

[52]. If one combines the results of the four largest published series, there is a 73% sensitivity and 96% specificity for the diagnosis of adrenal adenoma using a threshold value of 10 HU (Fig. 3) [52]. Unlike unenhanced CT attenuation values, enhanced CT values cannot accurately differentiate adrenal adenomas from nonadenomas [52].

Despite the impressive accuracy of unenhanced CT densitometry in characterizing an adrenal mass as an adenoma, its utility is clearly limited by the fact that most abdominal CT is performed with contrast enhancement, necessitating another examination at a later date to obtain an unenhanced scan. To address this limitation, we recently investigated the utility of obtaining a delayed adrenal CT scan 1 hour after routine enhanced abdominal CT demonstrated an adrenal mass [54]. The mean CT attenuation value of 41 adrenal adenomas (11 HU ± 13) was significantly lower (p < 0.001) than 10 adrenal metastases (49 HU ± 8.3). More importantly, there was very little overlap between the two groups. At a threshold value of 30 HU, the sensitivity/specificity ratio for the diagnosis of adrenal adenoma was 95% : 100%. If these results are confirmed with larger numbers and diverse etiologies of nonadenomas, this simple technique could be a practical way to characterize an adrenal incidentaloma.

274

Magnetic resonance imaging

There has been extensive investigation of MRI features of benign and malignant adrenal lesions. Initial studies using low field-strength magnets (0.35–0.5 T) suggested that adrenal adenomas had lower signal intensity on T2-weighted images than did nonadenomas [55–57]. This was reflected in a lower intensity ratio of adrenal tumor to adjacent liver or fat. Subsequent studies showed the separation between the two groups to be incomplete, with an overlap in about 20–30%. The overlap is even more extensive with higher field magnets; at 1.5 T the calculated T2 relaxation time of the tumor was found to be the most useful criterion, but even then some overlap between metastasis and adenoma is observed [58,59].

More recent MRI investigations have evaluated a number of different MRI sequences and techniques, including gradient echo sequences. The most promising of these approaches is chemical-shift imaging. Taking advantage of the different hydrogen-atom resonant-frequency peaks in water and triglyceride (lipid) molecules, this technique results in a decreased signal intensity (SI) of tissue containing both lipid and water compared with tissue without lipid. Previously used to identify fatty infiltration of the liver, this technique was described by Mitchell et al. [60] as an imaging method to detect the significant amount of lipid often present in adrenal adenomas and typically absent in most metastases and other nonadenomatous adrenal masses. Using breath-hold opposed-phase gradient echo imaging, Mitchell et al. [60] showed a relative loss of SI in 95% of adrenal adenomas and in none of the nonadenomatous lesions (Fig. 4). It should be noted that very few adrenocortical carcinomas have been assessed with opposed-phase chemical-shift MRI. Korobkin et al. [61] observed no decrease in relative SI in three carcinomas, but Schlund et al. [62] reported focal regions of SI loss in two cases which correlated with focal collections of macroscopic lipid in the resected specimen. Further experience with adrenocortical carcinomas is necessary to determine if the presence of uniform, rather than focal, areas of chemical-shift change will differentiate benign cortical adenomas from malignant cortical carcinomas.

Despite the growing number of reports that indicate opposed-phase chemical-shift imaging can accurately differentiate adrenal adenomas from nonadenomas, it is still uncertain whether to use quantitative or qualitative methods to assess the images. Tsushima et al. [63] and Bilbey et al. [64] reported 100% accuracy based on quantitative signal-intensity measurements. Korobkin et al. [61] compared quantitative to qualitative assessment of opposed-phase images in 46 adrenal masses. Only adenomas showed a visible decrease in relative signal-intensity ratio (100% specificity), with a sensitivity of 81%. At a quantitative relative SI loss of 12% compared with liver, specificity was 100% and sensitivity was 84%. Mayo-Smith et al. [65] described similar results using the spleen as the reference control organ, reporting that simple visual inspection was nearly identical to quantitative ratios.

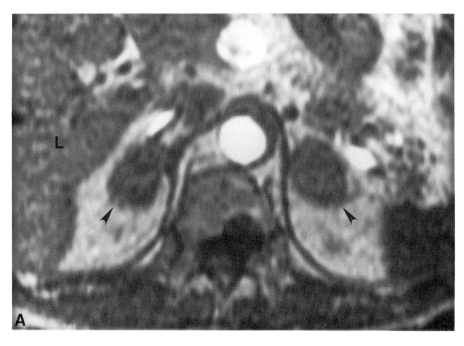

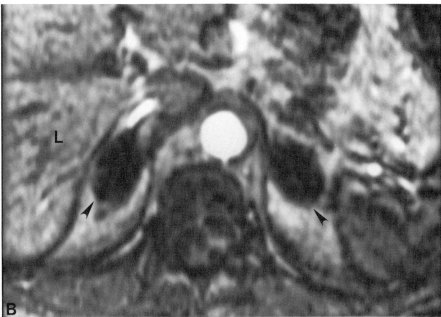

Figure 4. Bilateral adrenal adenomas. **A:** T1-weighted in-phase gradient echo MR shows adrenal masses (arrowheads) that are nearly isointense compared with liver (L). **B:** Out-of-phase image shows the masses (arrowheads) are now markedly hypointense compared with liver (L), highly suggestive of lipid-rich adenomas. (Reprinted with permission from Korobkin and Francis [9].)

276

Many authors have commented on the much greater potential applicability of an MRI characterization scheme based on simple visual analysis rather than quantitative formulas or ratios, regardless of how simple they may seem. The greater the operator-dependent interaction with the console to make measurements or calculations, the less the likely the method will be used [66]. Since qualitative methods appear to be as accurate as quantitative analysis [61,65,67], it seems likely that characterization of adrenal masses by opposed-phase chemical-shift MRI will be made often by simple visual analysis alone.

In order to combine the accuracies of unenhanced CT densitometry and chemical-shift MRI in differentiating benign from malignant adrenal masses, McNicholas et al. [68] developed an algorithm based on their study of 37 adrenal masses using both techniques. MRI adrenal SI normalized to spleen was used to calculate an adrenal-spleen ratio (ASR). The results of their study suggested that lesions of $\leq 0\,HU$ may be regarded as benign without further workup. Lesions with a density $>20\,HU$ are likely to be malignant and should be biopsied if the result will influence patient management. For CT-indeterminate lesions, chemical-shift MR should be obtained: An <70 indicates a benign mass, whereas an ASR >70 needs biopsy to confirm or exclude a metastasis. This report is the first of what will probably be many attempts to synthesize an effective algorithm for use of CT and chemical-shift MR to categorize adrenal masses.

CT and MRI correlations

Recent evidence suggests that the adrenal imaging features that are highly associated with benign adenomas on CT densitometry and chemical-shift MRI are manifestations of the same property, namely, the amount of intracytoplasmic lipid. Although many authorities have previously speculated on this possible association using anecdotal examples, a systematic and quantitative evaluation was lacking. In one recent study a correlation coefficient of 0.88 was found between unenhanced CT attenuation values and quantitative SI loss on out-of-phase chemical-shift MRI in 32 adrenal masses [69]. In addition, both techniques were indeterminate for a similar subset of benign lesions, suggesting that both techniques were measuring the same underlying property of benign adrenal masses.

To evaluate the relationship between lipid in adrenal adenomas and their CT attenuation values and chemical-shift MRI signal intensities, we recently assessed the percent of lipid-rich cortical cells in histologic sections from 26 surgically resected adenomas [70]. We found an inverse linear relationship between the percent of lipid-rich cortical cells in 13 hypersecreting and 13 nonhypersecreting adenomas and their unenhanced CT attenuation value (R^2 = 0.68, p = 0.0005). There was a similar inverse linear relationship to the change in relative MRI SI on opposed-phase chemical-shift images, using both quantitative ($R^2 = 0.83$, $p = 0.004$) and qualitative ($R^2 = 0.70$, $p = 0.019$) assessments. Our results suggest that the amount of intratumoral lipid accounts for the presence and degree of low CT attenuation and relative loss of opposed-phase MRI SI observed in many adrenal adenomas.

Radionuclide scintigraphy

The first radiocholesterol analog localization studies were performed in the late 1960s and early 1970s [35]. [^{131}I]-6-beta-iodomethyl-norcholesterol (NP59) and [^{75}Se]-selenomethyl-norcholesterol (Scintadren®) are the two agents in current clinical use. Steroid hormone-producing tissues, such as the adrenal cortex, ovarian corpora lutea, and the testicular Leydig cells, store cholesterol, which is the synthetic backbone from which all steroid hormones are synthesized. Eighty percent of cholesterol for adrenal steroidogenesis is from plasma low-density lipoproteins (LDL) and the remainder from de novo biosynthesis from acetate [34,71]. Twenty percent of the intravenously injected radiotracer is bound to LDL and a fraction undergoes cell-membrane LDL-receptor–mediated uptake into the adrenal cortex [33,35]. These radiocholesterol analogs are esterified and stored in intracellular lipid droplets and effectively trapped, because less than 4% are converted to measurable adrenal steroid hormone metabolites [33,35]. Calculated normal adrenal uptake of the injected dose ranges from 0.07% to 0.26% (mean 0.16%) for each gland. Uptake is positively influenced by ACTH stimulation and is negatively influenced by intravascular volume status and serum total and LDL cholesterol [34,35]. LDL receptors appear to be overexpressed in some adrenal tumors [72].

The usual NP59 dose is 1 mCi (37 MBq) administered intravenously [32]. Saturated potassium iodide solution (SSKI, one drop in any beverage three times per day), Lugol's solution, or another suitable iodine-containing preparation is begun 48 hours before NP59 injection and is continued for 14 days to block thyroidal uptake of free ^{131}I derived from in vivo deiodination. A laxative is used to decrease bowel background radioactivity, given the significant enterohepatic circulation and gastrointestinal excretion of NP59 (bisacodyl 10 mg orally two times daily beginning 2 days before imaging). Images are obtained by a gamma camera with a parallel-hole collimator interfaced with a dedicated, digital computer typically on days 5, 6, or 7 following NP59 administration ($\geq$50,000 counts/image). Additional images may be obtained daily or on alternate days for up to 3 weeks, but rarely are more than 1–2 days of imaging necessary.

The posterior view affords the best adrenal gland visualization and is often the only image necessary. The right adrenal gland is usually more cephalad and posterior than the left. Consequently, normal posterior images demonstrate equal or very slightly greater radiotracer accumulation in the right adrenal gland compared with the left, while the opposite is true for the anterior view [35]. A lateral view may assist in differentiating left adrenal gland radiotracer accumulation from hepatic activity, or right adrenal gland accumulation from gallbladder activity. NP59 and/or [^{75}Se]-selenomethylnorcholesterol is widely commercially available throughout the world as a routine imaging agent (especially in Europe). In the United States, NP59 is available as an investigational new drug (IND) and can be obtained on a regular basis from the University of Michigan Nuclear Pharmacy after filing an abbreviated Physician Sponsored IND Application with the U.S. Food and Drug Administration.

Adrenal scintigraphy is comparable with thyroid scanning to characterize lesions as nonfunctioning ('cold,' and possibly malignant) versus functioning ('hot,' and probably benign) [1]. Nonhypersecretory adrenocortical carcinomas, metastases, pheochromocytomas, and other space-occupying or destructive lesions (e.g., nonadenomas) demonstrate decreased, distorted, or absent radiocholesterol uptake in the affected adrenal gland (discordant image; see Fig. 2). Hormonally hypersecretory and nonhypersecretory adrenal adenomas, as well as a rare minority of hypersecretory adrenocortical carcinomas, demonstrate increased NP59 accumulation (concordant image; Fig. 5). Most hypersecretory adrenocortical carcinomas are inefficient tumors with respect to hormone synthesis and uptake of the radiolabeled hormone precursor (as are thyroid cancers). Thus, there is typically adrenal nonvisualization bilaterally with Cushing's syndrome caused by an adrenocortical carcinoma due to poor tumor radiotracer uptake and suppressed function of normal adrenocortical tissues [1].

With over 25 years of experience to date, in the setting of a normal bio-

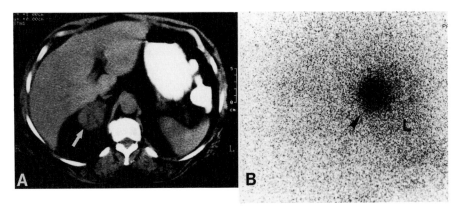

Figure 5. Adrenal adenoma. **A:** Contrast-enhanced abdominal CT demonstrates an inhomogeneous 5.3 × 4.7 cm right adrenal mass (arrow) and a normal left adrenal gland (not shown) with normal adrenal hormone secretion by routine testing. **B:** Posterior NP59 scan 5 days after radiotracer administration demonstrates a concordant image pattern with marked uptake within the right adrenal mass (arrowhead), normal liver (L) uptake, and suppressed uptake in the left adrenal gland.

chemical screening evaluation (and the absence of interfering medications, e.g., mitotane), NP59 avidity has been a 100% accurate predictor of benignity, while discordant imaging has been a 100% accurate predictor of a nonadenomatous lesion [1]. Similar accuracy has been reported with [^{75}Se]-selenomethyl-norcholesterol [73]. Symmetrical NP59 uptake bilaterally (normal, or nonlateralizing scan pattern) is seen in all periadrenal and pseudoadrenal masses. Unfortunately, nonlateralizing scans occur in some patients harboring both benign and malignant adrenal masses ≤2 cm. This fact is reflected in the decreased sensitivity and predictive value of a negative test for detecting nonadenomatous lesions reported in 220 nonhypersecretory unilateral adrenal incidentalomas of all sizes by Gross et al. [74]. Scintigraphic images were concordant in 159, discordant in 44, and nonlateralizing in 17 intra-adrenal masses, yielding a sensitivity of 72%, a specificity of 100%, an accuracy (diagnostic image) of 92%, a negative predictive value of 90%, and a positive predictive value of 100%. In a recent analysis of unilateral adrenal masses ≤3 cm, nonhypersecretory masses ≤1 cm, >1 to ≤2 cm, and >2 to ≤3 cm yielded diagnostic (e.g., lateralizing) images in 52%, 89%, and 100% of patients, respectively. Nonadenomatous lesions, including malignancies, >1 to ≤2 cm and >2 to ≤3 cm were present in 9% and 10% of patients, respectively [75]. Given its reasonably high sensitivity and favorable costs, adrenocortical scintigraphy may be the single most cost-effective diagnostic modality to characterize the adrenal incidentaloma [76].

Optimal follow-up for nonhypersecretory adrenal adenomas is not known. In a small number of documented instances, progression to frank Cushing's syndrome has occurred. We suggest a minimum of an annual complete history and physical examination. Overnight dexamethasone-suppression testing on an infrequent basis may also be reasonable. There are currently no data to support the use of serial NP59 scintigraphy.

As with scintigraphic imaging of functioning thyroid nodules, unilateral nonhypersecretory adrenal adenomas produce a range of patterns in remaining normal tissue from clear visualization to absent uptake (see Fig. 5) [1]. It is likely that NP59 uptake in normal tissue is reduced in these latter cases due to ACTH suppression (albeit incomplete or partial) by the functioning adenoma, suggesting autonomy and relative hypersecretion despite 'normal' biochemistry based on simple screening tests (such as the 24-hour UFC and 1-mg overnight DST). Presently, there is no evidence that these patients benefit from adrenalectomy unless clear biochemical evidence of Cushing's syndrome develops (with or without clinical features). Optimal follow-up for these patients is not known. A prudent approach may be 6-month follow-up history and physical examinations along with 1-mg overnight DST screening for 1 year, then annually for several years, and eventually decreasing the biochemical evaluation to every 2–5 years.

Adrenal masses are bilateral in 11–16% of incidentaloma cases [1,27]. Haab et al. reported six cases with bilateral masses and normal biochemical evaluations. Surgical pathology demonstrated bilateral metastases in two and bilateral adenomas in four [77]. In this setting, Gross et al. [78] considered visual NP59 uptake that is greater than equal to that in the contralateral adrenal gland and/or liver (as a normal reference tissue) to compatible with a benign process, while NP59 uptake markedly less than the contralateral adrenal gland and/or liver was compatible with a nonadenomatous lesion. Adrenal metastases were reported in 45% of cases, despite 59% of cases having pre-existing malignancies. Further, 7% had both a nonhypersecretory adrenal adenoma and a contralateral *smaller* metastasis. These findings suggest that NP59 scintigraphy may identify bilateral benign adrenal masses, as well as those toward which further evaluation should be directed. Clinical and bio-chemical evaluations in this setting remain critical given the likely increased presence of CAH and the uncommon occurrence of primary adrenal insuffi-ciency from bilateral destruction by solid tumor metastases, hematologic ma-lignancy, hemorrhage, infection, or granulomatous diseases.

Positron emission tomography

PET with 2-[fluorine-18]-fluoro-2-deoxy-D-glucose (FDG) has been used to characterize adrenal masses (1.5–10 cm in diameter; mean 2.8 cm) in 20 pa-tients with cancer [79]. PET tumor-to-background ratios [standardized uptake value (SUV)] correctly differentiated benign (0.2–1.2 SUV) from all malignant lesions (2.9–16.6 SUV). However, adrenal masses <1.5 cm were excluded, and the estimated spatial resolution is 1 cm (possibly less for lesions with intense FDG uptake). This remarkable separation of benign from malignant tumors has not yet been our experience (unpublished observation), nor has is been duplicated by others. Further, the SUV as a quantitative measure for this purpose has come under strong criticism [80]. Nevertheless, additional study is clearly warranted.

Percutaneous adrenal biopsy

Percutaneous adrenal biopsy is commonly used for the evaluation of adrenal masses detected by CT in patients with a known primary neoplasm and either no other evidence of metastatic disease or no other lesions more amenable to biopsy. A positive biopsy will usually place a patient into a nonsurgical treat-ment regimen, whereas a negative biopsy may allow for curative resection of the primary neoplasm. As with many endocrine tissues, histologic distinction between benign and well-differentiated primary malignancy of the adrenal gland is often difficult, with a reported cytologic sensitivity of only 54–86% [1]. Furthermore, it should be emphasized that if adrenal carcinoma is suspected and there is no evidence of metastastic disease, we consider percutaneous adrenal biospy relatively contraindicated because of the possibility of implan-tation of malignant cells in the retroperitoneum in a patient who may other-wise be potentially curable.

Percutaneous adrenal biopsies are usually performed with 20- to 22-gauge needles, although a larger caliber needle (18- or 19-gauge) can be used without increased morbidity [81]. Either a single-needle or coaxial technique can be used. For a right adrenal mass, either a posterior approach (in the prone or right lateral decubitus position) or a supine transhepatic approach (to help avoid a pneumothorax) is used. A left adrenal mass biopsy is usually more difficult because the posterior approach is often the only safe one available. Biopsy of a left adrenal mass from an anterior approach has a small, but not insignificant, risk of severe acute pancreatitis because the needle often traverses the pancreatic tail [82].

Bleeding and pneumothorax are the most common complications of percutaneous adrenal biopsy [83]. Less commonly observed is significant pain, fever, bacteremia, abdominal discomfort and nausea, needle-tract metastasis (Fig. 6), and severe acute pancreatitis [82–85]. Overall complication rates range from 8% to 12.7% when mild and self-limited events are included [84–87]. The rate is closer to 3% when only major complications are included, that is, those requiring hospitalization or therapeutic intervention [81,83].

Unlike percutaneous biopsy of many other abdominal masses, cytological assessment of aspirated specimens is usually sufficient, obviating the need for core biopsies. Adrenal masses are often quite small, and multiple biopsies of a single mass can be necessary for adequate sampling [84,88]. Silverman et al. [86] reported an 86% diagnostic result on initial biopsy. Bernardino et al. [89] similarly reported a correct diagnosis in 83% of their patients on initial biopsy. Four of their nine failures had repeat procedures, which yielded an overall accuracy of 90.6% when both biopsies were included. The overall accuracies of fine-needle aspiration biopsy of adrenal masses range from 80% to 100%, and with experienced cytopathologists the positive predictive value approaches 100% [1]. The false-negative rate (probability that a metastasis is present given a negative result) depends on the size of the adrenal mass. Silverman et al. [86] reported an overall negative predictive value of 91%, but this increased to 100% for masses ≥3 cm.

We routinely administer local anesthesia with 1% subcutaneous lidocaine for the biopsy procedure; intravenous sedation is rarely used. All patients have screening coagulation studies [prothrombin time (PT), partial thromboplastin time (PTT), and platelets] prior to the procedure and are questioned regarding a history of bleeding disorders. We have a cytopathologist present to review the material after each pass to determine if sufficient tissue was obtained for diagnosis in order to reduce the number of nondiagnostic procedures. Outpatients are typically monitored by a nurse for 4 hours and then discharged with appropriate instructions.

A positive biopsy is defined as the presence of malignant cells. A biopsy is considered consistent with an adrenal adenoma if it contains normal or benign-appearing adrenal cortical cells, no malignant cells, and the needle tip is demonstrated to be in the adrenal mass by cross-sectional imaging (almost always CT). A biopsy is considered insufficient, or nondiagnostic, if adrenal

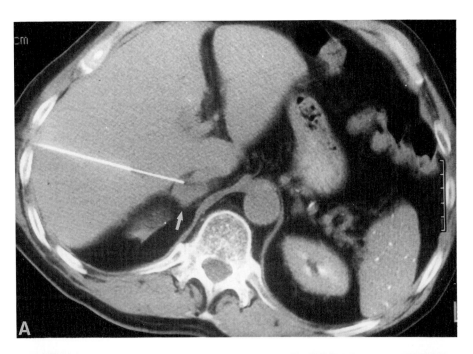

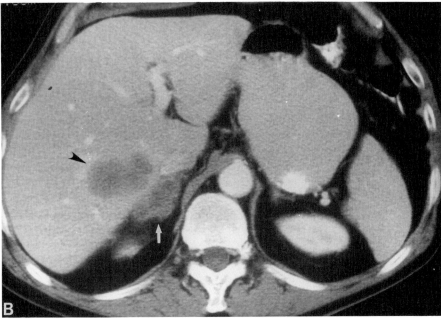

Figure 6. Needle-tract metastasis complicating percutaneous adrenal biopsy. **A:** Coaxial needle biopsy in a patient with lung cancer and an adrenal mass (arrow). The biopsy was positive for metastasis. **B:** A CT scan 5 months later shows a new solitary liver lesion (arrowhead) along the previous needle tract and an enlarging adrenal metastasis (arrow). (Reprinted with permission from Mody et al. [83].)

cortical cells and malignant cells are absent. Nondiagnostic aspiration biopsy rates have ranged from 6% to 12% [83,84,90].

Surgery

Currently, the adrenal mass discovered incidental to an imaging study obtained for a variety of reasons unrelated to suspected adrenal pathology is the most common problem referred to a surgeon for possible adrenalectomy. As noted earlier, all such patients require a careful biochemical assessment of the secretory activity of the mass before a rational decision can be made as to further management. With rare exception, we consider all patients with hypersecretory neoplasms as surgical candidates. These include patients with neoplasms secreting catecholamines, cortisol, mineralocorticoids, and rarely sex hormones. Rarely, patients are judged to be of an unacceptably high surgical risk. A small but promising literature is accruing that suggests the successful use of percutaneous ethanol injection therapy to treat hypersecretory adrenocortical adenomas in such patients [91,92]. Long-term studies will be needed before final conclusions may be drawn regarding the final efficacy and safety of the procedure, Venous retrograde adrenal gland ablation is not employed given reports of only temporary success, intense longlasting pain, and safety concerns [92]. Chemoembolization of adrenocortical carcinomas has been shown to slow tumor growth in otherwise inoperable patients [92].

Patients with pheochromocytomas are prepared for surgery with a 1- to 2-week course of alpha-adrenergic blockade starting with phenoxybenzamine (Dibenzyline) 10mg four times a day, with a doubling of the dose every other day until orthostatic hypotension has been noted. This serves as an endpoint for the dose escalation. Most patients are also given a beta blocker (e.g., Inderal 20mg) early on the morning of surgery with a sip of water. Our preferred surgical approach continues to be transabdominal through an upper abdominal bucket handle or chevron incision, which allows for the exposure of both adrenal glands and a retroperitoneal exploration for a possible occult extra-adrenal pheochromocytoma (paraganglioma). The right adrenal is exposed after mobilizing the right lobe of the liver medially and performing a Kocher maneuver. This allows an essentially 'on touch' technique of the tumor until the inferior phrenic vessels have been clipped and divided as well as the short central adrenal vein. The left adrenal is approached through the lesser sac after mobilizing the body and tail of the pancreas anteriorly, allowing direct exposure of the left renal and central adrenal veins. The latter is ligated and divided without tumor manipulation. This lateral and cephalic dissection allows exposure, clipping, and division of the inferior phrenic vessels, after which the adrenal gland can be manipulated without release of catecholamines. When the tumor has been excised, the contralateral adrenal gland is then palpated to rule out an occult tumor. The Kocher maneuver is extended to include the right colon and the retroperitoneum from the celiac axis to the pelvis to quickly facilitate exclusion of a coexistant paraganglioma.

Currently there are two alternative approaches to the small (<6 cm) incidental pheochromocytoma in the nonfamilial setting. These approaches are based on the assumption that current imaging using CT, MRI, and MIBG are nearly 100% reliable in confirming that a pheochromocytoma is singular and apparently benign. One is an open, unilateral posterior approach through the bed of the 12th rib, and the other is a minimally invasive laparoscopic procedure, either through the abdomen or most recently through the retroperitoneum [2,93–104]. Thus far, in experienced hands, these procedures appear to be safe and are gaining increasing acceptance and popularity. The obvious advantages of these alternative approaches are less disability and a shorter period of hospitalization. It is likely that the laparoscopic approach will be used with increasing frequency in the future, accepting the fact that the rare patient might have an overlooked, occult second lesion.

For patients with an aldosteronoma (and occasionally for primary aldosteronism secondary to markedly asymmetric bilateral adrenocortical hyperplasia), a unilateral adrenalectomy is performed with a posterior approach through the bed of the 12th rib. Again, an alternative procedure would be through a laparoscopic approach transabdominally or through the retroperitoneum. As experience is gained with the laparoscopic adrenalectomy, it is anticipated that this will be the procedure of choice for aldosteronomas.

We recommend unilateral adrenalectomy for patients with unilateral ACTH-independent Cushing's or pre-Cushing's syndrome. These patients require perioperative glucocorticoid stress therapy with rapid tapering to a maintenance dose of 30–35 mg of hydrocortisone per day. Many of these patients can be weaned from steroid replacement therapy after 3–6 months, but more prolonged adrenal suppression is not uncommon. The standard surgical approach in this group is posteriorly through the bed of the 12th rib. Here also, laparoscopic adrenalectomy for tumors <6 cm in diameter is becoming increasingly popular.

Nonhypersecretory adrenal masses that fail to concentrate NP59, or are considered nonadenomatous by a reliable anatomical imaging technique, are of concern because of the possibility of either primary adrenocortical carcinoma or metastatic disease to the adrenal gland. When the patient has a known previous malignancy and no other evidence of metastatic disease, percutaneous fine-needle aspiration cytology may be considered when the lesion is suspected to be a metastasis. Adrenalectomy should be considered in exceptional circumstances, such as in lung cancer and renal-cell carcinoma metastatic to the adrenal gland with no other detectable disease [2,105,106]. The adrenal appears to be the site of predilection for solitary metastases with this latter neoplasm, and a long-term tumor-free interval may result from its resection [7]. Further, a small literature exists suggesting the possibility of partial adrenalectomy with preservation of adrenal function in patients with bilateral adrenal involvement [107]. Adrenalectomy is indicated for suspected adrenocortical carcinoma. In selected patients with recurrent and/or extra-adrenal metastases, repeated surgical resection possibly offers extended palliation [108].

Conclusions

The optimal approach to the incidental adrenal mass remains highly controversial. We strongly emphasize biochemical screening for adrenal hormone hypersecretion in all patients. Size criteria lack utility because many adrenal adenomas are large, while some metastases and potentially curable adrenocortical carcinomas are small. Unenhanced CT attenuation values are currently the most useful CT measure to separate adrenal adenomas ($<$0–10 HU) from nonadenomatous lesions. Exciting preliminary data suggest that similar utility may be derived from 1-hour post-contrast attenuation values ($<$30 HU). Unlike routine MRI characteristics, MR chemical-shift imaging appears to contribute significantly toward characterization of adrenal masses by demonstrating the lipid-rich composition of most adrenal adenomas (and all myelolipomas) compared with the lipid-depleted nature of the vast majority of nonadenomatous lesions. NP59 scintigraphy has been 100% accurate in correctly characterizing all nonhypersecretory adrenal masses $>$2 cm in greatest diameter as either adenomas or nonadenomas, and offers accurate diagnoses in the majority of masses $\leq$2 cm. It may be the single most cost-effective diagnostic modality. However, NP59 is not commercially available in the United States, and the repeated visits for radiotracer injection and imaging are inconvenient.

One preliminary study on PET reported dramatic accuracy. However, this method has not been confirmed by others and must be considered investigational until further characterized. The frequent cytological difficulty of distinguishing benign from malignant endocrine tissues and the low, but appreciable, rate of complications limit the primary role of percutaneous adrenal biopsy. The procedure may be best utilized to further characterize an adrenal mass deemed nonadenomatous, or suspicious, by a noninvasive technique in a patient with a potentially respectable known extra-adrenal primary malignancy without evidence of other metastatic foci. The use of accurate noninvasive testing has greatly reduced the number of unnecessary surgical procedures. Adrenalectomy is generally reserved for unilateral hypersecretory processes and nonadenomatous lesions suspicious for adrenocortical carcinoma. Perioperative care of patients with pheochromocytomas and Cushing's syndrome remains critical. Open adrenalectomy techniques are the current standard of care and should be employed when malignancy is likely, given the need for intraoperative staging and the decreased risk of seeding malignant cells when the tumor is removed intact. Laparoscopic adrenalectomy is rapidly gaining favor and is likely to soon be the procedure of choice for most benign unilateral hypersecretory lesions.

References

1. Kloos RT, Gross MD, Francis IR, Korobkin M, Shapiro B. 1995. Incidentally discovered adrenal masses. Endocr Rev 16:460–484.
2. Kloos RT, Shapiro B, Gross MD. 1995. The adrenal incidentaloma. Curr Opin Endocrinol Diabetes 2:222–230.
3. Allard P, Yankaskas BC, Fletcher RH, Parker LA, Halvorsen RA Jr. 1990. Sensitivity and specificity of computed tomography for the detection of adrenal metastatic lesions among 91 autopsied lung cancer patients. Cancer 66:457–462.
4. Rubenstein SC, Benacerraf BR, Retik AB, Mandell J. 1995. Fetal suprarenal masses: Sonographic appearance and differential diagnosis. Ultrasound Obstet Gynecol 5:164–167.
5. Gicquel C, Bertagna X, Le Bouc Y. 1995. Recent advances in the pathogenesis of adrenocortical tumours. Eur J Endocrinol 133:133–144.
6. Haak HR, Fleuren GJ. 1995. Neuroendocrine differentiation of adrenocortical tumors. Cancer 75:860–864.
7. Barnes RD, Abratt RP, Cant PJ, Dent DM. 1995. Synchronous contralateral adrenal metastasis from renal cell carcinoma: A 7 year survival following resection. Aust N Z J Surg 65:540–541.
8. Higashiyama M, Doi O, Kodama K, Yokouchi H, Imaoka S, Koyama H. 1994. Surgical treatment of adrenal metastasis following pulmonary resection for lung cancer: Comparison of adrenalectomy with palliative therapy. Int Surg 79:124–129.
9. Korobkin M, Francis IR. 1995. Adrenal imaging. Semin Ultrasound CT MR 16:317–330.
10. Kasperlik-Zaluska AA, Migdalska BM, Zgliczynski S, Makowska AM, Kasperlik-Zauska AA. 1995. Adrenocortical carcinoma. A clinical study and treatment results of 52 patients. Cancer 75:2587–2591.
11. Favia G, Lumachi F, Carraro P, D'Amico DF. 1995. Adrenocortical carcinoma. Our experience. Minerva Endocrinol 20:95–99.
12. Boscaro M, Fallo F, Barzon L, Daniele O, Sonino N. 1995. Adrenocortical carcinoma: Epidemiology and natural history. Minerva Endocrinol 20:89–94.
13. Lenders JW, Keiser HR, Goldstein DS, Willemsen JJ, Friberg P, Jacobs MC, Kloppenborg PW, Thien T, Eisenhofer G. 1995. Plasma metanephrines in the diagnosis of pheochromocytoma [see comments]. Ann Intern Med 123:101–109.
14. Bravo EL. 1994. Evolving concepts in the pathophysiology, diagnosis, and treatment of pheochromocytoma. Endocr Rev 15:356–368.
15. Bravo EL, Gifford RW Jr. 1984. Current concepts. Pheochromocytoma: Diagnosis, localization and management. N Engl J Med 311:1298–1303.
16. Weinberger MH, Fineberg NS. 1993. The diagnosis of primary aldosteronism and separation of two major subtypes. Arch Intern Med 153:2125–2129.
17. Weigel RJ, Wells SA, Gunnells JC, Leight GS. 1994. Surgical treatment of primary hyperaldosteronism. Ann Surg 219:347–352.
18. Melby JC, Azar ST. 1993. Adrenal steroids and hypertension: New aspects. Endocrinologist 3:344–351.
19. Bravo EL. 1993. Primary aldosteronism: New approaches to diagnosis and management. Cleve Clin J Med 60:379–386.
20. Bunnag P, Tuck ML. 1995. Captopril test in the evaluation of primary aldosteronism. Endocrinologist 5:253–257.
21. Hoefnagel CA. 1994. Metaiodobenzylguanidine and somatostatin in oncology: Role in the management of neural crest tumours. Eur J Nucl Med 21:561–581.

22. Pujol P, Bringer J, Faurous P, Jaffiol C. 1995. Metastatic phaeochromocytoma with a long-term response after iodine-131 metaiodobenzylguanidine therapy. Eur J Nucl Med 22:382–384.

23. Elgazzar AH, Gelfand MJ, Washburn LC, Clark J, Nagaraj N, Cummings D, Hughes J, Maxon HR. 1995. I-123 MIBG scintigraphy in adults. A report of clinical experience. Clin Nucl Med 20:147–152.

24. Tenenbaum F, Lumbroso J, Schlumberger M, Mure A, Plouin PF, Caillou B, Parmentier C. 1995. Comparison of radiolabeled octreotide and meta-iodobenzylguanidine (MIBG) scintigraphy in malignant pheochromocytoma. J Nucl Med 36:1–6.

25. Maurea S, Lastoria S, Cuocolo A, Celentano L, Salvatore M. 1995. The diagnosis of nonfunctioning pheochromocytoma. The role of I-123 MIBG imaging. Clin Nucl Med 20:22–24.

26. Flecchia D, Mazza E, Carlini M, Blatto A, Olivieri F, Serra G, Camanni F, Messina M. 1995. Reduced serum levels of dehydroepiandrosterone sulphate in adrenal incidentalomas: A marker of adrenocortical tumour. Clin Endocrinol (Oxf) 42:129–134.

27. Ambrosi B, Peverelli S, Passini E, Re T, Ferrario R, Colombo P, Sartorio A, Faglia G. 1995. Abnormalities of endocrine function in patients with clinically 'silent' adrenal masses [see comments]. Eur J Endocrinol 132:422–428.

28. Terzolo M, Osella G, Ali A, Reimondo G, Borretta G, Magro GP, Luceri S, Paccotti P, Angeli A. 1995. Adrenal incidentaloma, a five year experience. Minerva Endocrinol 20:69–78.

29. Papanicolaou DA, Yanovski JA, Cutler GB, Chrousos GP, Nieman LK. 1994. A single midnight cortisol measurement discriminates Cushing syndrome from pseudoCushing states. 76th Annual Meeting of the Endocrine Society Program and Abstracts Book; June 15–18; Anaheim, CA The Endocrine Society Press, Bethesda, MD, p 518.

30. Crapo L. 1979. Cushing's syndrome: A review of diagnostic tests. Metabolism 28:955–977.

31. Suzuki H, Shibata H, Takita T, Wakino S, Ogishima T, Ishimura Y, Saruta T. 1994. Steroid contents and cortical steroidogenic enzymes in non-hyperfunctioning adrenal adenoma. Endocr J 41:267–274.

32. Thrall JH, Freitas JE, Beierwaltes WH. 1978. Adrenal scintigraphy. Semin Nucl Med 8:23–41.

33. Gross MD, Shapiro B. 1989. Scintigraphic studies in adrenal hypertension. Semin Nucl Med 19:122–143.

34. Gross MD, Valk TW, Swanson DP, Thrall JH, Grekin RJ, Beirewaltes WH. 1981. The role of pharmacologic manipulation in adrenal cortical scintigraphy. Semin Nucl Med 11:128–148.

35. Gross MD, Thrall JH, Beierwaltes WH. 1980. The adrenal scan: A current status report on radiotracers, dosimetry, and clinical utility. In Freeman LM, Weissmann HS, eds. Nuclear Medicine Annual 1980. New York: Raven Press, pp 127–175.

36. Aupetit-Faisant B, Blanchouin-Emeric N, Tenenbaum F, Battaglia C, Tabarin A, Amar J, Kuttenn F, Warnet A, Assayag M, Chamontin B. 1995. Plasma levels of aldosterone versus aldosterone precursors: A way to estimate the malignancy of asymptomatic and nonsecretory adrenal tumors: A French Retrospective Multicentric Study. J Clin Endocrinol Metab 80:2715–2721.

37. Osella G, Terzolo M, Borretta G, Magro G, Ali A, Piovesan A, Paccotti P, Angeli A. 1994. Endocrine evaluation of incidentally discovered adrenal masses (incidentalomas). J Clin Endocrinol Metab 79:1532–1539.

38. Del Monte P, Bernasconi D, Bertolazzi L, Meozzi M, Badaracco B, Torre R, Marugo M. 1995. Increased 17 alpha-hydroxyprogesterone response to ACTH in silent adrenal adenoma: Cause or effect? Clin Endocrinol (Oxf) 42:273–277.

39. Sciarra F, Tosti-Croce C, Toscano V. 1995. Androgen-secreting adrenal tumors. Minerva Endocrinol 20:63–68.

40. Palmer WE, Gerard-McFarland EL, Chew FS. 1991. Adrenal myelolipoma [clinical conference]. Am J Roentgenol 156:724.

288

41. Wolverson MK, Kannegiesser H. 1984. CT of bilateral adrenal hemorrhage with acute adrenal insufficiency in the adult. Am J Roentgenol 142:311–314.

42. Bowen AD, Keslar PJ, Newman B, Hashida Y. 1990. Adrenal hemorrhage after liver transplantation. Radiology 176:85–88.

43. Murphy BJ, Casillas J, Yrizarry JM. 1988. Traumatic adrenal hemorrhage: Radiologic findings. Radiology 169:701–703.

44. Spinelli C, Materazzi G, Berti P, Cecchi M, Morelli G, Miccoli P. 1995. Symptomatic adrenal myelolipoma: Therapeutic considerations. Eur J Surg Oncol 21:403–407.

45. Sanders R, Bissada N, Curry N, Gordon B. 1995. Clinical spectrum of adrenal myelolipoma: Analysis of 8 tumors in 7 patients. J Urol 153:1791–1793.

46. Johnson CD, Baker ME, Dunnick NR. 1985. CT demonstration of an adrenal pseudocyst. J Comput Assist Tomogr 9:817–819.

47. Wilson DA, Muchmore HG, Tisdal RG, Fahmy A, Pitha JV. 1984. Histoplasmosis of the adrenal glands studied by CT. Radiology 150:779–783.

48. Fishman EK, Deutch BM, Hartman DS, Goldman SM, Zerhouni EA, Siegelman SS. 1987. Primary adrenocortical carcinoma: CT evaluation with clinical correlation. Am J Roentgenol 148:531–535.

49. Dunnick NR, Heaston D, Halvorsen R, Moore AV, Korobkin M. 1982. CT appearance of adrenal cortical carcinoma. J Comput Assist Tomogr 6:978–982.

50. van Erkel AR, van Gils AP, Lequin M, Kruitwagen C, Bloem JL, Falke TH. 1994. CT and MR distinction of adenomas and nonadenomas of the adrenal gland. J Comput Assist Tomogr 18:432–438.

51. Lee MJ, Hahn PF, Papanicolaou N, Egglin TK, Saini S, Mueller PR, Simeone JF. 1991. Benign and malignant adrenal masses: CT distinction with attenuation coefficients, size, and observer analysis. Radiology 179:415–418.

52. Korobkin M, Brodeur FJ, Yutzy GG, Francis IR, Quint LE, Dunnick NR, Kazerooni EA. 1996. Differentiation of adrenal adenomas from nonadenomas using CT attenuation values. Am J Roentgenol 166:531–536.

53. Wilms GE, Baert AL, Kint EJ, Pringot JH, Goddeeris PG. 1983. Computed tomographic findings in bilateral adrenal tuberculosis. Radiology 146:729–730.

54. Brodeur FJ, Korobkin M, Francis IR, Quint LE, Dunnick NR. 1995. Delayed enhanced CT: A method of differentiating adrenal adenomas from nonadenomas (abstr). Radiology 197:185.

55. Reinig JW, Doppman JL, Dwyer AJ, Frank J. 1986. MRI of indeterminate adrenal masses. Am J Roentgenol 147:493–496.

56. Glazer GM, Woolsey EJ, Borrello J, Francis IR, Aisen AM, Bookstein F, Amendola MA, Gross MD, Bree RL, Martel W. 1986. Adrenal tissue characterization using MR imaging. Radiology 158:73–79.

57. Chang A, Glazer HS, Lee JK, Ling D, Heiken JP. 1987. Adrenal gland: MR imaging. Radiology 163:123–128.

58. Baker ME, Blinder R, Spritzer C, Leight GS, Herfkens RJ, Dunnick NR. 1989. MR evaluation of adrenal masses at 1.5 T. Am J Roentgenol 153:307–312.

59. Kier R, McCarthy S. 1989. MR characterization of adrenal masses: Field strength and pulse sequence considerations. Radiology 171:671–674.

60. Mitchell DG, Outwater EK, Matteucci T, Rubin DL, Chezmar JL, Saini S. 1995. Adrenal gland enhancement at MR imaging with Mn-DPDP. Radiology 194:783–787.

61. Korobkin M, Lombardi TJ, Aisen AM, Francis IR, Quint LE, Dunnick NR, Londy F, Shapiro B, Gross MD, Thompson NW. 1995. Characterization of adrenal masses with chemical shift and gadolinium-enhanced MR imaging. Radiology 197:411–418.

62. Schlund JF, Kenney PJ, Brown ED, Ascher SM, Brown JJ, Semelka RC. 1995. Adrenocortical carcinoma: MR imaging appearance with current techniques. J Magn Reson Imaging 5:171–174.

63. Tsushima Y, Ishizaka H, Matsumoto M. 1993. Adrenal masses: Differentiation with chemical shift, fast low-angle shot MR imaging. Radiology 186:705–709.

64. Bilbey JH, McLoughlin RF, Kurkjian PS, Wilkins GE, Chan NH, Schmidt N, Singer J. 1995. MR imaging of adrenal masses: Value of chemical-shift imaging for distinguishing adenomas from other tumors [see comments]. Am J Roentgenol 164:637–642.
65. Mayo-Smith WW, Lee MJ, McNicholas MM, Hahn PF, Boland GW, Saini S. 1995. Characterization of adrenal masses (<5 cm) by use of chemical shift MR imaging: Observer performance versus quantitative measures. Am J Roentgenol 165:91–95.
66. Reinig JW. 1991. Differentiation of hepatic lesions with MR imaging: The last word? [editorial]. Radiology 179:601–602.
67. Outwater EK, Siegelman ES, Radecki PD, Piccoli CW, Mitchell DG. 1995. Distinction between benign and malignant adrenal masses: Value of T1-weighted chemical-shift MR imaging. Am J Roentgenol 165:579–583.
68. McNicholas MM, Lee MJ, Mayo-Smith WW, Hahn PF, Boland GW, Mueller PR. 1995. An imaging algorithm for the differential diagnosis of adrenal adenomas and metastases. Am J Roentgenol 165:1453–1459.
69. Outwater EK, Siegelman ES, Shapiro MA. 1995. Correlation of CT and chemical shift MR imaging measurements of lipid in adrenal lesions (abstr). Radiology 197:184.
70. Korobkin MT, Giordano TJ, Brodeur FJ, Francis IR, Quint LE, Dunnick NR. 1995. Relationship between histologic lipid and CT and MR imaging findings in surgically resected adrenal adenomas (abstr). Radiology 197:185.
71. Orth DN, Kovacs WJ, deBold CR. 1991. The adrenal cortex. In Wilson JD, Foster DW, eds. Williams' Textbook of Endocrinology 8th ed. Philadelphia: WB Saunders, pp 489–619.
72. Nakagawa T, Ueyama Y, Nozaki S, Yamashita S, Menju M, Funahashi T, Kameda-Takemura K, Kubo M, Tokunaga K, Tanaka T. 1995. Marked hypocholesterolemia in a case with adrenal adenoma — enhanced catabolism of low density lipoprotein (LDL) via the LDL receptors of tumor cells. J Clin Endocrinol Metab 80:92–96.
73. Dominguez-Gadea L, Diez L, Bas C, Crespo A. 1994. Differential diagnosis of solid adrenal masses using adrenocortical scintigraphy. Clin Radiol 49:796–799.
74. Gross MD, Shapiro B, Francis IR, Glazer GM, Bree RL, Arcomano MA, Schteingart DE, McLeod MK, Sanfield JA, Thompson NW. 1994. Scintigraphic evaluation of clinically silent adrenal masses [see comments]. J Nucl Med 35:1145–1152.
75. Kloos RT, Gross MD, Shapiro B, Francis IR, Korobkin M, Thompson NW. 1996. The diagnostic dilemma of small incidentally discovered adrenal masses: A role for 131-I-b-iodomethyl-norcholesterol (NP59) scintigraphy. World J Surg, in press.
76. Dwamena BA, Kloos RT, Fendrick AM, Gross MD, Francis IR, Korobkin MT, Shapiro B. 1996. The adrenal incidentaloma: Decision and cost-effectiveness analyses of diagnostic management strategies (abstr). J Nucl Med 37:158P.
77. Haab F, Duclos JM, Julien J, Plouin PF. 1994. [Tumors of both adrenal glands. 12 consecutive cases]. Presse Med 23:511–514.
78. Gross MD, Shapiro B, Francis IR, Bree RL, Korobkin M, McLeod MK, Thompson NW, Sanfield JA. 1995. Incidentally discovered bilateral adrenal masses. Eur J Nucl Med 22:315–321.
79. Boland GW, Goldberg MA, Lee MJ, Mayo-Smith WW, Dixon J, McNicholas MM, Mueller PR. 1995. Indeterminate adrenal mass in patients with cancer: Evaluation at PET with 2-[F-18]-fluoro-2-deoxy-D-glucose. Radiology 194:131–134.
80. Keyes JW Jr. 1995. SUV: Standard uptake or silly useless value? J Nucl Med 36:1836–1839.
81. Welch TJ, Sheedy PF, Stephens DH, Johnson CM, Swensen SJ. 1994. Percutaneous adrenal biopsy: Review of a 10-year experience. Radiology 193:341–344.
82. Kloos RT, Gross MD, Shapiro B. 1994. Investigation of incidentally discovered, biochemically non-hypersecretory benign adrenal adenomas: A review of the current knowledge and areas for future investigation. Intern Med 2:9–15.
83. Mody MK, Kazerooni EA, Korobkin M. 1995. Percutaneous CT-guided biopsy of adrenal masses: Immediate and delayed complications. J Comput Assist Tomogr 19:434–439.

84. Candel AG, Gattuso P, Reyes CV, Prinz RA, Castelli MJ. 1993. Fine-needle aspiration biopsy of adrenal masses in patients with extraadrenal malignancy. Surgery 114:1132–1137.

85. Yankaskas BC, Staab EV, Craven MB, Blatt PM, Sokhandan M, Carney CN. 1986. Delayed complications from fine-needle biopsies of solid masses of the abdomen. Invest Radiol 21:325–328.

86. Silverman SG, Mueller PR, Pinkney LP, Koenker RM, Seltzer SE. 1993. Predictive value of image-guided adrenal biopsy: Analysis of results of 101 biopsies. Radiology 187:715–718.

87. Pagani JJ. 1983. Normal adrenal glands in small cell lung carcinoma: CT-guided biopsy. Am J Roentgenol 140:949–951.

88. Katz RL, Patel S, Mackay B, Zornoza J. 1984. Fine needle aspiration cytology of the adrenal gland. Acta Cytol 28:269–282.

89. Bernardino ME, Walther MM, Phillips VM, Graham SD Jr, Sewell CW, Gedgaudas-McClees K, Baumgartner BR, Torres WE, Erwin BC. 1985. CT-guided adrenal biopsy: Accuracy, safety, and indications. Am J Roentgenol 144:67–69.

90. Wadih GE, Nance KV, Silverman JF. 1992. Fine-needle aspiration cytology of the adrenal gland. Fifty biopsies in 48 patients. Arch Pathol Lab Med 116:841–846.

91. Rossi R, Savastano S, Tommaselli AP, Valentino R, Iaccarino V, Tauchmanova L, Luciano A, Gigante M, Lombardi G. 1995. Percutaneous computed tomography-guided ethanol injection in aldosterone-producing adrenocortical adenoma [see comments]. Eur J Endocrinol 132:302–305.

92. Regge D, Balma E, Lasciarrea P, Martina C, Serrallonga M, Gandini G. 1995. Interventional radiology of the adrenal glands. Minerva Endocrinol 20:15–26.

93. Mandressi A, Buizza C, Antonelli D, Chisena S, Servadio G. 1995. Retroperitoneoscopy. Ann Urol (Paris) 29:91–96.

94. Deans GT, Kappadia R, Wedgewood K, Royston CM, Brough WA. 1995. Laparoscopic adrenalectomy. Br J Surg 82:994–995.

95. Heintz A, Junginger T, Bottger T. 1995. Retroperitoneal endoscopic adrenalectomy. Br J Surg 82:215.

96. Hata M, Nakagawa K, Yanaihara H, Uchida A, Hayakawa K, Ohashi M, Ishikawa H. 1995. [Experience in seven cases of laparoscopic adrenalectomy]. Hinyokika Kiyo 41:507–510.

97. Mugiya S, Ishikawa A, Kageyama S, Ushiyama T, Hata M, Ohta N, Ohtawara Y, Suzuki K, Fujita K, Tajima A. 1995. [Adrenalectomy for nonfunctioning adrenal tumors–comparison between open and laparoscopic surgery, and indication for operation]. Hinyokika Kiyo 41:81–83.

98. Guazzoni G, Montorsi F, Bocciardi A, Da Pozzo L, Rigatti P, Lanzi R, Pontiroli A. 1995. Transperitoneal laparoscopic versus open adrenalectomy for benign hyperfunctioning adrenal tumors: A comparative study [see comments]. J Urol 153:1597–1600.

99. Schlinkert RT, van Heerden JA, Grant CS, Thompson GB, Segura JW. 1995. Laparoscopic left adrenalectomy for aldosteronoma: Early Mayo Clinic experience. Mayo Clin Proc 70:844–846.

100. Chapuis Y, Maignien B, Abboud B. 1995. [Adrenalectomy under celioscopy. Experience of 25 operations]. Presse Med 24:845–848.

101. Go H, Takeda M, Imai T, Komeyama T, Nishiyama T, Morishita H. 1995. Laparoscopic adrenalectomy for Cushing's syndrome: Comparison with primary aldosteronism. Surgery 117:11–17.

102. Walz MK, Peitgen K, Krause U, Eigler FW. 1995. [Dorsal retroperitoneoscopic adrenalectomy — a new surgical technique]. Zentralbl Chir 120:53–58.

103. Meurisse M, Joris J, Hamoir E, Hubert B, Charlier C. 1995. Laparoscopic removal of pheochromocytoma. Why? When? and Who? (reflections on one case report). Surg Endosc 9:431–436.

104. Pertsemlidis D. 1995. Minimal-access versus open adrenalectomy [editorial]. Surg Endosc 9:384–386.

105. Ayabe H, Tsuji H, Hara S, Tagawa Y, Kawahara K, Tomita M. 1995. Surgical management of adrenal metastasis from bronchogenic carcinoma. J Surg Oncol 58:149–154.
106. Piga A, Bracci R, Porfiri E, Cellerino R. 1995. Metastatic tumors of the adrenals. Minerva Endocrinol 20:79–83.
107. Schomer NS, Mohler JL. 1995. Partial adrenalectomy for renal cell carcinoma with bilateral adrenal metastases. J Urol 153:1196–1198.
108. Sakamoto K, Ariyoshi A, Okazaki M. 1995. Metastatic adrenocortical carcinoma treated by repeated resection: A case report of long-term survival over 18 years. Int J Urol 2:50–52.

14. Gastrin-producing tumors

Robert T. Jensen

Definition and classification

Strictly defined, gastrin-producing tumors include any tumor that produces gastrin. A gastrin-producing tumor in this strict definition would not be synonymous with the term *Zollinger-Ellison syndrome*. Gastrin can be detected in tumors by immunocytochemistry or by various molecular biological methods (in situ hybridization, PCR, Northern analysis, etc) and not cause any clinical syndrome or be associated with hypergastrinemia [1–4]. Whether hypergastrinemia and gastric hypersecretion are present or not, the tumor is still a gastrin-producing neoplasm. However, the diagnosis of Zollinger-Ellison syndrome is generally only made if the patient has the appropriate clinical findings (i.e., hypergastrinemia with simultaneous gastric acid hypersecretion), as discussed later. Strictly speaking a gastrin-producing tumor is synonymous with the term *gastrinoma*; however, generally the term *gastrinoma* is equated with Zollinger-Ellison syndrome. In this chapter this general usage will be retained. Therefore, a tumor in which gastrin is detected, without associated hypergastrinemia or gastric hypersecretion, would not be included in the general use of this term. Tumors that produce gastrin but are not associated with hypergastrinemia clinically present no unique hormonal features and thus clinically should be classified in a separate category than functional tumors (Table 1).

Because of the above-mentioned considerations, gastrin-producing neoplasms can be classified clinically into three categories (see Table 1). These different categories depend on whether Zollinger-Ellison syndrome is present or not and whether multiple endocrine neoplasia type I (MEN-I) is also present or not (see Table 1). Patients with Zollinger-Ellison syndrome with MEN-I differ clinically in their natural history, pathogenesis, and treatment from patients with Zollinger-Ellison syndrome without MEN-I [1,5], and therefore they are best considered in a separate clinical category (see Table 1). In this chapter, the discussion is almost entirely restricted to the clinical categories associated with the Zollinger-Ellison syndrome (see clinical categories I and II, Table 1) because these categories have the unique hormonal features that distinguish them from other pancreatic endocrine tumors (PETs)

Andrew Arnold (ed.) ENDOCRINE NEOPLASMS. 1997. Kluwer Academic Publishers. ISBN 0-7923-4354-9.

Table 1. Clinical classification of gastrin-producing neoplasms

---

I. Accompanied by the Zollinger-Ellison syndrome but not associated with multiple-endocrine neoplasia type-I (MEN-I) (sporadic form of Zollinger-Ellison syndrome — 75–80% of all Zollinger-Ellison syndrome cases)

II. Accompanied by the Zollinger-Ellison syndrome and MEN-I (familial form; 20–25% of all Zollinger-Ellison syndrome).

III. Not accompanied by the Zollinger-Ellison syndrome. Gastrin production demonstrated only in the tumor and not associated with hypergastrinemia and gastric-acid hypersecretion.

---

and carcinoid tumors. In addition, in this review the newer aspects of the tumor biology, diagnosis, and treatment of gastrin-producing tumors associated with Zollinger-Ellison syndrome are emphasized. Recent advances are emphasized because a number of recent papers of studies cover in detail various aspects of Zollinger-Ellison syndrome, including the disease in general [1,6,7], diagnosis [1,8,9], pathology [10], tumor localization [11–13], MEN-I with Zollinger-Ellison syndrome [14], medical treatment of the acid hypersecretion [9,15], medical treatment of the gastrinoma [9,16], and surgical treatment directed at the gastrinoma [6,17–19].

**Gastrin-producing neoplasms not associated
with Zollinger-Ellison syndrome**

Gastrin mRNA or various forms of gastrin peptides have been detected in bronchogenic carcinoma, acoustic neuromas, pheochromocytomas, ovarian carcinomas, colorectal carcinomas, and other pancreatic endocrine tumor syndromes than Zollinger-Ellison syndrome [2,20–23]. Normal and tumorous tissue give rise to identical cDNA clones [2], which suggests that the overexpression of the gastrin gene may be due to an alteration of the regulatory regions of the gene, such as in the 5′ untranslated region, resulting in an altered transcription rate or altered stability of the gene-specific mRNA. These results in colorectal carcinomas and ovarian carcinomas are of particular interest. In a recent study [3] either amidated gastrin, glycine-extended gastrin, or progastrin was detected in 12 ovarian serous cystadenocarcinomas, three ovarian nondifferentiated carcinomas, and five ovarian serous cystadenomas, mucinous cystadenomas, or follicular cysts. In 50% of the malignant ovarian tumors, significant concentrations of amidated gastrin were found. These results demonstrate that, in contrast to bronchogenic carcinomas, acoustic neuromas, and colon cancers, ovarian tumors can fully process the progastrin to the biologically active amidated form [2–4]. This result is particularly interesting because there are numerous case reports of Zollinger-Ellison syndrome occurring in patients with ovarian tumors [1–3,24], but hypergastrinemia does not occur in bronchogenic carcinoma, colorectal carcinoma, or acoustic neuromas [2].

In the case of colorectal tumors, the observation that these tumors contained gastrin mRNA or various forms of not fully processed gastrin has been of considerable interest [2,25,26]. Considerable experimental data exist demonstrating gastrin-related peptides can stimulate the growth of colorectal tumors and the development of these tumors [2,26–29]. Furthermore, a recent study reports increased proliferative rates of colonocytes in patients with Zollinger-Ellison syndrome [30]. However, the applicability of these results to human adenocarcinoma is unclear because epidemiological studies in patients with Zollinger-Ellison syndrome or pernicious anemia do not show a clear association of hypergastrinemia with colon cancer [2,26,29]. Recent studies demonstrate that many patients with colorectal carcinomas have detectable amounts of progastrin or elevated nonamidated gastrin levels in the circulation, regardless of *Helicobacter pylori* status [21,28,29]. These data, coupled with the recent demonstration that glycine-extended gastrin precursors can interact with a specific receptor, distinct from the CCK_B/gastrin receptor, to cause growth-promoting effects in AR 42J cells and Swiss 3T3 cells [31,32], further increase the possibility that a gastrin peptide might function as an autocrine or paracrine growth factor for colorectal cancers [25,26].

Gastrin-producing tumors associated with Zollinger-Ellison syndrome with or without MEN-I

General

Patients with Zollinger-Ellison syndrome without (see category I, Table 1) or with MEN-I (see category II, Table 1) share a number of common features, such as aspects of the clinical presentation, diagnosis, localization studies, and aspects of treatment. These common features are discussed together. The aspects in which patients with Zollinger-Ellison syndrome with MEN-I differ markedly from without MEN-I, including aspects of the clinical presentation, tumor localization, and treatment, are discussed in a separate section.

Zollinger-Ellison syndrome can be defined as a clinical syndrome caused by the ectopic release of gastrin by a gastrin-producing tumor (>99% in pancreas, duodenum, and surrounding lymph nodes), which results in hypergastrinemia, which, in turn, causes gastric acid hypersecretion (resulting primarily in peptic ulcer disease and malabsorption). The syndrome was originally described by Zollinger and Ellison in 1955 [33] in two patients with extreme gastric-acid hypersecretion, resulting in refractory peptic ulcer disease, satisfactorily treated only by total gastrectomy and a non–beta-islet cell tumor. Subsequent studies demonstrated these tumors released gastrin [1]. Although occasional reports have described PETs associated with gastric-acid hypersecretion but not releasing gastrin [34], at present no additional peptides or secretagogues have been isolated from such tumors. Therefore, at present gastrin is the only known peptide responsible for this syndrome with a pancreatic endocrine tumor.

Recent studies suggest that Zollinger-Ellison syndrome is more common relative to other pancreatic endocrine tumors than previously thought, but less common than some early studies suggested. It was originally proposed that the Zollinger-Ellison syndrome might occur in 0.1% of patients with duodenal ulcer disease [35]; however, studies show it has an incidence of 0.5 patients/million population/yr in Ireland, 1–3 patients/million/yr in Sweden, and 1 patient/million population/yr in Denmark [1,2]. Zollinger-Ellison syndrome was originally thought to be less common than insulinomas; however, in recent studies gastrinomas occur with equal [36] or greater [2] frequency than insulinomas, from 0.5 to 1.5 more commonly than nonfunctioning PETs or pancreatic polypeptide–producing tumors (Pomas), two to four times more frequently than VIPomas, and 8 to 15 times more common than glucagonomas or somatostatinomas. Therefore, gastrinomas are the most common symptomatic, malignant PET.

Clinical features

General. In most series, Zollinger-Ellison syndrome is slightly more common in males (60%), the mean age at the onset of symptoms is approximately 50 years (range 7–90 years), and 20–25% of patients have the MEN-I syndrome [1,8]. In almost all patients the initial and persisting symptoms are caused by the gastric acid hypersecretion [1,8,37]. Only late in the course of the disease in patients with widespread metastatic disease are symptoms caused by the gastrinoma per se [1,37]. Abdominal pain primarily caused by duodenal ulcer disease or reflux esophagitis is the most common symptom, occurring in >75% of patients, either alone or with diarrhea. The abdominal pain in most patients is clinically indistinguishable from that which occurs in patients with idiopathic peptic ulcer disease [1]. Diarrhea may be the sole presenting feature, and in several recent studies it is the second most common clinical feature, occurring alone in 9–20% of patients and with abdominal pain in 49–65% [1,8]. Esophageal symptoms are now frequently described, with 31% of patients having pyrosis and/or dysphagia as the initial symptom in one recent large series and 45–60% of patients having esophageal symptoms and/or esophageal lesions at presentation [1,8,38]. Patients with Zollinger-Ellison syndrome continue to present with complications of peptic ulcer disease, with recurrent upper gastrointestinal (UGI) bleeding, severe nausea and vomiting, and intestinal perforation reported in 10%, 31%, and 7% of patients in recent studies [39,40].

Patients with Zollinger-Ellison syndrome with MEN-I. MEN-I is an autosomal-dominant disorder characterized by tumors or hyperplasia of multiple endocrine organs, particularly the parathyroid glands, pancreas, pituitary, and, to a lesser degree, the adrenal gland [1,5]. The specific chromosomal defect remains unknown, although it has been localized by restriction fragment length polymorphism (RFLP) studies to chromosome 11q12–13 near the skeletal muscle glycogen phosphorylase locus (PYGM) [41,42]. The genetic alteration is discussed further under Pathogenesis in the next section.

Hypercalcemia due to primary hyperparathyroidism is the most common clinical abnormality in patients with MEN-I, occurring in 95–98% of patients [1,5,42]. Pancreatic endocrine tumors develop in 80–100% of patients [non-functional tumors or pancreatic polypeptide-producing tumors (PPomas)], with functional PETs developing in 50–80% of patients [1,5]. Gastrinomas are the most common functional PET, occurring in 54%, whereas insulinomas occur in 21%, glucagonomas in 3%, and VIPomas in 1% [1,5]. Pituitary adenomas occur in 16–100% and can cause symptoms due to local encroachment or hormone release. In various studies 41–76% are prolactinomas, 11–33% are associated with acromegaly, and Cushing's syndrome develops in 5–19% [5,43,44]. Patients with Zollinger-Ellison and MEN-I differed clinically from patients with the sporadic form of Zollinger-Ellison syndrome in that they present at an early age (43 vs. 48 years in one study) [18], most patients have hyperparathyroidism or pituitary disease at the time of the presentation of the Zollinger-Ellison syndrome, and the presence of the hypercalcemia can make it more difficult to control the gastric-acid hypersecretion [1,5,45].

Pathology, tumor biology, and pathogenesis

Pathology

Gastrinomas were originally reported to occur primarily [46,47] in the pancreas with a distribution of 4:1:4 in head:body:tail. In more recent studies only 30–50% occur in the pancreas [46,47]. In recent studies, 60–90% of gastrinomas occur in the gastrinoma triangle, an area formed by the junction of the cystic and common bile ducts superiorly, the junction of the second and third portions of duodenum inferiorly, and the junction of the neck and body of the pancreas medially [1,47,48]. The decreasing proportion of pancreatic gastrinomas is due to the increased use of careful exploration of the duodenum, which has resulted in an increased detection of duodenal gastrinomas [47]. Duodenal gastrinomas now comprise 45–60% of all tumors found at surgery in recent series [46,47,49]. Duodenal gastrinomas are distributed in a decreasing gradient proceeding distally, with 71% in the first portion of the duodenum, 21% in the second, 8% in the third, and 0% in the fourth [50].

Gastrinomas are increasingly found in lymph nodes in the pancreatic head area (19–40%) [49,51,52]. It is controversial whether gastrinomas can arise in lymph nodes or whether these all represent metastases from occult primaries [1,51]. The possibility of these being lymph-node primary gastrinomas is supported by studies that demonstrate cure postresection of a lymph-node tumor only [1,51], which in one study [51] occurred in 43% of such patients with a mean follow-up of 5.3 years. Furthermore, a recent study [53] has demonstrated 3% of patients without endocrine tumors possessed chromogranin B rests in abdominal lymph nodes, providing support that neuroendocrine arrests can occur in lymph nodes and may give rise to these nodal gastrinomas. A number of cases of ovarian tumor causing Zollinger-Ellison syndrome have been reported, primarily cystadenocarcinomas [1,54], and very rarely gastrinomas have been reported in the stomach, mesentery, and renal capsule [1].

In older studies 60–90% of gastrinomas were malignant, whereas in more recent studies 34% are associated with metastatic disease [1]. These older data suggest all gastrinomas should be considered potentially malignant [1]. Gastrinomas metastasize primarily to lymph nodes and the liver [1]. Increasingly, bone metastases [55] are being recognized as occurring exclusively in patients with liver metastases and far advanced disease [55].

Gastrinomas, like other PETs, are neuroendocrine neoplasms [10]. All neuroendocrine tumors have certain common features because they share the expression of various genes encoding certain makers and hormonal products, and have been classified as APUDomas (*A*mine *P*recursor *U*ptake and *D*ecarboxylation) [10]. General markers include chromogranin A and B, synaptophysin, neuron-specific enolase, 7B2, and epitope Leu-7 [10].

Histologically, gastrinomas usually contain uniform cuboidal cells with few mitoses and fine granular eosinophilic cytoplasm [1,10]. They can exist in trabecular, gyriform, or glandular patterns [1,10]. Similar to other neuroendocrine tumors [10,56], the biological behavior of the tumor cannot be reliably predicted from histological features, ultrastructural studies, or immunocytochemical studies. Neither the type of hormone released nor the aggressiveness can be predicted from these parameters. The only reliable criteria of malignancy is the presence of metastasis. The presence of vascular invasion is suggestive of malignancy [10].

The exact cell of origin of gastrinomas remains unclear [1]. Recent studies suggest duodenal and pancreatic gastrinomas may originate from a different cell type. Duodenal and pancreatic gastrinoma differ in biological behavior [1,46,57], and a recent study [58] supports the proposal that duodenal gastrinomas might arise from the ventral pancreatic bud tissue and pancreatic body/tail gastrinomas from the dorsal pancreatic bud tissue [57,58]. In this study [58] pancreatic polypeptide (PP) immunoreactivity, which is found primarily in pancreatic islets derived from the ventral pancreatic bud, was found in 80% of gastrinomas found to the right of the superior mesenteric artery (SMA) (n = 14) [58], which was significantly greater (p = 0.021) than the 0% of gastrinomas to the left of the SMA (n = 5) that had PP immunoreactivity [58].

On pathologic analysis, patients with Zollinger-Ellison syndrome with MEN-I differ from patients without MEN-I with Zollinger-Ellison syndrome in that patients with MEN-I contain large numbers of pancreatic microadenomas throughout the pancreas [1,59,60]. Some microadenomas produce multiple GI hormones according to immunocytochemical studies, with 80% producing PP [59,60], 60% somatostatin, 42% insulin, 33% gastrin, and 8% VIP in one study [60]; however, frequently no associated plasma peptide elevation is found. Recent studies [61–64] demonstrate that 60–80% of the gastrinomas in patients with MEN-I with Zollinger-Ellison syndrome occur in the duodenum. These gastrinomas are frequently multiple, and in one recent study 86% had metastasized to lymph nodes at the time of resection [63].

Tumor biology

Gastrinomas, like other PETs, in immunocytochemical studies frequently produce multiple GI peptides [1,65,66]. Gastrin is found in 80–100%, insulin in 30%, human pancreatic polypeptide in 35%, glucagon in 29%, and somatostatin in 21% [66]. Similarly, a plasma elevation of additional GI hormones other than gastrin occurs in 62% of patients with Zollinger-Ellison syndrome, with 44% having one additional and 18% two additional hormones elevated [66]. Plasma motilin levels were the most frequently elevated, in addition to plasma gastrin levels (29%), followed by human PP (27%), neurotensin (20%), and GRP (10%), whereas insulin, glucagon, and somatostatin were not elevated in any of the 45 patients with Zollinger-Ellison syndrome studied [66]. The presence of MEN-I did not affect whether or not a plasma elevation of another peptide was found [66]. Even though immunocytochemically other peptides associated with symptomatic syndromes are frequently found in gastrinomas (i.e., insulin, glucagon, somatostatin), the occurrence of a second symptomatic syndrome in patients with Zollinger-Ellison syndrome is relatively uncommon [66]. One study [67] in patients with various symptomatic PETs demonstrated that 7% developed a second symptomatic PET syndrome within a 34-month period. However, in 45 patients with Zollinger-Ellison syndrome, only one patient developed a secondary syndrome over a 10-year period, for a rate of two patients per 100 patients followed for 10 years [66], which is a relatively low rate.

Gastrinomas, similar to other PETs and carcinoid tumors, frequently synthesize and release chromogranin A and B, as well as the α and β subunits of human chorionic gonadotropin (α-HCG, β-HCG) [68,69]. Chromogranin A is elevated in the plasma in 100% of untreated patients (i.e., no somatostatin analogues, not postresection) with Zollinger-Ellison syndrome [68,69]. It has been proposed that plasma chromogranin levels can be used as a general marker for PETs [68]; however, chromogranin A is a 48-kD protein that is costored and coreleased with peptide hormones from many gut endocrine cells or tumors [1,68], including from antral G cells and gastric enterochromaffin-like cells (ECL cells). This latter point is important in patients with Zollinger-Ellison syndrome because these patients characteristically have ECL hyperplasia [70–72]. In one study it was concluded that the ECL cells, not the gastrinoma, were the principal source of chromogranin A in patients with Zollinger-Ellison syndrome [73].

However, a recent study measured both plasma chromogranin A levels and pancreastatin levels, with the latter being produced by the breakdown of chromogranin A in patients with Zollinger-Ellison syndrome [69], and demonstrated a significant correlation between the serum gastrin level and plasma pancreastatin levels ($r = 0.7$, $p < 0.002$) but no correlation between serum gastrin and plasma chromogranin A levels. This study [69] also concluded that the gastrinoma is not the main source of plasma chromogranin A in patients with Zollinger-Ellison syndrome, but that measurement of plasma pancreastatin levels likely did reflect activity of the gastrinoma. In one study [73] no correlation was found between the chromogranin A level and the presence of malignancy, whereas in another study [69] a weak correlation ($p = 0.04$) existed. α-Human chorionic gonadotropin (HCG) and β-HCG have been reported to be elevated in 41% and 30%, respectively, of patients with PETs including Zollinger-Ellison syndrome, and their presence has been correlated with malignancy [68]. However, in one study involving 30 patients with Zollinger-Ellison syndrome [74], 57% of patients with malignant tumors and 45% with benign tumors had elevated plasma α-HCG levels. Seven patients had elevated β-HCG plasma levels and 4 of the 7 patients had malignant disease. Normal levels can occur in the presence of malignancy and vice versa; therefore, it has been concluded that the usefulness of a level of α- or β-HCG in management is unclear [1].

Gastrinomas release, in addition to gastrin-17-I and gastrin-34, smaller and larger forms of gastrin, amino- and carboxy-terminal fragments, and carboxy-terminal glycine-extended forms [1,2,4]. Furthermore, post-translational processing may be altered in gastrinomas, leading to altered ratios of various fragments and increased amounts of gastrin precursors released [1,2,4,75,76]. Higher plasma progastrin levels have been reported in patients with metastatic gastrinomas in the liver [1,75] as well as a lower percentage of amidated gastrin of the total plasma gastrin immunoreactivity. Glycine-extended forms have been reported to predominate in benign disease [1,75]. Furthermore, the ratio of NH_2 to COOH-terminal gastrin fragments in the plasma in patients with Zollinger-Ellison syndrome is said to be predictive of the extent of gastrinoma. However, altered NH_2- to COOH-terminal ratios have not been found by all investigators, and because of the variability of the plasma levels of different gastrin fragments and precursors in different patients, it has been concluded that a single measurement of a progastrin product has little diagnostic meaning [4]. It has been proposed that a processing-independent gastrin analysis is more sensitive and may correlate better with malignancy [4].

Until recently, factors affecting the natural history of gastrinomas were largely unknown. In contrast to carcinoid tumors, the importance of the effect of gastrinoma location or size on malignant potential was unclear [1,43]. Furthermore, the effect of MEN-I on prognosis remained unclear [1]. A recent large study from the National Institutes of Health (NIH) [46] demonstrated

300

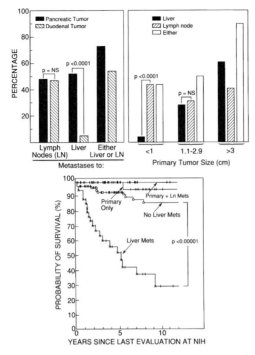

Figure 1. Effect of primary gastrinoma location or size on the frequency of metastases to the liver, lymph nodes, or both (top) and the survival of patients with Zollinger-Ellison syndrome (bottom). **Top**: Results on the left are from 83 patients with pancreatic (n = 42) or duodenal (n = 41) gastrinomas only. Results on the right are from 118 patients in whom primary tumors were localized and size of the primary (diameter) was assessed. Data are modified from Weber et al. [46]. **Bottom**: The data are plotted in the form of Kaplan-Meier curves. Results are from 36 patients with hepatic metastases and 149 patients without hepatic metastases. Results are shown from 31 patients who had a primary gastrinoma only, determined by surgical exploration, and 24 patients who had a primary gastrinoma with lymph-node metastases only, determined by surgical exploration. Data are modified from Weber et al. [46].

that the presence of liver metastases was highly dependent on both the size (p < 0.00001) and location (p < 0.00001) of the gastrinoma (Fig. 1). Pancreatic gastrinomas and large size (>3 cm) were associated with increased hepatic metastases (Fig. 1). Most duodenal gastrinomas were small (i.e., 92% ≤1 cm compared with 8% for pancreatic tumors), and therefore there were not sufficient large duodenal tumors or small pancreatic tumors to establish whether size and location were independent predictors [46]. In this study [46] the percentage of duodenal and pancreatic tumors with lymph-node metastases did not vary (see Fig. 1; i.e., they were 48% vs. 47%), and therefore the development of lymph-node metastases were not dependent on size or primary location. These data demonstrate duodenal and pancreatic gastrinomas are equally malignant (~50% metastasized to lymph nodes); however, they differ in the presence of more distal metastases and therefore

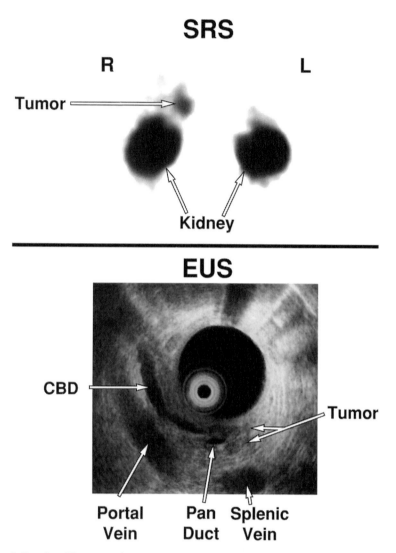

SRS

R   L

Tumor

Kidney

EUS

CBD

Tumor

Portal   Pan Splenic
Vein   Duct   Vein

Figure 2. Results of Somatostatin receptor scintigraphy (SRS) and endoscopic ultrasound localization of a gastrinoma in a patient with Zollinger-Ellison syndrome (NIH #1594011). SRS
localized a gastrinoma to the duodenum/pancreatic head area (arrow-labeled tumor), and
endoscopic ultrasound localized a gastrinoma in the pancreatic head (labeled tumor) situated
between the pancreatic duct (Pan duct) and common bile duct (CBD). The tumor was partially
obstructing the common bile duct, which is dilated.

their aggressiveness. This study demonstrated that a higher percentage of
patients without MEN-I presented initially with metastatic disease in the liver
compared with patients with MEN-I (6% vs. 22%, $p < 0.03$); however, the
percentage of patients with or without MEN-I who developed metastatic
disease during follow-up (9% vs. 5%, $p = 0.4$) and the survival in patients

without metastases initially was not significantly different (95% vs. 96%, 5 years) [46]. These data, coupled with other analyses, led the authors [46] to conclude that a higher proportion of patients with sporadic Zollinger-Ellison syndrome have an aggressive form of gastrinoma than do patients with Zollinger-Ellison syndrome and MEN-I.

In this large NIH study [46] in which the mean disease duration was 12.5 ± 0.6 years (range 1–35 years), the most important determinant of survival was the presence of liver metastases (see Fig. 1, bottom). In patients without liver metastases the 10-year survival was 90% (CI 82–95%), which was significantly greater (p < 0.0001) than the 30% (CI 14–52%) that occurred in patients with liver metastases. The presence or absence of lymph-node metastases had no effect on survival (see Fig. 1, bottom), similar to that reported in a number of smaller studies previously [1,77,78]. This excellent long-term survival, even with lymph-node metastases, has important implications for determining how aggressive one should be in the surgical treatment of the gastrinoma and is discussed further later. This recent NIH study [4] provided support for two distinct clinical forms of gastrinoma that had been proposed previously [77]. These two clinical forms have been called *benign* and *malignant* form [46,77], and these names are retained in Table 2; however, better names are *nonaggressive form* and *aggressive form* because patients with only lymph-node metastases have an excellent prognosis (nonaggressive course; Fig. 2); however, the gastrinoma is clearly malignant. Patients in whom the gastrinoma pursues an aggressive course (malignant form) comprise approximately one fourth of the patients, are more frequently female, are less likely to have MEN-I, have a short time from the onset of symptoms to the diagnosis, have primarily larger pancreatic gastrinomas with markedly elevated serum gastrin levels, and have a poor prognosis (Table 2). More aggressive disease has been shown [79] in a flow cytometry study to be associated with a higher mean S phase for the gastrinoma, a lower percentage of nontetraploid aneuploid, and a higher percentage multiple stem-line aneuploid [79] (see Table 2).

Despite these advances in the clinical classification of Zollinger-Ellison syndrome and in the value of flow cytometry in a group of patients [79], the major problem in the treatment of patients with gastrinoma is in developing methods that might be useful in an individual patient to predict tumor aggressiveness. Patients are now being seen earlier in their disease courses, and if predictive criteria could be developed, more appropriately aggressive treatment could be initiated earlier. At present, insights from studies of growth factors or molecular biologic studies of gene abnormalities are only beginning to be made, and it remains unclear how useful they will be. In most of the studies reported, patients with gastrinoma have been considered together with other malignant PETs (glucagonomas, VIPomas, nonfunctioning tumors, PPomas) and in some cases have been combined with carcinoid tumors.

Gastrinoma cells have been difficult to grow in culture from patients, and there are minimal data on the direct effect of growth factors on tumor growth.

Table 2. Comparison of clinical and laboratory characteristics of patients with a benign or malignant clinical course with gastrinoma

Characteristics[a]	Clinical course (% all patients)	
	Benign[b]	Malignant[b]
Percent of patients	76%	24%
Present with liver metastases	0%	19%
Develop liver metastases	0%	5%
Gender	Predominantly male (68%)	Predominantly female (67%)
MEN-I at initial evaluation	21%	Uncommon (6%)
Time from onset to diagnosis	Long (mean 5.9 yr)	Short (mean, 2.7 yr)
Serum gastrin level[c]	Moderately elevated (mean, 1711 pg/ml)	Very elevated (mean, 5157 pg/ml)
Size of primary tumor	Small (≤1 cm)	Large (>3 cm)
Location of primary tumor	Primarily duodenum (66%)	Primarily pancreatic (92%)
Survival at 10 years	Excellent (96%)	Poor (30%)
Flow cytometry of tumor	Low S phase (mean, 3.3)	High S phase (mean, 5.1)
	High % nontetraploid aneuploid (32%)	Low % nontetraploid aneuploid
	Multiple stem-line aneuploid rare	Multiple stem-line aneuploid frequent (25%)

[a] All characteristics were significantly different (p < 0.0001) between the two groups.
[b] The benign or nonaggressive course was not associated with the development of liver metastases (n = 140), whereas patients in whom the gastrinoma pursued a malignant or aggressive course had liver metastases either at the initial evaluation (n = 36) or developed liver metastases (n = 9) during follow-up.
[c] Normal serum gastrin level <100 pg/ml.
Data are modified from Weber et al. [46] from the study of 185 patients with Zollinger-Ellison syndrome. The flow cytometry data are modified from Metz et al. [79].

Various studies have demonstrated that PETs, including gastrinomas, similar to carcinoid tumors [80,81], frequently express both growth factors [PDGF, TGF-β_1, -β_2, and -β_3, and bFGF) as well as growth factor receptors (PDGF-α and -β receptor, EGF receptor). In addition, all gastrinomas, but not VIPomas or insulinomas, and 25% of nonfunctioning PETs, were found to express [82] the hyaluronate receptor, CD44 [81,82]. The expression of CD44 positivity in tumors correlated with a tendency to metastasize to lymph nodes (p = 0.005) as compared with CD44-negative tumors [82]. Each gastrinoma examined overproduced an alternatively spliced larger molecular variant of CD44 as compared with other PETs [82]. Various measures of cell proliferation in gastrinomas and other PETs have been shown to correlate with aggressiveness, including studies of the nucleolar organizer region-associated proteins, the level of expression of the Ki-67 antigen, and the level of expression of the proliferating cell nuclear antigen [83–85].

Numerous studies demonstrate various protooncogenes, and alterations in various tumor suppressor genes may play a role in the pathogenesis of some human malignancies [86,87], including some endocrine tumors [88,89]. Recently the protooncogene HER-2/*neu*, which is a member of the *erb*-β–like oncogene family that encodes a protein (p185[neu]) that has tyrosine kinase activity and is analogous to the EGF receptor, was examined in 11 gastrinomas [90]. It was found to be overexpressed (>twofold amplification) in all gastrinomas; however, in contrast to that reported by others in other tumors, the extent of amplification did not correlate with aggressiveness [89,90]. In contrast to the HER-2/*neu* oncogene, no alterations in K-*ras*, N-*ras*, H-*ras* were found in 23 gastrinomas in two studies [90,91]. In numerous studies only rarely have p53 mutations been detected in gastrinomas as well as in other PETs [89]. Loss of heterozygosity of the retinoblastoma gene has been reported in some endocrine tumors, such as parathyroid carcinomas [92], and in 20% of lung carcinoid cell lines [93]; however, there have been no studies on patients with gastrinomas [89].

Recently alterations in the expression of guanine nucleotide binding proteins have been reported in a number of endocrine tumors [89,94,95]. Alterations in the α chain of G_s, resulting in an inhibition of its GTPase activity causing the oncogene *gsp* [94], and of the α chain of G_{i2}, resulting in a putative oncogene *gip2* [95], are reported in pituitary and thyroid adenomas; however, in a recent study [96] no *gsp* or *gip2* mutations were found in two gastrinomas or nine insulinomas. However, the mRNA of the α subunit of G_s is reported [97] to be overexpressed up to 35-fold in an ACTHoma and an insulinoma but not in a gastrinoma, and therefore overexpression of G-protein subunits may be important in the unregulated hormone secretion by some PETs.

The tumor biology of gastrinomas in MEN-I is only briefly discussed because it has been reviewed recently [41,42,89,98]. The exact genetic defect in MEN-I remains unknown; however, it is known by restriction fragment length polymorphism (RFLP) studies to be located on chromosome 11q12–13 near the PYGM locus. These studies provide evidence that MEN-I is due to inactivation of a tumor suppressor gene at this location. Recently allelic losses on chromosome 11 have been reported to differ in different endocrine tumors in the same patient [99] and were not present in all tumors in patients with MEN-I, suggesting different mutation events may be involved in the pathogenesis of the different endocrine tumors in MEN-I. Recent studies provide evidence that loss of heterozygosity on chromosome 11 may also be important in the pathogenesis of sporadic gastrinomas and other sporadic PETs [41,89,100,101]. In one study [100], 5 of 11 sporadic gastrinomas had a loss of heterozygosity in this region, and in another study [101] of 39 sporadic PETs, 30% had a loss of heterozygosity in the region of the putative MEN-I gene. In an additional study [41], all 10 patients with MEN-I had allelic loss of the PET on chromosome 11q13; however, only 10 of 27 (32%) of sporadic tumors had an alteration on this chromosome.

Pathogenesis

All of the symptoms that patients with Zollinger-Ellison syndrome characteristically develop, except late in the course of the disease, are due to the massive gastric acid hypersecretion. Recent studies [102,103] demonstrate that gastric carcinoid tumors (ECLomas), which patients with MEN-I with Zollinger-Ellison syndrome develop with increased frequency [1,72,102,104,105], are also due to a loss of heterozygosity on chromosome 11q12–3 [1,37]. The chronic hypergastrinemia has a trophic effect on the gastric mucosa, causing parietal cell hyperplasia, with the result that patients with Zollinger-Ellison syndrome have a parietal cell mass four to six times normal [1,37]. This increased parietal cell mass results in increased gastric acid secretory capacity. The hypergastrinemia also stimulates acid secretion [37]. The result of these two effects of gastrin is that basal acid output (BAO) is increased and it is characteristically a higher percentage of the maximal acid output (MAO). Furthermore, because of the increased parietal cell mass, both the BAO and MAO are increased. The increased acid output results in peptic ulceration, and also frequently diarrhea, because of direct effects on the small intestinal mucosa and the low pH inactivates lipase and precipitates bile acids [1]. The hypergastrinemia per se does not cause effects on intestinal secretion because patients with Zollinger-Ellison syndrome are asymptomatic when the acid hypersecretion is controlled [1,37].

Differential diagnosis and diagnosis

General features that should suggest Zollinger-Ellison syndrome

The mean delay from the onset of the Zollinger-Ellison syndrome to diagnosis remains 3–6 years [1]. This delay occurs primarily because the Zollinger-Ellison syndrome is an uncommon condition (1–3 new cases/million population/yr), which, especially early in its course, mimics common conditions such as peptic ulcer disease (incidence of 230 new cases/100,000 population/yr [106]) and reflux esophagitis (3–4% of the population). Furthermore, most patients present with a duodenal ulcer, which is clinically and endoscopically indistinguishable from a routine peptic ulcer. There are certain clinical and laboratory features (Table 3), however, that should suggest Zollinger-Ellison syndrome. Zollinger-Ellison syndrome should be particularly suspected in a patient with peptic ulcer disease (PUD) with diarrhea, which is rarely present in patients with idiopathic PUD now that antacids are not used. Zollinger-Ellison syndrome should also be particularly suspected if *H. pylori* is not present because *H. pylori* is present in 90–98% of idiopathic duodenal ulcers but only in <50% of patients with Zollinger-Ellison syndrome [9,107] (see Table 3). Similarly, >90% of PUD heals with eradication of *H. pylori* or with histamine H_2-receptor antagonists, and therefore failure to heal a duodenal ulcer with these treatments should lead to a suspicion of Zollinger-Ellison syndrome.

In various studies 30–65% of patients with Zollinger-Ellison syndrome present with diarrhea and in 7–20% of patients the diarrhea is the main symptom [1,8]. Therefore, in a patient with chronic diarrhea that persists

Table 3. Clinical and laboratory conditions that should lead to suspicion of Zollinger-Ellison syndrome

---

A. Clinical features
1. In patients with a duodenal ulcer
   a. No *H. pylori* present
   b. Presence of diarrhea
   c. Failure to heal with treatment of the *H. pylori* or with histamine H$_2$-receptor antagonists
   d. Presence of a pancreatic tumor
2. Multiple duodenal ulcers or ulcers in unusual locations
3. Severe peptic ulcer disease leading to a complication (perforation, intractability, bleeding)
4. Severe or resistant peptic esophageal disease
5. Chronic secretory diarrhea
6. Nephrolithiasis or endocrinopathies
7. Family history of nephrolithiasis or endocrinopathies, or peptic ulcer disease

B. Laboratory features in a patient with peptic ulcer disease that should suggest Zollinger-Ellison syndrome
1. Hypergastrinemia
2. Hypercalcemia
3. Endocrinopathy
4. Prominent gastric folds on UGI x-ray or at endoscopy

---

during fasting or decreases with gastric-acid antisecretory treatment, Zollinger-Ellison syndrome should be suspected. Later in the disease course, particularly, the PUD in patients with Zollinger-Ellison syndrome is more severe than routine PUD; therefore, any patient with multiple ulcers, ulcers in unusual locations, refractory disease, or complications of PUD, including refractory reflux symptoms or esophageal strictures, should be suspected of having Zollinger-Ellison syndrome [1,9] (see Table 3). In any patient with PUD found to have hypergastrinemia, the diagnosis of Zollinger-Ellison syndrome should be entertained. Similarly, prominent gastric folds are not common in patients with routine PUD, and if these are found by barium studies or UGI endoscopy, Zollinger-Ellison syndrome should be suspected. Any patient with PUD with a pancreatic tumor, especially if it is endocrine in origin, should be considered as possibly having Zollinger-Ellison syndrome. Lastly, because 20% of patients with Zollinger-Ellison syndrome have MEN-I, the presence of other endocrinopathies, a family history of other endocrinopathies, particularly nephrolithiasis, hypercalcemia, or other laboratory data suggesting endocrinopathies in a patient with PUD should raise the possibility of the Zollinger-Ellison syndrome (see Table 3).

Differential diagnosis and diagnosis of Zollinger-Ellison syndrome. If the diagnosis of Zollinger-Ellison is suspected, measurements of the fasting serum gastrin level and the gastric pH should be used to determine if the patient likely has Zollinger-Ellison syndrome [1,9,108]. Frequently, only the fasting gastrin level is initially measured. Fasting serum gastrin levels were reported

Table 4. Causes of chronic hypergastrinemia

A. Associated with gastric-acid hyposecretion/achlorhydria
   1. Pernicious anemia/atrophic gastritis
   2. Treatment with potent gastric-acid antisecretory agents (especially with H^+-K^+ ATPase inhibitors)
   3. Chronic renal failure (common)
   4. *H. pylori* infection
   5. Post gastric acid–reducing surgery
B. Associated with gastric acid hypersecretion
   1. Retained gastric antrum syndrome
   2. Chronic renal failure (rare)
   3. Antral G-cell hyperfunction/hyperplasia
   4. Gastric-outlet obstruction
   5. Short-bowel syndrome
   6. *H. pylori* infection
   7. Zollinger-Ellison syndrome

to be elevated in >98% of patients with Zollinger-Ellison syndrome, especially if drawn on at least two separate occasions [1]. Recently patients with Zollinger-Ellison syndrome with normal fasting gastrin have been described, making up 17% of the patients in one series [109,110]. Many of these patients, however, had positive secretin provocative tests (see later). In most series, >90% of patients with Zollinger-Ellison syndrome will have an elevated fasting serum gastrin; therefore, this remains the best single initial screening study. If the fasting serum gastrin level is elevated, then it should be repeated and gastric fluid pH measured at the same time. If the fasting gastrin level remains elevated and the gastric fluid pH is <2.5, then the patient may have Zollinger-Ellison syndrome. If the pH is >2.5, it is very unlikely that the hypergastrinemia is due to Zollinger-Ellison syndrome, and it is likely due to one of the other causes of hypochlorhydria or achlorhydria listed in Table 4.

One condition in this category that can be difficult to differentiate from Zollinger-Ellison syndrome and is now a frequent cause of hypergastrinemia is drug-induced hypergastrinemia. With the widespread use of potent acid-suppressant agents such as the H^+-K^+ ATPase inhibitors, omeprazole and lansoprazole, this is becoming an increasing problem. In recent studies 80–100% of patients treated long-term with omeprazole develop hypergastrinemia, and in some studies gastrin levels increase more than five times the normal level [9]. Therefore, if the patient is taking these drugs, the hypergastrinemia could either be drug-induced or caused by a gastric acid hypersecretory state that caused the symptoms that led to the patient being treated with these drugs. To differentiate these possibilities, H^+-K^+ ATPase inhibitors should be stopped for at least 7 days and histamine H_2 blockers for at least 30 hours prior to the determination of gastric pH. If the gastric pH fluid is <2.5 and the serum gastrin level is >1000 pg/ml (normal <100 pg/ml), the patient almost certainly has Zollinger-Ellison syndrome if the possibility of the retained gastric antrum syndrome (see later) can be excluded. Thirty percent of patients with Zollinger-Ellison syndrome fall into this category [72]. A number of conditions can cause moderate elevations of serum gastrin levels (101–999 pg/ml, normal <100 pg/ml) and a gastric pH <2.5 (see Table 4), and Zollinger-Ellison has to be distinguished from these conditions. Seventy percent of patients fall into this range, with their fasting gastrin levels between 101 and 999 pg/ml [72].

In patients with moderate serum gastrin elevations (101–999 pg/ml) with the gastric fluid pH < 2.5 or in whom Zollinger-Ellison syndrome is strongly suspected but fasting gastrin levels are normal, a gastric analysis to measure BAO and a secretin test should be performed [8,9]. Diagnostic criteria for BAO usually used are >15 mEq/hr for patients without previous acid-reducing surgery and >5 mEq/hr for those with previous acid-reducing surgery [1]. This will include 66–99% of patients with Zollinger-Ellison syndrome in different series and will exclude 90% of patients with duodenal ulcer disease [8,9]. These criteria, unfortunately, are not specific for Zollinger-Ellison syndrome and can occur in the conditions listed in Table 4 associated with gastric acid hypersecretion. To distinguish Zollinger-Ellison syndrome from these other conditions, a secretin provocative test should be performed measuring fasting gastrin levels before and 2, 5, 10, and 20 minutes post iv injection of secretin (2 clinical units/kg). A positive response is greater than a 200 pg/ml increase over the preinjection gastrin level, and this will occur in 87% of patients with Zollinger-Ellison syndrome [111]. This test has no reported false-positive responses in patients who are not achlorhydric. Thirteen percent of patients with Zollinger-Ellison syndrome will have a negative secretin test. One third of the patients with a negative secretin test will have a positive calcium infusion test [111], and many of the remainder will have positive imaging studies supporting a diagnosis of Zollinger-Ellison syndrome. If a patient has a negative secretin test and fits the other criteria for Zollinger-Ellison syndrome but has *H. pylori*, then the *H. pylori* should be treated and the patient reassessed post eradication of the *H. pylori*. Recent reports describe such patients who did not have Zollinger-Ellison syndrome but had hypergastrinemia and hyperchlorhydria, which was caused by the *H. pylori* infection [112,113].

Diagnosis of MEN-I with Zollinger-Ellison syndrome. Until recently the diagnosis of MEN-I in patients with Zollinger-Ellison syndrome was not generally thought to be difficult [1,5,9,108]. This was because it was generally accepted that 95–98% of patients with Zollinger-Ellison syndrome as part of the MEN-I syndrome had developed hyperparathyroidism or pituitary disease prior to the gastrinoma and, therefore, by measuring serum calcium levels and plasma PTH levels or pituitary function at the time of the diagnosis of Zollinger-Ellison syndrome, it would be easy to establish that it was part of the MEN-I syndrome. However, recent studies show that patients with MEN-I can initially present only with a PET or Zollinger-Ellison syndrome, and thus it may be difficult to distinguish patients with or without MEN-I [114,115]. In one study [114] of 28 patients with Zollinger-Ellison syndrome with MEN-I, one third of the patients initially presented with Zollinger-Ellison syndrome and only developed laboratory or clinical features of hyperparathyroidism or pituitary dysfunction later. Despite serial serum calcium levels, plasma PTH levels, and pituitary function studies in this one third of patients with Zollinger-Ellison syndrome, the diagnosis of MEN-I was not established until 12–264 months after the diagnosis of Zollinger-Ellison syndrome. These data strongly support the conclusion that when specific genetic tests for MEN-I become available, all patients with Zollinger-Ellison syndrome should be examined because of the effect of the MEN-I diagnosis on treatment and, perhaps, on family screening.

Management of the gastric hypersecretion

Medical management of gastric hypersecretion

The first goal in the management of patients with Zollinger-Ellison syndrome is to control the gastric acid hypersecretion. It is important that the gastric acid secretion be controlled before the diagnosis is completely established if the patient is acutely ill because acid-peptic complications can develop rapidly in these patients. It is now widely accepted that gastric acid hypersecretion should be treated medically in all patients with Zollinger-Ellison syndrome, except for the small percentage (<1%) who cannot or will not take regular oral gastric acid antisecretory agents [1,6,9,15,17]. The gastric acid antisecretory drugs of choice are now the H^+-K^+ ATPase inhibitors, either omeprazole or lansoprazole [9,15]. These agents have the advantage over the histamine H_2-receptor antagonists of being long acting, with the result that once or twice daily dosing is possible in almost every patient [1,15,116]. Recent studies demonstrate that omeprazole and lansoprazole have similar long durations of action ($t_{0.5}$, 35 hr) [15,117,118]. Patients have now been treated continuously for up to 9 years with omeprazole with no loss of efficacy, no drug-related side effects, and no patient requiring emergency surgery or developing a complication due to treatment [119].

In the past, various criteria have been proposed that represent adequate control of gastric acid hypersecretion [1,15,37,108,117,120]. However, now almost all use the criterion of reduction of gastric acid secretion to <10 mEq/hr for the hour prior to the next dose of gastric antisecretory drug [1,15,37,108,117,120]. In patients with previous Billroth II procedures or with severe reflux esophagitis symptoms and/or disease, gastric acid hypersecretion needs to be reduced to <5 mEq/hr and in some cases to <1 mEq/hr [1,15,38,121].

Many patients suspected of having Zollinger-Ellison syndrome are acutely ill at presentation, and parenteral gastric acid antisecretory therapy may be needed. Parenteral omeprazole is highly effective [122,123] but is not available in the United States, and, therefore, parenteral histamine H_2-receptor antagonists are required [15,117]. Any of the histamine H_2-receptor antagonists can be used, but the most extensive experience is with iv ranitidine [124] or cimetidine [125]. Typically, a bolus injection of 150 mg of ranitidine is given, followed by a continuous iv infusion starting a 1 mg/kg body weight/hr. If cimetidine is used, a threefold higher dose is needed. Acid secretion should be rechecked after several hours, and if acid secretion is not controlled (<10 mEq/hr), the ranitidine dose should be increased by 0.5 mg/kg/hr. The mean dose of ranitidine is 1 mg/kg/hr, with a range of 0.5–2.5 mg/kg/hr [124], and for cimetidine the mean dose is 1.9 mg/kg/hr with a range of 0.5–0.7 mg/kg/hr [125]. Patients with Zollinger-Ellison syndrome have had acid secretion controlled for up to 2 months without side effects [124,125].

In patients post–successful resection of the gastrinoma, gastric acid secretion decreases such that by 6 months postresection, MAO decreased by 40%, and BAO decreased by 75% [126]. Even with follow-up up to 4 years, 67% of patients post–curative resection remained mild gastric acid hypersecretors [BAO <30 mEq/hr, mean 14) and required low doses of ranitidine [126]. The cause for this continued mild hypersecretion remains unclear [126].

Surgical management of gastric-acid hypersecretion

Total gastrectomy should now be reserved for the rare patient who will not or cannot take regular oral medication [1,127]. At present a total gastrectomy is relatively safe in a patient with Zollinger-Ellison syndrome [128]. Overall operative mortality was 5.6% in 248 cases reported since 1980 and 2.4% for elective cases [128]. The morbidity is unclear but in some studies up to 50% have moderate to severe side effects [1]. In 1985 parietal cell vagotomy (PCV) at the time of the surgical exploration to remove the gastrinoma was recommended [129] because it produced a mean decrease in BAO of 41% and doses of antisecretory drugs were reduced by 40%. However, PCV only augmented the inhibitory effect of the histamine H_2-receptor antagonist, and no patient was able to discontinue antisecretory drugs [129]. With the subsequent availability of more potent histamine H_2-receptor antagonists and more recently, H^+-K^+ ATPase inhibitors, PCV was rarely used. However, a recent long-term follow-up of these patients [130] demonstrates 36% had been able to discontinue all antisecretory drugs, and 86% continued to have BAOs 80% reduced from the preoperative level. This led the authors to propose that PCV now be routinely used at the time of laparotomy. An editorial analysis of this study [131] agreed with this conclusion, pointing out the importance of drug expense, the value to the patients who were able to stop all drugs, and avoidance of the need for long-term H^+-K^+ ATPase treatment with a successful PCV.

Tumor localization

General

After control of the gastric acid secretion to adequately treat a patient with Zollinger-Ellison syndrome, the location and the extent of the gastrinoma needs to be established [1,13]. Localization of the tumor extent is essential to determine whether surgical resection of the primary tumor should be attempted, whether cytoreductive surgery for more extensive disease needs to be considered, or whether treatment directed against metastatic disease needs to be considered [1,13]. Location of the primary is important because these tumors are frequently small and multiple, and can be difficult to find at laparotomy.

Conventional imaging studies [ultrasound, CT scan, magnetic resonance imaging (MRI), selective abdominal angiography] and bone scanning have been the procedures mainly used in the past [1,13]. Functional localization studies measuring gastrin venous gradients, either by percutaneous transhepatic portal venous sampling (PVS) or after intra-arterial secretin injections, with hepatic venous sampling for gastrin levels, have also been used both to localize the primary tumor [12,132,133] and metastatic gastrinomas to the liver [134]. Recently two newer methods, endoscopic ultrasound [135,136] and radionuclide scanning after injection of radiolabeled octreotide [(^{111}In-DTPA-DPhe^1)octreotide; somatosatin receptor scintigraphy (SRS)] [137–140], are being increasingly used. Because greater than 90% of gastrinomas have somatostatin receptors, SRS has been reported to be a particularly sensitive method to image gastrinomas, as well as most other PETs [138,139,141]. It has been difficult to compare the sensitivities and specificities of these procedures because only some procedures are done in some studies, many studies have only small numbers of patients, and the patients may vary in disease extent in different studies. Recently a prospective NIH study [140] evaluated the sensitivity of conventional imaging studies (ultrasound, CT scan, MRI, selective angiography) and SRS in 80 consecutive patients with Zollinger-Ellison syndrome, allowing a direct comparison of the different methods. These data are included in Table 5 with data from other studies. From a clinical point of view, it is important to consider the abilities of the different modalities to image the primary gastrinoma separate from their ability to localize gastrinoma metastatic to the liver [1,140]. Primary tumors are imaged to determine potential respectability, whereas metastatic liver lesions are frequently imaged to determine the need for treatment directed against the tumor, to determine that exploratory laparotomy for cure is not indicated, and to assess the results of antitumor therapy.

In recent studies, such as the NIH study of 80 consecutive cases [140], ultrasound, CT scan, MRI, and angiography localized an extrahepatic lesion in less than 50% of cases, although their specificities remain high (Table 5). The SRS is more sensitive in most studies than any conventional imaging study (see

312

Table 5. Ability of localization methods to identify extrahepatic and hepatic gastrinomas

	Sensitivity (%)			Specificity (%)	
	1996 NIH study (140)	Literature		Literature	
		Mean	(range)	Mean	(range)
Extrahepatic lesions					
Ultrasound	9[a]	23	(21–28)	92	(92–93)
CT scan	31[a]	38	(0–59)	90	(83–100)
MR	30[a]	22	(20–25)	100	(100)
Angiography	28[a]	68	(35–68)	89	(84–94)
SRS	58	72	(58–77)	100	
Endoscopic ultrasound	—	70	(16–86)		
Intra-arterial secretin test	—	89	(55–100)		
PVS	—	68	(60–94)		
Intraoperative US	—	83	(75–100)		
Metastatic liver disease					
Ultrasound	46[a]	14	(14–63)	100	
CT scan	42[a]	54	(35–72)	99	(94–100)
MR imaging	71	63	(43–83)	92	(88–100)
Angiography	65[a]	62	(33–86)	98	(96–100)
SRS	92	97	(92–100)		
Intra-arterial secretin test	—	40			

[a] p < 0.05 compared with SRS alone.
SRS data from refs. 137, 139, and 140. Endoscopic US from refs. 135–137 and 142. Intra-arterial secretin test for liver metastases from ref. 134. Other imaging studies from refs. 1, 12, 13, 47, 52, 132, 139, 143, 145, and 147.
CT scan = computed tomographic scan; MRI = magnetic resonance imaging; SRS = somatostatin receptor scintigraphy using [^{111}In-DTPA-DPhe^1]octreotide; PVS = transhepatic portal venous for gastrin gradients; US = ultrasound.

Table 5), and in the recent NIH study it was equal in sensitivity for localizing an extrahepatic gastrinoma to all the conventional imaging studies combined. Figure 2 shows the results of SRS in a patient with a negative conventional imaging study in which the SRS localized a gastrinoma in the pancreatic head area. Endoscopic ultrasound has been reported to be particularly useful for identifying pancreatic gastrinomas [135,142] (see Table 5). In a recent comparative study [137] of 32 patients with Zollinger-Ellison syndrome, SRS detected a pancreaticoduodenal tumor in 56%, endoscopic ultrasound in 40%, and both together in 69%. In a recent study, endoscopic ultrasound detected 50% of duodenal gastrinomas, 75% of the pancreatic tumors, and 62% of the gastrinomas in lymph nodes [135]. Figure 2 illustrates the results of endoscopic ultrasound in which SRS had shown a lesion in the pancreatic head/duodenal area. Endoscopic ultrasound visualizes a pancreatic head gastrinoma that was partially obstructing the biliary duct.

Numerous studies demonstrate that the ability to localize duodenal gastrinomas may be particularly difficult. The ability of ultrasound, CT scan, and MRI to identify a gastrinoma is dependent on the size of the lesion [13]. With lesions <1 cm no tumors are generally seen, with a diameter of 1–3 cm

15–30% are seen, and with tumors >3 cm in diameter 95–100% are detected [13]. Therefore, conventional imaging studies miss most duodenal gastrinomas that are characteristically <1 cm. In two studies CT scan detected only 9% of duodenal tumors in one study [135], and in another study [47] of 35 patients with surgically proven duodenal gastrinomas, 55% of which had metastases to lymph nodes, the combination of ultrasound, CT scan, and MRI identified a tumor in only 15% of the patients, and angiography detected it in 47%. In

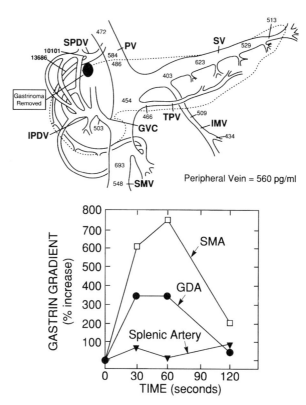

Figure 3. Results of portal venous sampling for gastrin (top) and intra-arterial secretin injection with hepatic venous gastrin sampling (bottom) in a patient with Zollinger-Ellison syndrome. **Top:** Serum gastrin concentrations at the indicated location. The peripheral venous gastrin concentration was 560 pg/ml. A positive gastrin gradient (>100%) of 2343% [(13,686–560/560)(100)] was found in the superior pancreaticoduodenal vein. **Bottom:** Hepatic venous gastrin levels expressed as a percentage of the preinjection level, after injection of secretin (75 clinical units) into the superior mesenteric, gastroduodenal, and splenic arteries. A positive gradient (>50 increase at 30 seconds, 105% at 1 minute [143]) is seen in the SMA and GDA. A duodenal wall gastrinoma was found at surgery in the area indicated in the top panel and supplied by the SMA and GDA in the bottom panel. Data are modified from Thom et al. [143]. PV = portal vein; SPDV = superior pancreaticoduodenal vein; SV = splenic vein; TPV = transverse pancreatic vein; IMV = inferior mesenteric vein; SMV = superior mesenteric vein; IPDV = inferior pancreaticoduodenal vein; GCV = gastrocolic vein.

many cases it is likely the angiogram was actually identifying lymph nodes, not the small duodenal tumor. These studies [135,142] suggest that both endoscopic ultrasound and SRS may miss more than 50% of all duodenal gastrinomas.

Functional studies measuring serum gastrin gradients are not dependent on tumor size. Recent studies demonstrate that hepatic venous sampling after a selective intra-arterial secretin study was more frequently positive than PVS (89% vs. 68%; see Table 5). With duodenal gastrinomas the intra-arterial secretin test was more frequently positive (78% vs. 28%) [143]. Similarly, in a recent study [47] on localizing duodenal gastrinomas, the intra-arterial secretin test was the most sensitive localization method (96%), which was greater than PVS (77%) and conventional imaging studies (52%). An example of an intra-arterial secretin test result and PVS in a patient with Zollinger-Ellison syndrome is shown in Figure 3. Both PVS and the intra-arterial secretin test were positive in this patient for the duodenum/pancreatic head area and at surgery a duodenal gastrinoma was found. It has been recently proposed that because of its increased sensitivity, ease of performance, and lower complication rate, the intra-arterial secretin test should replace PVS [12,143].

Functional localization has also been reported using injections of secretin into hepatic arteries and hepatic venous gastrin sampling to clarify equivocal liver lesions [134]. In a recent study [134], criteria were developed for a positive gradient in such a study and, although it had a lower sensitivity (41%) than CT (64%), ultrasound (64%), MRI (77%), or angiography (77%), the intra-arterial secretin test assisted in management in 22% of the patients. At present, functional localization studies are not routinely recommended [12]. In the case of extrahepatic lesions, functional studies localize only to the general area and not to specific structures within this area (i.e., pancreatic area, not duodenum). Because >70% of gastrinomas are in the pancreatic head area, the study is primarily of assistance in the 30% outside this area. A functional study should be particularly considered in two situations. First, if a proximal pancreaticoduodenectomy (Whipple) is planned if no tumor is found, then functional studies establish the presence of gastrinoma only in this area [12]. Secondly, if a patient has MEN-I and multiple tumors, functional localization will assist in excluding the 20% of gastrinomas outside the duodenum.

For imaging metastatic disease in the liver, the recent NIH study [140] confirms the results of a number of previous studies [138,139] that SRS is the single most sensitive modality (see Table 5). These studies demonstrate that SRS will identify greater than 90% of patients with Zollinger-Ellison syndrome with hepatic metastases (see Table 5), and in the NIH study [140] SRS was equal in sensitivity to the combination of all conventional studies for identifying patients with metastatic liver lesions (92% vs. 83%). It is important to realize that maximal sensitivity with SRS can only be obtained if SPECT (single photon emission computed tomographic scanning) is performed [144].

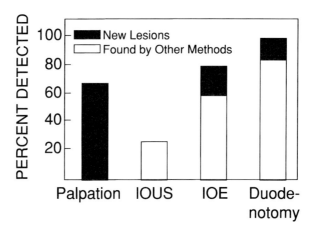

Figure 4. Intraoperative detection of duodenal gastrinomas. The ability of palpation (performed first), followed by intraoperative ultrasound (IOUS), followed by intraoperative endoscopy with transillumination (IOE) and duodenectomy to find a duodenal tumor in 42 consecutive patients with Zollinger-Ellison syndrome was studied. Gastrinomas were found in 95% of the patients, 30 of which had 36 duodenal tumors. Results are expressed as the percentage of the duodenal tumors found by the indicated method, with the black portion representing the percentage of new tumors found by the indicated method and the white area representing the percentage localized by the indicated method that had been found with the previous methods. Data are modified from Jensen and Fraker [6].

This is particularly true with liver lesions because they may be small, and it is unclear whether the lesions seen represent primary tumors or metastases. Recent improvements in MRI scanning have greatly increased its sensitivity, and especially if STIR sequences (short inversion-time inversion recovery sequences) are used, liver metastases are easily seen. The recent NIH study compared SRS with other imaging studies (see Table 5) [140], and the SRS and MRI had similar sensitivities (92% vs. 71%, p = 0.12). Therefore, if SRS is negative and the possibility of liver metastases is still of concern, MRI should be done.

If exploratory laparotomy is performed, three intraoperative procedures can help localize gastrinomas. Intraoperative ultrasound (IOUS) is particularly helpful for identifying pancreatic gastrinomas, localizing 91% of pancreatic gastrinomas but only 30% of duodenal gastrinomas [145,146]. The use of IOUS altered surgical management in 10% of cases in one study [146]. Transillumination of the duodenum at the time of surgery [147] will detect 20% more duodenal gastrinomas than palpation alone and is useful for planning the location of the duodenotomy in some cases [47,147] (see Fig. 3). Duodenotomy identifies 100% of all duodenal tumors, and a recent prospective study demonstrates it localizes 15% more duodenal gastrinomas than palpation, IOUS, and transillumination combined (Fig. 4). It is now recommended that IOUS and duodenotomy should be used in all Zollinger-Ellison syndrome cases during surgical exploration [17,145].

316

Treatment of the gastrinoma

*Treatment of the gastrinoma in patients with Zollinger-Ellison syndrome
without liver metastases or MEN-I*

Until recently, there was considerable difference of opinion about whether
all patients with Zollinger-Ellison syndrome without MEN-I or medical
contraindications to surgery should have surgical exploration [1,18,148–150].
This difference in opinion, in large part, was due to three different reasons
[1,149,151,152]. There was a lack of agreement on the natural history of
gastrinomas. There was a failure of any surgical studies to demonstrate for
patients with Zollinger-Ellison syndrome or any malignant PET that early
surgical removal of the primary tumor decreased the development of
metastases or extended survival. Finally, there was an uncertainty about long-
term cure rates postresection [1,149,151,152]. Within the last 2 years there
have been a number of studies that address these three concerns and support
the recommendation that all patients without metastatic liver disease, MEN-I,
or medical contraindications to surgery or limiting life expectancy should
undergo surgical exploration for possible cure [1,6,17,108].

First, a recent NIH study provides evidence for the first time that surgical excision decreases the rate of development of metastases [152]. In this
study only 3 of 98 patients (3) undergoing surgery for cure developed liver
metastases, whereas 6 of 26 patients (23%; $p < 0.0003$) not undergoing surgery
developed hepatic metastases (Fig. 5). Furthermore, two deaths due to metastatic disease occurred in the nonoperative group, and there were no disease-
specific deaths in the surgical group ($p = 0.085$) [152] (see Fig. 5). Although
this was not a readomized study, the groups were well matched for clinical
characteristics, time of onset to follow-up (15.4 vs. 14.0 years), and time since
diagnosis (9.4 vs. 7.7 years). The percentage of patients with MEN-I in the no-
operation group was numerically higher, but the difference was not significant
(35% vs. 15%, $p > 0.05$).

Secondly, at least three studies [46,130,152] now provide some long-term
follow-up data on patients with Zollinger-Ellison syndrome, either after undergoing surgical explorations (n = 120) or not (n = 28). The data from the
large NIH study [46] are particularly helpful because they provide evidence
that in 75% of patients (see Table 5) the gastrinoma pursues a relatively
benign nonaggressive course, whereas in 25% it has an aggressive course. At
present, unfortunately, as discussed in the tumor biology section, it is not
possible to predict which individual patient will be in the aggressive or
nonaggressive tumor group.

Lastly, data exist on short- and long-term cure rates. Presently gastrinomas
are found at surgery in >90% of cases, and in the most recent NIH study 60%
of patients were disease free immediately postoperative and 30% were disease
free at 5 years [151,153]. These results can only be obtained if a thorough
search of the duodenum is performed, including the routine use of

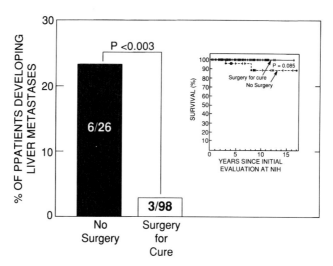

Figure 5. Effect of surgery for cure on development of hepatic metastases and survival in patients with the Zollinger-Ellison syndrome. The percentage of patients medically managed without surgical exploration for cure (n = 26) and the percentage of patients undergoing surgery for cure (n = 98) who developed hepatic metastases during follow-up (mean 7 years) are shown **Inset**: Survival in these two groups of patients. Data are from Fraker and Norton [152].

duodenotomy [6,47] (see Fig. 4). In a recent study [6] of 42 patients with Zollinger-Ellison syndrome in 95% of whom gastrinomas were found, 71% of the patients had duodenal tumors. Palpation alone found 65% of the duodenal tumors, intraoperative ultrasound localized no new duodenal tumors, endoscopic transillumination identified an additional 20%, and duodenotomy detected an additional 15% (see Fig. 4). These results demonstrate that routine duodenotomy should now be performed in all patients with Zollinger-Ellison syndrome undergoing exploratory laparotomy.

Treatment of the gastrinoma in patients with Zollinger-Ellison syndrome without liver metastases with MEN-I

Currently, there is no agreement on the best method to treat the gastrinoma in patients with MEN-I [1,5,43,148]. Until a few years ago it was recommended that these patients not undergo routine exploratory laparotomy because they were rarely cured by tumor enucleation [1,5,43,148]. In 1990 [64] 8 patients with Zollinger-Ellison syndrome and MEN-I were described, all of whom had only duodenal gastrinomas and in 4 of 6 patients with the gastrinoma excised, serum gastrin became normal. Based on these results [64], it was proposed that patients with Zollinger-Ellison syndrome with MEN-I should have surgical explorations to remove the duodenal tumors. Two recent studies have important findings commenting on this approach. In two studies [14,61,149] pancreatic gastrinomas were reported in 20% and 62% of patients with MEN-I and Zollinger-Ellison syndrome; therefore, gastrinomas do not exclusively occur in

318

the duodenum in these patients. In a recent prospective study [63], the ability to surgically cure patients with MEN-I and Zollinger-Ellison syndrome by careful duodenal exploration was assessed in 10 consecutive patients. All patients with MEN-I had gastrinomas found at exploration and 70% of patients had a duodenal gastrinoma, 20% a pancreatic gastrinoma, and 10% a gastrinoma in lymph nodes only [63]. No patient was cured. Failure to cure these patients was due to the fact that 86% of the duodenal gastrinomas had metastasized to the lymph nodes, 30% of patients had >20 duodenal gastrinomas, and enucleation of the pancreatic gastrinomas did not result in cure, suggesting there must be either retained metastases to lymph nodes or multiple primaries [63]. This study [63] clearly demonstrates these patients cannot be cured by gastrinoma enucleation alone. Some [154,155] have recommended Whipple resections be considered in patients with Zollinger-Ellison syndrome with MEN-I and in one study [155] three such patients remained cured for 7, 9, and 13 years postresection. At present this recommendation is not generally endorsed. The principal difficulty is that it remains unclear what the natural history of the PETs are in patients with MEN-I, and, therefore, it is unclear whether any surgical intervention prolongs survival. In the case of the Zollinger-Ellison syndrome, in which the symptoms of hypersecretion can be controlled effectively in all patients, the question of whether resection of the gastrinoma alone reduces the rate of metastatic disease and prolongs life remains unanswered.

Treatment of the gastrinoma in patients with Zollinger-Ellison syndrome with liver metastases

General

Although gastrinomas are, along with other malignant PETs, considered to be slow-growing tumors, in recent studies the 5-year survival of patients with metastatic disease is as low as 20% [1,43] (see Fig. 1). Furthermore, now that the gastric acid hypersecretion can be controlled medically or surgically in all patients, the natural history of the gastrinoma is increasingly becoming the primary determinant of survival [1,43]. There is thus an increasing need for effective treatment of metastatic gastrinomas. Chemotherapy, systematic removal of all resectable tumor (cytoreductive surgery), hormonal therapy with the long-acting somatostatin analogue octreotide, treatment with interferon, hepatic embolization alone or with chemotherapy (chemoembolization), and liver transplantation have all been advocated [1,16,19,156–160] (Table 6). Treatment with each of these modalities has recently been reviewed [156], including chemotherapy [16], cytoreductive surgery [159], vascular occlusion [160], liver transplantation [19], treatment with octreotide [161,162], and interferon [163] and thus is only briefly discussed here.

At present the role of each of these modalities in the treatment of patients

Table 6. Drug therapy for metastatic gastrinomas

Agent	Patients (no.)	Objective response (%)	Author	Year	Ref.
STZ	24	12 (50%)	Jensen et al.	(1983)	[37]
			Moertel et al.	(1980)	[167]
DTIC	5	0 (0%)	NIH	(1987)	
Etoposide	2	0 (0%)	Kelsen et al.	(1987)	[166]
CZT	4	1 (25%)	Moertel et al.	(1992)	[168]
Carboplatin	3	0 (0%)	Saltz et al.	(1993)	[165]
Etoposide + cisplatin	8	2 (25%)	Moertel et al.	(1991)	[176]
STZ + 5-FU	3	1 (33%)	Moertel et al.	(1980)	[167]
	10	8 (80%)	Mignon et al.	(1986)	[171]
	5	1 (20%)	Hofmann et al	(1973)	[172]
	22	1 (5%)	Ruszniewski et al.	(1991)	[173]
	11	5 (45%)	Moertel et al.	(1992)	[168]
CZT + 5-FU	12	3 (25%)	Bukowski et al.	(1992)	[169]
SZT + DOX	11	7 (64%)	Moertel et al.	(1992)	[168]
STZ or 5-FU + STZ (n = 17)	45	(42%)	Bonfils et al.	(1986)	[175]
STZ + 5-FU + DOX	10	4 (40%)	von Schrenck et al.	(1988)	[174]
Octreotide	9	1 (11%)	Kvols et al.	(1987)	[197]
	16	3 (19%)	Maton et al.	(1989)	[196]
	21	3 (14%)	Maton et al.	(1989)	[198]
	6	0 (0%)	Arnold et al.	(1993)	[162]
Interferon	4	2 (50%)	Eriksson et al.	(1986)	[188]
	11	0 (0%)	Pisegna et al.	(1993)	[187]

STZ = streptozotocin; DOX = doxorubicin; CZT = chlorozotocin; 5-FU = 5-fluorouracil; DTIC = dacarbazine.

with metastatic gastrinoma remains unclear [1,43,156]. This has occurred for a number of reasons. First, gastrinomas are usually combined in different series with other malignant PETs or carcinoid tumors, and it is not established that they respond similarly [1,43,156]. Secondly, because of their rarity, few systematic studies of different modalities in significant numbers of patients have been done (see Table 6). Lastly, there is no agreement on dosing frequency, dosage, and when therapy should be started, continued, or discontinued [1]. More importantly, there have been no placebo-controlled trials that clearly establish the benefit of any chemotherapy. Although different treatments have been compared with each other and the superiority of some has been shown, because of the variable course of different patients it still remains unclear how much advantage a given treatment has over no treatment.

Chemotherapy

In studies involving different types of PETs including gastrinomas, except for streptozotocin and chlorozotocin, single-agent chemotherapy has had low success rates [43,156,158,164]. Similar results are reported specifically in small

320

numbers of patients with gastrinomas with low response rates with carboplatin [165], etoposide [166], and DTIC (see Table 6). Streptozotocin [37,167] and chlorozotocin [168] alone have given response rates of 25–50% (see Table 6). Combinations of streptozotocin or chlorozotocin in patients with a variety of PETs have been evaluated in a number of studies [16,43,156,158,164,169]. In a prospective ECOG study [167], the combination of streptozotocin plus 5-fluorouracil was more effective than streptozotocin alone (63% vs. 40% response rate). A subsequent study by the same group [168] in patients with a variety of malignant PETs demonstrated that streptozotocin plus doxorubicin was superior to streptozotocin plus 5-fluorouracil or chlorozotocin alone (response rates of 69%, 45, and 30%, respectively). The median durations of tumor regression were 18 months, 14 months, and 17 months, respectively; however, the survival time for patients treated with the doxorubicin combination was longer [168].

Streptozotocin plus 5-fluorouracil [170–173], streptozotocin plus doxorubicin [168], and streptoxotocin plus both drugs [174] have been used in small numbers of patients with metastatic gastrinomas in various series (see Table 6). However, in two prospective studies involving only patients with metastatic gastrinoma [174,175], the response rates were lower than reported in the ECOG studies that involved patients with a number of different malignant PETs. In one study [174] involving 10 patients with metastatic gastrinomas increasing in size in the liver, the objective response (<25% decrease in tumor diameter) was 40% with streptozotocin, 5-fluorouracil, and doxorubicin. Furthermore, no complete remissions occurred, and there was no difference in the survival of responders versus nonresponders [174]. In another study of 21 patients with hepatic metastases with Zollinger-Ellison syndrome, only 5% (one patient) had an objective response (>50% decrease in size), whereas three patients had a transient, partial response (25–49% decrease in size) [162]. The combination of etoposide and cisplatin [176] is reported to give a response rate in 67% of anaplastic neuroendocrine tumors; however, the response rate in metastatic gastrinomas was 25% (see Table 6).

Hepatic embolization with or without chemotherapy

Hepatic embolization with or without chemotherapy has been recommended to be of value in small numbers of patients with metastatic gastrinomas and other PETs [43,156,160,177,178]. Because the liver derives only 20–25% of its blood supply from the hepatic artery and 75–80% from the portal vein, and because most PETs, including gastrinomas, are vascular with an arterial supply, hepatic artery embolization can be used if the portal vein is patient. In combined series of PETs, 68–100% of patients are reported to show improvement with this treatment [156]. In one large series [179] involving 111 patients, hepatic arterial occlusion with chemotherapy (doxorubicin plus dacarbazine or streptozotocin and 5-fluorouracil) resulted in an objective response in 80%

compared with 60% with occlusion alone. With occlusion alone the mean duration of the response was 4 months, and when chemotherapy was added it was 18 months.

Recently chemoembolization with doxorubicin in iodized oil combined with either sponge particles or gelatin powder has been reported to decrease tumor size in 57–100% of patients [156,177,178,180]. In a recent study [181] five patients with metastatic gastrinoma in the liver were treated with such a regimen. In contrast to 18 patients with carcinoid tumors in which symptoms of the carcinoid syndrome were controlled in 80% and the size of liver metastases decreased by 50% in one half of the patients, in patients with Zollinger-Ellison syndrome 60% (3 of 5 patients) had a minor response (n = 1) or stabilization (n = 2). The authors of this study [181] concluded that gastrinomas may be less responsive to chemoembolization than carcinoid tumors, although the experience was small.

Cytoreductive surgery

Systematic removal of all resectable tumor has been recommended in general for treating metastatic PETs [159,182–184]. A number of recent studies [182–185] and a recent review [159] have provided support for such an approach. In one study [183] involving 17 cases with potentially respectable PETs, in 80% of the cases tumor was completely resected and survival was 79% at 5 years. In this study [183] patients with extensive metastases had a 5-year survival of 28% and inoperable patients 28%, whereas patients with limited resections had a significantly prolonged surival (p = 0.02). In a second study [182] in 74 patients with potentially respectable disease, neuroendocrine hepatic metastases of different types, a hemihepatectomy, extended hepatectomy, or nonanatomic hepatic resection was done. Perioperative mortality was 2.7%, morbidity was 24%, and 4-year survival was 73%. Unfortunately only a small proportion of all patients with PETs fall into the potentially resectable category (i.e., 9% in one study [184] and 5% in another [183]). Such an approach has been advocated in patients with Zollinger-Ellison syndrome with potentially resectable metastatic disease [185,186]. In one study [185] 20% of patients with metastatic liver disease with Zollinger-Ellison syndrome were potentially resectable on imaging, each underwent hepatic resection, and two patients maintained normal serum gastrin levels postresection. These data, as well as experience with other PETs, suggest that if imaging studies determine the metastatic disease is confined to one liver lobe and the primary tumor is resectable, or if greater than 90% of the imaged tumor can be safely resected, surgical resection should be attempted.

Treatment with interferon

Interferon has been reported to be effective in both controlling symptoms and also in inhibiting further tumor growth of metastatic PETs in a number of

322

studies [43,156,163,187,188]. In a recent review [163] of a number of series involving 322 patients with various neuroendocrine tumors, 43% showed a biochemical response (>50% decrease in hormone levels) and 12% showed a decrease in tumor size with interferon. Of the 57 patients with PETs, 47% had a biochemical response and 12% a decrease in tumor size [163]. Disease stabilization was seen in 25% [163]. Interferon has been used in a small number of patients with metastatic gastrinoma [187,188]. In one recent study [187] of 11 patients with metastatic gastrinoma increasing in size in the liver treated with daily α interferon (5 million units/day), no patients had a decrease in tumor size but three patients (30%) had a stabilization of tumor size. These results and those in other metastatic PETs demonstrate that inteferon rarely causes a decrease in tumor size but has a tumoristic effect, stabilizing the metastatic disease in 25–30%. Whether interferon prolongs survival is not established.

Treatment with somatostatin analogs

In animal somatostatin analogs can inhibit tumor growth and the growth of transplanted insulinomas [156,189]. Greater than 90% of gastrinomas as well as other PETs, except insulinomas, possess somatostatin receptors [139,156,189–192] that mediate the action of somatostatin on these tumors. Two long-acting somatostatin analogs have been used in clinical studies, lanreotide and octreotide [192,193]. Recent studies provide evidence for five somatostatin receptor subtypes, and the actions of these two long-acting soma-tostatin analogs is primarily mediated by subtype 2 or 5 [190–192]. In a recent review of 66 patients treated with octreotide with metastatic neuroendocrine tumors, octreotide caused a decrease in tumor size in 12% of patients (eight patients); however, in other studies it caused a disease stabilization in 25–50% [156,162,194–198]. Similar studies have been performed on a small number of patients with metastatic gastrinoma [156,162,194,195]. These data suggest that long-acting somatostatin analogs likely have a tumorstatic effect in some patients with metastatic gastrinoma, but that they rarely have a tumoricidal effect, resulting in a decreasing tumor size. Whether these analogs will prolong life is not established. Long-acting somatostatin analogs will also inhibit acid secretion and decrease serum gastrin levels in Zollinger-Ellison syndrome patients [199]; however, in Zollinger-Ellison syndrome with the availability of highly effective oral gastric acid antisecretory agents, parenteral octreotide is rarely needed.

Liver transplantation

Liver transplantation has been performed in a small number of patients with metastatic PETs and with metastatic gastrinomas [19,157,200,201]. Each of these reports has small numbers of cases (<11 patients). All of these reports recommend liver transplantation be considered in selected cases, particularly in patients without extrahepatic disease. It appears from the small number of cases (n = 23) that long-term cure is uncommon, with recurrence to bone, lymph nodes, or liver being most common. At present it remains unclear which patients, if any, with metastatic gastrinoma or other PETs should undergo liver transplantation.

References

1. Jensen RT, Gardner JD. 1993. Gastrinoma. In Go VLW, DiMagno EP, Gardner JD, Lebenthal E, Reber HA, Scheele GA, eds. The Pancreas: Biology, Pathobiology and Disease. New York: Raven Press, pp 931–978.
2. Rehfeld JF, van Solinge WW. 1994. The tumor biology of gastrin and cholecystokinin. Adv Cancer Res 63:295–347.
3. van Solinge WW, Odum L, Rehfeld JF. 1993. Ovarian cancers express and process progastrin. Cancer Res 53:1823–1828.
4. Rehfeld JF, Bardram L. 1995. Prohormone processing and pancreatic endocrine tumors. In Mignon M, Jensen RT, eds. Endocrine Tumors of the Pancreas: Recent Advances in Research and Management. Frontiers of Gastrointestinal Research. Vol 23 Basel, Switzerland: S. Karger, pp 84–98.
5. Metz DC, Jensen RT, Bale AE, Skarulis MC, Eastman RC, Nieman L, Norton JA, Friedman E, Larrson C, Amorosi A, Brandi ML, Marx SJ. 1994. Multiple endocrine neoplasia type 1: Clinical features and management. In Bilezekian JP, Levine MA, Marcus R, eds. The Parathyroids. New York: Raven Press, pp 591–646.
6. Jensen RT, Fraker DL. 1994. Zollinger-Ellison syndrome: Advances in treatment of the gastric hypersecretion and the gastrinoma. JAMA 271:1–7.
7. Norton JA. 1994. Neuroendocrine tumors of the pancreas and duodenum. Curr Probl Surg 31:1–156.
8. Mignon M, Jais P, Cadiot G, Yedder D, Vatier J. 1995. Clinical features and advances in biological diagnostic criteria for Zollinger-Ellison syndrome. In Mignon M, Jensen RT, eds. Endocrine Tumors of the Pancreas: Recent Advances in Research and Management. Frontiers of Gastrointestinal Research. Vol 23 Basel, Switzerland: S. Karger, pp 223–239.
9. Weber HC, Orbuch M, Jensen RT. 1995. Diagnosis and management of Zollinger-Ellison syndrome. In Jensen RT, ed. Pancreatic Endocrine Tumors. Seminars in Gastrointestinal Diseases. Philadelphia: WB Saunders, pp 79–89.
10. Kloppel G, Schroder S, Heitz PU. 1995. Histopathology and immunopathology of pancreatic endocrine tumors. In Mignon M, Jensen RT, eds. Endocrine Tumors of the Pancreas: Recent Advances in Research and Management. Frontiers of Gastrointestinal Research. Vol 23 Basel, Switzerland: S. Karger, pp 99–120.
11. Gibril F, Reynolds JC, Doppman JL, Chen CC, Termanini B, Stewart CA, Jensen RT. 1995. Does the use of octreoscanning alter management in patients with Zollinger-Ellison syndrome: A prospective study (abstr)? Gastroenterology 108(Suppl 1):A356.
12. Strader DB, Doppman JL, Orbuch M, Fishbeyn VA, Benya RV, Jensen RT, Met DC. 1995. Functional localization of pancreatic endocrine tumors. In Mignon M, Jensen RT, eds. Frontiers of Gastrointestinal Research. Basel, Switzerland: S. Karger, pp 282–297.
13. Orbuch M, Doppman JL, Strader DB, Fishbeyn VA, Benya RV, Metz DC, Jensen RT. 1995. Imaging for pancreatic endocrine tumor localization: Recent advances. In Mignon M, Jensen RT, eds. Endocrine Tumors of the Pancreas: Recent Advances in Research and Management. Frontiers of Gastrointestinal Research. Vol 23 Basel, Switzerland: S. Karger, pp 268–281.
14. Mignon M, Cadiot G, Rigaud D, Ruszniewski P, Jais P, Lehy T, Lewin MJM. 1995. Management of islet cell tumors in patients with multiple endocrine neoplasia type 1. In Mignon M,

Jensen RT, eds. Endocrine Tumors of the Pancreas: Recent Advances in Research and Management. Frontiers of Gastrointestinal Research. Vol 23 Basel, Switzerland: S. Karger, pp 342–359.

15. Metz DC, Jensen RT. 1995. Advances in gastric antisecretory therapy in Zollinger-Ellison syndrome. In Mignon M, Jensen RT, eds. Endocrine Tumors of the Pancreas: Recent Advances in Research and Management. Frontiers of Gastrointestinal Research. Vol 23 Basel, Switzerland: S. Karger, pp 240–257.

16. Arnold R, Frank M. 1995. Systemic chemotherapy for endocrine tumors of the pancreas: Recent advances. In Mignon M, Jensen RT, eds. Endocrine Tumors of the Pancreas: Recent Advances in Research and Management. Frontiers of Gastrointestinal Research. Vol 23 Basel, Switzerland: S. Karger, pp 431–438.

17. Norton JA. 1994. Advances in the management of Zollinger-Ellison syndrome. Adv Surg 27:129–159.

18. Norton JA, Jensen RT. 1991. Unresolved surgical issues in the management of patients with the Zollinger-Ellison syndrome. World J Surg 15:151–159.

19. Azoulay D, Bismuth H. 1995. Role of liver surgery and transplantation in patients with hepatic metastases from pancreatic endocrine tumors. In Mignon M, Jensen RT, eds. Endocrine Tumors of the Pancreas: Recent Advances in Research and Management. Frontiers of Gastrointestinal Research. Vol 23 Basel, Switzerland: S. Karger, pp 461–476.

20. Walsh JH. 1994. Gastrin. In Walsh JH, Dockray GJ, eds. Gut Peptides. New York: Raven Press, pp 75–121.

21. Kochman ML, DelValle J, Dickinson CJ, Boland CR. 1992. Post-translational processing of gastrin in neoplastic human colonic tissues. Biochem Biophys Res Commun 189:1165–1169.

22. Mukai K, Grotting JC, Greider MH, Rosai J. 1982. Retrospective study of 77 pancreatic endocrine tumors using the immunoperoxidase method. Am J Surg Pathol 6:387–399.

23. Martensson H, Bottcher G, Sundler F, Nobin A. 1990. Localization and peptide content of endocrine pancreatic tumors. Ann Surg 212:607–614.

24. Maton PN, Mackem SM, Norton JA, Gardner JD, O'Dorisio TM, Jensen RT. 1989. Ovarian carcinoma as a cause of Zollinger-Ellison syndrome. Natural history, secretory products and response to provocative tests. Gastroenterology 97:468–471.

25. Dickinson CJ. 1995. Relationship of gastrin processing to colon cancer [editorial]. Gastroenterology 109:1384–1388.

26. Rehfeld JF. 1995. Gastrin and colorectal cancer: A never-ending dispute? [Editorial]. Gastroenterology 108:1307–1310.

27. Townsend CM Jr, Ishizuka J, Thompson JC. 1993. Gastrin trophic effects on transplanted colon cancer cells. In Walsh JH, eds. Gastrin. New York: Raven Press, pp 407–417.

28. Ciccotosto GD, McLeish A, Hardy KJ, Shulkes A. 1995. Expression, processing, and secretion of gastrin in patients with colorectal carcinoma. Gastroenterology 109:1142–1153.

29. Orbuch M, Venzon DJ, Lubensky IA, Weber HC, Gibril F, Jensen RT. 1996. Prolonged, hypergastrinemia does not increase the frequency of colonic neoplasia in patients with Zollinger-Ellison syndrome. Dig Dis Sci 41:604–613.

30. Sobhani I, Lehy T, Laurent-Puig P, Cadiot G, Ruszniewski P, Mignon M. 1993. Chronic endogenous hypergastrinemia in humans: Evidence for a mitogenic effect on the colonic mucosa. Gastroenterology 105:22–30.

31. Seva C, Dickinson CJ, Yamada T. 1994. Growth-promoting effects of glycine-extended progastrin. Science 265:410–412.

32. Singh P, Owlia A, Espeijo R, Dai B. 1995. Novel gastrin receptors mediate mitogenic effects of gastrin and processing intermediates of gastrin on Swiss 3T3 fibroblasts. Absence of detectable cholecystokinin CCK-A and CCK-B receptors. J Biol Chem 270:8429–8438.

33. Zollinger RM, Ellison EH. 1955. Primary peptic ulcerations of the jejunum associated with islet cell tumors of the pancreas. Ann Surg 142:709–728.

34. Chey WY, Chang TM, Park HJ, Lee KY, Escoffery R, Chen YF, Shah AN, Hamilton D, You CH, Menguy R. 1984. Non-gastrin secretagogue in ulcerogenic tumors of the pancreas. Ann Intern Med 101:7–13.

35. Grossman MI. 1966. Gastrin. Berkeley, CA: University of California Press.
36. Tjon AT, Jansen JB, Falke TH, Roelfsema F, Griffioen G, van den Sluys Veer A, Lamers CB. 1989. MR, CT, and ultrasound findings of metastatic vipoma in pancreas. J Comput Assist Tomogr 13:142–144.
37. Jensen RT, Gardner JD, Raufman JP, Pandol SJ, Doppman JL, Collen MJ. 1983. Zollinger-Ellison syndrome: Current concepts and management. Ann Intern Med 98:59–75.
38. Miller LS, Vinayek R, Frucht H, Gardner JD, Jensen RT, Maton PN. 1990. Reflux esophagitis in patients with Zollinger-Ellison syndrome. Gastroenterology 98:341–346.
39. Waxman I, Gardner JD, Jensen RT, Maton PN. 1991. Peptic ulcer perforation as the presentation of Zollinger-Ellison syndrome. Dig Dis Sci 16:19–24.
40. Jensen RT, Maton PN. 1992. Zollinger-Ellison syndrome. In Gustavsson S, Kumar D, Graham DY, eds. The Stomach. London: Churchill Livingstone, pp 341–374.
41. Bale AE. 1994. Molecular mechanisms of neoplasia in multiple endocrine neoplasia type 1-related and sporadic tumors of the pancreatic islet cells. Endocrinol Metab Clin North Am 23:109–115.
42. Skogseid B, Oberg K. 1995. Genetics of multiple endocrine neoplasia type 1. In Mignon M, Jensen RT, eds. Endocrine Tumors of the Pancreas: Recent Advances in Research and Management. Frontiers of Gastrointestinal Research. Vol 23 Basel, Switzerland: S. Karger, pp 60–69.
43. Norton JA, Levin B, Jensen RT. 1993. Cancer of the endocrine system. In DeVita VT Jr, Hellman S, Rosenberg SA, eds. Cancer: Principles and Practice of Oncology. Philadelphia: J.B. Lippincott pp 1333–1435.
44. Maton PN, Gardner JD, Jensen RT. 1986. Cushing's syndrome in patients with Zollinger-Ellision syndrome. N Engl J Med 315:1–5.
45. Norton JA, Cornelius MJ, Doppmann JL, Maton PN, Gardner JD, Jensen RT. 1987. Effect of parathyroidectomy in patients with hyperparathyroidism, Zollinger-Ellison syndrome and multiple endocrine neoplasia Type I: A prospective study. Surgery 102:958–966.
46. Weber HC, Venzon DJ, Lin JT, Fishbein VA, Orbuch M, Strader DB, Gibril F, Metz DC, Fraker DL, Norton JA, Jensen RT. 1995. Determinants of metastatic rate and survival in patients with Zollinger-Ellison syndrome: A prospective long-term study. Gastroenterology 108:1637–1649.
47. Sugg SL, Norton JA, Fraker DL, Metz DC, Pisegna JR, Fishbeyn V, Benya RV, Shawker TH, Doppman JL, Jensen RT. 1993. A prospective study of intraoperative methods to diagnose and resect duodenal gastrinomas. Ann Surg 218:138–144.
48. Stabile BE, Morrow DJ, Passaro E Jr. 1984. The gastrinoma triangle: Operative implications. Am J Surg 147:25–31.
49. Howard TJ, Zinner MJ, Stabile BE, Passaro E Jr. 1990. Gastrinoma excision for cure. A prospective analysis. Ann Surg 211:9–14.
50. Thom AK, Norton JA, Axiotis CA, Jensen RT. 1991. Location, incidence and malignant potential of duodenal gastrinomas. Surgery 110:1086–1093.
51. Arnold WS, Fraker DL, Alexander HR, Weber HC, Jensen RT. 1994. Apparent lymph node primary gastrinoma. Surgery 116:1123–1130.
52. Norton JA, Doppman JL, Collen MJ, Harmon JW, Maton PN, Gardner JD, Jensen RT. 1986. Prospective study of gastrinoma localization and resection in patients with Zollinger-Ellison syndrome. Ann Surg 204:468–479.
53. Perrier ND, Batts KP, Thompson GB, Grant CS, Plummer TB. 1995. An immunohistochemical survey for neuroendocrine cells in regional pancreatic lymph nodes: A plausible explanation for primary nodal gastrinomas? Surgery 118:957–965.
54. Bonfils S, Bader JP. 1970. The diagnosis of Zollinger-Ellison syndrome with special reference to the multiple endocrine adenomas. In Jerzy-Glass GB, ed. Progressive Gastroenterology, Vol. 2. New York: Grune & Stratton, pp 332–336.
55. Barton JC, Hirschowitz BI, Maton PN, Jensen RT. 1986. Bone metastases in malignant gastrinoma. Gastroenterology 91:1179–1185.

56. Jensen RT, Norton JA. 1995. Endocrine tumors of the pancreas. In Yamada T, Alpers BH, Owyang C, et al., eds. Textbook of Gastroenterology, 2nd ed. Philadelphia: J.B. Lippincott, pp 2131–2166.

57. Howard TJ, Sawicki MP, Stabile BE, Watt PC, Passaro E Jr. 1993. Biologic behavior of sporadic gastrinoma located to the right and left of the superior mesenteric artery. Am J Surg 165:101–105.

58. Howard TJ, Sawicki M, Lewin KJ, Steel B, Bhagavan BS, Cummings OW, Passaro E Jr. 1995. Pancreatic polypeptide immunoreactivity in sporadic gastrinoma: Relationship to intraabdominal location. Pancreas 11:350–356.

59. Kloppel G, Willemar S, Stamm B, Hacki WH, Heitz PU. 1986. Pancreatic lesions and hormonal profile of pancreatic tumors in multiple endocrine neoplasia type I. An immuno-cytochemical study of nine patients. Cancer 57:1824–1832.

60. Thompson NW, Lloyd RV, Nishiyama RH, Vinik AI, Strodel WE, Allo MD, Eckhauser FE, Talpos G, Mervak T. 1984. MEN I pancreas: A histological and immunohistochemical study. World J Surg 8:561–574.

61. Ruszniewski P, Podevin P, Cadiot G, Marmuse JP, Mignon M, Vissuzaine C, Bonfils S, Lehy T. 1993. Clinical, anatomical, and evolutive features of patients with the Zollinger-Ellison syndrome combined with type I multiple endocrine neoplasia. Pancreas 8:295–304.

62. Donow C, Pipeleers-Marichal M, Schroder S, Stamm B, Heitz PU, Kloppel G. 1991. Surgical pathology of gastrinoma: Site, size, multicentricity, association with multiple endocrine neoplasia type 1, and malignancy. Cancer 68:1329–1334.

63. MacFarlane MP, Fraker DL, Alexander HR, Norton JA, Jensen RT. 1995. A prospective study of surgical resection of duodenal and pancreatic gastrinomas. Surgery 118:973–980.

64. Pipeleers-Marichal M, Somers G, Willems G, Foulis A, Imrie C, Bishop AE, Polak JM, Hacki WH, Stamm B, Heitz PU, Kloppel G. 1990. Gastrinomas in the duodenums of patients with multiple endocrine neoplasia type 1 and the Zollinger-Ellison syndrome. N Engl J Med 322:723–727.

65. Heitz PU, Kasper M, Polak JM, Kloppel G. 1982. Pancreatic endocrine tumors. Hum Pathol 13:263–271.

66. Chiang HC, O'Dorisio TM, Huang SC, Maton PN, Gardner JD, Jensen RT. 1990. Multiple hormone elevations in patients with Zollinger-Ellison syndrome: Prospective study of clinical significance and of the development of a second symptomatic pancreatic endocrine tumor syndrome. Gastroenterology 99:1565–1575.

67. Wynick D, Williams SJ, Bloom SR. 1988. Symptomatic secondary hormone syndromes in patients with established malignant pancreatic endocrine tumors. N Engl J Med 319:605–607.

68. Eriksson B. 1995. Tumor markers for pancreatic endocrine tumors, including chromogranins, HCG-alpha and HCG-beta. In Mignon M, Jensen RT, eds. Endocrine Tumors of the Pancreas: Recent Advances in Research and Management. Frontiers of Gastrointestinal Research. Vol 23 Basel, Switzerland: S. Karger, pp 121–131.

69. Syversen U, Mignon M, Bonfils S, Kristensen A, Waldum HL. 1993. Chromogranin A and pancreastatin-like immunoreactivity in serum of gastrinoma patients. Acta Oncol 32:161–165.

70. Willems G. 1995. Trophic action of gastrin on specific target cells in the gut. In Mignon M, Jensen RT, eds. Endocrine Tumors of the Pancreas: Recent Advances in Research and Management. Frontiers of Gastrointestinal Research. Vol 23 Basel, Switzerland: S. Karger, pp 30–44.

71. Lehy T, Cadiot G, Mignon M, Ruszniewski P, Bonfils S. 1992. Influence of multiple endocrine neoplasia type 1 on gastric endocrine cells in patients with the Zollinger-Ellison syndrome. Gut 33:1275–1279.

72. Jensen RT. 1993. Gastrinoma as a model for prolonged hypergastrinemia in man. In Walsh JH, ed. Gastrin. New York: Raven Press, pp 373–393.

73. Stabile BE, Howard TJ, Passaro E Jr, O'Connor DT. 1990. Source of plasma chromogranin A elevation in gastrinoma patients. Arch Surg 125:451–453.

327

74. Bardram L, Agner T, Hagen C. 1988. Levels of alpha subunits of gonadotropins can be increased in Zollinger-Ellison syndrome, both in patients with malignant tumors and apparently benign disease. Acta Endocrinol (Copenh) 118:135–141.

75. Bardram L. 1990. Progastrin in serum from Zollinger-Ellison patients. An indicator of malignancy? Gastroenterology 98:1420–1426.

76. Kothary PC, Fabri PJ, Gower W, O'Dorisio TM, Ellis J, Vinik AI. 1986. Evaluation of NH2-terminus gastrins in gastrinoma syndrome. J Clin Endocrinol Metab 62:970–974.

77. Stabile BE, Passaro E Jr. 1985. Benign and malignant gastrinoma. Am J Surg 49:144–150.

78. Delcore R Jr, Cheung LY, Friesen SR. 1988. Outcome of lymph node involvement in patients with Zollinger-Ellison syndrome. Ann Surg 206:291–298.

79. Metz DC, Kuchnio M, Fraker DL, Venzon DJ, Jaffe G, Jensen RT, Stetler-Stevenson M. 1993. Flow cytometry and Zollinger-Ellison syndrome: Relationship to clinical course. Gastroenterology 105:799–813.

80. Oberg K. 1994. Expression of growth factors and their receptors in neuroendocrine gut and pancreatic tumors, and prognostic factors for survival. Ann NY Acad Sci 733:46–55.

81. Chaudhry A, Oberg K. 1995. Expression of growth factor peptides and adhesion molecules in endocrine pancreatic tumors. In Mignon M, Jensen RT, eds. Endocrine Tumors of the Pancreas: Recent Advances in Research and Management. Frontiers of Gastrointestinal Research. Vol 23 Basel, Switzerland: S. Karger, pp 132–146.

82. Chaudhry A, Gobl A, Eriksson B, Skogseid B, Oberg K. 1994. Different splice variants of CD44 are expressed in gastrinomas but not in other subtypes of endocrine pancreatic tumors. Cancer Res 54:981–986.

83. Bordi C, Viale G. 1995. Analysis of cell proliferation and tumor antigens of prognostic significance in pancreatic endocrine tumors. In Mignon M, Jensen RT, eds. Endocrine Tumors of the Pancreas: Recent Advances in Research and Management. Frontiers of Gastrointestinal Research. Vol 23 Basel, Switzerland: S. Karger, pp 45–59.

84. Ruschoff J, Willemer S, Brunzel M, Trautmann ME, Frank M, Arnold R, Kloppel G. 1993. Nucleolar organizer regions and glycoprotein-hormone alpha-chain reaction as markers of malignancy in endocrine tumours of the pancreas. Histopathology 22:51–57.

85. Pelosi G, Zamboni G, Doglioni C, Rodella S, Bresaola E, Iacono C, Serio G, Iannucci A, Scarpa A. 1992. Immunodetection of proliferating cell nuclear antigen assesses the growth fraction and predicts malignancy in endocrine tumors of the pancreas. Am J Surg Pathol 16:1215–1225.

86. Weinberg RA. 1994. Oncogenes and tumor suppressor genes. CA Cancer J Clin 44:160–170.

87. Knudson AG. 1993. Antioncogenes and human cancer. Proc Natl Acad Sci USA 90:10914–10921.

88. Arnold A. 1994. Molecular mechanisms of parathyroid neoplasia. Endocrinol Metab Clin North Am 23:93–107.

89. Weber HC, Jensen RT. 1996. Pancreatic endocrine tumors and carcinoid tumors: Recent insights from genetic and molecular biologic studies. In Dervenis C, Thieme G, eds. Advances in Pancreatic Diseases: Molecular Biology, Diagnosis and Treatment. Stuttgart, Germany: Verlag Publishing, pp 55–75.

90. Evers BM, Rady PL, Sandoval K, Arany I, Tyring SK, Sanchez RL, Nealon WH, Townsend CM, Thompson JC. 1994. Gastrinomas demonstrate amplification of the HER-2/neu proto-oncogene. Ann Surg 219:596–604.

91. Yashiro T, Fulton N, Hara H, Yasuda K, Montag A, Yashiro N, Straus F, Ito K, Aiyoshi Y, Kaplan EL. 1993. Comparison of mutations of ras oncogene in human pancreatic exocrine and endocrine tumors. Surgery 114:758–764.

92. Cryns VL, Thor A, Xu HJ, Hu SX, Wierman ME, Vickery AL, Benedict WF, Arnold A. 1994. Loss of the retinoblastoma tumor-suppressor gene in parathyroid carcinoma. N Engl J Med 330:757–761.

93. Lai SL, Brauch H, Knutsen T, Johnson BE, Nau MM, Mitsudomi T, Tsai CM, Whang-Peng

J, Zbar B, Kaye FJ, Gazdar AF. 1995. Molecular genetic characterization of neuroendocrine lung cancer cell lines. Anticancer Res 15:225–232.

94. Landis CA, Masters SB, Spada A, Pace AM, Bourne HR, Vallar L. 1989. GTPase inhibiting mutations activate the alpha chain of Gs and stimulate adenylyl cyclase in human pituitary tumours. Nature 340:692–696.

95. Lyons J, Landis CA, Harsh G, Vallar L, Grunewald K, Feichtinger H, Duh QY, Clark OH, Kawasaki E, Bourne HR. 1990. Two G protein oncogenes in human endocrine tumors. Science 249:655–659.

96. Vessey SJR, Jones PM, Wallis SC, Schofield J, Bloom SR. 1994. Absence of mutations in the Gsα and Gi2α genes in sporadic parathyroid adenomas and insulinomas. Clin Sci 87:493–497.

97. Zeiger MA, Norton JA. 1993. Gs alpha — identification of a gene highly expressed by insulinoma and other endocrine tumors. Surgery 114:458–462.

98. Larsson C, Weber G, Teh BT, Lagercrantz J. 1994. Genetics of multiple endocrine neoplasia type 1. Ann NY Acad Sci 733:453–463.

99. Beckers A, Abs R, Reyniers E, De Boulle K, Stevenaert A, Heller FR, Kloppel G, Meurisse M, Willems PJ. 1994. Variable regions of chromosome 11 loss in different pathological tissues of a patient with the multiple endocrine neoplasia type 1 syndrome. J Clin Endocrinol Metab 79:1498–1502.

100. Sawicki MP, Wan YJ, Johnson CL, Berenson J, Gatti R, Passaro E Jr. 1992. Loss of heterozygosity on chromosome 11 in sporadic gastrinomas. Hum Genet 89:445–449.

101. Eubanks PJ, Sawicki MP, Samara GJ, Gatti R, Nakamura Y, Tsao D, Johnson C, Hurwitz M, Wan YJ, Passaro E Jr. 1994. Putative tumor-suppressor gene on chromosome 11 is important in sporadic endocrine tumor formation. Am J Surg 167:180–185.

102. Cadiot G, Laurent-Puig P, Thuille B, Lehy T, Mignon M, Olschwang S. 1993. Is the multiple endocrine neoplasia type 1 gene a suppressor for fundic argyrophil tumors in the Zollinger-Ellison syndrome?. Gastroenterology 105:579–582.

103. Debelenko LV, Emmert-Buck MR, Zhuang Z, Jensen RT, Liotta LA, Lubensky IA. 1996. Frequent allelic deletions of MEN-I genelocus (11q13) in gastric ECL-cell carcinoids in patients with Zollinger-Ellison Syndrome (ZES) and MEN-I. Am J Clin Pathol, in press.

104. Lehy T, Mignon M, Cadiot G, Elouaer-Blanc L, Ruszniewski P, Lewin MJ, Bonfils S. 1989. Gastric endocrine cell behavior in Zollinger-Ellison patients upon long-term potent antisecretory treatment. Gastroenterology 96:1029–1040.

105. Rindi G, Luinetti O, Cornaggia M, Capella C, Solcia E. 1993. Three subtypes of gastric argyrophil carcinoid and the gastric neuroendocrine carcinoma: A clinicopathologic study. Gastroenterology 104:994–1006.

106. Grossman M. 1981. Peptic Ulcer: A Guide for the Practicing Physician. Chicago: Year Book Medical.

107. Metz DC, Weber C, Orbuch M, Strader DB, Gibril F, Jensen RT. 1994. *Helicobacter pylori* (Hp) infection and acid output in Zollinger-Ellison syndrome (ZES): A prospective study (abstr). Gastroenterology 106:A138.

108. Wolfe MM, Jensen RT. 1987. Zollinger-Ellison syndrome: Current concepts in diagnosis and management. N Engl J Med 317:1200–1209.

109. Zimmer T, Stolzel U, Bader M, Fett U, Foss HD, Riecken EO, Rehfeld JF, Wiedenmann B. 1995. Brief report: A duodenal gastrinoma in a patient with diarrhea and normal serum gastrin concentrations. N Engl J Med 333:634–636.

110. Jais P, Mignon M. 1995. Normal serum gastrin concentration in gastrinoma [letter]. Lancet 346:1421–1422.

111. Frucht H, Howard JM, Slaff JI, Wank SA, McCarthy DM, Maton PN, Vinayek R, Gardner JD, Jensen RT. 1989. Secretin and calcium provocative tests in the Zollinger-Ellison syndrome: A prospective study. Ann Intern Med 111:713–722.

112. Metz DC, Weber HC, Orbuch M, Strader DB, Lubensky IA, Jensen RT. 1995. *Helicobacter pylori* infection: A reversible cause of hypergastrinemia and hyperchlorhydria which can mimic Zollinger-Ellison syndrome. Dig Dis Sci 40:153–159.

113. el-Omar EM, Penman ID, Ardill JE, Chittajallu RS, Howie C, McColl KE. 1995. *Helicobacter pylori* infection and abnormalities of acid secretion in patients with duodenal ulcer disease. Gastroenterology 109:681–691.

114. Benya RV, Metz DC, Venzon DJ, Fishbeyn VA, Strader DB, Orbuch M, Jensen RT. 1994. Zollinger-Ellison syndrome can be the initial endocrine manifestation in patients with multiple endocrine neoplasia-type 1. Am J Med 97:436–444.

115. Shepherd JJ, Challis DR, Davies PF, McArdle JP, Teh BT, Wilkinson S. 1993. Multiple endocrine neoplasm, type 1: Gastrinomas, pancreatic neoplasms, microcarcinoids, the Zollinger-Ellison syndrome, lymph nodes, and hepatic metastases. Arch Surg 128:1133–1142.

116. Frucht H, Maton PN, Jensen RT. 1991. Use of omeprazole in patients with the Zollinger-Ellison syndrome. Dig Dis Sci 36:394–404.

117. Metz DC, Pisegna JR, Fishbeyn VA, Benya RV, Jensen RT. 1993. Control of gastric acid hypersecretion in the management of patients with Zollinger-Ellison syndrome. World J Surg 17:468–480.

118. Metz DC, Pisegna JR, Ringham GL, Feigenbaum KM, Koviack PD, Maton PN, Gardner JD, Jensen RT. 1993. Prospective study of efficacy and safety of lansoprazole in Zollinger-Ellison syndrome. Dig Dis Sci 38:245–256.

119. Metz DC, Strader DB, Orbuch M, Koviach PD, Feigenbaum KM, Jensen RT. 1993. Use of omeprazole in Zollinger-Ellison: A prospective nine-year study of efficacy and safety. Aliment Pharmacol Ther 7:597–610.

120. Raufman JP, Collins SM, Pandol SJ, Korman LY, Collen MJ, Cornelius MJ, Feld MK, McCarthy DM, Gardner JD, Jensen RT. 1983. Reliability of symptoms in assessing control of gastric acid secretion in patients with Zollinger-Ellison syndrome. Gastroenterology 84:108–113.

121. Maton PN, Frucht H, Vinayek R, Wank SA, Gardner JD, Jensen RT. 1988. Medical management of patients with Zollinger-Ellison syndrome who have had previous gastric surgery: A prospective study. Gastroenterology 94:294–299.

122. Vinayek R, Frucht H, London JF, Miller LS, Stark HA, Norton JA, Cederberg C, Jensen RT, Gardner JD, Maton PN. 1990. Intravenous omeprazole in patients with Zolling-Ellison syndrome undergoing surgery. Gastroenterology 99:10–16.

123. Vinayek R, Amantea MA, Maton PN, Frucht H, Gardner JD, Jensen RT. 1991. Pharmacokinetics of oral and intravenous omeprazole in patients with the Zollinger-Ellison syndrome. Gastroenterology 101:138–147.

124. Vinayek R, Hahne WF, Euler AR, Norton JA, Jensen RT. 1993. Parenteral control of gastric hypersecretion in patients with Zollinger-Ellison syndrome. Dig Dis Sci 38:1857–1865.

125. Saeed ZA, Norton JA, Frank WO, Young MD, Maton PN, Gardner JD, Jensen RT. 1989. Parenteral antisecretory drug therapy in patients with Zollinger-Ellison syndrome. Gastroenterology 96:1393–1402.

126. Pisegna JR, Norton JA, Slimak GG, Metz DC, Maton PN, Jensen RT. 1992. Effects of curative resection on gastric secretory function and antisecretory drug requirement in the Zollinger-Ellison syndrome. Gastroenterology 102:767–778.

127. Bonfils S, Jensen RT, Malagelada J, Stadil F. 1989. Zollinger-Ellison sydrome management: A protocol for strategy. Gastroenterol Int 2:9–15.

128. Thompson JC, Lewis BG, Wiener I, Townsend CM Jr. 1983. The role of surgery in the Zollinger-Ellison syndrome. Ann Surg 197:594–607.

129. Richardson CT, Peters MN, Feldman M, McClelland RN, Walsh JH, Cooper KA, Willeford G, Dickerman RM, Fordtran JS. 1985. Treatment of Zollinger-Ellison syndrome with exploratory laparotomy, proximal gastric vagotomy, and H$_2$-receptor antagonists. A prospective study. Gastroenterology 89:357–367.

130. McArthur KE, Richardson CT, Barnett CC, Smerud MJ, Eshaghi N, McClelland RN, Feldman M. 1996. Laparotomy and proximal gastric vagotomy in Zollinger-Ellison syndrome: Results of a 16-year prospective study. Am J Gastroenterol 91:1104–1111.

131. Jensen RT. 1996. Acid-reducing surgery in, aggressive resection out. Am J Gastroenterol, 91:1067–1070.

330

132. Miller DL, Doppman JL, Metz DC, Maton PN, Norton JA, Jensen RT. 1992. Zollinger-Ellison syndrome: Technique, results and complications of portal venous sampling. Radiology 182:235–241.

133. Imamura M, Takahashi K. 1993. Use of selective arterial secretin injection test to guide surgery in patients with Zollinger-Ellison syndrome. World J Surg 17:433–438.

134. Gibril F, Doppman JL, Chang R, Weber HC, Termanini B, Jensen RT. 1996. Metastatic gastrinomas: Localization with selective arterial injection of secretin. Radiology 198:77–84.

135. Ruszniewski P, Amouyal P, Amouyal G, Grange JD, Mignon M, Bouch O, Bernades P. 1995. Localization of gastrinomas by endoscopic ultrasonography in patients with Zollinger-Ellison syndrome. Surgery 117:629–635.

136. Ruszniewski P, Amouyal P, Amouyal G, Cadiot G, Mignon M, Bernades P. 1995. Endocrine tumors of the pancreatic area: Localization by endoscopic ultrasonography. In Mignon M, Jensen RT, eds. Endocrine Tumors of the Pancreas: Recent Advances in Research and Management. Frontiers of Gastrointestinal Research. Vol 23 Basel, Switzerland: S. Karger, pp 258–267.

137. de Kerviler E, Cadiot G, Lebtahi R, Faraggi M, le Guludec D, Mignon M. 1994. Somatostatin receptor scintigraphy in forty-eight patients with the Zollinger-Ellison syndrome. Eur J Nucl Med 21:1191–1197.

138. Krenning EP, Kwekkeboom DJ, Bakker WH, Breeman WAP, Kooij PPM, Oei HY, van Hagen M, Postema PTE, de Jong M, Reubi JC, Visser TJ, Reijs AEM, Hofland LJ, Koper JW, Lamberts SWJ. 1993. Somatostatin receptor scintigraphy with [^{111}In-DTPA-D-Phe^1]-and [^{123}I-Tyr^3]-octreotide: The Rotterdam experience with more than 1000 patients. Eur J Nucl Med 20:716–731.

139. Krenning EP, Kwekkeboom DJ, Oei HY, de Jong RJB, Dop FJ, Reubi JC, Lamberts SWJ. 1994. Somatostatin-receptor scintigraphy in gastroenteropancreatic tumors. Ann NY Acad Sci 733:416–424.

140. Gibril F, Reynolds JC, Doppman JL, Chen CC, Venzon DJ, Termanini B, Weber HC, Stewart CA, Jensen RT. 1996. Somatostatin receptor scintigraphy: A prospective study of its sensitivity compared to other imaging modalities in detecting primary and metastatic gastrinomas. Ann Intern Med 125:26–34.

141. Ur E, Bomanji J, Mather SJ, Britton KE, Wass JA, Grossman AB, Besser GM. 1993. Localization of neuroendocrine tumours and insulinomas using radiolabelled somatostatin analogues, ^{123}I-Tyr^3-octreotide and ^{111}In-pentatreotide. Clin Endocrinol 38:501–506.

142. Thompson NW, Czako PF, Fritts LL, Bude R, Bansal R, Nostrant TT, Scheiman JM. 1994. Role of endoscopic ultrasonography in the localization of insulinomas and gastrinomas. Surgery 116:1131–1138.

143. Thom AK, Norton JA, Doppman JL, Chang R, Miller DL, Jensen RT. 1992. Prospective study of the use of intraarterial secretin injection and portal venous sampling to localize duodenal gastrinomas. Surgery 112:1002–1008.

144. Corleto VD, Scopinaro F, Angeletti S, Materia A, Basso N, Polettini E, Annibale B, Schillaci O, D'Ambra G, Marignani M, Gualdi G, Bordi C, Passaro EJ, Delle Fave G. 1996. Somatostatin receptor localization of pancreatic endocrine tumors. World J Surg 20:241–244.

145. Norton JA. 1995. Surgical treatment of islet cell tumors with special emphasis on operative ultrasound. In Mignon M, Jensen RT, eds. Endocrine Tumors of the Pancreas: Recent Advances in Research and Management. Frontiers of Gastrointestinal Research. Vol 23 Basel, Switzerland: S. Karger, pp 309–332.

146. Norton JA, Cromack DT, Shawker TH, Doppman JL, Comi R, Gorden P, Maton PN, Gardner JD, Jensen RT. 1988. Intraoperative ultrasonographic localization of islet cell tumors. A prospective comparison to palpation. Ann Surg 207:160–168.

147. Frucht H, Norton JA, London JF, Vinayek R, Doppman JL, Gardner JD, Jensen RT, Maton PN. 1990. Detection of duodenal gastrinomas by operative endoscopic transillumination: A prospective study. Gastroenterology 99:1622–1627.

148. Jensen RT. 1994. Zollinger-Ellison syndrome: Past, present, and future controversies. Yale J Biol Med 67:195–214.

149. Hirschowitz BI. 1995. Clinical course of nonsurgically treated Zollinger-Ellison syndrome. In Mignon M, Jensen RT, eds. Endocrine Tumors of the Pancreas: Recent Advances in Research and Management. Frontiers of Gastrointestinal Research. Vol 23 Basel, Switzerland: S. Karger, pp 360–371.

150. McCarthy DM. 1980. The place of surgery in the Zollinger-Ellison syndrome. N Engl J Med 302:1344–1347.

151. Fishbeyn VA, Norton JA, Benya RV, Pisegna JR, Venzon DJ, Metz DC, Jensen RT. 1993. Assessment and prediction of long-term cure in patients with Zollinger-Ellison syndrome: The best approach. Ann Intern Med 119:199–206.

152. Fraker DL, Norton JA, Alexander HR, Venzon DJ, Jensen RT. 1994. Surgery in Zollinger-Ellison syndrome alters the natural history of gastrinoma. Ann Surg 220:320–330.

153. Norton JA, Doppman JL, Jensen RT. 1992. Curative resection in Zollinger-Ellison syndrome: Results of a 10-year prospective study. Ann Surg 215:8–18.

154. Delcore R, Friesen SR. 1994. The place for curative surgical procedures in the treatment of sporadic and familial Zollinger-Ellison syndrome. Curr Opin Gen Surg, pp 69–76.

155. Stadil F. 1995. Treatment of gastrinomas with pancreatoduoenectomy. In Mignon M, Jensen RT, eds. Endocrine Tumors of the Pancreas: Recent Advances in Research and Management. Frontiers of Gastrointestinal Research. Vol 23 Basel, Switzerland: S. Karger, pp 333–341.

156. Fraker DL, Jensen RT. 1996. Pancreatic endocrine tumors. In DeVita VT, Hellman S, Rosenberg SA, eds. Cancer: Principles and Practice of Oncology. 5th Edition. Philadelphia: J.B. Lippincott, in press.

157. Jensen RT. 1995. Pancreatic endocrine tumors. Curr Opin Gastroenterol 11:423–429.

158. Oberg K. 1993. The use of chemotherapy in the management of neuroendocrine tumors. Endocrinol Metab Clin North Am 22:941–952.

159. Nagorney DM, Que FG. 1995. Cytoreductive hepatic surgery for metastatic gastrointestinal neuroendocrine tumors. In Mignon M, Jensen RT, eds. Endocrine Tumors of the Pancreas: Recent Advances in Research and Management. Frontiers of Gastrointestinal Research. Vol 23 Basel, Switzerland: S. Karger, pp 416–430.

160. Arcenas AG, Ajani JA, Carrasco CH, Levin B, Wallace S. 1995. Vascular occlusive therapy of pancreatic endocrine tumors metastatic to the liver. In Mignon M, Jensen RT, eds. Endocrine Tumors of the Pancreas: Recent Advances in Research and Management. Frontiers of Gastrointestinal Research. Vol 23 Basel, Switzerland: S. Karger, pp 439–450.

161. Arnold R, Benning R, Neuhaus C, Rolwage M, Trautmann ME. 1992. Gastro-enteropancreatic endocrine tumors: Effect of Sandostatin on tumor growth. The German Sandostatin Study Group. Metabolism 41(Suppl 2):116–118.

162. Arnold R, Neuhaus C, Benning R, Schwerk WB, Trautmann ME, Joseph K, Bruns C. 1993. Somatostatin analog sandostatin and inhibition of tumor growth in patients with metastatic endocrine gastroenteropancreatic tumors. World J Surg 17:511–519.

163. Eriksson B, Oberg K. 1995. Interferon therapy of malignant endocrine pancreatic tumors. In Mignon M, Jensen RT, eds. Endocrine Tumors of the Pancreas: Recent Advances in Research and Management. Frontiers of Gastrointestinal Research. Vol 23 Basel, Switzerland: S. Karger, pp 451–460.

164. Moertel CG. 1987. Karnofsky memorial lecture. An odyssey in the land of small tumors. J Clin Oncol 5:1502–1522.

165. Saltz L, Lauwers G, Wiseberg J, Kelsen D. 1993. A phase II trial of carboplatin in patients with advanced APUD tumors. Cancer 72:619–622.

166. Kelsen D, Fiore J, Heelan R, Cheng E, Magill G. 1987. Phase II trial of etoposide in APUD tumors. Cancer Treat Rep 71:305–307.

167. Moertel CG, Hanley JA, Johnson LA. 1980. Streptozotocin alone compared with streptozotocin plus fluorouracil in the treatment of advanced islet-cell carcinoma. N Engl J Med 303:1189–1194.

168. Moertel CG, Lefkopoulo M, Lipsitz S, Hahn RG, Klaassen D. 1992. Streptozotocin-doxorubicin, streptozotocin-flourouracil or chlorozotocin in the treatment of advanced islet cell carcinoma. N Engl J Med 326:519–523.

169. Bukowski RM, Tangen C, Lee R, Macdonald JS, Einstein AB Jr, Peterson R, Fleming TR. 1992. Phase II trial of chlorozotocin and fluorouracil in islet cell carcinoma: A Southwest Oncology Group study. J Clin Oncol 10:1914–1918.
170. Broder LE, Carter SK. 1973. Pancreatic islet cell carcinoma. II. Results of therapy with streptozotocin in 52 patients. Ann Intern Med 79:108–118.
171. Mignon M, Ruszniewski P, Haffar S, Rignaud D, Rene E, Bonfils S. 1986. Current approach to the management of tumoral process in patients with gastrinoma. World J Surg 10:703–710.
172. Hofmann JW, Fox PS, Wilson SD. 1973. Duodenal wall tumors and the Zollinger-Ellison syndrome. Surgical management. Arch Surg 107:334–339.
173. Ruszniewski P, Hochlaf S, Rougier P, Mignon M. 1991. [Intravenous chemotherapy with streptozotocin and 5-fluorouracil for hepatic metastases of Zollinger-Ellison syndrome. A prospective multicenter study in 21 patients]. Gastroenterol Clin Biol 15:393–398.
174. von Schrenck T, Howard JM, Doppman JL, Norton JA, Maton PN, Smith FP, Vinayek R, Frucht H, Wank SA, Gardner JD, Jensen RT. 1988. Prospective study of chemotherapy in patients with metastatic gastrinoma. Gastroenterology 94:1326–1334.
175. Bonfils S, Ruszniewski P, Haffar S, Laucournet H. 1986. Chemotherapy of hepatic metastases (HM) in Zollinger-Ellison syndrome (ZES) (abstr). Report of a multicentric analysis. Dig Dis Sci 31:510S.
176. Moertel CG, Kvols LK, O'Connell MJ, Rubin J. 1991. Treatment of neuroendocrine carcinomas with combined etoposide and cisplatin. Evidence of major therapeutic activity in the anaplastic variants of these neoplasms. Cancer 68:227–232.
177. Carrasco CH, Chuang VP, Wallace S. 1983. Apudomas metastatic to the liver: Treatment by hepatic artery embolization. Radiology 149:79–83.
178. Perry LJ, Stuart K, Stokes KR, Clouse ME. 1994. Hepatic arterial chemoembolization for metastatic neuroendocrine tumors. Surgery 116:1111–1117.
179. Moertel CG, Johnson CM, McKusick MA, Martin JK Jr, Nagorney DM, Kvols LK, Rubin J, Kunselman S. 1994. The management of patients with advanced carcinoid tumors and islet cell carcinomas. Ann Intern Med 120:302–309.
180. Stokes KR, Stuart K, Clouse ME. 1993. Hepatic arterial chemoembolization for metastatic endocrine tumors. J Vasc Intervent Radiol 4:341–345.
181. Ruszniewski P, Rougier P, Roche A, Legmann P, Sibert A, Hochlaf S, Ychou M, Mignon M. 1993. Hepatic arterial chemoembolization in patients with liver metastases of endocrine tumors. A prospective phase II study in 24 patients. Cancer 71:2624–2630.
182. Que FG, Nagorney DM, Batts KP, Linz LJ, Kvols LK. 1995. Hepatic resection for metastatic neuroendocrine carcinomas. Am J Surg 169:36–43.
183. Carty SE, Jensen RT, Norton JA. 1992. Prospective study of aggressive resection of metastatic pancreatic endocrine tumors. Surgery 112:1024–1031.
184. McEntee GP, Nagorney DM, Kvols LK, Moertel CG, Grant CS. 1990. Cytoreductive hepatic surgery for neuroendocrine tumors. Surgery 108:1091–1096.
185. Norton JA, Sugarbaker PH, Doppman JL, Wesley RA, Maton PN, Gardner JD, Jensen RT. 1986. Aggressive resection of metastatic disease in selected patients with malignant gastrinoma. Ann Surg 203:352–359.
186. Zollinger RM, Ellison EC, Fabri PJ, Johnson J, Sparks J, Carey LC. 1980. Primary peptic ulcerations of the jejunum associated with islet cell tumors. Twenty-five-year appraisal. Ann Surg 192:422–430.
187. Pisegna JR, Slimak GG, Doppman JL, Strader DB, Metz DC, Fishbeyn VA, Benya RV, Orbuch M, Fraker DL, Norton JA, Maton PN, Jensen RT. 1993. An evaluation of human recombinant alpha interferon in patients with metastatic gastrinoma. Gastroenterology 105:1179–1183.
188. Eriksson B, Oberg K, Alm G, Karlsson A, Lundqvist G, Andersson T, Wilander E, Wide L. 1986. Treatment of malignant endocrine pancreatic tumors with human leucocyte interferon. Lancet 2:1307–1309.
189. Scarpignato C. 1995. Somatostatin analogues in the management of endocrine tumors of the pancreas. In Mignon M, Jensen RT, eds. Endocrine Tumors of the Pancreas: Recent Ad-

vances in Research and Management. Frontiers of Gastrointestinal Research. Vol 23 Basel, Switzerland: S. Karger, pp 385–414.

190. Reubi JC, Laissue J, Waser B, Horisberger U, Schaer JC. 1994. Expression of somatostatin receptors in normal, inflamed, and neoplastic human gastrointestinal tissues. Ann NY Acad Sci 733:122–137.

191. Bruns C, Weckbecker G, Raulf F, Kaupmann K, Schoeffter P, Hoyer D, Lubbert H. 1994. Molecular pharmacology of somatostatin-receptor subtypes. Ann NY Acad Sci 733:138–146.

192. Lamberts SWJ, van der Lely AJ, de Herder WW, Hofland LJ. 1996. Octreotide. N Engl J Med 334:246–254.

193. Anthony L, Johnson D, Hande K, Shaff M, Winn S, Krozely M, Oates J. 1993. Somatostatin analogue phase I trials in neuroendocrine neoplasms. Acta Oncol 32:217–233.

194. Saltz L, Trochanowski B, Buckley M, Heffernan B, Niedzwiecki D, Tao Y, Kelsen D. 1993. Octreotide as an antineoplastic agent in the treatment of functional and nonfunctional neuroendocrine tumors. Cancer 72:244–248.

195. Arnold R, Frank M, Kajdan U. 1994. Management of gastroenteropancreatic endocrine tumors: The place of somatostain analogues. Digestion 55:107–113.

196. Maton PN, Gardner JD, Jensen RT. 1989. Use of the long-acting somatostatin analog, SMS 201-995 in patients with pancreatic islet cell tumors. Dig Dis Sci 34:28S–39S.

197. Kvols LK, Buck M, Moertel CG, Schutt AJ, Rubin J, O'Connell MJ, Hahn RG. 1987. Treatment of metastatic islet cell tumors with somatostatin analogue. Ann Intern Med 107:162–168.

198. Maton PN. 1989. The use of the long-acting somatostatin analogue, octreotide acetate, in patients with islet cell tumors. Gastroenterol Clin North Am 18:897–922.

199. Ellison EC, O'Dorisio TM, Woltering EA, Sparks J, Mekhjian HS, Fromkes JJ, Carey LC. 1986. Suppression of gastrin and gastric acid secretion in the Zollinger-Ellison sundrome by long-acting somatostatin (SMS 201-995). Scand J Gastroenterol 21(Suppl 119):206–211.

200. Dousset B, Houssin D, Soubrane O, Boillot O, Baudin F, Chapuis Y. 1995. Metastatic endocrine tumors: Is there a place for liver transplantation?. Liver Transplant Surg 1:111–117.

201. Routley D, Ramage JK, McPeake J, Tan KC, Williams R. 1995. Orthotopic liver transplantation in the treatment of metastatic neuroendocrine tumors of the liver. Liver Transplant Surg 1:118–121.

15. Insulinoma and other islet-cell tumors

F. John Service

Historical aspects

The recognition of islet-cell tumors of the pancreas histologically preceded their clinical identification by many decades. In the case of insulinoma, its existence was predicted from the occurrence of 'insulin reactions' in nondiabetic persons [1]; in the case of other islet-cell tumors, their existence (glucagonoma, somatostatinoma, VIPoma, PPoma) followed the development of the ability to measure in the circulation the polypeptides that were secreted in excess. In most (somatostatinoma, glucagonoma, VIPoma) but not (PPoma) all instances, a clinical syndrome could be identified with the elevated levels of specific polypeptides.

Insulinomas derive from beta cells, glucagonoma from alpha cells, and somatostatinoma from delta cells of the pancreatic islets. The cells of origin of VIP and pancreatic polypeptide (HPP) have not been identified [2]. The first reports of patients either with the clinical syndromes associated with these disorders or with the association of polypeptide hypersecretion in the presence of an islet-cell tumor were insulinoma in 1927 [3], glucagonoma in 1966 [4], VIPoma in 1958 [5], and somatostatinoma in 1977 [6,7]. Because PPoma appears not to be a distinct entity (elevated levels of HPP may be seen in islet-cell tumors which secrete predominantly another polypeptide), it was not recognized until approximately the mid-1970s [2]. Gastrinoma is discussed in Chapter 14.

Epidemiologic and demographic features

These tumors are rare. During the period 1970–1985 an effort was made to identify all pancreatic endocrine tumors in a well-defined population of 1.5 million persons living in Northern Ireland. Forty-nine were identified, 21 of which were insulinomas, 13 were gastrinomas, 11 were islet-cell tumors of unknown type, 2 were VIPomas, 1 was glucagonoma, and 1 was an adrenocorticotrophic hormone (ACTH)-producing malignant islet-cell tumor [8]. From a population-based study conducted in Olmsted County, Minnesota, the inci-

Andrew Arnold (ed.) ENDOCRINE NEOPLASMS. 1997. Kluwer Academic Publishers. ISBN 0-7923-4354-9.

Table 1. Demographic features of islet-cell tumors

	Age[a] (yr)	Gender (% F)	Size[a] (cm)	Malignant (%)	Multiple (%)	MEN-I (%)	Clinical syndrome
Insulinoma [9,13]	47 (8–82)	59	1.5 (0.4–8)	5.8	8.9	7.6	+
Glucagonoma [2]	52 (19–73)	58	5 (1–35)	70	2–4	Rare	+
VIPoma [2]	47 (5–79)	65	3 (1–20)	90	15–20	4	+
Somatostatinoma [2]	53 (38–84)	67	5 (2–10)	71	10	45	+
PPoma	51 (20–74)	50	5.6 (0.7–15)	43	5	18–44	−

[a] Median or mean, range in parentheses.

dence of insulinoma was found to be 1 case per 250,000 person-years [9]. Although these results reflect the occurrence of insulinoma in persons with primarily Northern European heritage, insulinomas have been observed in African-Americans and Hispanic-Americans. The occurrence of other islet-cell tumors is an order of magnitude less than insulinoma. In other studies, which unfortunately are at risk for referral bias, 48–50% of islet-cell tumors were insulinomas, 22–30% gastrinomas, 10–15% VIPomas, and 5–10% assorted types, including glucagonomas, somatostatinomas, and PPomas [10,11]. The demographic features of these tumors are shown in Table 1.

Clinical syndromes

The major actions of insulin, glucagon, VIP, and somatostatin are shown in Table 2.

Insulinoma

These tumors lack the normal feedback control on insulin secretion exerted by circulating glucose concentrations. As a consequence of the continuous leakage of insulin, patients are at risk for hypoglycemia the longer they go without food. Because these tumors respond to the stimulatory effect of rising concentrations of nutrients in the circulation after food ingestion, some patients experience hypoglycemia postprandially. The frequency of symptoms is highly variable among patients: major symptoms arising from neuroglycopenia usually occur less frequently, but, on the other hand, are more memorable than those of the autonomic type. All patients with insulinoma eventually develop symptoms of the neuroglycopenic type. Studies done in normal and diabetic persons identified these as dizziness, confusion, tiredness, difficulty speaking, headache, and inability to concentrate [12]. Among 60 patients with insulinoma, 85% had various combinations of diplopia, blurred vision, sweating, palpitations, and weakness; 80% had confusion or abnormal behavior; 53% had amnesia or coma; and 12% had generalized seizures [13]. Unfortunately, none of these symptoms is specific for hypoglycemia.

It is essential, therefore, to confirm the presence of hypoglycemia by measuring plasma glucose during the occurrences of symptoms. A reflectance meter glucose measurement is inadequate to confirm hypoglycemia with confidence. Whipple's recommendation to biochemically confirm the existence of hypoglycemia during the occurrence of symptoms and the amelioration of symptoms by correction of the low glucose concentration (Whipple's triad) is a good rule to follow in the establishment of the presence of a hypoglycemic disorder [14]. If a patient is observed while symptomatic, blood should be obtained for plasma insulin, C-peptide, proinsulin, sulfonylurea, and betahydroxybutyrate. Correction of hypoglycemia can be achieved by an intravenous injection of 1 mg glucagon. These data obtained during a spontaneous episode of hypoglycemia or at the termination of a prolonged supervised fast (occurrence of symptoms and plasma glucose ≤45 mg/dl) permit an accurate diagnosis.

The detection of any of the beta-cell polypeptides in the circulation while a patient is hypoglycemic probably represents abnormal beta-cell function. Our criteria for insulinoma are plasma insulin ≥6 µU/ml, C-peptide ≥200 pmol/l, and proinsulin ≥5 pmol/l [15]. Insulin to glucose (or vice versa) ratios are useless for the diagnosis of insulinoma [16]. Betahydroxybutyrate is suppressed to <2.7 mmol/l, and the plasma glucose increases by ≥25 mg/dl over 30

Table 2. Major actions

Insulin	Glucagon	VIP[a]	Somatostatin[b]
Decreases hepatic glucose production	Stimulates glycogenolysis and gluconeogenesis	Stimulation of intestinal pancreatic and biliary secretion	Generalized inhibition of hormonal release
Increases glucose utilization	Decreases plasma amino acids	Stimulation of colonic potassium secretion	Inhibition of gastric emptying, pancreatic exocrine secretion, gallbladder emptying, gut motility, and nutrient absorption
		Stimulation of bone resorption	
		Decreased GI transit time	
		Inhibition of gastric-acid secretion	
		Inhibition of gallbladder contraction	
		Vasodilation	
		Glycogenolysis	

[a] Data from Anderson and Bloom [28].
[b] Data from Grier [25].

minutes after the injection of glucagon in insulinoma or other conditions in which hypoglycemia is mediated by insulin, for example, insulin factitial hypoglycemia [15] (Fig. 1). It is important to recognize that most methods for measuring second-generation sulfonylureas are insensitive. New liquid-chromatographic mass-spectroscopy methodology is in development for the detection of these drugs. It is essential, therefore, to examine a patient's medication personally or via a pharmacist for the purpose of correctly identifying all drugs because dispensing error (sulfonylurea in the place of the intended drug) is a common cause of hypoglycemia [15].

In many instances, the diagnosis of insulinoma is straightforward if the biochemical and hormonal determinations have been conducted on specimens collected under appropriate circumstances. In other instances, test results are ambiguous or inconclusive. Additional testing or repeated testing may be in order. The C-peptide suppression test [17] and tolbutamide test [18] are useful adjunctive diagnostic procedures. In the extraordinarily rare circumstance of a negative 72-hour fast in a patient with insulinoma, a correct diagnosis may

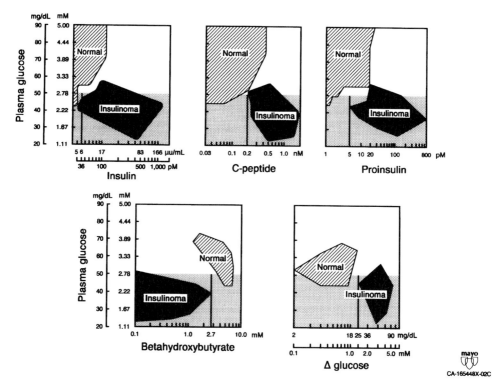

Figure 1. Distribution of plasma concentrations of insulin, C-peptide, and proinsulin at the end of the supervised fast in relation to the concurrent plasma and betahydroxybutyrate and glucose response to the intravenous glucagon glucose concentration in normal persons and patients with insulinoma. Criteria for diagnosis are represented by the vertical lines. (Reprinted from Service [15], with permission.)

338

depend on a positive C-peptide suppression or tolbutamide test. Patients who relate neuroglycopenic symptoms following food ingestion should be studied during and after ingestion of a mixed meal. Reproduction of hypoglycemic symptoms and an associated low plasma glucose concentration warrants further evaluation for possible insulinoma.

Patients with insulinoma appear to be healthy. Unless a patient is known to have MEN-I or has had a prior pancreatic exploration, the physical examination is normal. Insulinomas occur in persons of all walks of life, including health care workers, in whom the suspicion of factitial hypoglycemia is high. Insulinomas have been removed from pregnant women [19]. The tumors occur with an even distribution throughout the pancreas and are found in extrapancreatic locations in extremely rare instances [19].

Glucagonoma

Unlike insulinoma, in which the pathogenetic polypeptide causes symptoms early in the course of the disease, the presumed initial biochemical disturbance of glucagonoma, that is, mild hyperglycemia, is nonspecific and, therefore, does not trigger a search for elevated glucagon concentrations. Should all persons with newly discovered hyperglycemia have a plasma glucagon level measured? Probably not, because the tumor frequency was found to be 0.8% in ~1400 adult autopsies [20]. Diabetes may precede the diagnosis of glucagonoma by a decade or more. Unfortunately, therefore, the tumor does not manifest itself to such a degree that clinical recognition is feasible until it is sufficiently large or metastatic to cause mechanical symptoms or the degree and duration of hyperglucagonemia have been sufficient to cause severe metabolic disturbances and their sequelae.

Glucagonomas are usually larger than insulinomas and have a higher likelihood of malignancy. These tumors occur more often in the body and tail of the pancreas than in the head [21]. The glucagonoma syndrome includes mild diabetes, a pathognomonic dermatitis (migratory necrolytic erythema), angular stomatitis, vulvovaginitis, glossitis, hypoaminoacidemia, weight loss, normochromic normocytic anemia, propensity to venous thrombosis, and mental status change [2]. The dermatitis is likely to be related to the hypoaminoacidemia because the former is often improved by correction of the latter. The rash has a characteristic histologic appearance. It has a predilection for the groin, perineum, and lower abdomen but may occur elsewhere. Most, but not all, patients have the characteristic rash; for those who do not, the diagnosis of glucagonoma early in the course of the disease is largely by serendipity. The rash waxes and wanes, and various areas of involvement may be at differing stages of its evolution. Histological features include subcorneal separation due to vesicles that have developed in the superficial epidermis and areas of focal parakeratosis [22].

In a recently compiled review of a single institution's experience, the largest series (n = 21) of patients with the glucagonoma syndrome were described.

Seventy-one percent experienced weight loss, 67% had necrolytic migratory erythema, 38% had diabetes mellitus, 29% had cheilosis or stomatitis, and 29% had diarrhea. There was an almost equal gender incidence (10 F, 11 M). Symptoms other than diabetes or typical skin rash led to the diagnosis in 33% of the patients. All patients had metastatic disease at diagnosis. Abdominal CT scanning was positive in 86% of the patients. Median and range serum glucagon levels were 1400 (range, 84–14,300 pg/ml; normal, ≤60 pg/ml). Serum glucagon levels were higher in those patients with necrolytic migratory erythema and diabetes [23]. Elevated glucagon concentrations may be observed in other malignant endocrine tumors. In a review that spanned the period 1988–1993 at the same institution, 71 patients had serum glucagon levels twice the upper limit of normal and a malignant neuroendocrine tumor. Sixty-nine percent of the patients had tumors that secreted one or more peptides in addition to glucagon, for example, gastrin, insulin, HPP, ACTH, vasoactive intestinal polypeptide (VIP), calcitonin, and serotonin (5HIAA) [24]. Provocative tests are not necessary when the degree of hyperglucagonemia is extreme.

VIPoma

Most VIPomas occur in the pancreas, especially the tail, but may occur along the autonomic chain or in the adrenals (histologically, ganglioneuroma, ganglioblastomas, or neuroblastomas) in children [2,25]. The clinical syndrome of VIPoma is *w*atery *d*iarrhea, *h*ypokalemia, hypochlorhydria, and *a*cidosis (WDHA). The water diarrhea is secretory in type and may reach >3 L/day. It persists during periods of no nutrient intake. Some patients experience hyperglycemia, flushing, and hypercalcemia. Other peptides may be elevated in this syndrome, such as HPP, Peptide histidine methionine (PHM), calcitonin, and prostaglandin E (PGE).

Diarrhea may be constant or intermittent. The stool is rich in electrolytes. Fluid and electrolyte imbalance can lead to lethargy muscle weakness, cramps, nausea, and vomiting. The hypokalemia can cause abnormalities in renal function. Severely dehydrated patients are at risk for renal failure. A 24-hour stool volume <700 ml excludes the diagnosis [26]. A plasma VIP level >200 pg/ml is strongly suggestive of VIPoma. In one series, the average VIP level was ~1000 pg/ml, with the lowest being 255 pg/ml [27].

Somatostatinoma

The clinical syndrome arising from this tumor is diabetes, cholelithiasis, hypochlorhydria, and steatorrhea. Sixty-eight percent of these tumors arise in the pancreas (primarily the head), 19% occur in the duodenum, and 3% each in the ampulla of Vater and small bowel [29]. Diagnosis is made by finding a plasma somatostatin level greatly in excess of normal (≤100 pg/ml). Values may be 100- to 200-fold greater than normal. Patients with the triad of neurofibromatosis, pheochromocytoma, and somatostatinoma have been reported; this may be a novel multiple endocrine neoplasia (MEN) syndrome [30].

PPoma

Because there is no clinical syndrome associated with elevated HPP concentrations and the latter may be observed in islet-cell tumors that secrete other polypeptides and PP levels have not been systematically measured in nonfunctioning islet-cell tumors, a clear delineation of this as a nosologic entity has not been developed [2].

Localization

Because of their small size and low frequency of malignancy and, therefore, low frequency of metastases, insulinomas present the greatest challenge for localization. Despite their being the most frequently occurring pancreatic endocrine tumors, insulinomas are rare. Therefore, only a few tertiary-care centers have the opportunity to determine the effectiveness of various localization procedures. Transhepatic portal venous sampling for insulin [31,32] and arterial stimulation venous sampling for insulin [33] have the disadvantage of being invasive and limited to merely regionalizing the tumor, rather than providing precise localization. Celiac axis arteriography with magnification and subtraction, computed tomography, and magnetic resonance imaging have not achieved the degree of sensitivity in localization reached by ultrasonography, especially intraoperative ultrasound [33]. Octreotide scanning has been disappointing in the localization of insulinomas [34].

Considering the high degree of success in localization from a combination of intraoperative ultrasound and manual palpation by a skilled surgeon experienced in insulinoma surgery, a role for invasive preoperative localization procedures such as endoscopic ultrasonography seems to be in limbo. Nevertheless, an accurate noninvasive preoperative localization procedure does provide a certain comfort level to the surgeon. Perhaps spiral CT may displace or match preoperative ultrasonography [32]. Because glucagonomas, VIPomas, and somatostatinomas are relatively large and frequently are metastatic, they often are readily identified by CT scanning, transabdominal ultrasonography, or arteriography [2,29,34]. Radionuclide imaging, such as that with octreoscan, may be positive should the pancreatic islet-cell tumor contain somatostatin receptors on their cell membranes.

Treatment

Surgical

Every patient diagnosed as having an islet-cell tumor deserves a surgical consultation. In the case of insulinoma, where most patients have a single benign tumor, a cure can be expected with surgical extirpation of the tumor [35,9]. Because these tumors are rare, they should be operated on in tertiary referral centers by surgeons experienced with this type of surgery. This admonition is reinforced for patients who have had a failed initial pancreatic exploration. The cure rate for even these patients is high if the surgery is conducted by an experienced surgeon [36]. Blind pancreatic resection for an occult insulinoma should be discouraged.

In the instances of malignant islet-cell tumors, which by definition have metastatic disease, surgical debulking of the tumor is worthwhile. Debulking reduces the tumoral burden and thereby makes control of symptoms easier and may facilitate the effectiveness of tumoricidal therapy. Such an approach, although palliative, is to be recommended because of the rather indolent behavior of these tumors [37].

Medical

Medical treatment of functioning islet-cell tumors involves the control of symptoms and tumoricidal therapy. Because of the unique biochemical effects of the various polypeptides secreted from islet-cell tumors, control of symptoms requires an approach peculiar to that tumor. Treatment of hypoglycemic symptoms requires elevation of the low plasma glucose out of the hypoglycemic range. This can be achieved by parenteral administration of glucose or glucagon, or if feasible, oral administration of free carbohydrates. Preventative measures include frequent feeding and the use of diazoxide. Less effective or infrequently used medications are phenytoin sodium (Dilantin), propranolol, verapamil, or glucagon [15]. Somatostatin, a generalized inhibitor of polypeptide hormone release, should be effective in the treatment of islet-cell tumors. Unfortunately, its success in control of hyperinsulinemia from insulinoma is poor [38].

The dermatitis associated with glucagonoma improves with parenteral administration of amino acids. Octreotide in doses from 150 to 1500 µg/day is also an effective treatment for skin rash [39]. The most pressing need for patients with VIPoma is fluid volume replacement and correction of electrolyte and acid-base disturbance. There is a significant risk for dehydration, hypokalemia, and ultimately death from chronic renal failure. Intestinal absorption can be improved by use of glucocorticoids, angiotensin II and α_2-adrenergic agonists. Indomethacin, adenylate cyclase inhibitor, phenothiazines, propranolol, lithium carbonate, calcium-channel blockers, and opiates inhibit intestinal secretion [25]. Octreotide is particularly effective for the treatment of VIPoma [2]. The dose may be initiated at 100–150 µg sc q8h and increased by 50-µg increments per dose to 200 µg q8h if needed. Once effective control of symptoms has been achieved, the dose may be reduced [40]. There is no palliative pharmacotherapeutic agent for somatostatinoma [2].

Antitumor

Initiation of antitumor therapy for residual metastatic disease following surgical debulking depends on the degree of tumor burden and the degree of symptoms. A conservative approach is warranted because malignant islet-cell tumors run an indolent course [41].

Streptozotocin produces tumor regression in approximately 30% of patients. Randomized trials have shown an improved regression rate (45%) from a combination of fluorouracil and streptozotocin, compared with the latter alone and even a better regression rate (69%) from a combination of doxorubicin and streptozotocin [41]. In addition to the drugs noted earlier, dacarbazine (DTIC) may be particularly effective for metastatic glucagonoma [42]. DTIC, human leukocyte interferon, and doxorubicin (Adriamycin) in combination with streptozotocin have been used in a small number of patients with VIPoma [42].

Because the liver is the predominant organ involved with metastatic islet-cell carcinoma, treatment directed at removing disease from that organ is warranted. With modern surgical techniques, it may be possible to remove solitary metastases. In situations where there is diffuse hepatic involvement, an approach to devitalize metastases needs to be considered. This can be done by hepatic artery occlusion or embolization because metastatic tissue viability is dependent on hepatic arterial inflow, whereas hepatocytes can survive through portal venous blood flow alone. In a randomized study of 47 patients with islet-cell carcinoma metastatic to the liver, objective tumor regressions were observed in 43% of patients who underwent hepatic artery occlusion alone and in 78% of patients who underwent hepatic artery occlusion plus chemotherapy. The latter was initiated 3–4 weeks after the occlusion procedure, first with doxorubicin, then dacarbazine, and 1 month later with streptozotocin and fluorouracil. Hormonal regression was greater than tumor regression regardless of the hormone produced [41].

Survival

For patients with insulinoma, over 90% of whom have benign tumors, overall survival is excellent. We observed in 224 patients whose initial pancreatic exploration was both successful at the removal of the insulinoma and was also conducted at the Mayo Clinic, a normal survival (91% vs. expected 89%) rate over 45 years of follow-up (Fig. 2). Incidentally, the recurrence rate was 21% in patients with the MEN-I syndrome, but only 7% in patients without the MEN-I syndrome. In the small number of patients (n = 13) with malignant insulinoma, the survival at 10 years was 29% versus an expected survival of 88% [9].

Among patients with a heavy hepatic tumor burden from metastatic islet-cell carcinoma, the median survival tumor was 9 months in patients treated

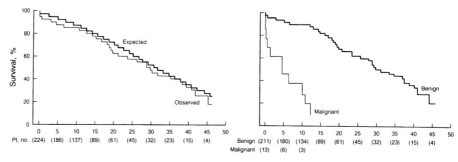

Pt. no. (224) (186) (137) (89) (61) (45) (32) (23) (15) (4)

Benign (211) (180) (134) (89) (61) (45) (32) (23) (15) (4)
Malignant (13) (6) (3)

Years after diagnosis

Figure 2. Survival of the total cohort (n = 224) of patients with insulinoma contrasted with that expected (**left**) and with that in patients with benign (211) insulinoma and malignant (n = 13) insulinoma (**right**) observed over 45 years of follow-up.

with hepatic artery occlusion alone and 35 months for those treated with hepatic artery occlusion and chemotherapy [41]. Among 27 patients with malignant islet-cell tumors (insulinoma = 13, VIPoma = 8, glucagonoma = 4, somatostatinoma = 2), the median survival was 151 months for insulinoma, 103 months for VIPoma, and 50 months for glucagonoma [10]. The median survival among 59 patients with a variety of malignant islet-cell tumors, both functional and nonfunctional was 6.7 years [43].

References

1. Harris S. 1924. Hyperinsulinism and dysinsulinism. JAMA 83:729–733.
2. Delcore R, Friesen SR. 1994. Gastrointestinal neuroendocrine tumors. J Am Coll Surg 178:187–211.
3. Wilder RM, Allan FN, Power MH, Robertson HE. 1927. Carcinoma of the islets of the pancreas: Hyperinsulinism and hypoglycemia. JAMA 89:348–355.
4. McGavran MH, Unger RH, Recant L, Polk HC, Kilo C, Levin ME. 1966. A glucagon-secretory alpha-cell carcinoma of the pancreas. N Engl J Med 274:1408–1413.
5. Verner JV, Morrison AB. 1958. Islet cell tumor of the pancreas with peptic ulceration diarrhea and hypokalemia. Am J Med 25:375–380.
6. Ganda OP, Weir GC, Soeldner JS, Legg MA, Chick WL, Patel YC. 1977. Somatostatinoma: A somatostatin-containing tumor of the endocrine pancreas. N Engl J Med 96:963–967.
7. Larsson L-I, Hirsch MA, Holst JJ, Ingemansson S, Kuhl C, Jensen SL, Lundquist G, Rehfeld JF, Schwartz TW. 1977. Pancreatic somatostatinoma: Clinical features and physiological implications. Lancet 1:66–68.
8. Watson RGP, Johnston CF, O'Hare MMT, Anderson JR, Wilson BG, Collins JSA, Sloan JM, Buchanan KD. 1989. The frequency of gastrointestinal endocrine tumours in a well-defined population — Northern Ireland 1970–1985. Q J Med 72:647–657.
9. Service FJ, McMahon MM, O'Brien PC, Ballard DJ. 1991. Functioning insulinoma — incidence, recurrence, and long-term survival of patients: A 60-year study. Mayo Clin Proc 66:711–719.
10. Grama D, Eriksson B, Mårtensson H, Cedermark B, Ahrén B, Kristoffersson A, Rastad J, Öberg K, Åkerström G. 1992. Clinical characteristics, treatment and survival in patients with pancreatic tumors causing hormonal syndromes. World J Surg 16:632–639.

344

11. Perry RR, Vinik AI. 1995. Diagnosis and management of functioning islet cell tumors. J Clin Endocrinol Metab 80:2273–2278.
12. Hepburn DA, Deary IJ, Frier BM, Patrick AW, Quinn JD, Fisher BM. 1991. Symptoms of acute insulin-induced hypoglycemia in humans with and without IDDM: Factor-analysis approach. Diabetes Care 14:949–957.
13. Service FJ, Dale AJD, Elveback LR, Jiang NS. 1976. Insulinoma: Clinical and diagnostic features of 60 consecutive cases. Mayo Clin Proc 51:417–429.
14. Whipple AO. 1938. The surgical therapy of hyperinsulinism. J Int Chir 3:237–276.
15. Service FJ. 1995. Hypoglycemic disorders. N Engl J Med 332:1144–1152.
16. Service FJ. 1983. Clinical presentations and laboratory evaluation of hypoglycemic disorders in adults. In Service FJ, ed. Hypoglycemic Disorder. Pathogenesis, Diagnosis and Treatment. Boston: GK Hall, pp 73–95.
17. Service FJ, O'Brien PC, Kao PC, Young WF. 1992. C-peptide suppression test: Effects of gender, age, and body mass index; implications for the diagnosis of insulinoma. J Clin Endocrinol Metab 74:204–210.
18. McMahon MM, O'Brien PC, Service FJ. 1989. Diagnostic interpretation of the intravenous tolbutamide test for insulinoma. Mayo Clin Proc 64:1481–1488.
19. Service FJ, van Heerden JA, Sheedy PF. 1983. Insulinoma. In Service FJ, ed. Hypoglycemic Disorders. Pathogenesis, Diagnosis and Treatment. Boston: GK Hall, pp 111–128.
20. Grimelius L, Wilander E. 1980. Silver stains in the study of endocrine cells of the gut and pancreas. Invest Cell Pathol 3:3.
21. Leichter S. 1980. Clinical and metabolic aspects of glucagonoma. Medicine 59:100–113.
22. Kahan RS, Perez-Figaredo RA, Neumanis A. 1977. Necrolytic migratory erythema: Distinctive dermatosis of the glucagonoma syndrome. Arch Dermatol 113:792–797.
23. Wermers RA, Fatourechi V, Wynne AG, Kvols LK, Lloyd R. 1996. The glucagonoma syndrome: Clinical and pathological features in 21 patients. Medicine 75:53–63.
24. Wermers RA, Fatourechi V, Kvols LK. 1996. The clinical spectrum of hyperglucagonemia associated with malignant neuroendocrine tumors. Mayo Clin Proc 71:1030–1038.
25. Grier JF. 1995. WDHA (Watery Diarrhea, Hypokalemia, Achlorhydria) syndrome: Clinical features, diagnosis, and treatment. South Med J 88:22–24.
26. Mekhjian HS, O'Dorisio TM. 1987. VIPoma syndrome. Semin Oncol 14:282–291.
27. O'Dorisio TM, Mekhjian HS. 1984. VIPoma syndrome. In Cohen S, Soloway RD, eds. Contemporary Issues in Gastroenterology. Edinburgh: Churchill Livingstone, p 101.
28. Anderson JV, Bloom SR. Endocrine pancreatic tumours: Diagnosis clinical syndromes and medical management. In Preece PE et al., eds. Cancer of Bile Ducts and Pancreas. Philadelphia: Saunders, pp 233–272.
29. Bieligk S, Jaffe BM. 1995. Islet cell tumors of the pancreas. Surg Clin North Am 75:1025–1040.
30. Griffith DFR, Williams GT, Williams ED. 1987. Duodenal carcinoid tumors, pheochromocytoma and neurofibromatosis: Islet cell tumor, pheochromocytoma and the Von Hippel-Lindau complex: Two distinctive neuroendocrine syndromes. Q J Med 64:769–782.
31. Glowniak JV, Shapiro B, Vinik AI, Glaser B, Thompson NW, Cho KJ. 1982. Percutaneous transhepatic venous sampling of gastrin: Value in sporadic and familial islet-cell tumors and G-cell hyperfunction. N Engl J Med 307:293–297.
32. Pedrazzoli S, Pasquali C, Miotto D, Feltrin G-P, Petrin P. 1987. Transhepatic portal sampling for preoperative localization of insulinomas. Surg Gynecol Obstet 165:101–106.
33. Doppman JL, Chang R, Fraker DL, Norton JA, Alexander HR, Miller DL, Collier E, Skarulis MC, Gorden P. 1995. Localization of insulinomas to the regions of the pancreas by intra-arterial stimulation with calcium. Ann Intern Med 123:269–273.
34. King CMP, Reznek RH, Dacie JE, Wass JAH. 1994. Imaging islet cell tumours. Clin Radiol 49:295–303.
35. Rothmund M, Angelini L, Brunt LM, Farndon JR, Geelhoed G, Grama D, Herfarth C, Kaplan EL, Largiader F, Morino F, Peiper H-J, Proye C, Roher H-D, Ruckert K, Kummerle F, Thompson NW, Van Heerden JA. 1990. Surgery for benign insulinoma: An international review. World J Surg 14:393–399.

345

36. Thompson GB, Service FJ, van Heerden JA, Carney JA, Charboneau JW, O'Brien PC, Grant CS. 1993. Preoperative insulinomas 1927–1992. An institutional experience. Surgery 114:1196–1206.

37. Grant CS. 1993. Surgical management of malignant islet cell tumor. World J Surg 17:498–503.

38. Arnold R, Franke M, Kajdan U. 1994. Management of gastroenteropancreatic endocrine tumors: The place of somatostatin analogues. Digestion 55(Suppl 3):109–113.

39. Wynick D, Hammond PJ, Bloom SR. 1993. The glucagonoma syndrome. Clin Dermatol 11:93–97.

40. Harris AG, O'Dorisio TW, Woltering EA, Anthony LB, Burton FR, Geller RB, Grendell JH, Levin B, Redfern JS. 1995. Consensus statement: Octreotide dose titration in secretory diarrhea. Dig Dis Sci 40:1464–1473.

41. Moertel CG, Johnson CM, McKusick MA, Martin JK, Nagorney DM, Kvols LK, Rubin J, Kanselman S. 1994. The management of patients with advanced carcinoid tumors and islet cell carcinomas. Ann Intern Med 120:302–309.

42. Modlin IM, Lewis JJ, Ahlman H, Bilchik AJ, Kumar RR. 1993. Surg Gynecol Obste 176:507–518.

43. Eriksson B, Oberg K, Skogseid B. 1989. Neuroendocrine pancreatic tumors. Acta Oncol 28:373–377.

16. Persistent hyperinsulinemic hypoglycemia of infancy

Pamela M. Thomas and Gilbert J. Cote

Persistent hyperinsulinemic hypoglycemia of infancy (PHHI), also known as familial hyperinsulinism and nesidioblastosis, is a disorder of glucose homeostasis characterized by unregulated hyperinsulinemia and profound hypoglycemia. Although rare, this disorder is the most common cause of persistent hyperinsulinemia in children. Description of PHHI as a unique clinical syndrome began 25 years ago with the association of nesidioblastosis, defined as the budding of isolated endocrine cells and islets from pancreatic duct cells, and severe infantile hypoglycemia [1]. Recent findings have elucidated the molecular cause for hyperinsulinemia in some families with this disorder, providing additional insight into the regulation of insulin secretion.

Pancreatic development

While frequently viewed as a single organ, discussion of pancreatic development is commonly divided into the two separate functional identities of this gland, exocrine and endocrine. This discussion focuses on the endocrine aspects of pancreatic development because they are most relevant to the topic of this chapter. Detailed description of the functional development of the exocrine pancreas, as well as embryological development of the whole pancreas, can be found elsewhere [2,3]. Our understanding of human pancreatic development is a continually evolving process, with much of this knowledge based on a combined extrapolation of data obtained from comparative morphology, animal models, and the study of pancreatic disorders [4,6]. In humans there is general consensus that the rudiments of the pancreas originate as dorsal and ventral outgrowths of the abdominal foregut beginning in fifth week of embryonic life. As development continues, these structures are rotated into proximity, allowing a fusion of the larger dorsal bud with the smaller ventral outgrowth into a single glandular structure by the seventh week of gestation. The dorsal portion will ultimately give rise to the tail and body of the adult gland, while the ventral portion develops into the head and uncinate process.

Andrew Arnold (ed.) ENDOCRINE NEOPLASMS. 1997. Kluwer Academic Publishers. ISBN 0-7923-4354-9.
All rights reserved.

At the microscopic level, most of the pancreas is comprised of primitive pancreatic tubules at the time of initial formation of the pancreas. It is not until between the 9th and 10th weeks of gestation that the appearance of endocrine cells is noted. In the mature pancreas the islet of Langerhans is comprised of four major cell types: the alpha cell (glucagon-producing), beta cell (insulin-producing), delta cell (somatostatin-producing), and PP cell (pancreatic-polypeptide producing). The order of cell appearance remains somewhat unresolved. An examination of 20 human embryos by Like and Orci in 1972 was able to detect the first appearance of alpha cells by 9 weeks, which was soon followed the appearance of delta cells and later beta cells at 10.5 weeks [7]. These observations were made using simple light and electron microscopy, and have been subject to reinterpretation as immunohistochemical and molecular genetic approaches have advanced.

Clark and Grant in 1983 were able to identify all cell types by 9 weeks gestation using immunostaining methods [8]. This observation is somewhat clouded by an incomplete understanding of the progenitor cell pathways followed during development. Recent studies in mice suggest that widespread immunostaining at this developmental stage may originate from precursor cells expressing multiple peptides, in which colocalization of two or more islet peptide hormones has been observed. Additional studies using RNA-PCR suggest that, while untranslated, mRNA for all four major peptide hormones is present in a common precursor islet cell [9,10]. As the pancreas continues to develop, peptide hormone expression must be specifically repressed as endocrine cell differentiation occurs. In humans all four hormone-producing cells are readily recognizable in well-formed islets by the 16th week of gestation.

An interesting feature of the developing mammalian pancreas is the biphasic developmental islets originally noted by Langerhans in lambs and calves [5]. During the first 2 weeks following birth, a peculiar type of large islets (visible to the eye) exists in these animals. However, these islets rapidly degenerate and are ultimately replaced by a second generation of cells. Examination of human fetal and newborn pancreas suggests a similar degeneration. Early histologic studies by Liu and Potter in 1962 suggested that the primary islets that formed around the primitive pancreas had a defined life span [11]. The cells in these islets reached maturity during the fifth month of gestation, after which they underwent a degeneration process. These islets were then replaced by a second generation of islets, which began formation during the third month of gestation. The generation of the primary islet-cell population is likely to continue through birth because there is a notable decrease in the percentage of islet cells observed at birth (~10%), infancy (~7%), and through adulthood (~2%) [5]. A disruption of this degenerative process is hypothesized to play a role in PHHI [12].

Clinical and pathological aspects of PHHI

Prompt recognition and treatment of this disorder is critical because uncorrected hypoglycemia in the newborn period is associated with permanent damage to the developing central nervous system. In the neonatal period, the presence of hypoglycemia leads to jitteriness, hypotonia, poor feeding, cyanosis, seizure, or sudden death [13]. Increased adiposity, due to persistent hyperinsulinemia, may be noted during an otherwise normal physical examination.

Hypoglycemia in neonates, infants, and children may be classified according to the duration of symptoms and organized into transient and persistent categories (Table 1). Traditionally, neonatal forms of hypoglycemia have referred to those with onset in the first 72 hours of life, and infantile and childhood forms with onset after 72 hours [14]. Transient forms of hypoglycemia usually correct within 3–7 days of life and require glucose infusions near the maintenance glucose production rate of approximately 6 mg/kg/min to maintain normoglycemia [15]. In general, persistent forms of hypoglycemia are both more protracted and severe than transient forms. Hypoglycemia due to hyperinsulinemia most commonly begins during the first year of life in pediatric patients, although it may occur at any age [14]. The

Table 1. Differential diagnosis of hypoglycemia in children

   I.   Transient neonatal hypoglycemia
        Infants of diabetic mothers (transient neonatal hyperinsulinemia)
        Prematurity
        Small for gestational age
        Systemic disease, septicemia, asphyxia
        Erythroblastosis fetalis
        Beckwith-Wiedemann syndrome
  II. Persistent hypoglycemia of the infant or child
        Hyperinsulinemia
          PHHI
            Beta-cell adenoma
            Exogenous insulin abuse
            Sulfonylurea use
        Hormone deficiency
          Growth hormone
          Cortisol
          Glucagon
          Panhypopituitarism
        Inborn error of metabolism
          Glycogen storage diseases
          Fat metabolism disorders
          Amino-acid metabolism disorders
        Ketotic hypoglycemia
        Reye's syndrome
        Intoxication (salicylate, ethanol)

Table 2. Characteristics of persistent hyperinsulinemic hypoglycemia or infancy

Inappropriate elevation of serum insulin despite the presence of hypoglycemia
Increased glucose utilization rate (requires glucose infusion >15 mg/kg/min to maintain euglycemia)
Nonketotic hypoglycemia
Glycemic response to glucagon

Table 3. Treatment of hyperinsulinism

Intravenous glucose infusion to maintain euglycemia
Medical therapy
Diaxozide
Octreotide
Surgical therapy
Near-complete pancreatectomy

complete differential diagnosis of childhood hypoglycemia has been extensively reviewed elsewhere [14,15].

The diagnostic features of PHHI are related to the unregulated production of insulin (Table 2). Hyperinsulinemia leads to hypoglycemia by increasing the rate of glucose utilization and by inhibiting endogenous glucose production. In the normal state, plasma insulin levels fall as blood glucose levels decrease. Repetitive glucose/insulin ratios of less than 2.6, obtained during an episode of hypoglycemia, are considered diagnostic for hyperinsulinemia [16]. However, many clinicians are hesitant to rely solely on such a ratio, especially in the case of preterm infants who routinely may have glucose levels of <40 mg/dl without suppressed insulin levels. In this case glucose utilization rates are not elevated and obesity, indicative of longstanding hyperinsulinemia, is lacking [16]. Insulin action inhibits the production of ketone bodies. Therefore, nonketotic hypoglycemia is the rule in hyperinsulinemic states. The other diagnostic category associated with nonketotic hypoglycemia is disorders of fat metabolism, including carnitine deficiency and fatty-acid acyl CoA dehydrogenase deficiency. Insulin levels will not be elevated in either of these disorders during episodes of hypoglycemia. Lastly, hyperinsulinemia leads to an increase in glycogen storage in the liver. Appropriate mobilization of glycogen during hypoglycemia is inhibited by hyperinsulinemia. Release of liver glycogen reserves is responsible for the elevations in blood glucose that occur following glucagon administration in PHHI.

Once the presence of hyperinsulinemia has been established, determination of the etiology follows. The most difficult distinction to make is the preoperative diagnosis of an islet-cell adenoma versus the diffuse hyperplasia of islet-cell tissue seen in PHHI. This distinction becomes important for the operative management of these disorders. Islet-cell adenomas, although reported, occur rarely in children [14]. When the diagnosis of an islet-cell adenoma is made, evaluation for other endocrine abnormalities, including hyperparathyroidism, hypergastrinemia, and pituitary tumor, should be

350

sought to establish whether the multiple endocrine neoplasia (MEN) type I syndrome might be present. No familial cases of isolated islet-cell adenomas in children have been reported. Plasma insulin levels following fasting or in response to secretagogues do not predict the underlying pancreatic pathology [14]. Use of ultrasonography and radionucleotide scanning have been found to be helpful in making the distinction between adenoma and PHHI [14,16].

Those with the Beckwith-Wiedemann syndrome, an overgrowth syndrome characterized by exomphalos, macroglossia, visceromegaly, gigantism, and ear-lobe creases, exhibit hyperinsulinemic hypoglycemia in approximately half of cases [17]. The hypoglycemia is usually transient in nature but may be persistent. The relationship between PHHI and Beckwith-Wiedemann syndrome, if any, remains to be determined.

Drug-related causes of hyperinsulinemia are very rare in the infant and child. A measurement of C-peptide level discriminates endogenous from exogenous hyperinsulinemia. In the case of factitious hyperinsulinemia, injected insulin, which lacks the C-peptide fragment, would lead to suppression of both insulin secretion and C-peptide levels in the affected individual. Sulfonylurea abuse produces hyperinsulinemia by stimulation of insulin secretion from pancreatic islet beta cells. Sudden onset of nonketotic hypoglycemia unrelated to fasting requires careful attention to possible drug intoxication. Toxicology screens are available for the detection of the presence of sulfonylureas.

For individuals affected with PHHI, prompt recognition, treatment, and rapid resolution of hypoglycemia are imperative to prevent permanent damage to the developing central nervous system [16] (*Table 3*). The effects of hyperinsulinemia, including hypoglycemia, suppressed gluconeogenesis, and inhibition of fatty-acid metabolism, deprive the brain of all energy substrates. Maintenance of normal glucose levels can be difficult. Glucose infusions of more than 15 mg/kg/min are frequently required to maintain normoglycemia [13], presenting practical problems with intravenous delivery of the required solutions. Central line placement is often required for the delivery of hypertonic solutions used to avoid volume overload. Prolonged use of such methods predisposes affected individuals to infection, venous sclerosis, and hepatomegaly [18].

Medical therapy for the treatment of hyperinsulinemia is often only temporizing, but when successful serves to avoid surgery. Diazoxide is the medial option for which the most experience has been gained. This nondiuretic benzothiadiazine was originally marketed for the treatment of hypertension. As a side effect, it was noted to produce hyperglycemia. While its mode of action has yet to be fully elucidated, it is known that diazoxide inhibits insulin secretion from pancreatic islet beta cells by stimulating membrane ATP-sensitive potassium (K_{ATP}) channels [19]. The binding site for diazoxide is separate on the membrane from that of stimulators of insulin secretion, the sulfonylurea agents [19]. Dose ranges of 5–20 mg/kg/day of diazoxide have been utilized [13,18,20].

Diazoxide has been documented as most effective in those initially presenting with hyperinsulinemia weeks to months after birth [18], although there has been success with treating those presenting within the first days of life [20]. Side effects of this medication include hypertrichosis, fluid retention, and heart failure. These side effects are not always dose related, and there is evidence that those with more severe disease more frequently develop side effects [20]. In seven patients with PHHI and cardiorespiratory failure attributed to diazoxide therapy studied by Abu-Osba et al., symptoms of cardiorespiratory failure resolved within 2–4 days after diazoxide was discontinued [20].

In an attempt to identify alternative medical therapies for the treatment of PHHI, other possibilities have been explored. Two hormones produced by the pancreatic islets, glucagon and somatostatin, have been investigated. Over the short term, both raise plasma glucose levels in this condition. Prolonged use of long-acting analogs of glucagon has not been successful [21]. Better experience has been obtained with a long-acting analog of somatostatin, octreotide. Two reports investigating octreotide use over 5 and 7 years revealed that only 25–50% of those studied had resolution of hypoglycemia, and many of those responsive to octreotide had undergone prior pancreatic surgery [22,23]. Delivery of this drug is difficult, requiring subcutaneous injection three to four times daily. Concerns regarding long-term use of octreotide are present due to the inhibitory effects it has on growth hormone, thyrotropin and pancreatic exocrine secretion and subsequent possible adverse affects on growth and nutrition [18]. Most authors agree that octreotide use is beneficial for the short-term management of hyperinsulinemia to achieve normoglycemia and euvolemia prior to operative intervention. Long-term use of octreotide remains controversial [21].

Current medical therapy does not lead to resolution of hypoglycemia in at least half of cases of hyperinsulinemia [24]. Surgery becomes the final solution in these cases. Aggressive and early control of hypoglycemia may result in avoidance of psychomotor retardation and neurologic dysfunction in those affected with PHHI [24,25]. Near-complete (95%) pancreatectomy is the procedure of choice to prevent recurrence of hypoglycemia [26]. While over the short term patients who have undergone 95% pancreatectomy have demonstrated few ill effects [27,28], there is now evidence that pancreatic insufficiency may become problematic in this group following puberty [29].

Of interest, some cases of PHHI have been reported to resolve [30]. Over the course of years, disease responsive to medical therapy can abate to the point of withdrawal of medical therapy and not require pancreatectomy. However, careful scrutiny of these reports is required because asymptomatic hypoglycemia may occur and results in damage to the central nervous system [24]. In addition, long-term follow-up has revealed that those affected with PHHI exhibit abnormal insulin secretion several years after clinical remission; the islet-cell defect responsible for PHHI in infancy does not resolve completely despite the resolution of symptomatic hypoglycemia [29].

Confusion remains in the histopathologic definition of PHHI. Morphologic findings in children affected with this disorder have included nesidioblastosis, described as a diffuse or disseminated proliferation of islet cells in close proximity to pancreatic ducts, islet-cell hyperplasia, islet-cell hypertrophy, multifocal ductulo-insular proliferation, and diffuse or focal islet-cell adenomatosis [31]. Upon review of 26 affected families, Thornton et al. found that histologic changes were not consistent among the affected individuals within a family. This led to the prediction that an abnormality of regulation of the beta cells is genetically determined, but that specific histopathological changes are not [32]. In addition, nesidioblastosis has been observed in normal control infants and young children, indicating that this finding is not pathognomonic for PHHI [31,33]. Several authors have described enlarged beta-cell nuclei in specimens obtained from individuals affected with PHHI, and this finding has been suggested as a possible morphologic criterion to differentiate focal from diffuse processes; although large nuclei have also been observed in adenomas, they appear to be present only in the focal lesion [34]. This finding of enlarged nuclei may be reflective of the increased activity of the beta cell due to unregulated production of insulin.

Genetic basis of PHHI

Recognition of familial forms of PHHI occurred following reports of affected siblings [35,36]. Inheritance in most cases is in an autosomal recessive pattern [32,37,38]. While the incidence of PHHI in a randomly mating Western population has been estimated at 1 per 50,000 live births [16], the incidence has been established as 1 per 2675 in a Saudi Arabian population in which 50% of matings were consanguineous [35]. The increased incidence present in inbred populations is consistent with autosomal recessive inheritance. A milder form of PHHI, which appears to be inherited in an autosomal dominant fashion, has been described in a small number of families [39].

The availability of well-characterized families with apparent autosomal recessive inheritance allowed the use of a combination of genetic linkage analysis and the candidate gene approach to identify a gene responsible for PHHI. PHHI was linked by Glaser et al. to a 6.6-centiMorgan (cM) interval on chromosome 11p in 15 independent families, 12 of which were Ashkenazi Jews [37]. Subsequent analysis revealed evidence for a founder effect in the Ashkenazi Jew ethnic population [40].

Using the homozygosity gene-mapping strategy, we confirmed and narrowed the assignment of Glaser et al. [38]. The homozygosity gene-mapping strategy is based on the premise that a rare disease in the affected progeny of a consanguineous mating is due to inheritance of two identical copies of the disease gene from the common ancestor, a situation termed *homozygosity by descent* [41]. In addition, regions flanking the disease gene, calculated to be of a median length of 28 cM in first-cousin matings, will be homozygous by

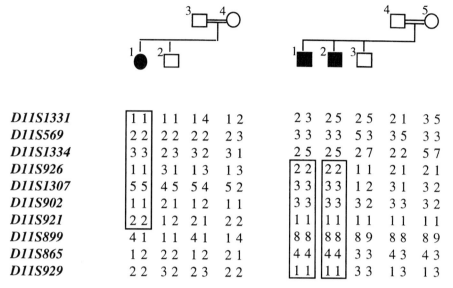

D11S1331	1 1	1 1	1 4	1 2	2 3	2 5	2 5	2 1	3 5
D11S569	2 2	2 2	2 2	2 3	3 3	3 3	5 3	3 5	3 3
D11S1334	3 3	2 3	3 2	3 1	2 5	2 5	2 7	2 2	5 7
D11S926	1 1	3 1	1 3	1 3	2 2	2 2	1 1	2 1	2 1
D11S1307	5 5	4 5	5 4	5 2	3 3	3 3	1 2	3 1	3 2
D11S902	1 1	2 1	1 2	1 1	3 3	3 3	3 2	3 3	3 2
D11S921	2 2	1 2	2 1	2 2	1 1	1 1	1 1	1 1	1 1
D11S899	4 1	1 1	4 1	1 4	8 8	8 8	8 9	8 8	8 9
D11S865	1 2	2 2	1 2	2 1	4 4	4 4	3 3	4 3	4 3
D11S929	2 2	3 2	2 3	2 2	1 1	1 1	3 3	1 3	1 3

Figure 1. Simplified pedigrees and genotypes on chromosome 11, in the region of homozygosity, of members of two families affected with PHHI. Regions of homozygosity in affected children are boxed. In both families the parents are second cousins. Note that within each family the parents share the same disease allele haplotype, which presumably is derived from their common ancestor. Comparison of the regions of homozygosity in these two families allow boundaries for PHHI to be placed between the chromosome 11 markers D11S1334 and D11S899. These data were obtained as part of the homozygosity mapping analysis for PHHI [38], and similar figures appear elsewhere.

descent in most cases. Other regions of the genome will also be homozygous by descent, but such regions will vary among affected children. For an informative, tightly linked marker, the calculations of Lander and Botstein revealed that three first-cousin matings, each with a single affected offspring, will provide a LOD score >3.0, the accepted threshold for linkage [41]. Ten or more nonrelated nuclear families with affected pairs of siblings would be required to generate a similar score. Study of progeny of five consanguineous families of Saudi Arabian origin using this approach allowed placement of PHHI to a 5-cM interval on chromosome 11p14–15.1, between markers D11S1334 and D11S899 [38] (Fig. 1). Subsequent analysis narrowed the PHHI locus to an estimated 0.8-cM interval between markers D11S926 and D11S928 on chromosome 11p15.1 [40].

In vitro studies of pancreatic islet beta cells isolated from individuals affected with PHHI have suggested a defect in glucose-regulated insulin secretion [13,42]. Current models of insulin secretion propose that, as a result of glucose metabolism, increases in the intracellular ATP/ADP ratio in pancreatic beta cells inhibit ATP-sensitive potassium (K_{ATP}) channels, leading to beta-cell membrane depolarization, opening of voltage-gated calcium channels, and ultimately an increase in exocytosis of insulin [43] (Fig. 2). This

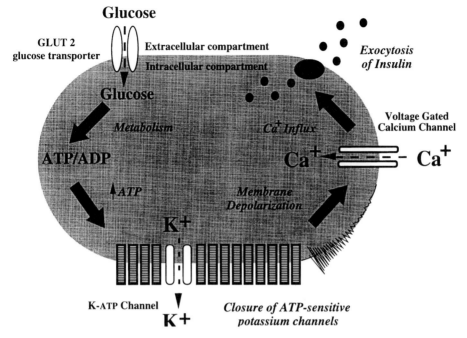

Figure 2. A schematic drawing of events hypothesized to lead to insulin secretion by pancreatic islet beta cells. Alterations in intracellular ATP level leads to closure of ATP-sensitive potassium channels. Subsequent membrane depolarization, opening of voltage-gated calcium channels, and exocytosis of insulin follows.

paradigm sets the pancreatic islets apart from other tissue systems because a metabolic signal, rather than an agonist-receptor signal, must be transduced to result in insulin secretion [44]. Therefore, candidate genes for PHHI included those involved in the beta-cell glucose-sensing mechanism and insulin secretion. Assignment of the PHHI locus to chromosome 11p excluded known genes involved in beta-cell function, including the glucokinase, islet glucose transporter, and glucagon-like peptide-1 receptor loci, as candidates for PHHI [45].

The high-affinity sulfonylurea receptor (SUR) [46], a subunit of the beta-cell K_{ATP} channel [47], was considered as a candidate for the PHHI gene based on its role as a modulator of insulin secretion. Certain sulfonamide antibiotics, used during World War II to treat typhoid fever, were noted to cause hypoglycemic symptoms [48]. Shortly thereafter, derivatives of these antibiotics were used as a treatment for diabetes [48]. The hypoglycemic action of sulfonylureas results from direct inhibition of pancreatic beta-cell K_{ATP} channels analogous to that produced by elevation of intracellular ATP levels [49]. The beta-cell high-affinity sulfonylurea receptor was cloned following purification of a 140-kD protein that demonstrated the pharmacological and biochemical characteristics of the sulfonylurea receptor [46].

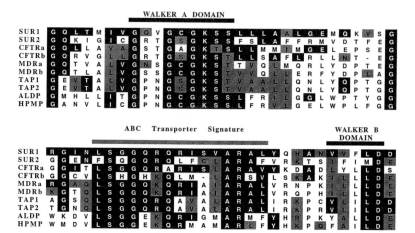

Figure 3. Alignment of portions of the first and second nucleotide-binding folds (NBF) of the human sulfonylurea receptor (SUR 1 and SUR 2) and corresponding portions the NBFs of other ATP-binding cassette family members. Black shading illustrates identity with another family member, and gray shading illustrates conservative amino-acid changes. The Walker A and B motifs of the NBF are marked. The single-letter amino-acid code is used. Similar alignments have occurred elsewhere [50]. CFTR = cystic fibrosis transmembrane conductance regulator; MDR1 = multidrug-resistant gene product; TAP = peptide transporters 1 and 2; ALDP = adrenoleukodystrophy protein, HPMP = human peroxisomal membrane protein.

The SUR is classified as a member of the ATP-binding cassette superfamily due to the presence of two nucleotide-binding fold (NBF) consensus sequences (Fig. 3) [46]. This class of molecules, also known as ABC transporters, is involved in selective transport of substrate across the cell membrane against a concentration gradient using ATP hydrolysis as an energy source. Although each transporter is specific for a given substrate, the spectrum of substrates pumped by family members is diverse and includes amino acids, sugars, inorganic ions, polysaccharides, and peptides [50]. The substrate for the SUR has not been elucidated. Well-known members of this family include the multidrug resistance proteins and the cystic fibrosis transmembrane conductance regulator (CFTR) [50]. Mutations in the CFTR have been shown to cause the autosomal-recessive disorder cystic fibrosis, and the more frequent and severe disease alleles are located in the regions of the two NBFs [51].

Localization of the human homolog of the SUR gene to chromosome 11p15.1 [45], the previously defined site of the PHHI locus, provided us with the necessary impetus to begin mutational analysis of this gene. The initial search for mutations in the SUR gene identified two mutations that affected RNA processing [45], (Fig. 4B). Both occurred within RNA splice-site consensus sequences located in the NBF-2 coding region. The first of these mutations causes skipping of the third exon of the NBF-2 region in the SUR mRNA transcript. This exon-skipping event results in disruption of the NBF-2 consensus sequence, due to a 109 base-pair (bp) deletion and associated framed shift,

356

SUR Mutations Occuring in NBF Domains

A. NBF-1 Domain

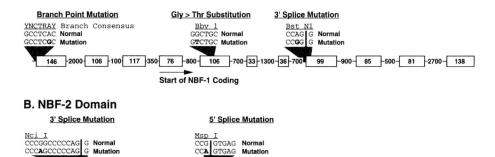

Figure 4. Location of mutations in the SUR that disrupt the first (NBF-1) (**A**) and second (NBF-2) (**B**) nucleotide-binding fold regions of the SUR gene in individuals affected with familial PHHI. This schematic drawing depicts the genomic organization of the NBF-1 and NBF-2 regions of the SUR. Solid rectangles represent exons that are arbitrarily labeled for identification with numbers indicating exon size for NBF-1 and with the letters α to φ for NBF-2. The numbers between rectangles represent intronic sizes. The predicted effects of each mutation are discussed in the text.

with inclusion of a premature stop 24 codons later. The second mutation was identified in the 3′ splice site sequence preceding the first exon of the NBF-2 region (see Fig. 4). In the presence of this splice-site mutation, three cryptic 3′ splice sites were used in place of the wild-type splicing pattern, resulting in a 7-bp addition, a 20-bp deletion, or a 30-bp deletion in the first exon of the NBF-2 region. The first mutation destroys an *Msp*I restriction endonuclease site and the second an *Nci*I site, providing a convenient means for testing for their presence. Eight of nine families identified with the first mutation were of eastern Saudi Arabian origin, and haplotype analysis with markers closely linked to the SUR supports a founder effect for this mutation (PMT, unpublished data).

Three additional mutations have been identified in the region of the NBF-1 of the SUR (see Fig. 4A) [52]. Two of these mutations affect RNA processing of the SUR precursor transcript. Exon-skipping events result in either a frame shift and the introduction of a premature stop codon (branch-point mutation) or an inframe deletion of 33 amino acids from the central coding region of the NBF-1 region (3′ splice-site mutation). A third point mutation located in the highly conserved sequence encoding the Walker A motif of the NBF-1 region (see Fig. 3) emphasized the importance of NBF-1 in the function of the SUR.

The patient population used for linkage analysis and subsequent mutation detection was purposefully selected as a homogeneous group of severely affected individuals with classical clinical presentation and a clear autosomal-recessive inheritance pattern of disease. The identified mutations do not represent the full spectrum of SUR mutations in individuals affected with PHHI, because we have identified several families that exhibit linkage to chromosome 11p15.1 yet demonstrate none of the described mutations. By analogy to individuals affected with cystic fibrosis and adrenoleukodystrophy, both of which are caused by mutations in ATP-binding cassette superfamily members, the spectrum of mutations in familial PHHI may be very large [51,53]. Before prenatal diagnosis or genetic counseling may be considered for this disorder, further study of simplex and multiplex families is necessary to establish the frequency of the identified and other mutations in a variety of ethnic groups and to assess the degree of genetic homogeneity for the disease.

Molecular pathophysiology of disease

The resting membrane potential of pancreatic islet beta cells is set by potassium channels. A link between the metabolic state of the cell and membrane electrical events is created by the inhibition of K_{ATP} channels by ATP; as intracellular ATP level increase, inhibition of K_{ATP} channels progressively increases, leading to cell depolarization. The SUR is closely associated with K_{ATP} channels in beta cells; however, no intrinsic channel activity has been demonstrated for it [46].

Demonstration that loss of function mutations in the SUR lead to PHHI implicates SUR as a regulator of channels. A similar model has been created for CFTR and other ATP-binding cassette family members, proposing that these proteins may be regulators of channels and pumps [54]. This model for SUR is supported by the cloning and initial characterization of Kir6.2, a new member of the inward rectifier potassium channel family [55]. Like SUR, Kir6.2 cannot conduct ions when expressed alone. However, when expressed with SUR, ion-channel activity and pharmacological sensitivities characteristic of the K_{ATP} channel are reconstituted. The definition of the K_{ATP} channel complex now includes at least the two members Kir6.2 and SUR, although the nature and stoichometry of this interaction remain to be defined (Fig. 5). It is unknown how the potassium-selective pore is formed. In addition, the binding site for the potassium-channel opener diazoxide, a pharmacological agent used in the treatment of PHHI, is also unknown. This model for the K_{ATP} channel complex implies that mutations in Kir6.2, which is located also on chromosome 11p15.1 approximately 4 kb 3' of the SUR locus [55], may be found in those affected with PHHI.

The finding of mutations in the SUR in individuals affected with PHHI also underscores the importance of SUR in the normal regulation of insulin secretion (Fig. 6). The observation that individuals heterozygous for the mutation have no obvious clinical symptoms is consistent with a model of ATP-sensitive channels put forth by Cooke et al. This model, similar to the 'spare

358

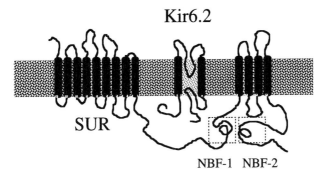

Kir6.2

Figure 5. Schematic of the beta-cell K_{ATP} channel, which is now known to be composed of at least the sulfonylurea receptor (SUR) and the inward rectifier Kir6.2. This schematic is based on computer modeling of the two genes and is modeled after a similar depiction presented elsewhere [58].

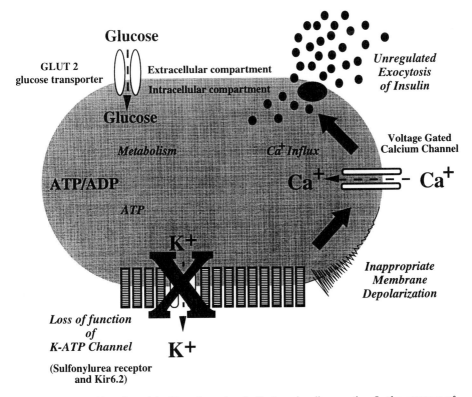

Figure 6. Loss of function of the K_{ATP} channel and effects on insulin secretion. In the presence of mutations in the SUR, or possibly Kir6.2, the link between metabolism and insulin secretion is lost because ATP-sensitive potassium (K_{ATP}) channels are unresponsive to alterations in intracellular ATP levels. This leads to inappropriate channel closure, membrane depolarization, opening of voltage-gated calcium channels, and ultimately unregulated exocytosis of insulin.

receptor' model, states that only a few channels need be open at any one time to control membrane potential in the physiologic voltage range [56]. Complete loss of function of the SUR leads to PHHI; however, 50% function does not lead to recognized clinical symptoms. Now that the identity of the beta cell K_{ATP} channel has been elucidated, at least in part, it may become possible to clarify the mechanisms by which diazoxide and somatostatin function to resolve hypoglycemia in PHHI. This, in turn, may ultimately lead to more specific strategies for the treatment of hyperinsulinemia. The mutations described may provide tools for the dissection of these signal-transduction pathways. The role of the SUR in other disorders of insulin secretion remains to be clarified.

Finally, many questions have yet to be explored regarding possible roles for the SUR in the normal developmental process. It remains unknown whether the histopathological changes noted in PHHI represent changes in islet growth due specifically to loss of function of the SUR or merely reflect the presence of prolonged and excessive insulin secretion. It can be hypothesized that PHHI represents a prolongation of the fetal developmental state in which insulin levels are elevated above those of the postnatal state and are poorly responsive to postnatal nutritional signals. In the prenatal state, insulin's role is as a growth factor, and the majority of glucose homeostasis is regulated by the maternal-fetal-placental unit [42,57]. It is plausible that SUR may play a prominent role in the regulation of prenatal insulin secretion and islet development.

References

1. Brown RE, Young RB. 1970. A possible role for the exocrine pancreas in the pathogenesis of neonatal leucine-sensitive hypoglycemia. Am J Dig Dis 15:65–72.
2. Lebenthal E, Lev R, Lee PC. 1986. Prenatal and postnatal development of the human exocrine pancreas. In Go VLW et al., eds. The Exocrine Pancreas, Biology, Pathobiology and Diseases. New York: Raven Press, pp 33–43.
3. McLean JM. 1979. Embryology of the pancreas. In Howat HT, Sarles H, eds. The Exocrine Pancreas. London: Saunders, pp 2–14.
4. Cruickshank AH, Benbow EW. 1995. Pathology of the Pancreas, 2nd ed. London: Springer Press, pp 13–27.
5. Falkmer S. 1995. Origin of the parenchymal cells of the endocrine pancreas: Some phylogenetic and ontogenetic aspects. In Mignon M, Jensen RT, eds. Endocrine Tumors of the Pancreas. Frontiers of Gastrointestinal Research. Basel: Karger, pp 2–29.
6. Hoet JJ, Reusens B, Remacle C. 1995. Anatomy, development and pathology of pancreatic islets. In DeGroot LJ, ed. Endocrinology, 3rd ed. Philadelphia: Saunders, pp 1277–1295.
7. Like AL, Orci L. 1972. Embryogenesis of the human pancreatic islets: A light and electron microscopic study. Diabetes 21:511–534.
8. Clark A, Grant AM. 1983. Quantitative morphology of endocrine cells in human fetal pancreas. Diabetologica 25:31–35.
9. Teitelman G, Alpert S, Polak JM, Martinez A, Hanahan D. 1993. Precursor cells of the mouse endocrine pancreas coexpress insulin, glucagon and the neuronal proteins tyrosine hydroxylase and neuropeptide Y, but not pancreatic polypeptide. Development 118:1031–1039.

10. Upchurch BH, Aponte GW, Leiter AB. 1994. Expression of peptide YY in all four islet cell types in the developing mouse pancreas suggests a common peptide YY-producing progenitor. Development 120:245–252.
11. Liu HM, Potter EL. 1962. Development of the human pancreas. Arch Pathol 74:439–452.
12. Shermeta DW, Mendelsohn G, Haller JA. 1980. Hyperinsulinemic hypoglycemia of the neonate associated with persistent fetal histology and function of the pancreas. Ann Surg 191:182–186.
13. Aynsley-Green A, Polak JM, Bloom SR, Gough MH, Keeling J, Ashcroft SJH, Turner RC, Baum JD. 1981. Nesidioblastosis of the pancreas: Definition of the syndrome and the management of the severe neonatal hyperinsulinaemic hypoglycaemia. Arch Dis Child 56:496–508.
14. Haymond MW. 1989. Hypoglycemia in infants and children. Endocrinol Metabo Clin North Am 18:211–252.
15. Schiffrin A, Colle E. 1989. Hypoglycemia. In Collu R, Ducharme JR, Guyda HJ, eds. Pediatric Endocrinology, 2nd ed. New York: Raven Press.
16. Bruining GJ. 1990. Recent advances in hyperinsulinism and the pathogenesis of diabetes mellitus. Curr Opin Pediatr 2:758–765.
17. Martinez R, Martinez-Carboney R, Ocampocampos R, Rivera H, Castillo J, Cuevas A, Martin Manrique MC. 1992. Wiedemann-Beckwith syndrome: Clinical, cytogenetical and radiological observations in 39 new cases. Genet Counsel 3:67–76.
18. Worden FP, Freidenberg G, Pescovitz OH. 1994. The diagnosis and management of neonatal hyperinsulinism. Endocrinologist 4:196–204.
19. Ashcroft SJH, Ashcroft FM. 1990. Properties and functions of ATP-sensitive K-channels. Cell Signal 2:197–214.
20. Abu-Osba YK, Manasra KB, Mathew PM. 1989. Complications of diazoxide treatment in persistent neonatal hyperinsulinism. Arch Dis Child 64:1496–1500.
21. Daneman D, Ehrlich RM. 1993. The enigma of persistent hyperinsulinemic hypoglycemia of infancy. J Pediatr 123:573–675.
22. Thornton PS, Alter CA, Katz LEL, Baker L, Stanley CA. 1993. Short- and long-term use of octreotide in the treatment of congenital hyperinsulinism. J Pediatr 123:637–943.
23. Glaser B, Hirsch HJ, Landau H. 1992. Persistent hyperinsulinemic hypoglycemia of infancy: Long-term octreotide treatment without pancreatectomy. J Pediatr 123:644–650.
24. Baker L, Thornton PS, Stanely CA. 1991. Management of hyperinsulinism in infants. J Pediatr 119:755–757.
25. Jacobs DG, Haka-Ikse K, Wesson DE, Filler RM, Sherwood G. 1986. Growth and development in patients operated on for islet cell dysplasia. J Pediatr Surg 21:1184–1189.
26. Gough MH. 1984. The surgical of hyperinsulinism in infancy and childhood. Br J Surg 71:75–78.
27. Dunger DB, Burns C, Ghale GK, Muller DPR, Spitz L, Grant DB. 1988. Pancreatic exocrine and endocrine function after subtotal pancreatectomy for nesidioblastosis. J Pediatr Surg 23:112–115.
28. Schonau E, Deeg KH, Huemmer HP, Akcetin YZ, Bohles HJ. 1991. Pancreatic growth and function following surgical treatment of nesidioblastosis in infancy. Eur J Pediatr 150:550–553.
29. Leibowitz G, Glaser B, Higazi AA, Salameh M, Cerasi E, Landau H. 1995. Hyperinsulinemic hypoglycemia of infancy in clinical remission: High incidence of diabetes mellitus and persistent β-cell dysfunction at long-term follow-up. J Clin Endocrinol Metab 80:386–392.
30. Horev S, Ipp M, Levey P, Daneman D. 1991. Familial hyperinsulinism: Successful conservative management. J Pediatr 119:717–720.
31. Jaffe R, Hashida Y, Yunis EJ. 1980. Pancreatic pathology in hyperinsulinemic hypoglycemia of infancy. Lab Invest 42:356–365.
32. Thornton PS, Sumner AE, Ruchelli ED, Spielman RS, Baker L, Stanley CA. 1991. Familial and sporadic hyperinsulinism: Histopathologic findings and segregation analysis support a single autosomal recessive disorder. J Pediatr 199:721–724.

33. Rahier J. 1989. Relevance of endocrine pancreas nesidioblastosis to hyperinsulinemic hypoglycemia. Diabetes Care 12:164–166.
34. Rahier J, Falt K, Muntefering H, Becker K, Gepts W, Falkmer S. 1984. The basic structural lesion of persistent neonatal hypoglycemia with hyperinsulinism: Deficiency of pancreatic D cells or hyperactivity of B cells? Diabetologia 26:282–289.
35. Mathew PM, Young JM, Abu-Osba YK, Mulhern BD, Hammoudi S, Hamdan JA, Sa'di AR. 1988. Persistent neonatal hyperinsulinism. Clin Pediatr 3:148–151.
36. Glaser B, Phillip M, Carmi R, Lieberman E, Landau H. 1990. Persistent hyperinsuliemic hypoglycemia of infancy: Autosomal recessive inheritance in 7 pedigrees. Am J Med Genet 37:511–515.
37. Glaser B, Chiu KC, Anker R, Nesforowicz A, Landau H, Ben-Bassat H, Shlomai Z, Kaiser N, Thornton PS, Stanley CA, Spielman RS, Gogolin-Ewens K, Cerasi E, Baker L, Rice J, Donis-Keller H, Permutt MA. 1994. Familial hyperinsulinism maps to chromosome 11p14–15.1, 30 cM centromeric to the insulin gene. Nature Genet 7:185–188.
38. Thomas PM, Cote GJ, Hallman DM, Mathew PM. 1995. Homozygosity mapping, to chromosome 11p, of the gene for familial persistent hyperinsulinemic hypoglycemia of infancy. Am J Hum Genet 56:416–421.
39. Thornton PS, Glaser B, Herold K, Chiu KC, Satin-Smith MS, Permutt MA, Baker L, Stanley CA. 1995. Familial hyperinsulinism inherited in an autosomal dominant form differs clinically and genetically from the more common autosomal recessive form. Society for Pediatr Res 37 (suppl):100A.
40. Glaser B, Chiu KC, Liu L, Anker R, Nestorowicz A, Cox NJ, Landau H, Kaiser N, Thornton PS, Stanley CA, Cerasi E, Baker L, Donis-Keller H, Permutt MA. 1995. Recombinant mapping of the familial hyperinsulinism gene to an 0.8 cM region on chromosome 11p15.1 and demonstration of a founder effect in Ashkenazi Jews. Hum Mol Genet 5:879–886.
41. Lander ES, Botstein D. 1987. Homozygosity mapping: A way to map human recessive traits with the DNA of inbred children. Science 236:1567–1570.
42. Kaiser N, Corcos AP, Tur-Sinai A, Ariav Y, Glaser B, Landau H, Cerasi E. 1990. Regulation of insulin release in persistent hyperinsulinaemic hypoglycaemia of infancy studied in long-term culture of pancreatic tissue. Diabetologia 33:482–488.
43. Ashcroft FM. 1988. Adenosine 5'-triphosphate-sensitive potassium channels. Ann Rev Neurosci 11:97–118.
44. MacDonald MJ. 1990. Elusive proximal signals of B-cells for insulin secretion. Diabetes 39:1461–1466.
45. Thomas PM, Cote GJ, Wohllk N, Haddad B, Mathew PM, Rabl W, Aguilar-Bryan L, Gagel RF, Bryan J. 1995. Mutations in the sulfonylurea receptor gene in familial persistent hyperinsulinemic hypoglycemia of infancy. Science 268:426–429.
46. Aguilar-Bryan L, Nichols CG, Wechsler SW, Clement JP, Boyd AE, Gonzalez G, Herrera-Sosa H, Nguy K, Bryan J, Nelson DA. 1995. Cloning of the β-cell high-affinity sulfonylurea receptor: A regulator of insulin secretion. Science 268:423–426.
47. Ashcroft SJ, Ashcroft FM. 1992. The sulfonylurea receptor. Biochim Biophys Acta 1175:45–59.
48. Boyd AE, Aguilar-Bryan L, Bryan J, Kunze DL, Moss L, Nelson DA, Rajan AS, Raef H, Xiang H, Yaney GC. 1991. Sulfonylurea signal transduction. Recent Progr Horm Res 47:299–317.
49. Ashcroft SJH, Niki I, Kenna S, Weng L, Skeer J, Coles B, Ashcroft FM. 1993. The β-cell sulfonylurea receptro. In Ostenson CG, et al. New Concepts in the Pathogenesis of NIDDN. New York: Plenum Press.
50. Higgins CF. 1992. ABC transporters: From microorganisms to man. Annu Rev Cell Biol 8:67–113.
51. Tsui LC. 1992. The spectrum of cystic fibrosis mutations. Trends Genet 8:392–398.
52. Thomas PM, Wohllk N, Huang E, Kuhnle U, Rabl W, Gagel RF, Cote GJ. 1996. Inactivation of the first nucleotide-binding fold of the sulfonylurea receptor, and familialpersistent hyperinsulinemic hypoglycemia of infancy. Am J Hum Genet 59:510–518.

362

53. Ligtenberg MJL, Kemp S, Sarde C-O, van Geel BM, Kleijer WJ, Barth PG, Mandel JL, van Oost BA, Bolhins PA. 1995. Spectrum of mutations in the gene encoding the adrenoleukodystrophy protein. Am J Hum Genet 56:44–50.

54. Higgins CF. 1995. The ABC of channel regulation. Cell 82:693–696.

55. Inagaki N, Gonoi T, Clement JP, Namba N, Inazawa J, Gonzalez G, Anguilar-Bryan L, Seino S, Bryan J. 1995. Reconstitution of I-KATP: An inward rectifier subunit plus the sulfonylurea receptor. Science 270:1166–1170.

56. Cook DL, Satin LS, Ashford MLJ, Hales CN. 1988. ATP-Sensitive K channels in pancreatic B-cells; spare-channel hypothesis. Diabetes 37:495–498.

57. Otonkoski T, Andersson S, Simell O. 1993. Somatostatin regulation of β-cell function in the normal human fetuses and in neonates with persistent hyperinsulinemic hypoglycemia. J Clin Endocrinol Metab 76:184–188.

58. Philpson LH. 1995. ATP-Sensitive K-channels: Paradigm lost, paradigm regained. Science 270:1159.

17. Somatostatin analogs and receptors
Diagnostic and therapeutic applications

L.J. Hofland and S.W.J. Lamberts

Somatostatin and somatostatin receptors

The widely distributed small cyclic peptide hormone somatostatin (SS) plays an important regulatory role in the function of multiple target organs, including the brain, pituitary, gastrointestinal tract, and the pancreas [1,2]. It has a mainly inhibitory role in these organ systems on neurotransmission and secretion processes [1,2]. High-affinity membrane receptors for the two molecular forms of somatostatin (i.e., SS-14, consisting of 14 amino acids, and SS-28, an NH_2-terminally extended form of SS-14, [3]) have been found in most of the target organs of this important regulatory peptide hormone [4,5]. In addition to the above-mentioned role of SS, the peptide may have inhibitory effects on the proliferation of normal and tumorous cells in experimental models [5,6].

Recently, five different somatostatin receptor (SSR) subtypes have been cloned and characterized [7–11]. These receptor subtypes — named sst_1, sst_2, sst_3, sst_4, and sst_5 [12] — are localized on different chromosomes [13–16] and have a distinct expression pattern in the different target organs (Table 1). Interestingly, one target organ may express multiple SSR subtypes. The precise functional role of the different SSR subtypes in each of these target organs remains to be elucidated. The different SSR subtypes are all coupled to G-proteins [7–11] and are linked to multiple cellular effector systems, including inhibition of adenylyl cyclase activity, stimulation of phosphotyrosine phosphatases, and inhibition of Ca^{2+}-influx (Table 1). In addition, in COS-7 cells expressing sst_{1-5}, all subtypes are linked to a stimulatory effect on phospholipase C and Ca^{2+} mobilization, with a rank order of potency of $sst_5 > sst_2 > sst_3 > sst_4 > sst_1$ [17], although a recent study by Buscail et al. [18] showed in Chinese hamster ovary (CHO) cells expressing sst_5 that receptor activation resulted in an inhibition of cholecystokinin-induced intracellular Ca^{2+} mobilization.

Somatostatin analogs

The very short half-life of native SS in the circulation (less than 3 minutes) has limited its use for therapeutic purposes [1,19]. Therefore, several structural

Andrew Arnold (ed.) ENDOCRINE NEOPLASMS. 1997. Kluwer Academic Publishers. ISBN 0-7923-4354-9.
All rights reserved.

Table 1. Tissue distribution and coupling to second messenger systems of the five cloned SSR subtypes

sst subtype	Tissue distribution	2nd messenger coupling
sst$_1$	Brain, pituitary, lung, stomach, jejunum, kidney,pancreas, liver	Adenylyl cyclase ↓ Phosphotyrosine phosphatase ↑ Phospholipase C/Ca^{2+} mobilization ↑
sst$_2$	Brain, pituitary, kidney	Adenylyl cyclase ↓ Phosphotyrosine phosphatase ↑ Ca^{2+} influx ↓ Phospholipase C/Ca2$^+$ mobilization ↑
sst$_3$	Brain, pituitary, pancreas	Adenylyl cyclase ↓ Phospholipase C/Ca^{2+} mobilization ↑
sst$_4$	Brain, lung	Adenylyl cyclase ↓ Phospholipase C/Ca^{2+} mobilization ↑
sst$_5$	Brain, pituitary, heart, adrenals, placenta, small intestine, muscle	Adenylyl cyclase ↓ Phospholipase C/Ca^{2+} mobilization ↑[a]/↓[b]

[a] Data from Akbar et al. [17].
[b] Data from Buscail et al. [18].
Adapted from refs. 9, 30, and 88 and data from refs. 17, 18, 40, and 42.

analogs of SS have been developed via step-by-step modification of the parental SS molecule [20–24]. So far three of these analogs, which are all octapeptide analogs of somatostatin, are in clinical use and/or studies. The amino-acid sequences of these analogs, that is, octreotide (Sandostatin, SMS 201-995), BIM-23014 (Lanreotide), and RC-160 (Vapreotide, Octastatin), are shown in Figure 1. Octreotide contains the sequence residues 7–10 of SS, Phe-Trp-Lys-Thr, essential for receptor binding, in which D-Trp was substituted for Trp. BIM-23014 and RC-160 are Tyr^3/Val^6-substituted analogs, which have been suggested to produce a more selective action on growth hormone (GH) secretion [21–24]. In addition to these differences in amino-acid composition with octreotide, BIM-23014 and RC-160 have substitutions at positions 1 (DβNal for DPhe) and 8 [Trp for Thr(ol)] of the molecule, respectively see (Fig. 1).

Interestingly, the five cloned SSR subtypes show a distinct pharmacological binding profile of these SS analogs currently available for clinical use in comparison with that of native SS. This is shown in Table 2. Both SS-14 and SS-28 bind with high affinities, in the nanomolar range, to all SSR subtypes. Octreotide, BIM-23014, and RC-160 have comparable binding profiles and bind with a high affinity to sst$_2$ and sst$_5$ only, and show low or no affinity to sst$_3$, sst$_1$, and sst$_4$, respectively [7–11,25]. Previous data have suggested that RC-160 may have a more selective action on tumor cell growth in comparison to octreotide [26]. In addition, receptor binding studies with membrane preparations of human breast and ovarian cancers and of certain human pancreatic adenocarcinomas provided evidence for a significant higher affinity of RC-160 for SS-14 binding sites in comparison with that of octreotide [27].

366

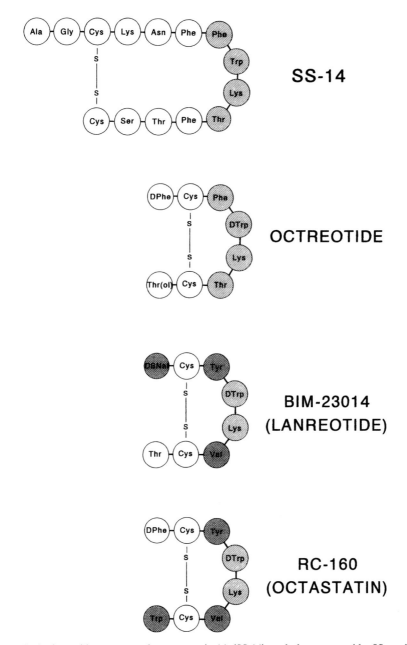

Figure 1. Amino-acid sequence of somatostatin-14 (SS-14) and the octapeptide SS analogs octreotide, lanreotide, and octastatin. The hatched circles represent the amino acids essential for SSR (sst$_2$ and sst$_5$) binding. The crosshatched circles represent amino acids of lanreotide and octastatin that differ from octreotide.

Table 2. Pharmacological binding profiles of SS-14, SS-28, and the octapeptide SS analogs octreotide, BIM-23014 (Lanreotide), and RC-160 (Vapreotide, Octastatin) to the five cloned SSR subtypes

	Affinity constant (K_i) in nM				
sst Subtype	SS-14	SS-28	Octreotide	BIM-23014	RC-160
sst_1	1.1	2.2	>1000	>1000	>1000
sst_2	1.3	4.1	2.1	1.8	5.4
sst_3	1.6	6.1	4.4–31.6[a]–35[b]	43.0	30.9
sst_4	0.5	1.1	>1000	66.0	45.0
sst_5	0.9	0.1	5.6	0.6	0.7

[a] Data from Kubota et al. [39].
[b] Data from Bruns et al. [7].
Data are derived from refs. 25, 39, and 7.
[a,b] Values represent IC_{50} values (nM).

Another study pointed to a significant difference in the potency of inhibition of growth hormone (GH) release by octreotide and BIM-23014, on the one hand, and of RC-160, on the other hand [28]. RC-160 was significantly more potent in inhibiting GH release by cultured normal rat anterior pituitary cells and human GH-secreting pituitary adenomas in comparison with the two other octapeptide SS analogs, although those GH-secreting pituitary adenomas that were unresponsive to octreotide and BIM-23014 were unresponsive to RC-160 as well [28]. In agreement with this latter observation, Janson et al. [29] showed in patients with carcinoids that those tumors that showed no binding of octreotide in in vivo SSR scintigraphy did not respond to therapy with RC-160 or BIM-23014. In summary, in agreement with the comparable pharmacological binding profiles of the three octapeptide SS analogs to the five SSR subtypes, it seems that no major differences can be expected among the therapeutic effects of octreotide, BIM-23014, and RC-160. On the other hand, recent preliminary data from our group suggest that there may be a place for newly developed SSR-subtype–selective SS analogs in the treatment of those tumors that are unresponsive to octreotide, BIM-23014, or RC-160 therapy. We have found that hormone secretion by certain human insulinomas, clinically nonfunctioning pituitary adenomas, and prolactinomas is unresponsive to octreotide, whereas SS-14 and/or SS-28 significantly inhibit hormone secretion [L.J. Hofland, unpublished; 30].

Somatostatin receptor (subtype) expression in human tumors

Many neuroendocrine tumors, often originating from SS target tissues, express a high density of SS receptors [31–33]. These include pituitary adenomas, islet-cell tumors, carcinoids, paragangliomas, pheochromocytomas, small-cell

368

lung cancers, and medullary thyroid carcinomas, but also breast cancers and malignant lymphomas [34]. Earlier studies by Reubi et al. [31–33] pointed to the existence of SSR subtypes in certain subgroups of human tumors. SS-receptor autoradiographic studies showed the absence of binding of [^{125}I-Tyr^3] octreotide in a small subgroup of human insulinomas, carcinoids, medullary thyroid carcinomas, ovarian cancers, and GH-secreting pituitary adenomas, while in the same tumors binding sites for iodinated [Tyr^{11}]SS-14 or [LTT]SS-28 were present [31–33]. This differential binding between octreotide and SS-14/SS-28 ligands in insulinomas and other subgroups of SSR-positive tumors again suggests that new SSR-subtype–selective analogs can be developed for the treatment of patients with tumors carrying SSR of this particular subtype.

The recent cloning of the five SSR subtypes also provided tools to study their expression in human tumors. SSR subtype expression in different types of human cancers has now been studied using in situ hybridization [35,36], RNAse protection assays, and the reverse transcriptase polymerase chain reaction (RT-PCR) [37–43]. These first studies indicate that the majority of human tumors express multiple SSR subtypes at the same time, although there is a considerable variation in SSR-subtype expression between the different tumor types and among tumors of the same type.

Table 3 summarizes the currently available data. From this table it is clear that sst$_2$ is most abundantly expressed in all types of tumors of different origins. It must be pointed out that studies on SSR subtype expression in whole-tissue homogenates using very sensitive techniques such as PT-PCR might overestimate the real level of expression in tumor cells due to the

Table 3. Summary of literature data of SSR subtype expression in different types of human tumors

Tumor type	Somatostatin receptor subtype mRNA expression				
	sst$_1$	sst$_2$	sst$_3$	sst$_4$	sst$_5$
Pituitary tumor					
Somatotroph	11/25 (4)	27/28 (4)	11/25 (4)	1/22 (3)	19/22 (3)
Lactotroph	16/19 (3)	12/19 (3)	6/17 (3)	1/17 (3)	12/17 (3)
Nonfunctioning	9/24 (3)	18/24 (3)	10/23 (3)	3/23 (3)	11/23 (3)
Corticotroph	5/9 (3)	6/9 (3)	2/8 (3)	0/7 (3)	6/7 (3)
Islet-cell tumor	10/12 (3)	10/12 (3)	9/12 (3)	6/7 (2)	1/7 (2)
Carcinoid	19/27 (3)	21/27 (3)	10/27 (3)	7/16 (2)	0/1 (1)
Pheochromocytoma	11/11 (2)	11/11 (2)	8/11 (2)	8/11 (2)	8/11 (2)
Renal cell cancer	11/13 (2)	13/13 (2)	0/13 (2)	6/12 (1)	Not done
Breast cancer	33/52 (2)	52/52 (2)	34/50 (2)	16/46 (1)	Not done
Meningioma	0/10 (1)	10/10 (1)	0/10 (1)	Not done	Not done
Neuroblastoma	0/6 (1)	6/6 (1)	1/6 (1)	Not done	Not done

Values are expressed as the number of positive tumors over the total number of tumors investigated; values in brackets represent the number of studies included. Data are derived from refs. 35 and 37–43.

detection of receptor mRNA in tumor-related structures such as vessels and stroma. This was clearly illustrated by two recent studies by Reubi et al. [36,44]. First, these investigators showed that peritumoral veins of various types of human cancer expressed SSR [44]. Secondly, they demonstrated the preferential expression of sst_1 in primary prostate cancers, whereas normal and hyperplastic prostates were shown to mainly express the sst_2 subtype in the smooth muscles of the stroma but not in the glandular cells [36]. These observations may also have consequences for the therapeutic and diagnostic application of SS analogs, which are discussed later.

The functional significance of the presence of the different SSR-subtype mRNAs in human tumors remains to be established. The few available clinical data suggest that the sst_2 subtype is involved in mediating the antihormonal effects of octreotide. Greenman and Melmed [37] found that tumors of two acromegalic patients who responded to therapy with octreotide exclusively expressed sst_2. It must be mentioned, however, that it is difficult to fully exclude the involvement of other SSR subtypes (sst_{3-5}) because these were not investigated in this study. In addition, Kubota et al. [39] observed an absent response of 5-HIAA excretion to octreotide therapy in a patient with a carcinoid tumor lacking sst_2 expression, while a patient with a sst_2-expressing glucagonoma responded to octreotide with lowered plasma glucagon levels. Finally, in vitro studies provided evidence for the involvement of sst_2 in the inhibition of GH secretion by SS [45].

Somatostatin receptor scintigraphy and radiotherapy

A wide variety of human SSR-positive tumors can be visualized in vivo using the technique of SSR scintigraphy. After the injection of [^{123}I-Tyr^3] octreotide or [^{111}In-DTPA-D-Phe^1] octreotide, SSR-positive tumors show a high 'uptake' of radioactivity, which can be visualized using a gamma camera [46,47]. This method is now used as a diagnostic tool in many hospitals, and Krenning recently reviewed the Rotterdam experience with more than 1000 patients [48]. As indicated earlier, octapeptide SS analogs preferentially bind to sst_2 and to a lesser extent to the sst_5 subtype (see Table 2). Fortunately, in the vast majority of human SSR-positive tumors, sst_2 is predominantly expressed (see Table 3). This may explain the high sensitivity of the technique of SSR-scintigraphy, which probably visualizes the sst_2 and sst_5 subtypes. SSR-subtype–selective SS analogs with specificity to the other subtypes (sst_1, sst_3 or sst_4) and that can be radiolabeled, might be interesting for the visualization of those (small) subgroups of SSR-positive tumors to which octapeptide analogs like octreotide do not bind (see earlier) discussion. The recent observation that human prostate cancer cells express sst_1 but not sst_2 [36] is of particular interest in this respect. Human prostate cancer might therefore also be a potential target for novel SS analogs specific for SSR subtypes, other than sst_2 and sst_5, both in terms of therapy and diagnosis.

370

Radiotherapy of SSR-positive tumors with radiolabeled SS-analogs has recently been carried out with some success in a patient with an inoperable, metastasized glucagonoma [49]. This case report showed that radiotherapy with Auger and conversion electron-emitting [^{111}In-DTPA-D-Phe^1] octreotide transiently lowered circulating glucagon levels, while a small but significant decrease in total abdominal tumor volume was observed. When radiotherapy with radiolabeled SS analogs is considered, it is important to establish whether the radioligand is actually internalized by the tumor cells, a process that might bring the radioisotope closer to its target, the DNA. We recently showed that the iodinated octapeptide SS-analog [Tyr^3] octreotide is rapidly internalized by mouse AtT20 pituitary tumor cells and by primary cultures of human GH-secreting pituitary tumor cells [50]. Preliminary results show that primary cultures of other SSR-positive human tumors (i.e., carcinoids, paragangliomas, islet-cell tumors, as visualized by SSR scintigraphy) also internalize a high amount of [^{125}I-Tyr^3] octreotide (L.J. Hofland et al., unpublished).

As has already been discussed, octreotide has a high affinity for only sst$_2$ and sst$_5$. Again, the vast majority of human SSR-positive tumors express the sst$_2$ subtype, thereby providing the possibility of carrying out radiotherapy of these tumors. However, some subgroups of SSR-positive tumors [31–33], as well as human prostate cancers, do not express sst$_2$ but do express other SSR subtype(s) such as sst$_1$ [36]. It seems important, therefore, to establish which of the five SSR subtypes is involved in receptor-mediated internalization of SS (analogs). Unfortunately, no stable SSR-subtype–selective SS analogs, other than octapeptide analogs such as octreotide, lanreotide, and octastatin that bind to the same SSR subtypes, are available at present. Studies on the internalization of SS in cells transfected with the different SSR-subtype genes may also help to answer this question. Our preliminary results show that the human sst$_2$ subtype is involved in this process (Fig. 2). This figure shows that hsst$_2$-transfected COS-1 cells internalize [^{125}I-Tyr^3] octreotide, in contrast to 'control' cells, which showed no specific accumulation of the radioligand.

It is also important to establish which factor(s) (up)regulate SSR expression or the expression of particular SSR subtypes. With this information it may become possible to improve the results of SSR scintigraphy or to increase the potential effects of radiotherapy with radiolabeled SS analogs. In this respect a recent study by Berelowitz et al. [51,52], who showed that sst$_{1,3,4, and 5}$ mRNAs increased dramatically in rat GH$_3$ pituitary tumor cells exposed to 1 μM SS for up to 48 hours while sst$_2$ exhibited a biphasic response, is of interest. Our studies in AtT20 and human GH-secreting pituitary adenoma cells showed that low doses of octreotide increased the internalization of [^{125}I-Tyr^3] octreotide, possibly by recruitment of cellular SSRs to the outer tumor cell membrane [50]. In vivo studies in rats also pointed to a bell-shaped function of the injected mass of the uptake of [^{111}In-DTPA-D-Phe^1] octreotide in SS-receptor–positive organs. In agreement with this, Dörr et al. [53] demonstrated an improved visualization of carcinoid liver metastases with

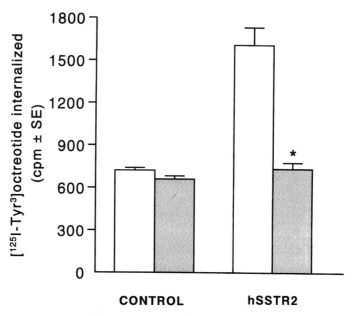

Figure 2. Internalization of [^{125}I-Tyr^3] octreotide by hsst$_2$-transfected COS-1 cells. COS-1 cells were transiently transfected with an expression vector containing the cDNA encoding the hsst$_2$ (kind gift of Dr. GI Bell). After 72 hours the transfected cells were incubated for 4 hours with [^{125}I-Tyr^3] octreotide without (open bars) or with (hatched bars) excess (1 μM) unlabeled octreotide. Thereafter, the amount of internalized radioactivity was determined by the acid-washing method, as described previously [50]. *p < 0.01 versus control cells (transfected with expression vector

[^{111}In-DTPA-D-Phe^1] octreotide in patients during octreotide therapy. Further studies on the regulation of SSR expression in tumor cells are needed, however. Also, studies directed at investigating the effects of drugs (i.e., interferons, glucocorticoids) on SSR (-subtype) expression seem important for a better understanding of the results of SSR scintigraphy in patients treated with these agents. Öberg et al. [54] have shown that interferon-alpha treatment of patients with carcinoid tumors may improve the sensitivity of the tumor cells to octreotide. By using the combination of octreotide and alpha-interferon, patients who were previously resistant to either octreotide alone or to alpha-interferon alone demonstrated biochemical responses with complete biochemical remissions in 4 out of 22 patients (18%) and partial remissions in 13 out of 22 patients (59%), although no significant tumor reduction was observed [54].

Treatment of hormone-secreting tumors with SS analogs

The two main actions of SS analogs on SSR-positive tumor cells represent inhibition of secretions and inhibition of cell proliferation [1,5,6]. Both actions have implications for the treatment of patients with SSR-positive tumors with SS analogs. The potent antihormonal effect of octapeptide SS analogs such as octreotide accounts for the successful treatment of patients with GH-secreting pituitary tumors. A double-blind randomized study in 115 acromegalic patients showed normalization of GH and IGF-I levels in 53% and 68% of the patients, respectively [55]. In about half of the patients, a slight tumor-size reduction is observed [19,55]. This tumor size reduction is reversible and probably reflects a decrease in the size of the individual tumor cells via an increased GH breakdown [56], because no major effects on GH synthesis have been observed [57–59]. Another, non–pituitary-mediated, clinically beneficial effect of octreotide in acromegalic patients is its stimulatory effect on circulating IGF binding protein 1 (IGFBP-1) levels [60]. IGFBP-1 inhibits the biological effects of IGF-1 at target cells. An interesting, recently developed form of SS analogs is the slow-release formulations. Both octreotide and lanreotide have been introduced in sustained-release formulations. Early results indicate that an effective reduction of serum GH levels can be achieved when administered intramuscularly at 4- to 6-week or 10- to 14-day intervals, respectively [61,62].

Also, the majority of TSH-secreting and clinically nonfunctioning pituitary adenomas express SSR [63,64] (see Table 3). Octreotide treatment of patients with TSH-secreting pituitary tumors results in lowered TSH levels and normalization of T4 levels in 73% of patients [63]. Therapy with octreotide of patients with clinically nonfunctioning pituitary tumors seldomly results in tumor-size reduction, although a rapid improvement of visual-field defects is sometimes observed within days after initiation of treatment [65]. This is suggested to be a direct effect of octreotide via SSRs in the optic nerve or retina. Octreotide seems not of benefit in the treatment of patients with ACTH-secreting pituitary adenomas and prolactinomas [19]. However, as indicated in Table 3, subtypes other than sst_2 and sst_5 are expressed in these types of pituitary adenomas and may provide a target for new SSR-subtype–selective SS analogs.

The majority of islet-cell tumors and carcinoids also express SSRs [31–33] (see Table 3). Octreotide treatment of patients with metastatic carcinoids, VIPomas, gastrinomas, insulinomas, and glucagonomas results in a rapid improvement of clinical symptomatology, such as diarrhea, dehydration, flushing attacks, hypokalemia, peptic ulceration, hypoglycemic attacks, and necrolytic skin lesions, respectively [66–68]. In some of these patients (about 20%) octreotide treatment may also induce tumor shrinkage [66]. The most important clinical effect of octreotide therapy in these patients seems to be an improvement in the quality of life [66–68]. A major problem in the treatment of patients with islet-cell tumors and carcinoids with octreotide is that the inhibition of the secretion of tumor-related hormones is transient. Most patients become insensitive to octreotide treatment within weeks to months [69]. This desensitization to octreotide therapy probably reflects an outgrowth of SSR-negative clones, althouth downregulation of SSR expression also may play a role [5,70]. This is in sharp contrast to GH-secreting pituitary adenomas, which do not 'escape' from octreotide therapy, even after 10 years of continuous treatment [19,71]. Perhaps the potency to 'upregulate' their SSR expression may play a role in this behavior [50,72]. Finally, while most insulinomas express receptors capable of binding SS-14 and SS-28, in about half of them no binding sites for octreotide are observed [5], suggesting that these tumors lack sst_2 and sst_5 expression. Again, other SSR-subtype–selective SS analogs that may be developed in the near future may be of value in the treatment of patients harboring this type of tumor.

Oncologic application of SS analogs

Experimentally, SS and SS analogs inhibit the growth of a wide variety of SSR positive, as well as some SSR-negative tumors in vitro and in vivo in animal tumor models. This has been reviewed extensively [5,6,73]. SS may have an inhibitory effect on tumor cell growth via a number of different mechanisms that are summarized in Figure 3. An indirect tumor growth inhibition may be achieved via the inhibition of tumor growth-promoting circulating hormones (GH, insulin, gastrointestinal hormones) or growth factors, and/or possibly via a stimulatory effect on IGFBP-1 levels [60]. Another indirect mode of action of antitumor effect of SS analogs may be based on its potential influence on tumor blood supply. A direct inhibitory effect of SS analogs on angiogenesis has been demonstrated, whereas Reubi et al. [44] recently showed a high density of SS receptors on veins in the peritumoral zone of several types of malignant tumors, such as colon cancer, small-cell lung cancer, breast cancer, renal-cell cancer, and malignant lymphomas. Thirdly, tumor growth inhibition by SS analogs may be achieved via the inhibition of local paracrine- and/or autocrine-secreted stimulatory growth factors. SS and SS analogs can also modulate the activity of immune cells [74]. At present, it is difficult to predict the final influence of the immune-modulatory effect of SS (analogs) on tumor growth in vivo. Finally, direct SSR-mediated antiproliferative effects on SSR-positive tumor cells may result in a reduction of tumor growth in vivo.

Direct antiproliferative effects of SS and SS analogs can be mediated via different intracellular signaling systems. Both cAMP-dependent and-independent mechanisms have been suggested [75–78], while stimulation of phosphotyrosine phosphatase activity may play an important role in the inhibition of growth factor–stimulated cell growth [18,26,79]. Recent important data suggest that the sst_2 and sst_5 subtypes, but not sst_1, sst_3 and sst_4, are involved in the direct inhibition of cell proliferation via the phosphatase and inositol phospholipid/calium pathways, respectively [18]. The predominant expression of sst_2 in human SSR-positive tumors suggests a potential therapeutic role for SS analogs in the control of tumor growth.

However, despite the overwhelming evidence that SS and SS analogs are able to inhibit tumor growth in vitro and in vivo in experimental models, the

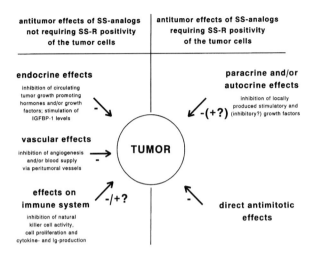

POTENTIAL MECHANISMS OF ACTION OF ANTITUMOR
EFFECTS OF SOMATOSTATIN ANALOGS

antitumor effects of SS-analogs
not requiring SS-R positivity
of the tumor cells

antitumor effects of SS-analogs
requiring SS-R positivity
of the tumor cells

endocrine effects

inhibition of circulating
tumor growth promoting
hormones and/or growth
factors; stimulation of
IGFBP-1 levels

**paracrine and/or
autocrine effects**

inhibition of locally
produced stimulatory and
-(+?) (inhibitory?) growth factors

vascular effects

inhibition of angiogenesis
and/or blood supply
via peritumoral vessels

TUMOR

**effects on
immune system**

-/+?

inhibition of natural
killer cell activity,
cell proliferation and
cytokine- and Ig-production

-

**direct antimitotic
effects**

only).

Figure 3. Schematic representation of the possible mechanisms of tumor growth-inhibitory effects of SS analogs.

limited number of clinical trials so far using SS analogs in oncology, either alone or in combination with other types of treatment such as chemotherapy and/or endocrine treatment, are rather disappointing. No response or a partial response to therapy with octapeptide SS analogs has been observed in a number of phase I and II trials, including in patients with prostate, breast, and pancreatic cancer [80–84]. In addition, octreotide treatment only transiently inhibits tumor growth in a subset of patients with metastatic carcinoids [66]. Combined treatment with interferon-alpha seems to be of benefit in this group of patients [54]. Moreover, at present a prospective trial comparing the values of adjuvant tamoxifen versus tamoxifen in combination with octreotide for breast cancer is being carried out in the United States. Octreotide may enhance the tamoxifen-induced suppression of IGF-I gene expression, resulting in lowered circulating IGF-I levels [85,86].

Malignant lymphomas have been shown to express SSR [34]. While the functional significance of the presence of SSRs on normal and tumorous lymphoid cells is not fully established yet, an interesting recent study demonstrated efficacy of treatment with a low dose of cotreotide in 56 patients with lymphoproliferative disorders [87]. Partial remissions were found in patients with low-grade non-Hodgkin's lymphoma and cutaneous T-cell lymphoma, while no remissions were observed in patients with chronic lymphocytic leukemia.

Several explanations may be given for the relatively poor effects of SS-analog therapy in oncology thus far: (1) Several types of human cancers show a heterogeneous expression of SS receptors, which may result in the outgrowth of SS-receptor–negative cells after SS-analog therapy. (2) The objective of inhibiting circulating growth-promoting hormones and/or growth factors may be hampered by the local adaptation of normal SSR-positive cells to the inhibitory effect of SS analogs [88]. (3) SS may inhibit natural killer cell activity [89], lymphoid cell proliferation, and cytokine and immunoglobulin production [74]. These latter, immune-inhibitory effect, may interfere with the body's defense mechanisms against tumor growth (see Fig. 3). (4) A possible inhibitory effect of SS analogs on the secretion of locally produced growth inhibitory factors might counteract the beneficial effects on the secretion of growth-stimulatory factors (see Fig. 3). In cultured human meningiomas a simulatory effect of octreotide on cell proliferation was found [90]. In this study, octreotide inhibited adenylate cyclase activity, possibly resulting in inhibition of the secretion of negative growth-regulatory factors, such as interleukin-6 [91]. Finally, the number of SS receptors on tumor cells may also determine the efficacy of SS analogs on cell proliferation [77].

In summary, the value of SS-analog therapy in oncology awaits the results of ongoing clinical trials. Higher dosages of SS analogs may well be needed to control tumor growth in comparison with those needed for the control of tumor-related hormone hypersecretions. Also, the development of novel SSR-subtype–selective analogs may provide new tools for the treatment of those patients with tumors carrying SS receptors to which the octapeptide SS analogs currently available for clinical use do not bind. In this respect, the recent observation of the presence of sst_1, but not sst_2, in human prostate cancer seems of particular interest.

Summary and outlook

SS analogs such as octreotide are used successfully in the treatment of patients with SSR-positive neuroendocrine tumors. Treatment with the current generation of octapeptide SS analogs available for clinical use (octreotide, lanreotide, and octastatin) often results in a rapid improvement of clinical symptomatology caused by overproduction of tumor-related hormones, whereas tumor-size reduction is observed much less frequently. At present, the major effect of SS analogs in the treatment of patients with neuroendocrine tumors is an (transient) improvement in the quality of life. An interesting recent development is the availability of sustained-release formulations of lanreotide and octreotide, which effectively control serum GH levels in acromegalic patients when administered intramuscularly in 2- or 4- to 6-week intervals, respectively. Despite the significant inhibitory effects of this generation of SS analogs on the growth of tumors of various origins in animal models, no major effects of SS-analog therapy on tumor growth have yet been observed clinically. Possibly, combined treatment with chemotherapy and/or other forms of endocrine treatment (i.e., antiestrogens) may help to increase the efficacy of SS analogs in oncology.

Five SSR subtypes (sst_{1-5}) have been cloned. The sst_2 subtype is most predominantly expressed in the majority of SSR-positive tumors. This subtype seems to be involved in the inhibition of hormone secretion, as well as in the inhibition of cell proliferation. Some subgroups of SSR-positive tumors do not express sst_2, however. These tumors may comprise targets for therapy with novel SS analogs, other than the current generation of octapeptide SS analogs, which have a high affinity for sst_2 and sst_5 only. Human prostate cancer, which selectively expresses the sst_1 subtype, is an interesting novel target in this respect.

The predominant expression of sst_2 in human SSR-positive tumors may also explain the high sensitivity of the technique of SSR scintigraphy, in which a radiolabeled sst_2-selective SS analog is used ($[^{111}In$-DTPA-D-Phe$^1]$octreotide). Most neuroendocrine tumors express a high density of SSR. This high SSR density on tumor cells opens the possibility of performing radiotherapy with radiolabeled SS analogs. The development of novel SSR-subtype–selective SS analogs that can be radiolabeled seems to be needed for diagnostic and radiotherapeutic applications in certain groups of tumors such as prostate cancer.

References

1. Guillemin R, Gerich JE. 1976. Somatostatin: Physiological and clinical significance. Ann Rev Med 27:379–388.
2. Guillemin R. 1978. Peptides in the brain: The new endocrinology of the neuron. Science 202:390–402.
3. Pradayrol L, Jörnvall H, Mutt V, Ribet A. 1980. N-terminally extended somatostatin: The primary structure of somatostatin-28. FEBS Lett 109:55–58.
4. Patel YC, Murthy KK, Escher EE, Banville D, Spiess J, Srikant CB. 1990. Mechanism of action of somatostatin: An overview of receptor function and studies of the molecular characterization and purification of somatostatin receptor proteins. Metabolism 39:63–69.
5. Lamberts SWJ, Krenning EP, Reubi JC. 1991. The role of somatostatin and its analogs in the diagnosis and treatment of tumors. Endocr Rev 12:450–482.
6. Schally AV. 1988. Oncological applications of somatostatin analogues. Cancer Res 48:6977–6985.
7. Bruns C, Weckbecker G, Raulf F, Kaupmann K, Schoeffter P, Hoyer D, Lubbert H. 1994. Molecular pharmacology of somatostatin-receptor subtypes. In Wiedeman B, Kvols LK, Arnold R, Riecken EO, eds. Molecular and Cell Biological Aspects of Gastroenteropancreatic Neuroendocrine Tumor Disease. Ann NY Acad Sci 733:138–146.
8. Hoyer D, Lubbert H, Bruns C. 1994. Molecular pharmacology of somatostatin receptors. Arch Pharmacol 350:441–453.
9. Hofland LJ, Visser-Wisselaar HA, Lamberts SWJ. 1995. Somatostatin analogs: Clinical application in relation to human smatostatin receptor subtypes. Biochem Pharmacol 50:287–297.
10. Patel YC, Greenwood MT, Panetta R, Demchyshyn L, Niznik H, Srikant CB. 1995. The somatostatin receptor family. Life Sci 57:1249–1265.
11. Reisine T, Bell GI. 1995. Moleculr biology of somatostatin receptors. Endocr Rev 16:427–442.

12. Hoyer D, Bell GI, Berelowitz M, Epelbaum J, Feniuk W, Humphrey PPA, O'Carroll A-M, Patel YC, Schonbrunn A, Taylor JE, Reisine T. 1995. Classification and nomenclature of somatostatin receptors. Trends Pharmacolo Sci 16:86–88.

13. Yamada Y, Stoffel M, Espinosa R III, Xiang K-S, Seino M, Seino S, Le Beau MM, Bell GI. 1993. Human somatostatin receptor genes: Localization to human chromosomes 14, 17, and 22 and identification of simple tandem repeat polymorphisms. Genomics 15:449–452.

14. Panetta R, Greenwood MT, Warszynska A, Demchyshyn LL, Day R, Niznik HB, Srikant CB, Patel YC. 1994. Molecular cloning, functional characterization, and chromosomal localization of a human somatostatin receptor (somatostatin receptor type 5) with preferential affinity for somatostatin-28. Mol Pharmacol 45:417–427.

15. Demchyshyn LL, Srikant CB, Sunahara RK, Kent G, Seeman P, van Tol HHM, Panetta R, Patel YC, Niznik HB. 1993. Cloning and expression of a human somatostatin-14-selective receptor variant (somatostatin receptor 4) located on chromosome 20. Mol Pharmacol 43:894–901.

16. Corness JD, Demchyshyn LL, Seeman P, van Tol HHM, Srikant CB, Kent G, Patel YC, Niznic HB. 1993. A human somatostatin receptor (SSTR3), located on chromosome 22, displays preferential affinity for somatostatin-14 like peptides. FEBS Lett 321:279–284.

17. Akbar M, Okajima F, Tomura H, Majid MA, Yamada Y, Seino S, Kondo Y. 1994. Phospholipase C activation and Ca^{2+} mobilization by cloned human somatostatin receptor subtypes 1–5, in transfected COS-7 cells. FEBS Lett 348:192–196.

18. Buscail L, Estève J-P, Saint-Laurent N, Bertrand V, Reisine T, O'Carroll, Bell G-I, Schally AV, Vaysse N, Susini C. 1995. Inhibition of cell proliferation by the somatostatin analogue RC-160 is mediated by somatostatin receptor subtypes SSTR2 and SSTR5 through different mechanisms. Proc Natl Acad Sci USA 92:1580–1584.

19. Lamberts SWJ. 1988. The role of somatostatin in the regulation of anterior pituitary hormone secretion and the use of its analogs in the treament of human pituitary tumors. Endocr Rev 9:417–436.

20. Bauer W, Briner U, Doepfner W, Haller R, Huguenin R, Marbach P, Petcher TJ, Pless J. 1982. SMS 201-995: A very potent and selective octapeptide analogue of somatostatin with prolonged action. Life Sci 31:1133–1140.

21. Cai R-Z, Szoke B, Lu R, Fu D, Redding TW, Schally AV. 1986. Synthesis and biological activity of highly potent octapeptide analogs of somatostatin. Proc Natl Acad Sci USA 83:1896–1900.

22. Cai R-Z, Karashima T, Guoth J, Szoke B, Olsen D, Schally AV. 1987. Superactive octapeptide somatostatin analogues containing tryptophan at position 1. Proc Natl Acad Sci USA 84:2502–2506.

23. Parmar H, Bogden A, Mollard M, de Rougé B, Phillips RH, Lightman SL. 1989. Somatostatin and somatostatin analogues in oncology. Cancer Res Treat 16:95–115.

24. Heiman ML, Murphy WA, Coy DH. 1987. Differential binding of somatostatin agonists to somatostatin receptors in brain and adenohypophysis. Neuroendocrinology 45:429–436.

25. Patel YC, Srikant CB. 1994. Subtype selectivity of peptide analogs for all five cloned human somatostatin receptors (hsstr 1–5). Endocrinology 135:2814–2817.

26. Liebow C, Reilly C, Serrano M, Schaly AV. 1989. Somatostatin analogues inhibit growth of pancreatic cancer by stimulating tyrosine phosphatase. Proc Natl Acad Sci USA 86:2003–2007.

27. Srkalovic G, Cai R-Z, Schally AV. 1990. Evaluation of receptors for somatostatin in various tumors using different analogs. J Clin Endocrinol Metab 70:661–669.

28. Hofland LJ, van Koetsveld PM, Waaijers M, Zuyderwijk J, Lamberts SWJ. 1994. Relative potencies of the somatostatin analogs octreotide, BIM-23014, and RC-160 on the inhibition of hormone release by cultured human endocrine tumor cells and normal rat anterior pituitary cells. Endocrinology 134:301–306.

29. Janson ET, Westlin J-E, Eriksson B, Ahlström H, Nilsson S, Öberg K. 1994. [^{111}In-DTPA-D-Phe^1] octreotide scintigraphy in patients with carcinoid tumors: The predictive value for somatostatin analogue treatment. Eur J Endocrinol 131:577–581.

378

30. Hofland LJ, Lamberts SWJ. 1996. Somatostatin receptors and disease: Role of receptor subtypes. In Sheppard MC, Franklyn JA, eds. Surface Membrane Receptors and Disease. Baillière's Clin Endocrinol Metab 10:163–176.

31. Reubi JC, Laissue J, Krenning E, Lamberts SWJ. 1992. Somatostatin receptors in human cancer: Incidence, characteristics, functional correlates and clinical implications. J Steroid Biochem Mol Biol 43:27–35.

32. Reubi JC, Krenning E, Lamberts SWJ, Kvols L. 1992. In vitro detection of somatostatin receptors in human tumors. Metabolism 41:104–110.

33. Reubi J-C, Laissue J, Waser B, Horisberger U, Schaer J-C. 1994. Expression of somatostatin receptors in normal, inflamed and neoplastic human gastrointestinal tissues. In Wiedeman B, Kvols LK, Arnold R, Riecken EO, eds. Molecular and Cell Biological Aspects of Gastroenteropancreatic Neuroendocrine Tumor Disease. Ann NY Acad Sci 733:122–137.

34. Reubi JC, Waser B, van Hagen PM, Lamberts SWJ, Krenning EP, Gebbers JO, Laissue JA. 1992. In vitro and in vivo detection of somatostatin receptors in human malignant lymphomas. Int J Cancer 50:895–900.

35. Reubi JC, Schaer JC, Waser B, Mengod G. 1994. Expression and localization of somatostatin receptor SSTR1, SSTR2, and SSTR3 messenger RNAs in primary human tumors using in situ hybridization. Cancer Res 54:3455–3459.

36. Reubi J-C, Waser B, Schaer J-C, Markwalder R. 1995. Somatostatin receptors in human prostate and prostate cancer. J Clin Endocrinol Metab 80:2806–2814.

37. Greenman Y, Melmed S. 1994. Heterogeneous expression of two somatostatin receptor subtypes in pituitary tumors. J Clin Endocrinol Metab 78:398–403.

38. Greenman Y, Melmed S. 1994. Expression of three somatostatin receptor subtypes in pituitary adenomas: Evidence for preferential SSTR5 expression in the mammosomatotroph lineage. J Clin Endocrinol Metab 79:724–729.

39. Kubota A, Yamada Y, Kagimoto S, Shimatsu A, Imamura M, Tsuda K, Imura H, Seino S, Seino Y. 1994. Identification of somatostatin receptor subtypes and an implication for the efficacy of somatostatin analogue SMS 201-995 in treatment of human endocrine tumors. J Clin Invest 93:1321–1325.

40. Panetta R, Patel YC. 1995. Expression of mRNA for all five human somatostatin receptors (hSSTR1-5) in pituitary tumors. Life Sci 56:333–342.

41. Epelbaum JE, Bertherat J, Prevost G, Kordon C, Meyerhof W, Wulfsen I, Richter D, Plouin P-F. 1995. Molecular and pharmacological characterization of somatostatin receptor subtypes in adrenal, extraadrenal, and malignant pheochromocytomas. J Clin Endocrinol Metab 80:1837–1844.

42. Miller GM, Alexander JM, Bikkal HA, Katznelson L, Zervas N, Klibansky A. 1995. Somatostatin receptor subtype gene expression in pituitary adenomas. J Clin Endocrinol Metab 80:1386–1392.

43. Vikić-Topić S, Raisch KP, Kvols LK, Vuk-Pavlović S. 1995. Expression of somatostatin receptor subtypes in breast carcinoma, carcinoid tumor, and renal cell carcinoma. J Clin Endocrinol Metab 80:2974–2979.

44. Reubi J-C, Horisberger U, Laissue J. 1994. High density of somatostatin receptors in veins surrounding human cancer tissue: Role in tumor-host interaction? Int J Cancer 56:681–688.

45. Raynor K, Murphy WA, Coy DH, Taylor JE, Moreau J-P, Yasuda K, Bell GI, Reisine T. 1993. Cloned somatostatin receptors: Identification of subtype-selective peptides and demonstration of high affinity binding of linear peptides. Mol Pharmacol 43:838–844.

46. Bakker WH, Krenning EP, Breeman WAP, Kooij PPM, Reubi J-C, Koper JW, de Jong M, Lameris JS, Visser TJ, Lamberts SWJ. 1991. In vivo use of a radioiodinated somatostatin analogue: Dynamics, metabolism and binding to somatostatin receptor positive tumors in man. J Nucl Med 32:1184–1189.

47. Krenning EP, Bakker WH, Kooij PPM, Breeman WAP, Oei HY, de Jong M, Reubi J-C, Visser TJ, Bruns C, Kwekkeboom DJ, Reijs AEM, van Hagen PM, Koper JW, Lamberts SWJ. 1992. Somatostatin receptor scintigraphy with [^{111}In-DTPA-D-Phe^1]-octreotide in man: Metabolism, dosimetry and comparison with [^{123}I-Tyr^3]-octreotide. J Nucl Med 33:652–658.

379

48. Krenning EP, Kwekkeboom DJ, Bakker WH, Breeman WAP, Kooij PPM, Oei HY, van Hagen M, Postema PTE, de Jong M, Reubi JC, Visser TJ, Reijs AEM, Hofland LJ, Koper JW, Lamberts SWJ. 1993. Somatostatin receptor scintigraphy with [^{111}In-DTPA-D-Phe^1]- and [^{123}I-Tyr^3]-octreotide: The Rotterdam experience with more than 1000 patients. Eur J Nucl Med 20:716–731.

49. Krenning EP, Kooy PPM, Bakker WHB, Breeman WAP, Postema PTE, Kwekkeboom DJ, Oei HY, de Jong M, Visser TJ, Reijs AEM, Lamberts SWJ. 1994. Radiotherapy with a radiolabeled somatostatin analog [^{111}In-DTPA-D-Phe^1]-octreotide: A case history. In Wiedeman B, Kvols LK, Arnold R, Riecken EO, eds. Molecular and Cell Biological Aspects of Gastroenteropancreatic Neuroendocrine Tumor Disease. Ann NY Acad Sci 733:496–506.

50. Hofland LJ, van Koetsveld PM, Waaijers M, Zuyderwijk J, Breeman WAP, Lamberts SWJ. 1995. Internalization of the radioiodinated somatostatin analog [^{125}I-Tyr^3] octreotide by mouse and human pituitary tumor cells: Increase by unlabeled octreotide. Endocrinology 136:3698–3706.

51. Bruno JF, Xu Y, Berelowitz M. 1994. Somatostatin regulates somatostatin receptor subtype mRNA expression in GH$_3$ cells. Biochem Biophys Res Commun 202:1738–1743.

52. Berelowitz M, Xu Y, Song J, Bruno JF. 1995. Regulation of somatostatin receptor mRNA expression. In Chadwick DJ, Cardew G, eds. Somatostatin and its Receptors. Ciba Foundation Symposium 190. Chichester, UK: Wiley & Sons, pp 111–126.

53. Dörr U, Räth U, Sautter-Bihl M-L, Guzman G, Bach D, Adrian H-J. 1992. Improved visualization of carcinoid liver metastases by indium-111 pentreotide scintigraphy following treatment with cold somatostatin analogue. Eur J Nucl Med 20:431–433.

54. Öberg K, Eriksson B, Janson ET. 1994. The clinical use of interferons in the management of neuroendocrine gastroenteropancreatic tumors. In Wiedeman B, Kvols LK, Arnold R, Riecken EO, eds. Molecular and Cell Biological Aspects of Gastroenteropancreatic Neuroendocrine Tumor Disease. Ann NY Acad Sci 733:471–479.

55. Ezzat S, Snyder PJ, Young WF, Boyajy LD, Newman C, Klibanshi A, Molitch ME, Boyd AE, Shealer L, Cook DM, Malarkey WB, Jackson I, Vance ML, Thorner MO, Banhan A, Frahmen LA, Melmed S. 1992. Octreotide treatment of acromegaly. Ann Intern Med 117:711–718.

56. Asa SL, Felix I, Singer W, Kovacs K. 1990. Effects of somatostatin on somatotroph adenomas of the human pituitary: An in vitro functional and morphological study. Endocr Pathol 1;228–235.

57. Davis JRE, Wilson EM, Vidal ME, Johnson AP, Lynch SS, Sheppard MC. 1989. Regulation of growth hormone secretion and messenger ribonucleic acid accumulation in human somatotropinoma cells in vitro. J Clin Endocrinol Metab 69:704–708.

58. Levy A, Lightman SL. 1988. Quantitative in-situ hybridization histochemistry studies on growth hormone (GH) gene expression in acromegalic somatotrophs: Effects of somatostatin, GH-releasing factor and cortisol. J Mol Endocrinol 1:19–26.

59. Hofland LJ, Velkeniers B, van der Lely AJ, van Koetsveld PM, Kazemzadeh M, Waaijers M, Hooghe-Peters, Lamberts SWJ. 1992. Long-term in-vitro treatment of human growth hormone (GH)-secreting pituitary adenoma cells with octreotide causes accumulation of intracellular GH and mRNA levels. Clin Endocrinol 37:240–248.

60. Ezzat S, Ren S-G, Braunstein GD, Melmed S. 1991. Octreotide stimulates insulin-like growth factor binding protein-1 (IGFBP-1) levels in acromegaly. J Clin Endocrinol Metab 73:441–443.

61. Fløgstad AK, Halse J, Haldorsen T, Lancranjan I, Marbach P, Bruns C, Jervell J. 1995. Sandostatin LAR in acromegalic patients: A dose-range study. J Clin Endocrinal Metab Clin Endocrinol Metab 80:3601–3607.

62. Marek J, Hana V, Kresk M, Justova V, Catus F, Thomas F. 1994. Long-term treatment of acromegaly with the slow-release somatostatin analogue lanreotide. Eur J Endocrinol 131:20–26.

63. Chanson P, Weintraub BD, Harris AG. 1993. Octreotide therapy for thyroid-stimulating hormone-secreting pituitary adenomas. A follow-up of 52 patients. Ann Intern Med 119:236–240.

64. de Bruin TWA, Kwekkeboom DJ, Van't Verlaat JW, Reubi J-C, Krenning EP, Lamberts SWJ, Croughs RJM. 1992. Clinically nonfunctioning pituitary adenoma and octreotide response to long term high dose treatment, and studies in vitro. J Clin Endocrinol Metab 75:1310–1317.

65. Warnet A, Timsit J, Chanson P, Guillausseau PJ, Zamfirescu F, Harris AG, Derome P, Cophignon J, Lubetzki J. 1989. The effect of somatostatin analogue on chiasmal dysfunction from pituitary macroadenomas. J Neurosurg 71:687–690.

66. Kvols LK, Moertel CG, O'Connell MJ. 1986. Treatment of the malignant carcinoid syndrome, evaluation of a long-acting somatostatin analogue. N Engl J Med 315:5663–5666.

67. Kvols LK, Buck M, Moertel CG, Schutt AJ, Rubin J, O'Connel HJ, Hahn RG. 1987. Treatment of metastatic islet cell carcinoma with a somatostatin analogue (SMS 201-995). Ann Intern Med 107:162–168.

68. O'Dorisio TM. 1986. Neuroendocrine disorders of the gastro-entero pancreatic system. Clinical applications of the somatostatin analogue SMS 201-995. Am J Med 81:1–101.

69. Wynick D, Anderson JV, Williams SJ, Bloom SR. 1989. Resistance of metastatic pancreatic endocrine tumours after long-term treatment with the somatostatin analogue octreotide (SMS 201-995). Clin Endocrinol 30:385–388.

70. Lamberts SWJ, Pieters GFFM, Metselaar HJ, Ong GL, Tan HS, Reubi J-C. 1988. Development of resistance to a long-acting somatostatin analogue during treatment of two patients with metastatic endocrine pancreatic tumours. Acta Endocrinol (Copenh) 119:561–566.

71. Melmed S, Dowling RH, Frohman L, Ho K, Lamberts SWJ, LaMont JT, Sassolas G, Schoenfield L, Snyder PJ, Wass JAH. 1994. Consensus statement: Benefits versus risks of medical therapy for acromegaly. Am J Med 97:468–473.

72. Berelowitz M. 1995. Editorial: The somatostatin receptor — a window of therapeutic opportunity? Endocrinology 136:3695–3697.

73. Weckbecker G, Raulf F, Stolz B, Bruns C. 1993. Somatostatin analogs for diagnosis and treatment of cancer. Pharmacol Ther 60:245–264.

74. van Hagen PM, Krenning EP, Kwekkeboom DJ, Reubi J-C, van de Anker-Lugtenburg PJ, Löwenberg B, Lamberts SWJ. 1994. Somatostatin and the immune and haematopoetic system; a review. Eur J Clin Invest 24;91–99.

75. Viguerie N, Tahiri-Jouti N, Ayral AM, Cambillau C, Scemama JL, Bastie MJ, Knuhtsen S, Esteve JP, Pradayrol L, Susini C, Vaysse N. 1989. Direct inhibitory effects of a somatostatin analog, SMS 201-995, on AR4-2J cell proliferation via pertussis toxin-sensitive guanosine triphosphate-binding protein-independent mechanism. Endocrinology 124;1017–1025.

76. Chou CK, Ho LT, Ting LP, Hu CP, Su TS, Chang WC, Suen CS, Huang MY, Chang C. 1987. Selective suppression of insulin-induced proliferation of cultured human hepatoma cells by somatostatin. J Clin Invest 79:175–178.

77. Hofland LJ, van Koetsveld PM, Wouters N, Waaijers M, Reubi J-C, Lamberts SWJ. 1992. Dissociation of antiproliferative and antihormonal effects of the somatostatin analogue octreotide on 7315b pituitary tumor cells. Endocrinology 131:571–577.

78. Qin Y, Ertl T, Groot K, Horvath J, Cai R-Z, Schally AW. 1995. Somatostatin analog RC-160 inhibits growth of CFPAC-1 human pancreatic cancer cells in vitro and intracellular production of cyclic adenosine monophosphate. Int J Cancer 60:694–700.

79. Buscail L, Delescque N, Estève J-P, Saint-Laurent N, Prats H, Clerc P, Robberecht P, Bell GI, Liebow C, Schally AV, Vaysse N, Susini C. 1994. Stimulation of tyrosine phosphatase and inhibition of cell proliferation by somatostatin analogues: Mediation by human somatostatin receptor subtypes SSTR1 and SSTR2. Proc Natl Acad Sci USA 91:2315–2319.

80. Maulard C, Richaud P, Droz JP, Jessueld D, Dufour-Esquerré, Housset M. 1995. Phase I-II study of the somatostatin analogue lanreotide in hormone-refractory prostate cancer. Cancer Chemother Pharmacol 36:259–262.

81. Figg WD, Thibault A, Cooper MR, Reid RR, Headlee D, Dawson N, Kohler DR, Reed E, Sartor O. 1995. A phase I study of the somatostatin analogue somatuline in patients with metastatic hormone-refractory prostate cancer. Cancer 75:2159–2164.
82. Rosenberg L, Barkun AN, Denis MH, Pollak M. 1995. Low dose octreotide and tamoxifen in the treatment of adenocarcinoma of the pancreas. Cancer 75:23–28.
83. Bootsma AH, van Eijck CHJ, Hofland LJ, Lamberts SWJ. 1995. The clinical significance of somatostatin receptor expression in human breast cancer. Endocr Related Cancer 2:281–292.
84. Vennin PH, Peyrat JP, Bonneterre J, Louchez MM, Harris AG, Demaille A. 1989. Effect of the long-acting somatostatin analogue SMS 201-995 (Sandostatin) in advanced breast cancer. Anticancer Res 9:153–156.
85. Huynh H, Pollak M. 1994. Enhancement of tamoxifen-induced suppression of insulin-like growth factor I gene expression and serum level by a somatostatin analogue. Biochem Biophys Res Commun 203:253–259.
86. Pollak M. 1990. Effect of tamoxifen on serum insulin-like growth factor I levels in stage I breast cancer patients. J Natl Cancer Inst 32:1693–1696.
87. Witzig TE, Letendre L, Gerstner J, Schroeder G, Maillard JA, Colon-Otero G, Marschke RF, Windschitl HE. 1995. Evaluation of a somatostatin analog in the treatment of lymphoproliferative disorders: Results of a phase II north central cancer treatment group trial. J Clin Oncology 13:2012–2015.
88. Lamberts SWJ, van der Lely A-J, de Herder WW, Hofland LJ. 1996. Drug therapy: Octreotide. N Engl J Med 334:246–254.
89. Sirianni MC, Annibale B, Fais S, Delle Fave G. 1994. Inhibitory effect of somatostatin-14 and some analogues on human natural killer cell activity. Peptides 15:1033–1036.
90. Koper JW, Markstein R, Kohler C, Kwekkeboom DJ, Avezaat CJJ, Lamberts SWJ, Reubi J-C. 1992. Somatostatin inhibits the activity of adenylate cyclase in cultured human meningioma cells and stimulates their growth. J Clin Endocrinol Metab 74:543–547.
91. Todo T, Adams EF, Rafferty B, Fahlbusch R, Dingermann T, Werner H. 1994. Secretion of interleukin-6 by human meningioma cells: Possible autocrine inhibitory regulation of neoplastic cell growth. J Neurosurg 81:384–401.

18. Multiple endocrine neoplasia type I
Clinical genetics and diagnosis

Britt Skogseid

Multiple endocrine neoplasia type I (MEN-I) is a well-characterized hereditary syndrome with occurrence of primary hyperparathyroidism (HPT)
in combination with pancreatic-duodenal endocrine and anterior pituitary
tumors. Other endocrine lesions, such as adrenocortical proliferation;
thymic, bronchial, and gastric carcinoids; as well as thyroid adenomas,
colloid goiters, differentiated thyroid carcinoma, and lipomas, are over-
represented in MEN-I. MEN-I is also referred to as Wermer's syndrome,
because an autosomal-dominant inheritance pattern with high penetrance
was first recognized by Wermer in 1954 [1]. Biochemical and genetic
screening techniques for MEN-I have been developed, and gene carriers
can be identified prior to presentation of an overt disease [2,3]. The
pancreatic and duodenal endocrine tumors exhibit a propensity to malignant
progression [4,5], while the other two classical MEN-I lesions almost
invariably are benign but nevertheless may lead to considerable endocrine
morbidity [6–10]. Early diagnosis and timely treatment instituted in order to
avoid malignancy and endocrine morbidity comprise an increasing concern in
MEN-I.

The vastly diverging strategies for diagnosis and intervention in MEN-I
at different referral centers reflect the lack of controlled studies and
consensus with respect to management policy. This situation, however,
seems to be a challenge to endocrine oncology in general. Rare prospective
studies [3,11] and some comprehensive retrospective reports [7–10,12]
consequently form the currently meager basis for clinical treatment of MEN-
I patients and kindreds. The number of reports on MEN-I nevertheless
is substantial compared with its low prevalence, which probably relates to
the complexity of the disease and its engagement of several aspects of endocrinology as well as oncology and genetics. Increased understanding of
MEN-I tumorigenesis, diagnostics, and treatment will most certainly affect
mangement consensus of the more common sporadic counterparts to
the different MEN-I lesions. In this chapter clinical features, current genetic
and biochemical diagnostics, as well as treatment options for MEN-I are
highlighted.

Andrew Arnold (ed.) ENDOCRINE NEOPLASMS. 1997. Kluwer Academic Publishers. ISBN 0-7923-4354-9.

Clinical characteristics

General aspects

Diagnosis of MEN-I in possible probands necessitates the recognition of at least two of the three lesions classically associated with the syndrome, while only one of them is required for individuals belonging to established MEN-I kindreds. Distinct features of MEN-I are the multiplicity of organ involvement, the multicentricity of tumors within the affected organs [13–15], as well as the complex pattern of clinical signs of these tumors [9] and their sometimes temporally variable profile of hormone excess [3,16]. Clinical presentation of MEN-I is thus highly inconsistent due mainly to differences in the tumor involvement and the nature and quantity of their secreted hormones. There may be different histologic processes within a given organ such that a microadenoma in one part of the pancreas can be accompanied by discrete or gross, and eventually malignant, tumors in another portion [4,13,17]. Some kindreds demonstrate a propensity for specific patterns of organ involvement, profile of peptide excess, and thereby associated clinical syndromes [3,18], as well as differences in the malignant course of the MEN-I trait [3].

The incidence of MEN-I has not been satisfactorily established because prospective, long-term, population-based studies are lacking. Prevailing prevalence estimations, based on published reports, suggest values in the range of 2–20 per 100,000 persons, which probably represents an underestimate because of the only moderate level of general awareness of the disease [6]. The clinically overt MEN-I syndrome usually is diagnosed during the fourth and fifth decades of life [7,19], which represents a considerable delay due to the mild and uncharacteristic symptoms seen for many years after the biochemically detectable onset [3]. Lesions associated with hormone excess may remain truly asymptomatic for many years. Nonfunctioning tumors of the endocrine pancreas and pituitary gland can present themselves through symptoms resulting from the tumor expansion alone. Furthermore, it can take years from detection of the presenting lesion to the development of a full-scale syndrome, and indeed also to the recognition of malignant transformation by means of demonstrable metastases.

Thorough screening studies, however, have demonstrated that the MEN-I trait is biochemically detectable virtually two decades prior to clinically overt disease [3,11]. The mean age at which negative results convert to positive is 14–18 years, and all individuals who are gene carriers can be biochemically identified prior to their midtwenties. It is also evident that any of the MEN-I endocrine lesions could be the presenting organ involvement [3]. Follow-up of a MEN-I carrier constitutes a life-long commitment, and skipped generations of MEN-I are essentially nonexistent.

Pituitary lesion

The MEN-I pituitary lesion is commonly detected during the fourth decade of life, is often multicentric, and may consist of microadenomas [7,14,19]. Although nonfunctioning tumors exist, most tumors are endocrinologically functional and predominantly hypersecrete prolactin, growth hormone, or corticotrophin, sometimes in combination. These lesions cause classical symptoms due to the hormone excess and the tumor expansion itself. Thus far no published data can establish the value of early diagnosis and presymptomatic treatment of the MEN-I pituitary disease, but nevertheless we advocate an active search for these lesions by means of biochemical screening because our experience is that early diagnosis may enable successful therapy prior to the development of irreversible metabolic disturbances and local tumor complications. Apoplexy caused by hemorrage in the pituitary or invasive tumor growth comprise uncommon causes of death in MEN-I patients [6,20]. Clinically detectable anterior pituitary gland involvement seems less prevalent (16–42%) than the other classical involvements [3,7,12,18,19]. Autopsy studies, however, reveal these tumors in about 65–100% of patients [8,10,20]. This discrepancy could support the necessity to improve biochemical screening programs for the pituitary involvement of MEN-I by adding dynamic endocrine tests as well as a radiological tumor search with computed tomography, magnetic resonance imaging, and the rarely available positron emission tomography to the program. On the other hand, previous analyses may suffer from biased over-representation of patients presenting the complete triad of MEN-I lesions [21]. Taken together, these diverging frequencies indicate a limited clinical significance of pituitary lesions merely detected at autopsy.

Parathyroid lesion

Parathyroid involvement is the most common MEN-I lesion. Both autopsy and screening studies of MEN-I substantiate about a 90% prevalence of HPT [3,6–8,10,12,18,19]. HPT of MEN 1 is now rarely accompanied by severe complications, and symptoms are mild and thus contribute only marginally to the mortality of these patients [6,20]. The disease is more or less invariably multiglandular in character, and evolution of the parathyroid pathology is asynchronous [22]. These tumors possibly consist of monoclonal lesions [23,24], but this has been less clearly established for the minimally enlarged parathyroid glands [25]. Very rare patients demonstrate a single enlarged gland, and in these instances the unusual propensity for recurrent HPT after parathyroid surgery may be less striking [26]. Critical interpretation of the parathyroid cell proliferation is difficult and, analogous to the situation with sporadic parathyroid diseases, differentiation between an adenoma and hyperplasia constitutes a classical controversy among pathologists.

Visualization of the parathyroid lesion by ultrasound or other radiological and scintigraphic techniques should be expected to require substantial gland enlargement, and exhibits unsatisfactory sensitivity and specificity for the purpose of diagnosing HPT. Diagnosis depends only on biochemical analysis and screening with albumin-corrected total calcium and intact PTH in serum. HPT in MEN-I can be detected as early as 12 years of age, with the average age of detection being 19 years [3,11,12]. In contrast to the implications of retrospective analyses, HPT alone or in combination with other lesions was the presenting MEN-I involvement in only half of prospectively diagnosed family members [3]. Although the number of individuals was limited, this finding supports the poor yield when using calcium and PTH determinations alone in screening programs directed toward early detection of the MEN-I trait. The true clinical benefit accrued from early detection of HPT in MEN-I remains to be firmly established.

Pancreatic endocrine lesion

The pancreatic involvement in MEN-I is the second most common lesion, and the reported prevalence in clinical screening varies between 30% and 75% [3,7,12,19] and approaches 80% in necropsy analyses [8,10]. All patients with pancreatic endocrine involvement of MEN-I should be expected to harbor multiple pancreatic lesions. These lesions usually consist of mixtures of microadenomas (Fig. 1) and macroadenomas [4,13,17], while nesidioblastosis (ductal cell proliferation; see Fig. 1) is considerably less prevalent. It remains controversial whether or not true islet-cell hyperplasia exists in the MEN-I pancreas [13]. Malignant disease caused by detectable metastases is seen in approximately 50% of MEN-I patients with pancreatic involvement [3,6,8,12], although local lymph-node metastases alone need not carry a poor prognosis. Submucosal, usually multiple, carcinoids of the duodenum can be found in about half of patients with pancreatic endocrine tumors [5].

Although usually minute in size, these carcinoids may be malignant and may produce serotonin, gastrin, or somatostatin. The pancreatic neoplasms characteristically express multiple immunoreactivity for a variety of tumor markers, which encompass pancreatic polypeptide (PP), glucagon, insulin, somatostatin, gastrin, vasoactive intestinal polypeptide (VIP), and neurotensin with decreasing frequency [13]. Consistent with this complex peptide expression, MEN-I patients with pancreatic involvement almost invariably display a multitude of elevated tumor markers in the circulation [3,7], but one hormone usually predominates and eventually causes a specific clinical syndrome. MEN-I pancreatic tumor patients may, however, remain asymptomatic for decades [3]. The different syndromes associated with islet-cell tumors are thoroughly discussed in specific chapters elsewhere in this issue. The most frequent syndromes associated with the MEN-I pancreatic involvement are the Zollinger-Ellison syndrome due to hypergastrinemia and the hypoglycemic syndrome due to insulinomas. Other peptides that fre-

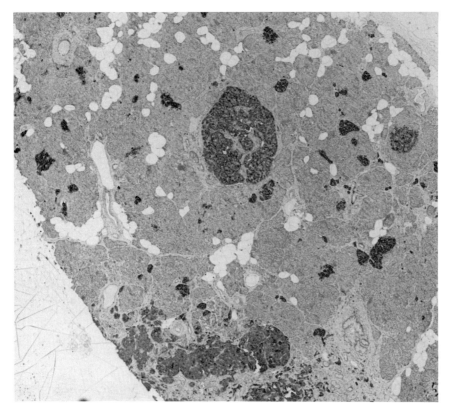

Figure 1. MEN-I pancreatic specimen stained with chromogranin A antiserum, revealing minimal disease of the pancreas, that is, microadenomas and normal islets.

quently occur in excess alone or in combinations are chromogranins, PP, VIP, glucagon, somatostatin, and calcitonin. Intraindividual shifts of syndromes have been demonstrated during longitudinal follow-up [3,16], and metastases may express other peptides than the primary tumor.

Early diagnosis of MEN-I pancreatic tumors is based on biochemical screening alone, and it has been substantiated that an unequivocal rise in pancreatic tumor markers precedes radiological detection of these lesions by at least 5 years [3,27,28] (Fig. 2). In the clinical routine and retrospective reports, pancreatic involvement usually is demonstrated during the fifth decade of life [7,5,12,19]. In contrast, systematic prospective assessment shows that these lesions are detectable at a mean age of 25 years (range, 16–38 years) [3]. These young pancreatic endocrine tumor patients were almost invariably asymptomatic (90%). In comparison, 75% of the nonprospectively detected patients in the same kindreds suffered from endocrine morbidity related to their pancreatic tumors. Prospective analysis of pancreatic MEN-I involvement also revealed the necessity of including markers of pancreatic endocrine tumors in the biochemical evaluation of relatives of individuals with MEN-I.

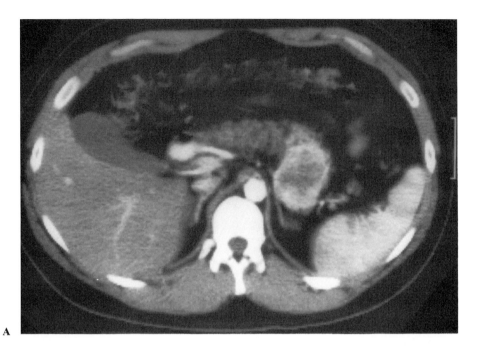

A

B

Figure 2

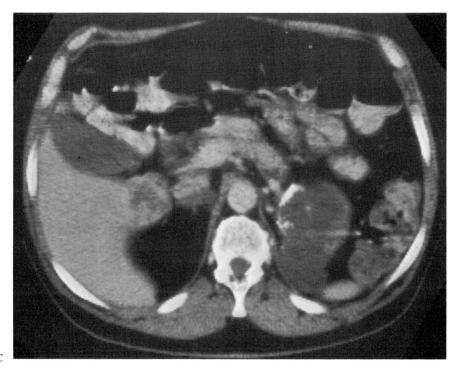

C

Figure 2. Abdominal CT scan of three MEN 1 patients. **A:** An asymptomatic 25-year-male displayed a large tumor (5cm in diameter) in the pancreatic tail after several years of observed normal basal marker levels but with an enhanced PP response to a meal at screening. Postoperative follow-up for 10 years has failed to show malignant disease. **B:** Elevated PP level was the only sign of pancreatic involvement in this asymptomatic 55-year-old male. CT reveals a huge PPoma of the pancreas and liver metastases, as well as an enlarged left adrenal (3cm). **C:** This 50-year-old male suffered from Zollinger-Ellison syndrome. CT scan failed to demonstrate the multiple pancreatic tumors (range, 0.5–1.5cm in diameter) as well as the lymph-node metastases. Both adrenals were enlarged. The left adrenal was 10cm in diameter due to a benign degenerative cyst, and the right displayed nodular hyperplasia (3cm in diameter).

Apart from the observation that these tumors could be clinically diagnosed in 75% of all the MEN-I–affected individuals, the pancreatic endocrine involvement actually constituted the most common presenting lesion within the previously unrecognized MEN-I gene carriers. A total of 43% of these individuals displayed lesions of the endocrine pancreas as their primary sign of MEN-I and another 29% of them demonstrated onset of the lesion and primary HPT simultaneously [3].

The consequences of the malignant potential of the endocrine pancreatic tumors comprise important causes of death in this syndrome [3,4,7,20]. Because of the recent development of fairly efficient symptomatic therapy (discussed later) death of MEN-I patients with pancreatic endocrine tumors now most often depends on tumor progression per se.

Thymic, bronchial, and gastric foregut carcinoids have been reported in a substantial proportion of MEN-I–affected individuals [8,10,12]. The biological behavior of these tumors has not been reported to differ from sporadic counterparts. Thus, they should primarily be regarded as potentially malignant lesions. Thyroid adenomas, colloid goiters, differentiated thyroid carcinoma, and lipomas are also over-represented in MEN-I [6,8–10].

About one third of MEN-I carriers demonstrate adrenocortical enlargements [8,29]. The abnormal adrenals are almost invariably nonhypersecreting and consist of diffuse to nodular adrenocortical hyperplasia and histologically benign to atypical adenomas [29,30]. The patients exhibit a normal hypothalamicpituitary-adrenal hormonal axis [29]. Furthermore, statistical analyses fail to indicate a connection between pituitary enlargement and adrenocortical proliferations [29]. Adrenocortical carcinoma is uncommon in MEN-I, but may develop exceedingly rapidly after several years of stable hyperplastic disease in combination with symptoms of adrenocortical hormone excess [29]. All MEN-I patients with the adrenocortical lesion have also displayed pancreatic endocrine tumors, preferentially accompanied by insulin and proinsulin excess. These findings have led to the suggestion that adrenocortical proliferation in MEN-I could be regarded as a secondary phenomenon of the pancreatic lesion and not a primary effect of the inactivated MEN-I gene [29].

Genetics

Mapping of MEN-I locus

Genetic studies leading to mapping of the MEN-I gene to chromosome 11q13 began with the assumption that tumorigenesis involved loss of function of a tumor suppressor gene according to the two-hit model proposed by Knudson [31]. He postulated that predisposition to inherited cancer, such as retinoblastoma, is passed through generations by constitutionally heterozygous carriers harboring minor genetic alterations such as point mutations or minor insertions/deletions (first hit), and that tumor development requires a somatic mutation, which eliminates the normal gene function. The second mutation could represent a point mutation, chromosome deletion, somatic recombination, or loss of a chromosome. Because the elimination of both copies of the gene is a requisite for tumor development, these genes are called *tumor suppressor genes*. Moreover, on a per-cell basis they act in a recessive manner, whereas the tumor susceptibility trait is dominantly transmitted. If MEN-I tumors result from unmasking of a recessive mutation, detection of the chromosomal alteration representing the second hit would enable identification of the chromosome containing the gene subjected to the first hit. Restriction fragment length polymorphism (RFLP) markers have been used to compare pancreatic endocrine tumor genotypes of MEN-I patients with then corresponding constitutional genotypes, and allele losses in the form of large deletions were found on chromosome 11 [2]. The retained alleles were derived from the affected MEN-I parent, whereas the lost alleles were inherited from the unaffected parent. These findings corroborate the hypothesis that the MEN-I gene constitutes a tumor suppressor gene located on chromosome 11. Subsequently, RFLP analyses in families linked MEN-I to markers close to the centromeric part of chromosome 11, and the gene for skeletal muscle glycogen phosphorylase (PYGM) on band q13 gave the highest LOD score [2]. Other groups have later confirmed these findings [23,31], and additional linked markers have been identified [32].

Tumor deletions

The observation that 50–60% of MEN-I associated parathyroid tumors displayed allelic loss in chromosome 11 was simultaneously published by two independent groups [23,25], and this finding was later confirmed by others [24,33,34]. These losses invariably included the proposed MEN-I region and could encompass regions varying from the whole chromosome down to small or even discontinuous deletions. Inactivation of the MEN-I gene also seems important for tumorigenesis of sporadic parathyroid lesions, because one third of such adenomas have displayed loss of constitutional heterozygosity for the MEN-I locus [23–25]. This finding strengthens the suggestion that the MEN-I gene belongs to the tumor suppressor gene group.

Pancreatic endocrine tumors of MEN-I patients (insulinomas, PPomas, gastrinomas, and nonhypersecreting tumors) consistently lose heterozygosity for chromosome 11 markers according to various reports [29,33,34] that followed the initial observation in two insulinomas [2]. Furthermore, in families in which the haplotype carrying the MEN-I mutation has been established, analyses have confirmed that the retained allele is derived from the affected parent, while the wild-type allele is lost in the tumor [2,29,33]. Sporadic pancreatic endocrine tumors sometimes display loss of constitutional heterozygosity for the MEN-I locus [34,35]. MEN-I pancreatic endocrine tumors <0.5 cm in diameter have lost heterozygosity for the MEN-I gene [2], which indicates that this DNA alteration is an early event in pancreatic endocrine tumorigenesis. This contrasts with reports on minimal parathyroid lesions of MEN-I, which have failed to show loss of heterozygosity for the MEN-I locus [25]. A mitogenic factor trigging polyclonal parathyroid hyperplasia has been suggested to be the first event in MEN-I tumor formation [36]. These observations, although highly interesting, have not been confirmed.

Recent reports have either succeeded or failed in revealing allelic losses for the MEN-I locus in sporadic as well as MEN-I–associated pituitary tumors [24,34,37,38]. The rarity with which neurosurgery is indicated in MEN-I pituitary disease is reflected by the low number of hitherto examined tumors.

There is also the problem of dissecting pituitary tumors in order to minimize the risk that admixture of normal tissues prevents detection of allelic losses. Nevertheless, a growth hormone–secreting tumor of an MEN-I patient demonstrated a mutation in the Gs-α gene [39], which indicated a different pathogenesis than the other classical MEN-I lesions. Another study, however, of sporadic, growth hormone–producing tumors substantiated allele losses for the MEN-I locus in 5 of 13 neoplasias, 2 of which also displayed Gs-α mutations [40]. Allelic losses for chromosome 11 also have been shown in subsets of nonhereditary prolactinomas [24,38].

Allelic losses at the MEN-I locus also have been reported in a fundic enterochromaffin cell-like tumor (ECLoma) from a MEN-I patient suffering from the Zollinger-Ellison syndrome [41]. Furthermore, loss of constitutional heterozygosity has been revealed in an adrenocortical Conn tumor associated with MEN-I [30]. One adrenocortical carcinoma in an MEN-I patient showed loss of the wild-type allele for the MEN-I locus as well as allelic losses for markers surrounding the Wiedemann-Beckwith locus on 11p, and at chromosome 17p and 13q [29]. On the other hand, common (30–40% of MEN-I patients) benign and nonfunctioning adrenocortical proliferation (diffuse and nodular hyperplasia, adenoma) failed to show such losses, even in cases exhibiting characteristic alterations in their parathyroid and pancreatic lesions.

Attempts to clone the MEN-I gene

Positional cloning of the putative MEN-I gene–containing region requires restriction of the target region to a few million base pairs. By linkage analysis in large reference families of at least three generations, the relative order and genetic distance were determined for several anchor markers defining the MEN-I locus [42]. Identification of multiple meiotic recombinants for markers at or centromeric to the PGA locus, as well as for markers at or telomeric to the D11S97 locus, positioned the MEN-I gene within a 7-cM interval between PGA and D11S97 [43]. Additional polymorphic cosmid clones of chromosome 11q13 were isolated and sublocalized on a panel of radiation-reduced somatic cell hybrids. Physical mapping by pulse-gel electrophoresis, and deletion mapping of tumors narrowed the MEN-I gene–containing region to less than 900 kb (Fig. 3) [44,45]. Two cosmid clones closely related to PYGM and located within the 900-kb region were used for screening a cDNA library. Five different clones were obtained, and their localization to chromosome 11q13 was verified by hybridization to a hamster-hybrid panel. Sequence data showed that three of these cDNA clones were previously unknown, while the remaining two represented the identified genes of phospholipase C β 3 (PLC β 3) and the 13-KD FK 506 binding protein (FKBP2) [44]. The latter gene has been excluded as a candidate gene for MEN-I after mutation analysis in MEN-I kindreds.

PLC β 3, on the other hand, has been suggested as a strong candidate for the MEN-I gene, although no constitutional mutations in MEN-I families have

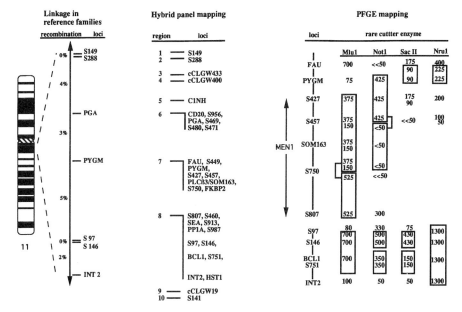

Figure 3. Mapping of the MEN-I locus by three strategies, genetic mapping, localization on a hybrid panel and physical mapping. (Reproduced with permission from the *Journal of Internal Medicine* 1995;238:249–253.)

been hitherto described. PLC β 3 is expressed in all normal tissues, and plays an important role in transmitting the transduction signal of the seven transmembrane domain receptor family by generating the second-messenger molecules inositol 1,4,5-triphosphate and diacylglycerol from phosphatidylinositol 4,5-biphosphate [46]. The human PLC β 3 gene is about 15 kb, contains 31 exons, and the transcript is 4.4 kb [47]. The putative promoter region of PLC β 3 conforms to the group of housekeeping promoters and lacks transcriptional regulatory sequences such as TATA and CAAT boxes. The rationale for suggesting that PLC β 3 is the MEN-I gene is based on the observed absence of the transcript in a sporadic insulinoma, a medullary thyroid carcinoma, a parathyroid adenoma, and a sporadic adrenocortical carcinoma, using Northern blots [44]. Furthermore, RNA in-situ hybridization shows lack of PLC β 3 expression in two of three MEN-I–associated pancreatic endocrine tumors, although the transcript is clearly present in the corresponding normal pancreatic tissue. On the other hand, in-situ hybridization on more than 10 MEN-I parathyroid adenomas indicated no discernible reduction in PLC β 3 expression [48]. MEN-I–associated adrenocortical proliferation also did not produce low levels of the PLC β 3 transcript, except in an adrenocortical carcinoma [49]. However, two of three MEN-I pituitary adenomas have demonstrated absent or very low PLC β 3 expression (unpublished data; Fig. 4).

Two of the three previously unidentified cDNA clones from the MEN-I locus are less likely to represent the elusive gene due to their expression

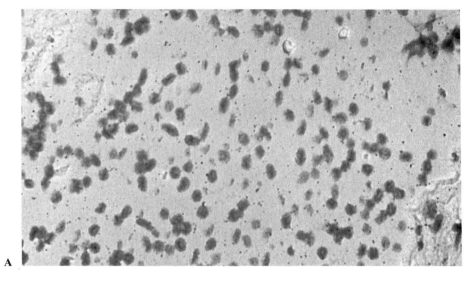

A

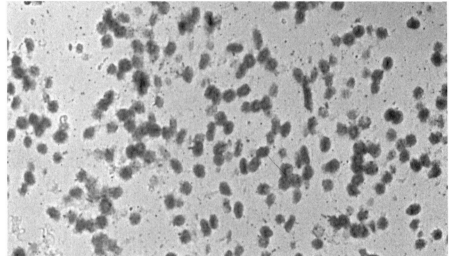

B

Figure 4

pattern [45]. The third cDNA, initially denoted pSOM 172, has been characterized and is now called the *phospholipase C β 3 Neighboring gene (PNG)*.
PNG is located head to head (5′ ends facing each other) upstream of PLC β 3.
The PNG gene spans 2.5 kb and contains four exons and three introns. Like
PLC β 3, the genomic organizaton of PNG suggests a housekeeping promoter
structure, and the head-to-head arrangement of these genes indicates interac-
tive transcriptional regulation [50].

The *fau* gene, located centromeric to PYGM but within the target region,

394

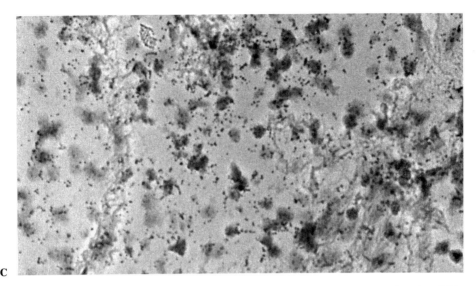

C

Figure 4. In situ RNA-RNA hybridization of a MEN 1 pituitary tumor. **A:** Expression of PLC β3 is low and grain count does not exceed the (**B**) background count (sense probe). **C:** hybridization with β actin.

has been excluded as the MEN-I gene by mutational analysis. Another recently characterized gene located telomeric and close to PYGM has been suggested to be the MEN-I gene by a Japanese group [51]. This gene, designated ZFM1, is widely expressed in endocrine organs and the predicted amino-acid sequence has properties that indicate DNA binding capacity. Furthermore, ZFM1 has significant structural similarities to parts of the Wilm's tumor suppressor gene. Loss of expression of ZFM1 in MEN-I–associated tumors or germline mutations, however, have not been established.

Diagnostic measures

In order to identify the MEN-I trait, this syndrome should at least be considered whenever managing patients with one of the classical MEN-I–associated lesions (young HPT patients or patients with a family history of an MEN-I lesion, all patients with recurrent HPT, all with pancreatic endocrine tumors, or patients with both a single MEN-I–associated lesion and adrenal enlargements). The current ignorance of this disease among physicians and surgeons, is reflected in the relatively late referral of index cases. General (but not uniform) opinion favors widespread and early screening for the trait in MEN-I kindreds despite the fact that prolonged survival after early detection has not been established. An important aspect in favor of screening relates to the existence of reasonable effective therapeutic regimens that are available for early-diagnosed endocrine lesions of the trait (see later discussion). Another

395

striking advantage of such a procedure is the possibility of excluding MEN-I gene carrier status in 50% of relatives, which otherwise has relied on the lag of disease-free period alone. Paradoxically, the screening procedure per se can offer relief from anxiety, which often prevails in MEN-I kindreds, even if the result indicates gene-carrier status, provided that expert care is offered without further delay. Moreover, there are efficient biochemical means of establishing at least parathyroid and pancreatic endocrine involvement, and most of the pituitary tumors at early and presymptomatic disease stages [3,7,11].

DNA-based diagnosis of MEN-I

In most cases it is possible to determine genetically the carrier status in MEN-I family members. Accurate identification of the haplotype for the chromosomal region carrying the MEN-I mutation generally requires RFLP and microsatellite polymorphism analysis of at least two affected family members [24,32,42,43]. The genotype of the offspring can then be settled by comparison. When only one affected family member can be genotyped, analysis of allele losses in the parathyroid or pancreatic endocrine tumors will enable haplotype identification [2,23,24,29]. Until the MEN-I gene has been cloned, reliable predictive testing of the MEN-I predisposition must use closely linked markers as well as markers flanking both sides of the MEN-I locus (see Fig. 3). If these markers are informative, genetic screening for the MEN-I trait should reach an accuracy of 99.5% [32]. Genetic analysis currently fails to establish carrier status in potential MEN-I probands. Until the MEN-I gene has been identified, recognition of probands involves a clinical search for two of the classical MEN-I lesions. Common examples of such individuals include referrals for recurrent parathyroid disease, especially if this is multiglandular in character; a family history of HPT; the presence of multifocal pancreatic lesions; and indices of adrenocortical proliferation or foregut carcinoids in patients with parathyroid, endocrine pancreatic, or pituitary involvement. This problem will disappear on identification of the MEN-I gene, which will permit carrier status to be established genetically.

Biochemical diagnostic measures

Genetically detected MEN-I individuals should undergo annual clinical testing (Table 1) from the onset of adolescence, although very rarely pancreatic and pituitary lesions may already be present in childhood. The penetrance of the disease is very high, probably complete, and follow-up of a MEN-I carrier is lifelong. Radiological examinations of the upper abdomen and pituitary gland may be performed every fifth year. If screening markers are inconsistently elevated, which indeed is rather common at the clinical onset of all tumor types, radiological examinations may have to be performed more often.

We believe that establishment of the diagnosis of MEN-I in a proband

Table 1. Extended investigation on clinical suspicion or genetic establishment of MEN-I carrier status

Annual biochemical workup
 Intact PTH, albumin-corrected total serum calcium
 Prolactin, somatomedin C, ACTH, cortisol
 Glucose, insulin, proinsulin, panceratic polypeptide, glucagon, gastrin, calcitonin, vasoactive
  intestinal peptide, serotonin, somatostatin,
 HCG-α and β, chromogranin
 Meal test with PP and gastrin analysis
 Pancreatic and pituitary stimulatory tests

Tumor visualization[a]
 Gastroduodenal endoscopy
 Endoscopic ultrasound
 Pancreatic, liver, retroperitoneal and adrenal examination by ultrasound, computed
  tomography, octreotide scanning
 Pituitary computed or magnetic resonance tomography

[a] Every fifth year, or more frequently with biochemical suspicion.

Table 2. Primary screening program for MEN-I[a]

Intact PTH, albumin-corrected total serum calcium
Prolactin, somatomedin C
Glucose, insulin, proinsulin, pancreatic polypeptide, glucagon, gastrin, chromogranin A
Meal test with PP and gastrin analysis

[a] Applied every third year in genetically unexamined individuals.

necessitates family examination. Until genetic screening becomes generally available, this biochemical examination should include all individuals older than age 15 years, and even the offspring of persons without a clear MEN-I history can have a mild form of the disease for decades with hardly any symptoms. Such programs should search for all the classical lesions of MEN-I and minimize the incidence of false-positive results (Table 2). The optimal interval between screening investigations of healthy individuals has not been assessed, but we have chosen to repeat the procedure every third year. Some investigators advocate annual investigations [7] and others have chosen a 5-year interval [19]. Family members passing through their mid-thirties without signs of any of the classical MEN-I lesions on repeated examination usually can be assigned a noncarrier status [2].

 Our current primary screening procedure (Table 2) has yielded about 10% false positives when compared with RFLP data [3,27]. When using the primary screening program, hypercalcemia and inappropriate intact serum PTH values recognize HPT amenable to treatment. It should be emphasized that ionized plasma calcium values may increase sensitivity for detection of HPT among younger MEN-I carriers [52]. Moreover, borderline serum calcium values and intermittent or mild hypercalcemia generally should be expected to be accompanied by normal intact PTH values, albeit in the upper reference range, in at least half of patients. In primary screening pituitary lesions are most readily recognized by prolactin and somatomedin C analysis. Pancreatic endocrine tumor diagnosis must be biochemically established, and radiology fails to localize lesions in half of patients [28]. Pancreatic involvement in young MEN-I patients is most consistently demonstrated by analyzing serum insulin, proinsulin, PP, as well as plasma glucagon and chromogranin A levels, which have exhibited sensitivities of 56%, 56%, 67%, 37%, and 60%, respectively [3,11]. Serum PP is an nonspecific marker of islet tumors, that should be applied in conjunction with other peptide markers for this involvement. Moreover, PP may vary with age and time within the same patient, so repeated measurement and standardization of values for age are necessary. Although chromogranin A is an unsatisfactory marker for the parathyroid lesion [53] and generally requires a rather massive burden of endocrine pancreatic tumors for elevation in MEN-I patients, it has proven to be a sensitive marker for pancreatic involvement (D Granberg, unpublished). On the other hand, there are several false-positive pitfalls to be considered when evaluating chromogranin A elevation, such as hypertension, impaired kidney function, stress, and inflamatory bowl disease. Moreover, the day-to-day variation in chromogranin A levels are substantial in tumor patients. Elevation of basal gastrin values generally indicates the presence of advanced pancreatic tumour involvement or duodenal carcinoids, and gastrin immunoreactivity generally has been confined to pancreatic lesions measuring centimeters in diameter [3–5,7,19]. Gastrin excess thus has been found in only one fifth of patients with pancreatic endocrine lesions detected by screening [3]. This biochemical marker usually becomes diagnostic during the fourth or fifth decades of life [5,19], and even then it has been elevated in only about two thirds of patients with pancreatic tumor involvement [3].

Early diagnosis of pancreatic endocrine tumors in MEN-I is enhanced by the use of a standardized meal stimulation test with measurements of serum PP and gastrin responses, and problems with the specificity and sensitivity of PP as a tumor marker have decreased [3,27]. During longitudinal analysis of asymptomatic and otherwise biochemically healthy MEN-I relatives with subsequently verified pancreatic endocrine involvement, this test was the single most sensitive marker and substantiated the presence of tumor in 75% of individuals, whose mean age was 25 years. Moreover, it yielded true positive pancreatic tumor detection in all the older and already diagnosed MEN-I patients independent of the diagnosis of PPoma, gastrinoma, insulinoma and proinsulinoma, VIPoma, neurotensinoma, somatostatinoma, glucagonoma, and 'nonfunctioning' pancreatic tumors [3,27]. This carbohydrate-rich and low-protein test meal is composed of milk, cereals, orange juice, bread, butter, cheese, and ham (560 kcal).

Blood samples are drawn immediately prior to, during, and 40 minutes after the 20-minute meal. An abnormal response to this meal is defined as a serum PP elevation exceeding the mean level of a control group by at least two standard deviations. Because healthy controls reveal postprandial PP increments just 100% above the basal value, PP elevations exceeding twice the upper reference limit for the immunoassay are regarded as abnormal and indicate the necessity for surveillance for tumor development. Doubling of the basal gastrin value, reaching twice above the upper reference limit, also serves as an indicator for such observation. False-positive stimulations due to the meal test have been found in about 10% of previously investigated individuals [3]. None of them, however, has shown concomitantly diagnostic elevations of both serum gastrin and PP levels. Moreover, the meal test substantiates that non-MEN-I carriers with achlorhydria and elevated basal gastrin levels display normal PP responses, but cannot be used to differentiate antral G-cell hyperplasia from pancreatic endocrine tumours. Simultaneous elevations of gastrin and PP responses to diagnostic levels consequently seem to yield absolute specificity for the presence of pancreatic tumor.

Extended endocrine investigation (see Table 1) should follow findings of abnormal tumor markers on primary biochemical screening (see Table 2). Surveillance for possible Cushing's syndrome should be performed by analysis of urinary cortisol and plasma ACTH and reassured by classical dynamic endocrine tests. In order to ascertain the diagnosis of pancreatic endocrine tumor, at least two independent tumor markers must be increasingly elevated on repeated analysis, separated in time by at least 6 months. Apart from repeating the primary examination, diagnostic studies should include basal calcitonin, vasoactive intestinal peptide, serotonin, and somatostatin values. Elevation of human chorionic gonadotrophin subunits (hCG) alpha and beta might be indicators for malignant transformation of neuroendocrine tumors [54], and should be evaluated regularly during follow-up of diagnosed pancreatic lesions. Classic dynamic challenges, such as 72-hour fasts, insulin, secretin, and atropine tests, might be necessary to functionally specify tumor subgroups. Patients should be screened with pancreatic tumor visualization, preferentially with endoscopic or cutaneous ultrasound, octreotide scanning [55], computed tomography, and/or magnetic resonance imaging at high resolution (1.5 Tesla), or positron emission tomography [56]. Many of these radiological investigations compliment each other and should be applied selectively. Although all radiological techniques display poor sensitivities for pancreatic tumor detection, except for intraoperative ultrasonography [28], the pancreas and liver should be imaged in order to reveal malignant disease or rare tumors not detectable by the screening program outlined.

Treatment

Details of MEN-I HPT management are highlighted elsewhere in this book. In general, the treatment of HPT of MEN-I is surgical, but the optimal timing and extent of the resection have not been determined in controlled studies. Primarily, it is important that the diagnosis is correctly established and that the surgeon is experienced in performing MEN-I parathyroid surgery. In many instances MEN-I parathyroid surgery is more difficult than surgery for sporadic HPT, because the obligatory identification of at least four parathyroid glands often requires exceptionally thorough exploration, especially in early, asymptomatic cases with only modestly enlarged glands. Surgical intervention, therefore, might be postponed for years in asymptomatic patients with equivocal hypercalcemia in order to reduce the risk of postoperatively persistent hypercalcemia. Re-exploration essentially carries the risk of additional morbidity because of difficulty in identifying critical structures embedded in scar tissue, and postoperative persistent hypercalcemia is more frequent following reoperation [57]. Unequivocal symptoms or signs of complications of HPT invariably warrant parathyroidectomy, even with only mild hypercalcemia, unless clear contraindications to operation prevail. There is generally no need for preoperative localization prior to primary explorations nor intraoperative ultrasonography [58].

Neck dissection should always be bilateral, supernumerary glands should be sought, and resection of the cervical thymus should be performed to remove the most common site of accessory parathyroid tissue. The most common resection procedure is subtotal parathyroidectomy, usually a 3–3.5 gland resection, leaving about 50 mg of tissue from the most normal-appearing gland in situ. The alternative is total parathyroidectomy with immediate autografting to the brachioradialis muscle of the nondominant forearm. This procedure usually is accompanied by transient hypoparathyroidism, requiring substitution therapy for up to 3–4 months until the graft produces sufficient parathyroid hormone. Up to one third of MEN-I patients may remain hypoparathyroid after this procedure [57], while the risk of persistent disease generally seems somewhat greater after subtotal resection. Postoperative follow-up of MEN-I HPT is lifelong.

Treatment of MEN-I–associated pituitary lesions includes surgery, radiation, and medication, and does not differ from the treatment of sporadic pituitary tumors. These aspects are thoroughly outlined elsewhere in this book. In summary, prolactinomas, which are the most common MEN-I pituitary manifestation, almost invariably are successfully treated with dopamine agonists, which most often normalize or decrease the prolactin levels and often also tumor size. On the other hand, this treatment is rarely curative and recurrences are common, so the drug often must be continued, even after normalization of the prolactin levels. Radiation therapy or neurosurgery are seldom warranted for these tumors. The first-line treatment for GH-secreting tumors is octreotide, which efficiently suppresses GH excess. Reduction of tumor size may also be achieved with long-term administration of octreotide. A substantial proportion of patients with acromegaly, however, ultimately require either surgical or radiation therapy. The rare corticotropinomas of MEN-I often are subjected to trans-sphenoidal resection, although radiation is an acceptable alternative for larger invasive tumors of this type. All patients with MEN-I pituitary tumors must be followed throughout life with repeated radiological and biochemical examination because relapses are common and may be associated with shifts in hormone excess.

The apparently prolonged longevity of MEN-I patients demands a therapeutic focus on the risk of malignancy of the pancreatic lesion. A principal management goal consequently includes cancer prevention without unnecessary induction of symptomatic endocrine and exocrine pancreatic insufficiency. Treatment of the pancreatic tumors always includes surgical considerations, despite the fact that its role is much debated; this is thoroughly discussed elsewhere in this book. In the absence of unequivocal evidence of malignancy, that is, clinically apparent metastases, all macroscopic tumors of the MEN-I pancreas should be regarded as potentially malignant. Tumor size and the profile of peptide excess, however, are not reliable indicators. In our experience, surgical removal of the asymptomatic pancreatic lesions in young MEN-I patients may lead to a substantial duration of cancer prevention, and essentially half of middle-aged patients with pancreatic involvement display gross or microscopic metastases from pancreatic tumors [59].

The most common operative procedure is distal pancreatic resection combined with intraoperative ultrasonography and bidigital palpation for enucleation of tumors in the pancreatic head and duodenal submucosa. Careful dissection of lymph nodes along the hepatic ligament and celiac trunk is warranted. Substantial rates of biochemical recurrence, accompany this management strategy. On the other hand, biochemical cure is not a prime motive for surgery. Time may be an important risk factor for the hitherto unknown mutagenetic events that cause the development of malignant pancreatic tumors. A recent uncontrolled study implies that when malignant transformation does develop, it may occur between one and three decades after the onset of biochemically detectable pancreatic involvement, and hypothetically a similar duration might be necessary to develop pancreatic endocrine malignancy after thorough exploration. Surgical reintervention preferentially should include tumor enucleation in the attempt to reduce the risk of pancreatic insufficiencies. Such active management with repeated biochemical examination and timely reintervention may be a realistic way to reach the goals of long-term prevention of malignancy plus satisfactorily maintained pancreatic function.

Occasionally, symptomatic therapy is of utmost importance in MEN-I pancreatic tumor management. Other chapters in this book elucidate the different syndromes associated with these tumors. In summary, omeprazole has had a major influence on MEN-I survival. Complications of gastrointestinal ulcers from gastrinomas, which comprised a substantial cause of death historically in MEN-I, can be avoided with liberal use of omeprazole. Furthermore, long-acting somatostatin analogues have significantly improved the quality of life for many MEN-I patients. They inhibit the secretion of different peptides hypersecreted by pancreatic tumors. Recently it has been noted that somatostatin analogues at high dosages may induce apoptosis (Öberg et al., personal communication) and perhaps also have antiproliferative effects. The drug generally is well tolerated, and side effects include malabsorption, cholestasis, and cholelithiasis.

Surgical ligation of the hepatic artery and embolization by interventional radiology reduce the tumor mass and levels of hormone excess from hepatic metastases. Adverse reactions to these treatments are tolerable, and other therapies, such as somatostatin analogs, interferon, and chemotherapy, may produce additive effects following the occlusion [60].

Despite the fact that essentially half of MEN-I patients with pancreatic endocrine tumors display malignant disease, either by means of liver metastases or mere local lymph-node metatases (which probably do not carry the same poor prognosis), systemic antitumoral and radiation therapies have not been comprehensively evaluated for MEN-I management. The effects of the latter, however, seem to be restricted to palliation of symptomatic metastases in the bone and skin, for example. Studies of systemic therapy for sporadic neuroendocrine tumors have been summarized in a recent review [61]. The combination of streptozocin with 5-fluorouracil or doxorubicin in malignant sporadic pancreatic endocrine tumors has sometimes demonstrated remarkable response rates of 40–69% [62]. Insulin- and VIP-producing tumors seem especially responsive to this combination therapy. On the other hand, etoposide and cisplatin combination therapy may be effective in poorly differentiated pancreatic neuroendocrine tumors (67% response rate), which contrasts with the meager response (7%) in well-differentiated islet-cell tumors and carcinoids [63].

Alpha-interferon has been widely used in the treatment of various malignant diseases, particularly in hematology. Solid tumors rarely seem to respond to interferon, however, with the possible exception of renal and colonic tumors and melanomas. Small series of patients with malignant pancreatic endocrine tumors, mostly sporadic, have been subjected to interferon treatment. Interferon blocks cell-cycle progression in the G0/G1 phase. Rather early (weeks) in treatment with interferon, a reduction of hormones can be monitored, whereas significant tumor reduction normally requires years. In our hands, alpha-interferon has produced a biochemical response in 51% and significant tumor reduction in 12% of patients with malignant sporadic and familial pancreatic endocrine tumors [64]. The median duration of these responses was 20 months. Furthermore, disease stabilization with apparent growth arrest was recorded in an additional 25% of patients, and persisted for 16 months. Patients with Verner-Morrison syndrome had the highest response rate (10 of 12 patients).

There is no clear correlation between dose and antitumoral response. The individual dose should be titrated to optimize compliance and to enable long-term treatment (years). Most adverse reactions are dose dependent and include flulike symptoms (initial 3–5 days), fatigue, low-grade weight loss, depression, mild impairment of liver and bone-marrow function, and autoimmune reactions. A usually tolerable maintenance dose is 5 million units of alpha-interferon three to five times per week subcutaneously. Interferon treatment may be combined with somatostatin analogs or chemotherapy. Future controlled multicenter studies are warranted in order to reach a consensus on the management of the rare MEN-I malignant pancreatic endocrine tumors.

MEN-I foregut carcinoids must be regarded as potentially malignant, and surgery should always be considered. Recurrent disease may respond to external radiation or indium-labeled octreotide (unpublished data). MEN-I adrenal proliferation should be evaluated as incidentalomas. Thus, lesions >3 cm in diameter may be considered for surgery. Moreover, adrenalectomy is warranted if the lesion grows or if the patient has symptoms or signs of hormonal excess. Radiological and biochemical follow-up of MEN-I adrenals is mandatory.

References

1. Wermer P. 1954. Genetic aspects of adenomatosis of endocrine glands. Am J Med 16:363–371.
2. Larsson C, Skogseid B, Öberg K, Nakamura Y, Nordenskiöld M. 1988. Multiple endocrine neoplasia type 1 gene maps to chromosome 11 and is lost in insulinoma. Nature 332:85–87.
3. Skogseid B, Eriksson B, Lundqvist G, Lörelius LE, Rastad J, Wide L, Wilander E, Öberg K. 1991. Multiple endocrine neoplasia type 1: A 10 years prospective screening study in four kindreds. J Clin Endocrinol Metab 73:281–287.
4. Grama D, Skogseid B, Wilander E, Eriksson B, Mårtensson H, Cedermark B, Ahrén B, Kristoffersson A, Rastad J, Öberg K, Åkerström G. 1992. Clinical presentation and surgical treatment. World J Surg 16:611–619.
5. Pipeleers-Marichal M, Somers G, Willems G, Foulis A, Imrie C, Bishop AG, Polak JM, Path FRC, Häcki WH, Stamm B, Heitz PU, Klöpper G. 1990. Gastrinomas of the duodenum of patients with multiple endocrine neoplasia type 1 and the Zollinger-Ellison syndrome. N Engl J Med 322:723–727.
6. Lips CJM, Vasen HFA, Lamers CBHW. 1984. Multiple endocrine neoplasia syndromes. Crit Rev Oncol Hematol 2:117–184.
7. Vasen HFA, Lamers CBHW, Lips CJM. 1989. Screening for the multiple endocrine neoplasia type 1 syndrome: A study of 11 kindreds in the Netherlands. Arch Intern Med 149:2717–2722.
8. Ballard HS, Frame B, Hartsock RJ. 1964. Familial multiple endocrine adenomatosis ulcer complex. Medicine (Baltimore) 43:481–516.
9. Brandi ML, Marx SJ, Aurbach GD, et al. 1987. Familial multiple endocrine neoplasia type 1: A new look at pathophysiology. Endocr Rev 8:391–405.
10. Eberle F, Grun R. 1981. Multiple endocrine neoplasia type 1 (MEN 1). Egreb Inn Med Kinderheilkd 46:75–149.
11. Lips CJ, Koppeschaar HPF, Berends MJH, Jansen-Schillhorn van Veen JM, Struyvenberg A, Van Vroonhoven ThJMV. 1992. The importance of screening for the MEN 1 syndrome: Diagnostic results and clinical mangement. Henry Ford Hosp Med J 40:171–172.
12. Sheppherd JJ. 1991. The natural history of MEN 1 which may be highly unrecognized rather than highly uncommon. Arch Surg 126:935–952.
13. Klöpper G, Willemer S, Stamm B, Häcki WH, Heitz PU. 1986. Pancreatic lesions and hormonal profile of pancreatic tumors in multiple endocrine neoplasia type 1. Cancer 57:1824–1832.
14. Sheithauer BW, Laws ER, Kovacs K, Horvath E, Randall RV, Carney JA. 1987. Pituitary adenomas of the multiple endocrine neoplasia type I syndrome. Semin Diagn Pathol 4:205–211.
15. Brandi ML. 1992. Parathyroid tumor biology in familial multiple endocrine neoplasia type 1: A model for cancer development. Henry Ford Hosp Med J 40:181–185.

16. Eriksson B, Arnberg H, Lindgren P-G, Lörelius LE, Magnusson A, Lundqvist G, Skogseid B, Wide L, Wilander E, Öberg K. 1990. Neuroendocrine pancreatic tumors: Clinical presentation, biochemical and histopathological findings in 84 patients. J Intern Med 228:103–113.

17. Thompson NW, Lloyd RV, Nishiyama RH, Vinik AI, Stodel WE, Allo MD, Eckhauser FE, Talpos G, Mervak T. 1984. MEN 1 pancreas. A histological and immunohistochemical study. World J Surg 8:561–574.

18. Farid NR, Bueler S, Russel NA, Mauron FB, Allerdice P, Smith HS. 1980. Prolactinomas in familial multiple endocrine neoplasia syndrome type 1. Am J Med 69:874–880.

19. Marx SJ, Vinik AI, Santen RJ, Floyd JC, Mills JL, Green J. 1986. Multiple endocrine neoplasia type I: Assessment of laboratory tests to screen for the gene in a large kindred. Medicine 65:226–241.

20. Wilkinson S, Teh BT, Davey KR, McArdle JP, Young M, Shepperd JJ. 1993. Cause of death in multiple endocrine neoplasia type 1. Arch Surg 128:683–690.

21. Majewski JT, Wilson SD. 1979. The MEA-I syndrome: An all or none phenomenon? Surgery 86:475–484.

22. Mallette LE. 1994. Management of hyperparathyroidism in the multiple endocrine neoplasia syndromes and other familial endocrinopathies. Endocrinol Metab Clin North Am 23:19–36.

23. Thakker RV, Bouloux P, Wooding C, Chotai K, Broad PM, Spurr NK, Besser GM, O'Riordan JLH. 1989. Association of parathyroid tumors in multiple endocrine neoplasia type 1 with loss of alleles on chromosome 11. N Engl J Med 321:218–224.

24. Byström C, Larsson C, Blomberg C, Sandelin K, Falkmer U, Skogseid B, Öberg K, Nordenskiöld M. 1990. Localization of the gene for multiple endocrine neoplasia type 1 to a small region within chromosome 11q13 by deletion mapping in tumors. Proc Natl Acad Sci USA 87:1968–1972.

25. Friedman E, Sakaguchi K, Bale AE, Falchetti A, Streeten E, Zimering MB, Weinstein LS, McBride OW, Nakamura Y, Brandi ML, Norton JA, Aurbach GD, Spiegel AM, Marx SJ. 1989. Clonality of parathyroid tumors in familial multiple endocrine neoplasia type 1. N Engl J Med 321:213–218.

26. Kraimps JL, Demeure M, Clark OH. 1992. Hyperparathyroidism in multiple endocrine neoplasia syndrome. Surgery 112:1080–1086.

27. Skogseid B, Öberg K, Benson L, Lindgren PG, Lörelius LE, Lundqvist G, Wide L, Wilander E. 1987. A standardized meal stimulation test of the endocrine pancreas for early detection of pancreatic endocrine tumors in multiple endocrine neoplasia type 1 syndrome: Five years experience. J Clin Endocrinol Metab 64:1233–1240.

28. Skogseid B, Grama D, Rastad J, Eriksson B, Lindgren PG, Ahlström H, Lörelius LE, Wilander E, Åkerström G, Öberg K. 1995. Operative tumor yield obviates preoperative pancreatic localization in multiple endocrine neoplasia type 1. J Intern Med 238:281–288.

29. Skogseid B, Larsson C, Lindgren PG, Kvanta E, Rastad J, Theodorsson E, Wide L, Wilander E, Öberg K. 1992. Clinical and genetic features of adremocortical lesions in multiple endocrine neoplasia type 1. J Clin Endocrinol Metab 75:76–81.

30. Beckers A, Abs R, Willems PJ, van der Auwera B, Kovacs K, Reznik M, Stevenaert A. 1992. Aldosterone-secreting adrenal adenoma as part of the multiple endocrine neoplasia type 1 (MEN 1): Loss of heterozygosity for polymorphic chromosome 11 deoxyribonucleic acid markers, including the MEN 1 locus. J Clin Endocrinol Metab 75:564–570.

31. Bale SJ, Bale AE, Stewart K, Dachowski L, McBried OW, Glaser T, Green JE, Mulvihill JJ, Brandi ML, Sakaguchi K, Aurbach GD, Marx SJ. 1989. Linkage analysis of multiple endocrine neoplasia type 1 with INT2 and other markers on chromosome 11. Genomics 4:320–322.

32. Larsson C, Calender A, Grimmond S, Giraud S, Haywarg NK, Teh B, Farnebo F. 1995. Molecular tools for presymptomatic testing in multiple endocrine neoplasia type 1. J Intern Med 238:239–244.

33. Radford DM, Ashley SW, Wells SA, Gerhard DS. 1990. Loss of heterozygosity of markers on chromosome 11 in tumors from patients with multiple endocrine neoplasia syndrome type 1. Cancer Res 50:6529–6533.

404

34. Bale AE, Norton JA, Wong EL, Fryburg JS, Maton PN, Oldfield EH, Streeten E, Aurbach GD, Brandi ML, Frideman E, Spiegel AM, Taggart RT, Marx SJ. 1991. Allelic loss on chromosome 11 in hereditary and sporadic tumors related to familial multiple endocrine neoplasia type 1. Cancer Res 51:1154–1157.

35. Patel P, O'Rahilly S, Buckle V, Nakamura Y, Turner RC, Wainscoat JS. 1990. Chromosome 11 allele loss in sporadic insulinoma. J Clin Pathol 43:377–378.

36. Zimering MB, Riley DJ, Thakker-Varia S, Walker AM, Lakshminaryan V, Shah R, Brandi ML, Ezzat S, Katzumata N, Friesen HG, Marx SJ, Eng J. 1994. Circulating fibroblast growth factor-like autoantibodies in two patients with multiple endocrine neoplasia type 1 and prolactinoma. J Clin Endocrinol Metab 79:1546–1552.

37. Yoshimoto K, Iwahana H, Kubo K, Saito S, Itakura M. 1991. Allele loss on chromosome 11 in a pituitary tumor from a patient with multiple endocrine neoplasia type 1. Jpn J Cancer Res 82:886–889.

38. Herman V, Drazin NZ, Gonsky R, Melmed S. 1993. Molecular screening of pituitary adenomas for gene mutations and rearrangements. J Clin Endocrinol Metabol 77:50–55.

39. Hsoi E, Yokogoshi Y, Yokoi K, Sano T, Saito S. A pituitary specific point mutation of codon 201 of the Gs alpha gene in a pituitary adenoma of a patient with multiple endocrine neoplasia (MEN) type 1. Endocrinol Jpn 39:319–324.

40. Thakker RV, Pook MA, Wooding C, Boscaro M, Scanarini M, Clayton RN. 1993. Association of somatotrophinomas with loss of alleles on chromosome 11 and with gsp mutations. J Clin Invest 91:2815–2821.

41. Cadiot G, Laurent-Puig P, Thuille B, Lehy T, Mignon M, Olschwang S. 1993. Is the multiple endocrine neoplasia type I gene a supressor for fundic argyrophil tumors in the Zollinger-Ellison syndrome? Gastroenterology 105:579–582.

42. Nakamura Y, Larsson C, Julier C, Byström C, Skogseid B, Wells S, Öberg K, Carlsson M, Taggart RT, O'Connel P, Leppert M, Lalouel JM, Nordenskjöld M, White R. 1989. Localization of the genetic defect in multiple endocrine neoplasia type 1 within a small region of chromosome 11. Am J Hum Genet 44:751–755.

43. Larsson C, Shepherd J, Nakamura Y, Blomberg C, Weber G, Werelius B, Hayward N, Teh B, Tokino T, Seizinger B, Skogseid B, Öberg K, Nordenskjöld M. 1992. Predictive testing for multiple endocrine neoplasia type 1 using DNA polymorphisms. J Clin Invest 89:1344–1349.

44. Weber G, Friedman E, Grimmond S, Hayward NK, Phelan C, Skogseid B, Gobl A, Zedenius J, Sandelin K, Teh BT, Carson E, White I, Öberg K, Shepherd J, Nordenskjöld M, Larsson C. 1994. The phospholipase C β3 gene located in the MEN 1 region shows loss of expression in endocrine tumors. Hum Mol Genet 3:1775–1781.

45. Lagercranz J, Larsson C, Grimmond S, Skogseid B, Gobl A, Friedman E, Carson E, Phelan C, Öberg K, Nordenskjöld M, Hayward NK, Weber G. 1995. Candidate genes for multiple endocrine neoplasia type 1. J Intern Med 238:245–248.

46. Jhon DY, Lee HH, Park D, Lee CW, Lee KH, Yoo OJ, Rhee SG. 1993. Cloning sequencing, purification, and Gq-dependent activation of phopholipase C-β3. J Biol Chem 68:6654–6661.

47. Lagercrantz J, Carson E, Phelan C, Grimmond S, Rose'n A, Dare'E, Nordenskjöld M, Hayward NK, Larsson C, Weber G. 1995. Genomic organization and complete cDNA sequence of the human phopholipase C b3 gene (PLC b3). Genomics 26:1–6.

48. Carling T, Ridefelt R, Gobl A, Hellman P, Öberg K, Larsson C, Juhlin C, Åkerström G, Rastad J, Skogseid B. 1995. Hyperparathyroidism of multiple endocrine neoplasia type 1. Candidate gene and parathyroid calcium sensor expressions. Surgery 118:924–930.

49. Skogseid B, Larsson C, Gobl G, Backlin K, Juhlin C, Åkerström G, Rastad J, Öberg K. 1995. Adrenal lesion in multiple endocrine neoplasia type 1. Surgery 118:1077–1082.

50. Lagerkrantz J, Carson E, Larsson C, Nordenskjöld M, Weber G. 1996. Isolation and characterization of a novel gene close to the human phophoinsitide-specific phopholipase C β3 gene on chromosome 11q13. Genomics 31:380–384.

51. Toda T, Iida A, Miwa T, Nakamura Y, Imai T. 1994. Isolation and characterization of a novel gene encoding nuclear protein at a locus (D11S636) tightly linked to multiple endocrine neoplasia type 1 (MEN 1). Hum Mol Genet 3:465–470.

405

52. Sheppherd JJ, Teh BT, Parameswaran V, David R. 1992. Hyperparathyroidism with normal albumin corrected total calcium in patients with multiple endocrine neoplasia type 1. Henry Ford Hosp Med J 40:186–190.

53. Nanes MS, O'Connor DT, Marx SJ. 1989. Plasma chromogranin A in primary hyperparathyroidism. J Clin Endocrinol Metab 69:950–955.

54. Öberg K, Wide L. 1981. HCG and HCG subunits as tumor markers in patients with endocrine pancreatic tumors and carcinoids. Acta Endocrinol (Copenh) 98:256–260.

55. Tiensuu Janson E, Westlin JE, Ahlström H, Eriksson B, Nilsson S, Åkerström G, Öberg K. 1993. Somatostatin receptor scintigraphy: Recent advances imaging endocrine pancreatic tumors. Diagn Oncol 3:45–48.

56. Ahlström H, Eriksson B, Bergström M, Bjurling P, Långström B, Öberg K. 1995. Pancreatic neuroendocrine tumors: Diagnosis with PET. Radiology 195:333–337.

57. Hellman P, Skogseid B, Juhlin C, Åkerström G, Rastad J. 1992. Findings of long-term results of parathyroid surgery in multiple endocrine neoplasia type. World J Surg 16:718–723.

58. Mallette LE, Malini S. 1989. The role of parathyroid ultrasonography in the management of primary hyperparathyroidism. Am J Med Sci 298:51–58.

59. Skogseid B, Öberg K, Juhlin C, Granberg D, Rastad J, Åkerström G. Surgery at asymptomatic pancreatic endocrine lesion in multiple endocrine neoplasia type 1. World J Surg, in press.

60. Moertel CG, Johnsson CM, McKusick MA, Martin JK Jr, Nagorney DN, Kvols LK, Rubin J, Kunselman S. 1994. The management of patients with advanced carcinoid tumors and islet cell carcinomas. Ann Int Med 120:302–309.

61. Öberg K. 1994. Endocrine tumors of the gastrointestinal tract: Systemic treatment. Anticancer Drugs 5:503–519.

62. Moertel CG, Lefkopoulo M, Lipsitz M, Hahn RG, Klassen D. 1992. Streptozocin-doxorubicin, streptozocin-fluorouracil or chlorozotocin in the treatment of advanced islet cell carcinoma. N Engl J Med 326:519–523.

63. Moertel CG, Kvols LK, O'Connell MJ, Rubin J. 1991. Treatment of neuroendocrine carcinoma with combined etoposide and cisplatin. Evidence of major therapeutic activity in the anaplastic variants of these neoplasms. Cancer 68:227–232.

64. Eriksson B, Öberg K. 1993. An update of the medical treatment of malignant endocrine pancreatic tumors. Acta Oncol 32:203–208.

19. Multiple endocrine neoplasia type I
Surgical therapy

Norman W. Thompson

The therapy of MEN-I is multifaceted in that surgical treatment in the individual patient is dependent on the phenotypic expression at the time of diagnosis. In many patients, the first clinical expression of the syndrome is hyperparathyroidism (HPT). In others, it may be a combination of manifestations, including a functional endocrine pancreatic syndrome and HPT, or a combination of HPT and a pituitary tumor such as a prolactinoma. Occasionally, an MEN-I patient may present with clinical manifestations in all three organs simultaneously. This discussion will be limited to the surgical management of the parathyroid and pancreatic components of the syndrome.

MEN-I hyperparathyroidism

More than 90% of all patients proven to have the MEN-I syndrome develop HPT, and most commonly hypercalcemia is the first biochemical finding detected in at-risk family members being screened for the disease. Although asymptomatic hypercalcemia may be encountered during the early teenage years, symptomatic disease usually is not diagnosed until the 20s or 30s [1–10]. These patients may have any of the symptoms and findings associated with primary HPT, including renal stones, which have been common in our experience. However, some are apparently completely asymptomatic when first diagnosed. Nevertheless, in some patients the disease may be severe and present as hypercalcemic crisis with serum calcium levels of 15 mg/dl or higher, a decrease in renal function, nausea, vomiting and dehydration, and impaired sensorium [11]. Progressive disease seems to be the rule, and there is general consensus that any patient with MEN-I HPT should undergo parathyroidectomy once the diagnosis is established based on hypercalcemia and elevated intact parathyroid hormone levels. The only controversy in surgical management is the specific operation for the disease [3,6,7,9,10].

Asymmetrical parathyroid enlargement caused by a nodular type of hyperplasia is typical of MEN-I [1–11]. Multiglandular disease is present in all

Andrew Arnold (ed.) ENDOCRINE NEOPLASMS. 1997. Kluwer Academic Publishers. ISBN 0-7923-4354-9.
All rights reserved.

MEN-I patients with HPT. Furthermore, it is assumed that up to 20% of patients will have a supernumerary (fifth) gland within the thymus that must be considered in the operative strategy [3,12,13]. Frequently one or more parathyroid glands may be normal in size and even in microscopic appearance from a limited biopsy. Only one or two parathyroid glands may be enlarged grossly, resulting in a false impression that the disease is caused by an adenoma or double adenoma. This may occur in the patient without a known family history or other manifestation of the MEN-I syndrome [6,12].

Two surgical procedures are widely used in treating MEN-I HPT. Both are based on the likelihood that persistent or recurrent hypercalcemia will occur if less than a subtotal parathyroidectomy is performed. One approach is to perform a total parathyroidectomy with excision of the cervically accessible thymus gland and autotransplantation of sufficient parathyroid tissue into a forearm muscle or another accessible location so that, should recurrence develop, reoperation using a local anesthetic could be performed on an outpatient basis [6,9]. This procedure has the potential for permanent hypoparathyroidism if the transplant tissue does not survive. Although this is infrequent in centers with expertise, it is estimated that the failure rate world-wide has been approximately 10%[3,7–10,12,14]. These patients all require replacement therapy with vitamin D and oral calcium until the graft functions adequately. Its advantage is that if the parathyroidectomy has been thorough, a second procedure in the neck can usually be avoided. The transplanted parathyroid tissue can be reduced under local anesthesia if there is a subsequent recurrence [3].

The second procedure is a subtotal parathyroidectomy with cervical thymectomy [3,5,7,12–14]. In this procedure, all parathyroid glands but one are excised. When all four glands are enlarged, a well-vascularized gland is partially resected, leaving a viable remnant weighing approximately 50–60 mg. When a normal-sized gland has been identified, regardless of its location, it is carefully preserved and marked with a metal clip for possible future identification. In the patient with four-gland enlargement, the smallest inferior gland is mobilized and trimmed to the desired size after carefully placing a metal clip across the gland. The resected portion is cut on the clip after packing the surrounding area to prevent possible implantation of hyperplastic parathyroid cells. The remnant with clip is then tacked with a stitch to the trachea so that it will be easily accessible should a recurrence caused by remnant hypertrophy subsequently develop.

We have preferred subtotal parathyroidectomy with cervical thymectomy in MEN-I patients because if performed correctly, it avoids permanent hypoparathyroidism and results in long-lasting eucalcemia in most patients [11–14]. Thirty-eight MEN-I patients with HPT were treated at the University of Michigan Medical Center between 1972 and 1996, and were available for follow-up studies ranging from 1 month to 24 years following parathyroidectomy. Twenty-seven patients had their primary operations at the University of Michigan. One of these patients in whom only three parathyroid glands were found at exploration had persistent hypercalcemia (3.7%). At re-operation, the missing left inferior parathyroid gland was found within the lower pole of the thyroid gland. Five patients developed recurrent hyperparathyroidism diagnosed at intervals of 2, 5, 8, 16, and 17 years after a subtotal parathyroidectomy and thymectomy (18.5%). Four of the patients were reoperated and were found to have remnant hypertrophy. Partial resection of the remnants have resulted in normocalcemic in each case. One patient suspected of having a middle mediastinal ectopic fifth parathyroid has not undergone reoperation.

Twenty-six out of the 27 patients became transiently hypocalcemic after their initial operations and most required dihydrotachysterol in addition to oral calcium supplements. Transient hypocalcemia also developed in reoperated patients as well. Only one patient has developed more longlasting hypocalcemia, and has required DHT and oral calcium daily for more than 1 year. This patient was a teenager in whom only two parathyroid glands were identified despite a complete exploration. She was left with a viable normalsized gland after excision of the enlarged gland and her thymus. After $1^1/_2$ years her replacement requirements are slowly decreasing.

A subset of this group of 27 patients consists of 9 who had synchronous primary HPT and neuroendocrine pancreatic and/or duodenal endocrine tumors. Each underwent a combined cervical and abdominal exploration, avoiding a second operative procedure. These patients, all explored between 1990 and 1995, are currently normocalcemic following subtotal parathyroidectomy and cervical thymectomy, with the exception of a 30-year-old male who has calcium levels that are just above the normal range 3 years after his operation. Each of these patients also underwent a distal pancreatectomy. Five patients with ZES also had duodenotomies and excision of submucosal gastrinomas. Based on the favorable results in this group, we recommend a combined approach for synchronous HPT and pancreatic disease, providing neither the neck nor abdominal procedure is a reoperative exploration. None of these combined procedures exceeded 5 hours in total operative time [14].

Eleven patients who were initially treated elsewhere underwent reoperative parathyroidectomies for persistent (n = 8) or recurrent disease (n = 3). A subtotal parathyroidectomy was accomplished in eight patients in whom one or more enlarged hyperplastic glands was excised. Each patient also had a cervical thymectomy. The three patients with recurrences were found to have hypertrophy of remnants that were trimmed to an estimated 50–60 mg. One out of the 11 patients has persistent hypercalcemia, and another has serum calcium levels at the upper limit of normal. All but one patient was temporarily hypocalcemic.

Thirty-three out of the 38 MEN-I patients are normocalcemic (87%). The four who have persistent or recurrent hypercalcemia are asymptomatic at the present time. However, it should be emphasized that 16 of these 34 patients required two operations (47%), 9 for persistent and 7 for recurrent disease. Remnant hypertrophy was the only cause of true recurrence in this group of patients and occurred at intervals ranging from 2 to 7 years after an initially successful operation. Reoperation for remnant recurrences was not difficult in cases in which the surgeon had carefully documented the location of the remaining gland. Annual follow-up of these patients is indicated for life because late recurrences can be anticipated and occurred in 19% of all patients in this series. We favor subtotal parathyroidectomy and thymectomy because if carefully performed this avoids permanent hypoparathyroidism, and in our own primary cases was associated with a long-term recurrence rate of only 18.5%. Most reoperations in this group were successful without any significant morbidity.

MEN-I: Pancreatic duodenal endocrine disease

Clinical manifestations of neuroendocrine disease of the pancreas and/or duodenum develop in about 70% of patients with MEN-I, even though almost all patients develop a diffuse endocrine dysplasia of the pancreas, consisting of islet-cell hyperplasia, microadenomatosis, and nesidioblastosis [4,15–21]. In addition to these findings, symptomatic MEN-I patients develop benign or malignant neoplasms, some of which are functional, causing a specific hormonal syndrome. The morbidity and mortality from MEN-I pancreatic disease is the result of the functional activity of a variety of tumors and/or their malignant behavior. The operative management of neuroendocrine disease in MEN-I patients is directly influenced by important findings that have been determined in recent years. The first is that patients with functional hormonal syndromes have one or more discrete tumors as the cause or the syndrome, rather than islet-cell hyperplasia, even though the diffuse changes or dysplasia of islet cells always accompany the tumors [17]. It became apparent that functional syndromes could be effectively treated if all gross tumors were excised without the necessity of performing a total pancreatectomy. Another finding is that in most patients with MEN-I Zollinger-Ellison syndrome (ZES), the most common functional tumors found are small gastrinomas arising within the duodenal wall [14–16,18–29]. Frequently these are accompanied by gross tumors elsewhere in the pancreas, which, based on immunochemical studies, have been found to be unrelated to the production of gastrin. More recently it has been discovered that duodenal gastrinomas, despite their small size, frequently metastasize to the peripancreatic and periduodenal lymph nodes but are accompanied by liver metastases in less than 10% of cases and only then after a long period without surgical intervention [4,23–36]. Finally, MEN-I pancreatic tumors, which were previously considered to be less malignant than those occurring sporadically, may be the cause of significant mortality as a result of liver metastases or local invasion [14–16,19,38–41].

Our surgical approach, developed over the past 15 years, is based on the premise that MEN-I patients with neuroendocrine disease of the pancreas or

410

duodenum can be cured of their syndrome or nonfunctional tumors, providing that the tumor has not metastasized to the liver and that the operation is extensive enough to excise all sites of disease [14,25–27]. An aggressive surgical approach is indicated because the incidence of malignancy is similar to that in patients with sporadic islet-cell tumors. Liver metastases are less common at the time of diagnosis, perhaps because of the younger age of patients at the time of diagnosis and the frequency of duodenal primary tumors in MEN-I ZES patients, which appear to have a less aggressive biological behavior than those that arise in the pancreas.

MEN-I: Nonfunctional tumors

In our experience the majority of patients with functional tumors have had other neuroendocrine tumors that were nonfunctional or secreting hormones that produce no identifiable syndrome. Additionally, some patients, estimated to represent 5–10% of MEN-I patients, have developed neuroendocrine tumors producing symptoms entirely related to their size, local invasion, or hepatic metastases. In these patients, the pancreatic tumor may become quite large and locally invasive before any symptoms develop. The presenting symptoms may include GI bleeding from portal hypertension, pain, or a palpable abdominal mass. The challenge in these cases is often technical, and their surgical management may require extensive procedures, such as pancreatoduodenectomy, extensive distal pancreaticectomy, and/or resection of a portion of the superior mesenteric or portal vein and replacement by either a vein or prosthetic graft [14]. Because such tumors can develop insidiously, it is our policy to perform periodic screening of the pancreas in all proven MEN-I patients. This can best done by endoscopic ultrasound rather than reliance on hormonal screening in asymptomatic patients.

Although a battery of hormonal assays may be obtained in the asymptomatic patient at periodic intervals, such studies have not been rewarding nor cost effective in our experience. Evaluation of levels of chromogranin A and pancreatic polypeptide (PP) might prove useful in the early detection of nonfunctional MEN-I neoplasms, but a sensitive assay for chromogranin is not widely available in the United States [16]. Chromogranins are secreted by virtually all pancreatic and duodenal neuroendocrine tumors, regardless of their secretion of other functional hormones, and elevated levels could be used as an indication for imaging or endoscopic ultrasound (EUS). Periodic octreotide scinticanning may also prove useful in MEN-I patients at risk, but as yet there have been no studies reported using this technique to follow asymptomatic MEN-I patients. Because of our favorable experience with EUS in evaluating the entire pancreas, we are currently using this procedure to follow asymptomatic patients annually after distal pancreatectomy [14]. We are also screening new MEN-I patients with EUS. How often the procedure should subsequently be repeated in those with initially negative findings is not known at the present time. Hopefully, prospective studies will eventually determine which study and at what interval will be most cost effective in detecting tumors at a stage when they can be easily resected or enucleated.

Functional neuroendocrine tumors

A variety of islet-cell tumors have been reported in MEN-I patients, including those causing hypersecretion of gastrin, insulin, glucagon, VIP, ACTH, somatostatin, growth hormone, and PTH. With the exception of ZES and hypoglycemia, clinical syndromes caused by other hormones are rare and will not be considered in further detail here.

Gastrinomas

The management of the ZE syndrome in association with MEN-I remains controversial. This is the most frequent syndrome detected in MEN-I and accounts for approximately 60% of the functional syndromes encountered. Our management is based on the facts that all gastrinomas, whether in the duodenum or the pancreas, have malignant potential or are malignant when detected and that surgical treatment can be successful in patients without liver metastases, providing that the operative procedure performed addresses all facets of the disease. We believe that all patients without liver metastases should be explored with the intent to cure the disease, usually without requiring either a Whipple procedure or total pancreatectomy. After the diagnosis of ZES is confirmed by elevated serum gastrin levels and a positive secretin stimulation test, either computed tomography (CT) or magnetic resonance imaging (MRI) is used to evaluate the liver for metastases and the adrenal glands for possible cortical tumors. For the past 3 years, the only other localization study that we performed is EUS, primarily to evaluate the head and the uncinate process of the pancreas [14]. Duodenal gastrinomas, present in the majority of these patients, are usually too small to be detected by any localization technique. Fewer than 10% of MEN-I ZES patients present with liver metastases. As a result, the great majority of these patients are considered candidates for exploration. The following principles are guidelines in all explorations for ZES in MEN patients:
1. A duodenotomy is performed and the wall of the duodenum is circumferentially palpated from the pylorus through its third portion. Small (<0.5 cm) gastrinomas are enucleated with closure of the mucosa afterward. Larger gastrinomas are excised with a full-thickness margin of duodenal wall.
2. Whenever a duodenal neuroendocrine (NE) tumor is detected, all peripancreatic lymph nodes are excised, including those along the common bile duct, the portal vein, and the hepatic artery to the celiac axis.

3. After full mobilization of the head and uncinate by an extended Kocher's maneuver, any palpable or ultrasonically identified tumor is enucleated.
4. A distal pancreatectomy, including the neck, body, and tail, preserving the spleen when possible, is routinely performed (Figs. 1 and 2).

Since 1978 we have explored 27 MEN-I patients with ZES with the intent to cure each individual. A duodenotomy was not routinely used until 1985, when it became apparent that most patients had small duodenal neuroendocrine tumors as well as other tumors in their pancreas. Furthermore, some of the earlier patients who had not had a distal pancreatectomy developed new tumors in the body or tail. Three subsequently underwent distal pancreatectomies for hypoglycemia (insulinomas). In each patient, all of the tumors in the duodenum and pancreas were characterized by immunohistological staining.

The location of proven gastrinomas in these 27 patients is shown in Table 1. Multiple gastrinomas within the duodenum were found in approximately 60% of all patients, and nearly 40% of these were associated with one or more lymph nodes containing neuroendocrine tumor metastases. Only one pancreatic neoplasm was associated with a single metastatic lymph node. This was from a 2 cm somatostatinoma arising in the body of the pancreas. This patient has had no evidence of recurrence during a 14-year follow-up. None of these patients has subsequently developed liver metastases after follow-up periods

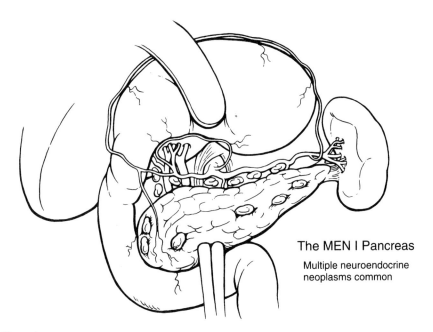

The MEN I Pancreas

Multiple neuroendocrine neoplasms common

Figure 1.

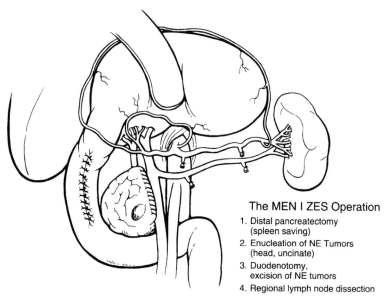

The MEN I ZES Operation

1. Distal pancreatectomy
   (spleen saving)
2. Enucleation of NE Tumors
   (head, uncinate)
3. Duodenotomy,
   excision of NE tumors
4. Regional lymph node dissection

Figure 2.

Table 1. MEN-I–Zollinger-Ellison syndrome

Duodenal gastrinomas	23/27	85%
Multiple duodenal gastrinomas	16/27	59%
	16/23 (69%)	
Malignant duodenal gastrinomas	09/23 (39%)	33%
Pancreatic gastrinomas	10/27	37%
Duodenal and pancreatic gastrinomas	06/27	22%
Pancreatic gastrinoma (only)	04/27	15%
Palpable neuroendocrine tumors in distal pancreas (initial operation)	24/27	89%

ranging from 6 months to 18 years. Two thirds of these patients became eugastrinemic, and the others had lowered basal serum gastrin levels and lower drug requirements to control hypersecretion of acid. Although only one third have been secretin stimulation negative, some patients with normal basal serum gastrin levels have been free of symptoms and have required no drug therapy for up to 18 years. One patient with three duodenal gastrinomas and three pancreatic neuroendocrine tumors was found to have multiple gastric carcinoids (ECL tumors) [42]. The two largest of these, measuring 1.5 cm in diameter, were excised at the time of her pancreatic duodenal exploration, but the remainder were left in situ. Subsequent to her operation, the serum gastrin levels have remained normal and there has been progressive regression of her remaining gastric lesions during the 1-year interval.

414

Because none of the patients who were not cured have developed liver metastases, they are periodically being re-evaluated and are considered potential candidates for re-exploration. Whether this decision should be based on EUS findings in the remaining head-uncinate or based on a progressively rising serum gastrin level has not yet been established.

Insulinomas

Approximately 15–20% of MEN 1 patients develop hypoglycemia as the only manifestation of their pancreatic neuroendocrine disease [14,16]. With few exceptions, sporadic insulinomas are solitary tumors, whereas insulinomas in MEN-I are likely to be multiple or associated with concomitant nonfunctional islet-cell tumors. Because the multiple tumors in MEN-I patients with hypoglycemia are not always insulinomas, their designation as such must be proven by immunohistological chemical staining. Whenever a presumed sporadic insulinoma patient is found to have multiple islet-cell tumors, a complete evaluation for MEN-I should be undertaken. Most of these patients will eventually be proven to have this syndrome [43,44].

Six patients with symptomatic insulinomas occurring in MEN-I patients were treated at the University of Michigan during the past 20 years. One additional patient, operated on elsewhere, underwent the enucleation of an insulinoma located in the tail of the pancreas when only 9 years of age. At that time there was no known family history of MEN-I and this was considered a sporadic tumor. She did well for the next 26 years. At 35 years of age she developed both hyperparathyroidism and ZES. When re-explored, two palpable neuroendocrine tumors were enucleated from the head and four were resected from the distal pancreas. Seven microgastrinomas were enucleated from the duodenum. In the other six patients, at least two or more insulinomas were excised in each. One patient, a 27-year-old male with a 7-cm pedunculated insulinoma arising from the neck of the pancreas, was treated by distal pancreatectomy. An additional insulinoma, as well as three other nonfunctioning neuroendocrine tumors, were found in the body and tail. The largest insulinoma was histologically malignant, and one contiguous lymph node contained metastatic disease that stained positive for insulin [14]. All seven patients are euglycemic at the present time, with follow-ups ranging from 1 to 18 years.

In our management plan for MEN-I insulinomas, after the diagnosis is confirmed biochemically during a 72-hour fast with appropriate glucose, insulin, and C-peptide levels, we proceed with EUS. This is the only localization study we currently use. Its purpose is to evaluate the head and uncinate process of the pancreas because the distal pancreas will be resected. It is important to obtain a serum gastrin as well because if the basal levels are elevated and a secretin stimulation test is positive, a duodenotomy should be done at the time of exploration in search for a small gastrinoma.

The operative procedure we perform is a distal pancreatectomy to the level of the superior mesenteric vein and enucleation of any neuroendocrine tumors in the head or uncinate process. A duodenotomy is performed only when the preoperative serum gastrin levels are elevated and a secretin test is positive. We have not encountered an extrapancreatic insulinoma, nor have they been reported in MEN-I patients. A lymphatic dissection is performed only in those patients with a concomitant duodenal gastrinoma or in the rare MEN-I patient with a malignant insulinoma suspected on the basis of size larger than 5 cm or local invasion.

Conclusions

Neuroendocrine tumors of the pancreas develop in more than 70% of patients with MEN-I and may cause significant morbidity or mortality. Their treatment is surgical when detected by imaging, biochemical screening, or biochemical confirmation of a hormonal syndrome. The objective in all patients is to detect and excise the tumor(s) before their malignant potential has been confirmed by hepatic metastases. In patients with functional syndromes caused by hypersecretion of a specific hormone, surgical treatment may be life saving (glucagonoma, VIPoma, or insulinoma) or may eliminate the need for expensive daily drug therapy (gastrinoma). These objectives need to be re-emphasized in MEN-I patients with ZES because many groups have excluded these patients for operation based on historical failures caused by previous inadequate knowledge of tumor pathophysiology.

Whether MEN-I patients with hypergastrinemia have a greater propensity to have concomitant neuroendocrine tumors in the pancreas is not known. The fact that virtually 100% of our patients had or developed neuroendocrine tumors in the body or tail of the pancreas is the basis for our recommendation that a distal pancreatectomy be performed routinely in the MEN-ZES operation. An alternative approach, which has been advocated by several authors, is to perform a pancreaticoduodenectomy, which would eliminate any neuroendocrine tumors in the duodenum, head, uncinate, and peripancreatic lymph nodes [45,46]. Any tumor in the remaining pancreatic body and/or tail could be enucleated. It is not unreasonable to assume that an even higher cure rate of the ZES could be achieved with this procedure. Whether the potential added morbidity and possible mortality associated with this operation is justifiable remains to be answered.

In those patients who are not cured after our procedure, we perform, a second-look procedure, which can be performed a year or so afterward with the reasonable assumption that a previously occult tumor or lymph node may have grown to detectable size. Another approach is to excise all duodenal tumors and to enucleate any pancreatic tumors without resecting the distal pancreas. Failures after this procedure would still be candidates for pancreaticoduodenectomy without resorting to a total pancreatectomy.

In patients without liver metastases, a total pancreatectomy, including any involved lymph nodes, would cure the MEN-I patient of pancreatic and duodenal neuroendocrine disease. However, the potential long-term side effects of this procedure in relatively young patients and the relative indolence of most neuroendocrine malignancies of MEN-I obviates the benefits gained and makes this procedure unacceptable in all but clearly identified MEN-I families with proven highly aggressive pancreatic malignancies [40].

Although our series is relatively small, several observations can be emphasized. The first is that the majority of the MEN-I–ZES patients can be rendered eugastrinemic if diagnosed and explored before liver metastases have developed. The second is that excision of tumors and lymph-node metastases, when present, may prevent the subsequent development of liver metastases. No patient in our series has developed liver metastases. These results encourage us to recommend pancreaticoduodenal exploration in all MEN-I–ZES patients without liver metastases. Most patients will obtain significant long-term benefits. Although it appears likely that the tumor mortality will be reduced by our management plan, this has not been proven unequivocally as yet based on the length of follow-up in our series and the lack of any reported controlled studies. Treatment with drug therapy alone until a tumor is imaged may eliminate the potential opportunity to cure many of these patients and offers an explanation as to why the results of others who follow this policy are so disappointing [15].

References

1. Block MA. 1991. Familial hyperparathyroidism and hyperparathyroidism associated with multiple endocrine neoplasia syndrome. In Cady B, Rossi RL, eds. Surgery of the Thyroid and Parathyroid Glands, 3rd ed. Philadelphia: W.B. Saunders.
2. Lamers CB, Froeling PG. 1979. Clinical significance of hyperparathyroidism in familial multiple endocrine adenomatosis type 1 (MEA I). Am J Med 66:422–424.
3. Malmaeus J, Benson L, Johansson H, Ljunghall S, Rastad J, Akerstrom G, et al. 1986. Parathyroid surgery in the multiple endocrine neoplasia type 1 syndrome: Choice of surgical procedure. World J Surg 10:668–672.
4. Shepherd JJ. 1991. The natural history of multiple endocrine neoplasia type 1. Arch Surg 126:935–946.
5. Block MA, Frame B, Jackson CF. 1978. The efficacy of subtotal parathyroidectomy for primary hyperparathyroidism due to multiple gland involvement. Surg Gynecol Obstet 147:1–5.
6. Light GS, Hensley MI. 1986. Management of familial hyperparathyroidism. Prog Surg 18:106–116.
7. Prinz RA, Gamvros OI, Sellu D, Lynn JA. 1981. Subtotal parathyroidectomy for primary chief cell hyperplasia of the multiple endocrine neoplasia type 1 syndrome. Ann Surg 193:26–29.
8. Rizzoli R, Green J III, Marx SJ. 1985. Primary hyperparathyroidism in familial multiple endocrine neoplasia type 1. Long-term follow-up of serum calcium levels after parathyroidectomy. Am J Med 78:467–474.

9. Wells SA Jr, Farndon JR, Dale JK, Leight GS, Dilley WG. 1980. Long term evaluation of patients with primary parathyroid hyperplasia managed by total parathyroidectomy and heterotopic autotransplantation. Ann Surg 192:451–458.

10. van Heerden JA, Kent RB III, Sizemore GW, Grant CS, ReMine WH, Kent RB. 1983. Primary hyperparathyroidism in patients with multiple endocrine neoplasia syndrome. Surgical experience. Arch Surg 118:533–536.

11. Allo M, Thompson NW. 1983. Hyperparathyroidism as a part of MEN 1 syndrome. In Kaplan EL, ed. Surgery of the Thyroid and Parathyroid Glands. Clinical Surgery International. Churchill Livingston, 177–192.

12. Thompson NW. 1983. The techniques of initial parathyroid exploration and reoperative parathyroidectomy. In Thompson NW, Vinik AI, eds. Endocrine Surgery Update. New York: Grune & Stratton, pp 365–383.

13. Thompson NW, Eckhauser FE, Harness JK. 1982. Anatomy of primary hyperparathyroidism. Surgery 92:814–822.

14. Thompson NW. 1995. The surgical management of hyperparathyroidism and endocrine disease of the pancreas in the multiple endocrine neoplasia type 1 patient. J Intern Med 238:269–280.

15. MacFarlane MP, Fraker DL, Alexander HR, et al. 1995. Perspective study of surgery resection of duodenal and pancreatic gastrinomas in multiple endocrine neoplasia type 1. Surgery 118:973–980.

16. Skogseid B, Grama D, Rastad J, et al. 1995. Operative tumor yield obviates preoperative pancreatic tumor localization in multiple endocrine neoplasia type 1. J Intern Med 238:281–288.

17. Thompson NW, Lloyd RB, Nishiyama RH, Vinik AI, Strodel WE, Allo MD, et al. 1984. MEN-1 pancreas: A histological and immunohistological study. World J Surg 8:561–574.

18. Shepherd JJ, Challis DR, Davies PF, McArdle JP, Teh BT, Wilkinson S, et al. 1983. Multiple endocrine neoplasia, type 1: Gastrinomas, pancreatic neoplasms, microcarcinoids, the Zollinger-Ellison syndrome, lymph nodes and hepatic metastases. Arch Surg 128:1133–1142.

19. Akerstrom G, Johansson H, Grama D. 1991. Surgical treatment of endocrine pancreatic lesions in MEN 1. Acta Oncol 30:541–545.

20. Mignon M, Rusziniewski P, Podevin P, et al. 1993. Current approach to the management of gastrinoma and insulinoma in adults with multiple endocrine neoplasia 1. World J Surgery 17:489–497.

21. Sheppard BC, Norton JA, Doppman JL, et al. 1989. Management of islet-cell tumors in patients with multiple endocrine neoplasia: A prospective study. Surgery 106:1108–1118.

22. Kloppel G, Willemer S, Stamm B, Hacki WH, Heitz PU. 1986. Pancreatic lesions and hormonal profile of pancreatic tumors in multiple endocrine neoplasia type 1: An immunocytochemical study of nine patients. Cancer 57:1824–1832.

23. Pipeleers-Marichal M, Somers G, Willems G, Foulis A, Imrie C, Bishop AE, et al. 1990. Gastrinoma in the duodenums of patients with multiple endocrine neoplasia type 1 and the Zollinger-Ellison syndrome. N Engl J Med 322:723–727.

24. Friesen SR. 1990. Are 'aberrant nodal gastrinomas' pathogenetically similar to 'lateral aberrant thyroid' nodules? Surgery 107:236–238.

25. Thompson NW. 1992. The surgical treatment of Zollinger-Ellison syndrome in sporadic and MEN 1 syndrome. Acta Chir Austriaca 24:82–87.

26. Donow C, Pipeleers-Marichal M, Schroder S. 1991. Surgical pathology of gastrinoma: Site, size, multicentricity, association with multiple neoplasia type 1 and malignancy. Cancer 68:1329–1334.

27. Thompson NW, Bondeson AG, Bondeson L, Vinik AI. 1989. The surgical treatment of gastrinoma in MEN-1 syndrome patients. Surgery 106:1081–1086.

28. Thompson NW, Pasieka J, Fukuuchi A. 1993. Duodenal gastrinomas, duodentomy and duodenal exploration in the surgical managment of Zollinger-Ellison syndrome. World J Surg 17:455–462.

29. Pipeleers-Marichal M, Donow C, Heitz PU, Kloppel G. 1993. Pathologic aspects of gastrinomas in patients with Zollinger-Ellison syndrome with and without multiple endocrine neoplasia type 1. World J Surg 17:481–488.
30. Delcore R Jr, Cheung LY, Frieson SR. 1990. Characteristics of duodenal wall gastrinomas. Am J Surg 160:621–624.
31. Thom AK, Norton JA, Axiotis CA, Jenson RT. 1991. Location incidence and malignant potential of duodenal gastrinomas. Surgery 110:1086–1093.
32. Bornman PC, Marks IN, Mee AS, Price S. 1987. Favorable response to conservative surgery for extra-pancreatic gastrinoma with lymph nodes metastases. Brit J Surg 74:198–201.
33. Imamura M, Kanda M, Takahashi K, Shimada Y, Miyahara T, Wagata T, et al. 1992. Clinicopathological characteristics of duodenal microgastrinomas. World J Surg 16:703–710.
34. Thompson NW, Vinik AI, Eckhauser FE. 1989. Microgastrinomas of the duodenum. A cause of failed operations for the Zollinger-Ellison syndrome. Ann Surg 209:396–404.
35. Delcore R, Herumreck AS, Friesen SR. 1989. Selective surgical management of correctable hypergastrinemia. Surgery 106:1094–1102.
36. Thompson NW. 1992. The surgical treatment of the endocine pancreas and Zollinger-Ellison syndrome in the MEN-1 syndrome. Henry Ford Hosp Med J 40:195–198.
37. Sugg SL, Norton JA, Fraker DL, Metz DC, Pisegna JR, Fishbeyne V, et al. 1993. A prospective study of intraoperative methods to diagnosis and resect duodenal gastrinomas. Ann Surg 218:138–144.
38. Cheruer JA, Sawyers JL. 1992. Benefit of resection of metastatic gastrinoma in multiple endocrine neoplasia type 1. Gastroenterology 102:1049–1053.
39. Norton JA, Doppman JL, Jensen RT. 1992. Curative resection in Zollinger-Ellison syndrome: Results of a 10 year prospective study. Ann Surg 215:8–18.
40. Tisell LE, Ahlman H, Jansson S, Grimelius L. 1988. Total pancreatectomy in the MEN-1 syndrome. Br J Surg 75:154–157.
41. van Heerden JA, Smith SL, Miller L. 1986. Management of the Zollinger-Ellison syndrome in patients with multiple endocrine neoplasia type 1. Surgery 100:971–976.
42. Solcia E, Capella C, Fiocca R, Rindi G, Rosai J. 1990. Gastric argyrophil carcoidosis in patients with Zollinger-Ellison syndrome due to type I multiple endocrine neoplasia. A newly recognized association. Am J Surg Pathol 14:503–513.
43. Pasieka JL, McLeod MK, Thompson NW, Burney RE. 1992. Surgical approach to insulinomas: Assessing the need for preoperative localization. Arch Surg 127:442–447.
44. Service FJ, McMahaon MM, O'Brien PC, Ballard DJ. 1991. Functioning insulinoma-incidence recurrence and long-term survival of patients: A 60-year study. Mayo Clin Proc 66:711–719.
45. Delcore, Friesen SR. 1992. The role of pancreatoduodenectomy of primary duodenal wall gastrinomas in patients with the Zollinger-Ellison syndrome. Surgery 112:1–8.
46. Imamura M, Takahashi K, Adachi H, Minematsu S, Shimada Y, Naito M, Suzuki T, et al. 1987. Usefulness of selective arterial secretion injection test for localization of gastrinoma in the Zollinger-Ellison syndrome. Ann Surg 205:230–236.

20. Multiple endocrine neoplasia type II

and familial medullary thyroid carcinoma
Impact of genetic screening on management

Robert F. Gagel

Clinical syndromes associated with multiple endocrine neoplasia type II (MEN-II)

Multiple endocrine neoplasia type IIA (MEN-IIA)

In 1961, Sipple provided the first description of the autosomal-dominant endocrine neoplasia syndrome that bears his name [1]. The clinical features of this syndrome, more clearly defined by Steiner [2], include bilateral and multicentric medullary thyroid carcinoma (MTC), unilateral or bilateral pheochromocytoma, and parathyroid neoplasia. Penetrance of individual tumor types is highest for MTC (90%), followed by unilateral (50%) or bilateral (25%) pheochromocytomas and parathyroid neoplasia (15–20%). Parathyroid disease is almost never seen as an initial manifestation in children, and prospectively screened children who have been treated by thyroidectomy between the ages of 6 and 18 years and followed for two decades have not developed hyperparathyroidism [3].

There are several shared features of the three neoplastic manifestations. First, hyperplasia precedes the development of tumors. For example, adrenal gland pheochromocytomas develop on a background of diffuse adrenal medullary hyperplasia, and multicentric pheochromocytomas develop on a background of adrenal medullary hyperplasia. Second, the process is multicentric. Foci of MTC or its precursor lesions are distributed throughout the thyroid gland. The greatest concentration of abnormal foci is at the normal location of the greatest number of C cells, which is at the junction of the upper one third and lower two thirds of the thyroid gland along a central superior-inferior axis. Finally, each of the cell types involved retain their differentiated function throughout the development of the neoplastic syndrome and produce the hormone that characterizes the cell type.

Variants of multiple endocrine neoplasia type II

Familial medullary thyroid carcinoma (FMTC). Approximately 20% of kindreds with MEN-IIA develop only MTC [4]. This designation is generally

Andrew Arnold (ed.) ENDOCRINE NEOPLASMS. 1997. Kluwer Academic Publishers. ISBN 0-7923-4354-9.

accorded to families in which there are 10 or more affected members crossing several generations who have only MTC. The 50% penetrance of pheochromocytoma and the lower penetrance of parathyroid disease make it possible to miscategorize an MEN-IIA family unless sufficient numbers of older family members are evaluated. It is important to differentiate between an MEN-II family in which insufficient numbers have been studied to identify all components and FMTC kindreds, because of the potential for inadequate screening for pheochromocytoma, a major cause of morbidity and sudden death in MEN-II.

Medullary thyroid carcinoma associated with FMTC tends to follow a less aggressive course than is found in MEN-IIA. Death related to metastatic disease does occur, but with a lower frequency than in MEN-IIA. It is not uncommon for multigeneration families with FMTC to exist in which only one or two family members are affected in each generation. Unless a careful family history is obtained, individual affected members are likely to be categorized as having sporadic MTC.

MEN II and Hirschsprung disease. A small number of families have been reported in which there is the association of classic MEN-IIA and a Hirschsprung phenotype [5].

MEN II and cutaneous lichen amyloidosis. Approximately 15 families world-wide have been described in which there is the association of classic MEN-IIA with a cutaneous skin lesion over the upper back [6,7]. Patients with this cutaneous manifestation present with an intermittent but intense pruritus, presumably causing the lichenoid skin lesion. There is no specific therapy for this skin lesion, although cutaneous administration of corticosteroids or capsaicin may reduce the pruritus.

Multiple endocrine neoplasia type IIB (MEN-IIB)

Although multiple endocrine neoplasia type-IIB was the first of the hereditary MTC syndromes to be identified [8], the current classification of this disorder evolved out of a series of studies performed more than 60 years later [9–11]. The key features of this MEN-II variant include MTC in all; unilateral or bilateral pheochromocytoma in 50%; characteristic neuromas (distinguished from neurofibromas) on the tongue, within the lips, and throughout the gastrointestinal tract; and several features of Marfan syndrome, including altered upper/lower body ratio; long, thin arms, legs, fingers, and toes; and pectus abnormalities. Medullary thyroid carcinoma develops early, and follows an aggressive course with widespread metastasis during the first or second decade of life. Death occurs most commonly during the third or fourth decade from metastatic MTC, although broader and more recent experience suggests that the disease may pursue a less aggressive course in some families, leading to a number of multigenerational families [12,13].

422

The pheochromocytomas associated with MEN-IIB are bilateral in 50%, rarely malignant, and do not differ substantially from those found in MEN-IIA. The gastrointestinal mucosal neuromas are a major cause of morbidity. Children may come to medical attention because of gastrointestinal difficulties, including constipation, profound diarrhea causing dehydration, or intestinal obstruction. It is important in these children to differentiate between an adynamic ileus caused by neuronal dysfunction, which may clear after several days, and an obstructive process. Exploratory surgery may aggravate rather than help the gastrointestinal dysfunction. Gastrointestinal difficulties may worsen throughout life. The diarrhea may be exacerbated by the presence of high levels of serum calcitonin secondary to metastatic MTC. The most effective treatment for the diarrhea, especially that caused by secretory products of MTC, is oral tincture of opium.

Genetics of multiple endocrine neoplasia type II

The availability of large and well-defined kindreds with MEN-IIA and smaller but equally well-defined kindreds with MEN-IIB made it possible to apply genetic mapping techniques to localize the causative gene. Reports from two groups localized the responsible gene to centromeric chromosome 10 in 1987 [14,15]. Efforts over the next 5 years further narrowed the region to proximal chromosome 10q and led to the identification of *ret* protooncogene mutations in 1993 [16,17].

ret *protooncogene*

Transformation of NIH 3T3 cells by a rearranged form of the *ret* protooncogene led to its discovery in 1986 [18,19]. The gene encodes a tyrosine kinase receptor that has several unique features, including an extracellular cadherin-like region, a cysteine-rich extracellular domain thought to be important for dimerization of the receptor, and an intracellular tyrosine kinase domain (Fig. 1).

A ligand for the *ret* receptor has recently been identified. Glial cell-derived neurotrophic factor (GDNF) is a transforming growth factor-beta–like peptide [20] important for promoting growth and development of certain classes of neurons. The high level of expression of this protein in regions of the brain, kidney, and enteric neuronal system led investigators to postulate GDNF as a ligand for the *ret* tyrosine kinase receptor. Recent reports provide substantial evidence for specific interaction of GDNF with the *ret* receptor and a new receptor, GDNFR-α, which forms a complex with ret [21,22].

Prior to the identification of mutations of *ret* in MEN-IIA, its oncogenic potential had been established in papillary thyroid carcinoma (PTC), a neoplasm of the thyroid follicular cell. At least three different rearrangements of

The *Ret* Proto-oncogene

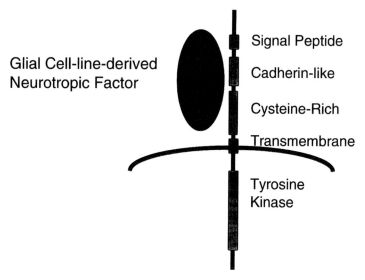

Glial Cell-line-derived
Neurotropic Factor

Signal Peptide

Cadherin-like

Cysteine-Rich

Transmembrane

Tyrosine
Kinase

Figure 1. Schemiatic diagram of the c-*ret* protooncogene. The *ret* protooncogene encodes a tyrosine kinase receptor. It has several distinctive featurs, including extracellular cadherin and cysteine-rich domains and an intracellular tyrosine kinase domain. The interaction of glial cell–derived neurotrophic factor (GDNF) with the *ret* receptor causes dimerization and auto-phosphorylation of the receptor and initiates a cascade of phosphorylation events. A second component of the receptor complex, GDNFR-α (not shown), has recently been identified (22).

ret have been identified in PTC in which the tyrosine kinase domain of *ret* is fused to a promoter sequence from another constitutively expressed gene (Fig. 2). Interestingly, all three rearrangements, given the names PTC1–3, occur in intron 10 of *ret*, immediately upstream of the transmembrane domain, and result in continuous activation of *ret*. In the United States and Europe, approximately 30–35% of PTCs express the PCT oncogene [23–25], whereas this rearrangement is rare in Japan [26]. Overexpression of the *ret* protooncogene has also been shown to cause transformation of several cell types when expressed in mice under the control of a ubiquitously expressed promoter sequence [27,28].

Role of the *ret* protooncogene in development. The *ret* protooncogene is expressed in developing neural crest, the developing kidney, C cells of the thyroid gland, the adrenal medulla, and components of the sympathetic sensory and enteric nervous system. Recent evidence for an important role of *ret* in normal enteric neuronal and kidney development has been provided by targetted disruption of the tyrosine kinase domain by homologous recombina-

424

tion in mice. Mice homozygous for the knockout have two prominent findings: They develop a phenotype indistinguishable from Hirschsprung disease and have a failure of normal kidney and ureteral development [29].

The recent identification of GDNF as a ligand for *ret* will undoubtedly lead to further elucidation of developmental events that direct the migration and differentiation of enteric neurons and neuroendocrine and kidney precursors from the neural crest [21,22]. Whether *ret* has additional ligands is unclear at present.

Mutations of the cysteine-rich extracellular domain of the ret *protooncogene in MEN-IIA*

Mutations of five codons of the *ret* protooncogene have been identified in MEN-IIA [17,30–32]. Each of the identified mutations converts a cysteine to another amino acid (Fig. 3, Table 1). The most common mutation, found in approximately 80% of all MEN-IIA kindreds, is a codon 634 mutation. The most common coding change at 634 is a cys634arg substitution, which accounts for approximately 50% of all mutations identified in MEN-IIA. Other common substitutions include cys634gly, cys634tyr, and cys634trp [17,30–32].

Sipple syndrome or MEN-IIA is most commonly associated with a cys634arg mutation [33], although other amino-acid substitutions are also

Genomic Organization of the *ret* Proto-oncogene

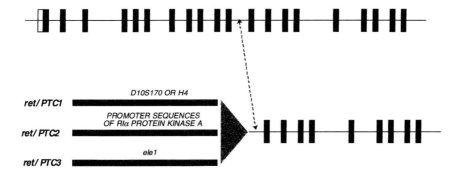

Ret Rearrangements in Papillary Thyroid Carcinoma

Figure 2. Papillary thyroid carcinoma rearrangements of the *ret* protooncogene. One of three rearrangements of the *ret* protooncogene results in continuous expression of the *ret* tyrosine kinase in approximately 30% of papillary thyroid carcinomas. These rearrangements are given the names *ret*/PTC1, *ret*/PTC2, and *ret*/PTC3. The breakpoint within the *ret* gene for each of these three rearrangements is in intron 11, just downstream of the coding sequence for the transmembrane domain.

Ret Proto-oncogene Mutations in MEN 2

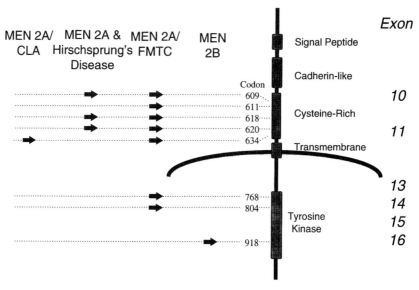

Figure 3. Mutations of the *ret* protooncogene associated with multiple endocrine neoplasia type II. The mutations of codons 609, 611, 618, 620 (all in exon 10), and 634 (exon 11) mutate a heavily conserved cysteine in the extracellular region of the *ret* receptor to another amino acid. There is considerable overlap in phenotype between mutations of these five codons. Mutations of codons 768 and 804 have been identified in a few families with familial medullary thyroid carcinoma. Germline mutations of codon 918 are found only in MEN-IIB.

observed. Mutations of codons 609, 611, 618, and 620 are less commonly found in association with classic MEN-IIA, although there is considerable overlap (see Fig. 3) [32]. There have been no reports of pheochromocytoma in association with a codon 609 mutation [32].

Mutations associated with variants of MEN-IIA

Familial medullary thyroid carcinoma is most commonly associated with mutations of exon 10, including codon 609, 611, 618, and 620 [32,34]. The most common mutation found in FMTC is a cys618ser substitution. A few families with FMTC have been found to have intracellular mutations at codon 768 and 804 [35,36], within the tyrosine kinase domain (see Fig. 3).

MEN-IIA with Hirschsprung disease. Mutations of codon 609 (cys609tyr), 618, and 620 have been identified in the Hirschsprung variant of MEN-IIA [30,32,37,38].

MEN-IIA and cutaneous lichen amyloidosis. All reported examples of MEN-IIA and cutaneous lichen amyloidosis have a codon 634 mutation with an

426

arginine, glycine, tyrosine, tryptophan, or phenylalanine substitution [39,40]. No other mutations of *ret* have been identified in these families.

Mutation of the intracellular tyrosine kinase domain in multiple endocrine neoplasia type-IIB

A single mutation at codon 918 (met918thr) has been identified in MEN-IIB at the site of the substrate recognition pocket [41]. Approximately 92–95% of individuals with MEN-IIB have a germline mutation at this codon. The mutation in the other 5–8% has not been identified, although the recent identification of GDNF as a ligand for *ret* and a second component of the receptor system, GDNF-α, provides obvious candidate genes for this group [21,22].

Mutations of the ret *protooncogene associated with sporadic medullary thyroid carcinoma*

Somatic *ret* protooncogene mutations in sporadic medullary thyroid carcinoma. Mutations of the *ret* protooncogene have been identified in approximately 25% of sporadic MTCs. The most common mutation is a codon 918 mutation (met918thr), the same coding change that causes MEN-IIB when

Table 1. Mutations of the *ret* protooncogene associated with MEN II and hereditary MTC

Affected codon	Amino-acid change normal→mutant	Nucleotide change normal→mutant	Clinical syndrome	Percentage of all MEN-II mutations
609	cys→arg	TGC→CGC	MEN-IIA/	0–1
	cys→tyr	TGC→TAC	FMTC	
611	cys→tyr	TGC→TAC	MEN-IIA/	2–3
	cys→trp	TGC→TGG	FMTC	
	cys→ser	TGC→AGC		
	cys→gly	TGC→GGC		
618	cys→arg	TGC→CGC	MEN-IIA/	
	cys→phe	TGC→TTC	FMTC	3–5
	cys→ser	TGC→TCC		
	cys→end	TGC→TGA		
	cys→arg	TGC→CGC		
620	cys→tyr	TGC→TAC	MEN-IIA/	
	cys→phe	TGC→TTC	FMTC	6–8
	cys→ser	TGC→TCC		
	cys→ser	TGC→AGC		
	cys→gly	TGC→GGC		
	cys→arg	TGC→CGC		
634	cys→tyr	TGC→TAC	MEN-IIA	80–90
	cys→phe	TGC→TTC		
	cys→ser	TGC→TCC		
	cys→trp	TGC→TGG		
768	glu→asp	GAG→GAC	FMTC	0–1
804	val→leu	GTG→TTG	FMTC	0–1
918	met→thr	ATG→ACG	MEN-IIB	10–20

it occurs as a germline mutation [38,42,43]. A small number of codon 634, 768, and 804 somatic mutations have been described in sporadic MTC. There is currently no definitive evidence that these mutations initiate transformation, but their frequency and the demonstrated transforming ability of the codon 918 mutation hint at an important role. Some evidence exists that MTCs with a somatic codon 918 mutation follow a more aggressive course than those without, although this observation was made in a small number of patients and has not been confirmed in a larger series [44].

Identification of germline *ret* protooncogene mutations in patients with apparent sporadic medullary thyroid carcinoma. The combined experience in over 200 patients has demonstrated the presence of germline mutations in approximately 6% of these patients. This finding was surprising, especially because some of these reports come from cancer centers that focus on the identification of hereditary malignancy [42–46]. What has become clear as a result of these studies is that hereditary MTC cannot be reliably detected by family history alone. In one report, 2 of 6 cases represented de novo mutations, and 2 of the other 4 resulted from kindreds in which family connectivity was lost through war and separation or by adoption [38]. A compilation of published mutations in sporadic MTC shows a broad spectrum of mutations in this group (Table 2).

Mutations of the ret *protooncogene associated with Hirschsprung disease*

Several genetic clues, such as the association of MEN-IIA and Hirschsprung disease [5], and the identification of a child with Hirschsprung disease with a proximal chromosome 10q deletion [47], led to the identification of a locus for

Table 2. Identification of germline mutations of the *ret* protooncogene in apparent sporadic medullary thyroid carcinoma

Study	Codons					Total examined	Percentage
	609	611	618	620	634		
Karolinska Hospital[a]					1	10	10
University of Cambridge[b]				1		67	1.5
University of Michigan[c]			1	1	3	21	24
University of Zurich[d]					2	16	12.5
MDACC[e]	2	1	1		2	101	6
Totals	2	1	2	2	8	215	7%

This information was obtained from the following publications:
[a] Zedenius et al. 1994. Hum Mol Genet 3:1259.
[b] Eng et al. 1995. Genes Chromosome Cancer 12:209.
[c] Decker et al. 1995. Surgery 118:257.
[d] Komminoth et al. 1995. Cancer 76:479.
[e] Wohllk et al. 1996. J Clin Endocrinol Metab 85:1113.

familial Hirschsprung, indistinguishable from familial MEN-II [48]. Following the identification of *ret* mutations in MEN-II, mutations were also identified in familial Hirschsprung disease [37,49]. Most of the described mutations are inactivating; however, a few at codons 609 and 620 are identical to those found in hereditary MTC [37]. These results suggest that either activating or inactivating mutations may result in abnormal migration of neurons from the neural crest to the developing gastrointestinal tract. A second Hirschsprung locus caused by point mutations of the endothelin beta receptor has been identified [50] and the *ret* ligand, GDNF, has thus become a candidate for mutational analysis [21,22].

Mechanism of oncogenesis

Overexpression of mutant *ret* cDNAs containing either codon 634 or 918 mutations in NIH 3T3 cells causes transformation of the cells and tumor formation in nude mice [51–53]. The extracellular codon 634 mutations are associated with increased dimerization of the receptor. It had been postulated that the cysteine-rich extracellular domain might play an important role in dimerization of the receptor based on the presence of a similar type of mutation in the epidermal growth factor receptor. In vitro studies with mutant ret, however, provide the first experimental evidence for receptor dimerization in the absence of ligand. Dimerization is associated with autophosphorylation of the receptor and phosphorylation of a subset of cellular proteins whose identity is unknown at this time. Connexin 43, a gap junction protein, is the only downstream effector implicated in the transformation process [51]. The codon 918 mutations cause autophosphorylation and activation of a different set of downstream proteins without receptor dimerization [52,53]. Finally, both mutations appear to cause activation of the receptor in a ligand-independent manner [52,53], although the effect of GDNF, a *ret* ligand, in these model systems has not been evaluated. Both types of mutations result in tumor formation when transformed cells are injected into nude mice. In one report there was the paradoxical result in which transformed cells expressing the codon 918 mutation grew more slowly when injected into nude mice than the cells expressing *ret* containing the codon 634 mutation [51]. This result was unexpected in view of the generally greater aggressiveness of tumors containing the codon 918 mutation [51]. This result may be explained by the use of a truncated 3′ alternatively processed form of *ret* in these studies that has a lower biological activity [54].

Possible strategies for modifying or reversing the effects of the mutant ret *protooncogene*

The identification of specific *ret* mutations associated with MEN-II makes it possible to perform genetic screening during pregnancy. Although feasible, abortion of an affected fetus is rarely considered by MEN-II family members in the United States. Family members have reasoned that a normal life span is possible if affected children are identified and treated early in life. Another approach that may be more acceptable to specific families, especially in those families in which MTC is aggressive, is the use of in vitro fertilization combined with preimplantation screening of the embryo [55]. This approach has been applied to other genetic diseases with some success, and the costs of this procedure, although high, are reasonable when compared with the costs of treatment of MEN-II over a lifetime. Although the rates of successful pregnancy are well below 50%, elimination of mutant *ret* from the germline and the resultant benefits to the family over several generations make this an attractive alternative.

The long lag period between birth and the development of cellular transformation in MEN-II, especially for the most common mutations of the extracellular cysteine-rich domain, suggest that a strategy to reduce *ret* activation by 70–80% might be effective in delaying the onset of malignancy by several decades or in preventing complete transformation. The extracellular location of these mutations makes it possible to envision strategies to inhibit dimerization of mutant *ret* without affecting the wild-type receptor. Another strategy is the selective destruction of mutant *ret* mRNA, an approach that would leave expression of the wild-type normal allele intact. Finally, it may be possible to modify the ligand. GDNF, to downregulate receptor activation. It is reasonable to believe that attempts will be made to develop such approaches over the next decade.

Clinical application of genetic information in the management of multiple endocrine neoplasia type II syndromes

The overall goal of screening for MEN-II is to identify gene carriers early in an attempt to modify the outcome of the disease. The two manifestations that are most life threatening are MTC and pheochromocytoma. There is compelling evidence for both that early intervention will positively affect outcome [3,56]. In contrast, parathyroid neoplasia occurs less frequently and is rarely a threat to life.

ret protooncogene testing

Critical elements of genetic testing. The identification of a genetic defect in a family will change individual family dynamics. Individuals will overnight acquire information that will change the course of their life. It is important that normal and affected family members be counseled about the impact of a positive or negative genetic test. This is best done in the context of a family meeting with multiple family members present, making it possible for family members to share questions and feelings following the meeting. The transmission of the genetic trait should be explained in simple terms, with a clear explanation of transmission of an autosomal-dominant trait. A pamphlet describing the key features in straightforward language has been helpful for the education of family members; they should be given multiple copies and encouraged to share this information with other family members (A copy of a *Guide for Hereditary Medullary Thyroid Carcinoma* may be obtained from the University of Texas M.D. Anderson Cancer Center Section of Endocrine Neoplasia and Hormonal Disorders Web Site at the following address: http//endrcr06.mda.uth.tmc.edu). Some family members may refuse to participate in discussions or screening efforts. It is important in these situations to recognize the right to privacy. At the same time, the health professional should make every effort to deliver information to potentially affected individuals. A written pamphlet, given to them by another family member, guarantees their privacy and makes them aware of the salient features of the syndrome. In many cases, recalcitrant family members will eventually join in screening and treatment once they are reassured it is in their best interest. Experience suggests that a long-term strategy of education and support is more likely to yield a positive outcome than initial dire predictions of a poor outcome.

Another issue of considerable concern in the United States is the impact of the identification of a genetic defect on an individual's insurability. Although some individual states have passed legislation prohibiting the use of genetic information to exclude individuals from health insurance, most have not. Until there is over-riding federal legislation, individual family members must decide when and how to determine whether they are gene carriers. It is important to balance the need for medical care against the impact that such information might have on insurability. In most cases the need for appropriate medical therapy will be paramount, but it may be appropriate to plan the timing of diagnostic procedures, including genetic testing, to minimize the insurance impact.

Obtaining samples. Samples should be collected from all first-degree relatives of a gene carrier with appropriate expansion of screening efforts if additional family members are identified. It is important to test each family member at least twice on separate blood draws. There are several reasons for this recommendation. Families frequently have similar names and may have blood samples drawn at the same sampling period, making a sample mixup possible. Perhaps the greatest error is one that causes samples from an affected and an unaffected family member to be switched [57]. Analysis of a second sample, obtained independently, will minimize the risk of a sampling or laboratory mixup.

Testing techniques. Several approaches to genetic testing are available through commercial testing facilities. (A list of commercial sources for genetic testing is available on the University of Texas M.D. Anderson Cancer Center

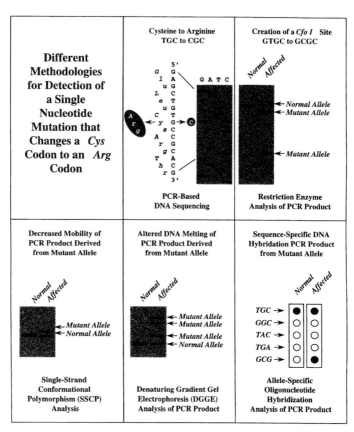

Different Methodologies for Detection of a Single Nucleotide Mutation that Changes a *Cys* Codon to an *Arg* Codon

Cysteine to Arginine
TGC to CGC

PCR-Based
DNA Sequencing

Creation of a *Cfo I* Site
GTGC to GCGC

← Normal Allele
← Mutant Allele

← Mutant Allele

Restriction Enzyme
Analysis of PCR Product

Decreased Mobility of
PCR Product Derived
from Mutant Allele

←Mutant Allele
←Normal Allele

Single-Strand
Conformational
Polymorphism (SSCP)
Analysis

Altered DNA Melting of
PCR Product Derived
from Mutant Allele

←Mutant Allele
←Mutant Allele
←Mutant Allele
←Normal Allele

Denaturing Gradient Gel
Electrophoresis (DGGE)
Analysis of PCR Product

Sequence-Specific DNA
Hybridation PCR Product
from Mutant Allele

TGC →
GGC →
TAC →
TGA →
GCG →

Allele-Specific
Oligonucleotide
Hybridization
Analysis of PCR Product

Figure 4. Different methodologies for detection of a single nucleotide mutation of the *ret* protooncogene. Five different techniques have been applied to the detection of mutations in multiple endocrine neoplasia type II and familial medullary thyroid carcinoma. This figure depicts results in an individual with a codon 634 cysteine (TGC) to arginine (CGC) mutation of the *ret* protooncogene. The **upper middle panel** shows the appearance of a sequencing band indicative of a G to C mutation at codon 634. The PCR-based sequencing technique shows both the normal and the mutant base at this codon. In the **upper right panel** is shown a *Cfo*I restriction enzyme analysis of the PCR product. In the normal individual without the mutation, treatment with the restriction enzyme results in only a single electrophoretic band. In the affected individual, there is a normal band and the appearance of two smaller bands representing the two fragments of the mutant allele. Single-strand conformational polymorphism (SSCP), shown in the **lower left panel**, is the third technique that can be used to identify a mutant allele. In this example the normal DNA sample has a single electrophoretic band, whereas there is separation of the mutant and normal alleles in the affected individual. The fourth technique used is denaturing gradient gel electrophoresis (DGGE), shown in the **lower middle panel**. The normal allele migrates as a single electrophoretic band, whereas the mutant allele shows a characteristic pattern that is specific for this particular mutation. Sequence-specific DNA hybridization is shown in the **lower right panel**. In this technique, a DNA oligonucleotide containing either the normal sequence or one of the mutations shown to the left of the figure is dotted onto a membrane. The PCR-amplified DNA from a normal subject (left) or an affected individual with a codon 634 cysteine (TGC) to arginine (CGC) mutation (right) is radiolabeled and then hybridized to the membrane using conditions in which a single-base mismatch will result in failure to hybridize. In the normal subject there is hybridization only to the oligonucleotide containing the normal TGC sequence, whereas the affected individual has both a normal (TGC) and mutant (CGC) allele. (Modified from Wohlllk et al. 1996. Application of genetic screening information to the management of medullary thyroid carcinoma and multiple endocrine neoplasia type 2. Endocrinol Metab Clini North Am 25:1–25.)

Section of Endocrine Neoplasia and Hormonal Disorders Web Site at the following address: http//endrcr06.mda.uth.tmc.edu). All techniques currently use DNA fragments generated by polymerase chain reaction (PCR) amplification of genomic DNA from tested individuals. Several analytic techniques have been applied to detect specific mutations, including direct DNA sequencing [58], denaturing gradient gel electrophoresis [59], restriction analysis of amplified products [30], and allele-specific hybridization [60] (Fig. 4). Each of these techniques has proved reliable for detection of the most common mutations causing MEN-II or FMTC.

Direct DNA sequencing of exons 10, 11, and 16 is the most commonly applied methodology. However, most commercial laboratories do not analyze for mutations outside these regions. Denaturing gradient gel electrophoresis is a sensitive and specific technique for the identification of differences between two *ret* alleles and will easily detect single base differences. In most cases a mutation will provide a specific electrophoretic profile. However, it is also possible that a polymorphism within the PCR fragment could create a similar electrophoretic profile, resulting in the misassignation of gene carrier status. Although the probability of such a polymorphism is low, some investigators believe that a positive result should be confirmed by DNA sequencing.

Restriction enzyme digestion is dependent upon the mutation creating or destroying a specific restriction site. This technique is not useful for initial screening, but once the specific mutation has been identified it provides a specific confirmatory technique. Allele-specific hybridization is rapid, specific, and economical. However, previously unrecognized nucleotide substitutions will not be identified unless the laboratory synthesizes all possible nucleotide changes at a particular codon. It is particularly useful for a rapid screen of a family with a known mutation and as a confirmatory methodology.

To ensure the greatest possible probability of correct assignation of gene carrier status, it is preferable to perform the analysis on separately obtained samples in two laboratories using different methodologies. Although this is frequently inconvenient, the probability of error will be lowest.

Perhaps the greatest difficulty occurs when germline transmission of MTC is proven but no *ret* protooncogene mutation is identified. Currently, 5–7% of kindreds are in this situation. Because most commercial laboratories test only for exon 10, 11, and 16 mutations, it is necessary to identify a research laboratory that will analyze regions of *ret* outside the most commonly mutated regions. It also seems likely that mutations of the ret ligand, GDNF [21,22,61], GDNFR-α, or a downstream effector protein could cause hereditary MTC.

Use of genetic information in the management of MEN-IIA

Management of medullary thyroid carcinoma. Three years have passed since the initial identification of genetic defects in MEN-II. During this period considerable information has accumulated on the clinical usefulness of genetic information. In a kindred with an identifiable *ret* mutation, individuals who have no genetic abnormality themselves are not at risk for development of MEN-II. After confirmation of a negative test result, it is appropriate to exclude these family members from further screening efforts.

Most adults who are gene carriers and have not been previously been treated for MTC will have signs of the disease, detectable by palpation, ultrasound examination, or an abnormal calcitonin response to pentagastrin testing. In most individuals, total thyroidectomy and central lymph-node dissection should be performed after exclusion of pheochromocytoma and hyperparathyroidism [3,62]. If a pheochromocytoma is detected, its management takes precedence.

The appropriate management of a gene carrier of advanced age is more controversial. The use of genetic testing has resulted in the identification of a small number of gene carriers older than 60 years with only abnormal calcitonin values and no other clinical evidence of disease. In most cases the decision to proceed with thyroidectomy in such a patient should be based on the expected longevity of the patient. For example, in a patient with significant coronary artery disease, it is likely that this will be life limiting rather than MTC. In such a patient, however, it will be important to exclude pheochromocytoma or hypercalcemia.

Two approaches have evolved for the management of children and teenagers who are gene carriers. The first is an extension of strategies that have been used for 20 years, which use annual pentagastrin stimulation of calcitonin release to detect an abnormal number of C cells [3,63]. The major advantage of this approach is the ability to defer total thyroidectomy until the pentagastrin test result becomes abnormal. This test is performed by the injection of 0.5 µg per kg body weight of pentagastrin intravenously with measurement of the serum calcitonin concentration initially and at 2, 5, and 10 minutes following the injection. This approach will generally identify affected children at an average age of 10–13 years. However, there have been false-positive tests, resulting in unnecessary thyroidectomies [57]. By combining genetic and pentagastrin testing, false-positive results will be eliminated.

A greater concern related to pentagastrin testing is the failure to identify C-cell abnormalities at the earliest stage. Approximately 50% of children diagnosed by pentagastrin testing had microscopic MTC rather than C-cell hyperplasia, which is a preneoplastic lesion [3,64]. In thyroidectomies performed during the past 2–3 years on individuals with positive genetic test results, over 50% had microscopic or macroscopic MTC, despite having a normal pentagastrin test [57,65–67]. These results demonstrate clearly the insensitivity of pentagastrin testing for the detection of premalignant abnormalities of the C cell. A small percentage (5–10%) of patients identified by pentagastrin testing have developed calcitonin abnormalities 15–20 years post-thyroidectomy, and there is at least one case in which metastatic MTC has been identified in a previously thyroidectomized child.

There are at least two possible mechanisms for the subsequent development of recurrent disease. The presence of microscopic MTC in 50% or more of the prospectively screened children suggests the possibility that metastasis may have been present at the time of primary surgery. A second possibility is the later transformation of residual C cells remaining after an incomplete thyroidectomy. It is known that total thyroidectomy is difficult, and it is plausible that continuous expression of *ret* in a few C cells over the 15 to 20-year follow-up period may have resulted in transformation. It is not possible at present to determine whether either of these two hypotheses is correct.

The second approach to the management of minors who are gene carriers is to perform a total thyroidectomy based solely on the results of genetic testing. The earliest age at which metastatic disease has been described in MEN-II is age 6 [68], suggesting that surgical removal of the thyroid gland at age 5 or 6 years would result in surgical cure. Performance of a total thyroidectomy at this age makes it unnecessary to perform preoperative pentagastrin testing. Although there is parental concern about thyroidectomy at this early age, the available experience suggests that thyroidectomy in these young children is well tolerated, and the risks of recurrent laryngeal nerve damage or hypoparathyroidism are no greater than in older children [57,65–67]. One group has been sufficiently concerned about the risks of hypoparathyroidism in young children to advocate early thyroidectomy combined with total parathyroid removal and transplantation to the nondominant arm [66]. This operative strategy is combined with central-node dissection, making it less likely that normal or metastatic C cells remain in the neck.

A major question is whether earlier thyroidectomy or the more aggressive approach with central lymph-node dissection and parathyroid transplantation will improve the cure rate. Available long-term data indicate that 90% of children followed for 15–20 years are cured by thyroidectomy based on pentagastrin testing [3], suggesting improvement by no more than 10% over a similar period. At present there are no compelling data to suggest that either approach is superior, although a decision based on genetic testing is clearly the most cost-effective approach to management. Kindreds with this disorder readily accept an approach that eliminates the costs and unpleasantness associated with the annual pentagastrin test, especially because there is the prospect that earlier intervention may improve cure rates.

Management of pheochromocytoma. The most important impact of genetic testing on the management of pheochromocytoma is the exclusion of 50% of family members from the screening process. Because pheochromocytomas are rarely malignant [69], removal should be postponed until symptoms of pheochromocytoma develop or there is evidence of abnormal catecholamine production. Annual measurement of urine catecholamines and metanephrines on a timed specimen (12 or 24 hour) provides a straightforward outpatient screening approach [3]. Basal or exercise-stimulated measurement of plasma catecholamines provides a second method for early detection of adrenomedullary abnormalities [70].

Magnetic resonance imaging (MRI) scans provide a sensitive technique for detection of small pheochromocytomas or an enlarged medulla, making it possible to remove a single pheochromocytoma through a flank incision. Examination of the contralateral adrenal gland at the time of surgical exploration rarely yields more information than MRI scanning. Metaiodobenzyl guanidine or octreotide scanning are sensitive methods for the detection of abnormalities but are probably unnecessary in most clinical situations because almost all pheochromocytomas in MEN-II occur in the adrenal medulla.

Appropriate alpha- and beta-adrenergic blockade should be employed prior to surgical exploration. In most cases, small pheochromocytomas can be removed safely without the major arrhythmias noted with larger pheochromocytomas in a previous era. One clinical situation of remaining concern is the pregnant woman with an undetected pheochromocytoma. Deaths related to catecholamine release during labor and delivery have been described [71], suggesting that all pregnant gene carriers should be screened routinely for pheochromocytoma during pregnancy.

Management of parathyroid neoplasia. Measurement of serum calcium should be performed annually or biannually in gene carriers. Prospective studies have demonstrated little parathyroid disease after 15–20 years of follow-up in children thyroidectomized in the first or second decade because of abnormal pentagastrin tests [3]. Whether longer follow-up will be associated with parathyroid neoplasia is unclear. Most surgeons perform a subtotal parathyroidectomy for treatment of hyperparathyroidism in hypercalcemic patients, although it may be appropriate to perform total parathyroidectomy with transplantation to the nondominant forearm in kindreds in which parathyroid disease has been a major problem [72].

Use of genetic information in the management of MEN-IIB

In children with phenotypic features of MEN-IIB, microscopic carcinoma with metastasis has been described during the first year of life [73]. It is appropriate to document gene carrier status by performance of a *ret* protooncogene analysis, but thyroidectomy should be performed during the first 6 months of life. It is prudent to consider performance of a central-node dissection at the time of primary surgery because of the high probability of metastatic disease in these children, even early in life. Other family members should also be tested for the presence of a codon 918 mutation because examples have been described in which the mucosal neuroma phenotype was incompletely penetrant [74].

ret protooncogene analysis in apparent sporadic MTC

The identification of germline *ret* protooncogene mutations in 6% of individuals with apparent sporadic MTC suggests that routine analysis for germline mutations involving codons 609, 611, 618, 620, 634, 768, and 804 should be performed. The most compelling reason for this recommendation is the twofold- or more multiplier effect observed when germline mutations have been detected. In one report the identification of six germline carriers led to the identification of an additional 11 gene carriers within these families [38].

An analysis comparing standard pentagastrin testing of first-degree relatives of an index case with *ret* protooncogene testing of the index case demonstrates that genetic testing is equivalent or slightly better than pentagastrin testing for the detection of hereditary medullary thyroid carcinoma, assuming 100% compliance with pentagastrin testing. A point of fact is that fewer than 50% of first degree relatives submit to pentagastrin testing, making it clear that genetic testing of index cases with apparent sporadic MTC is superior to pentagastrin testing [38].

Summary

The identification of *ret* protooncogene mutations in MEN-II and Hirschsprung disease has not only improved the clinical management of these genetic conditions but has also provided important information regarding mechanisms of transformation and neural crest development. An indication of how neural-crest cells migrate during embryonic life and the key processes involved in their differentiation now seems within reach. The continued pace of scientific discovery suggests that our understanding of and ability to prevent or treat hereditary and sporadic forms of MTC will continue to improve.

References

1. Sipple JH. 1961. The association of pheochromocytoma with carcinoma of the thyroid gland. Am J Med 31:163–166.
2. Steiner AL, Goodman AD, Powers SR. 1968. Study of a kindred with pheochromocytoma, medullary carcinoma, hyperparathyroidism and Cushing's disease: Multiple endocrine neoplasia, type 2. Medicine 47:371–409.
3. Gagel RF, Tashjian AH Jr, Cummings T, Papathanasopoulos N, Kaplan MM, DeLellis RA, Wolfe HJ, Reichlin S. 1988. The clinical outcome of prospective screening for multiple endocrine neoplasia type 2a: An 18-year experience. N Engl J Med 318:478–484.
4. Farndon JR, Leight GS, Dilley WG, Baylin SB, Smallridge RC, Harrison TS, Wells SA Jr. 1986. Familial medullary thyroid carcinoma without associated endocrinopathies: A distinct clinical entity. Br J Surg 73:278–281.
5. Verdy M, Weber AM, Roy CC, Morin CL, Cadotte M, Brochu P. 1982. Hirschsprung's disease in a family with multiple endocrine neoplasia type 2. J Pediatr Gastroenterol Nutr 1:603–607.
6. Nunziata V, Giannattasio R, di Giovanni G, D'Armiento MR, Mancini M. 1989. Hereditary localized pruritus in affected members of a kindred with multiple endocrine neoplasia type 2A (Sipple's syndrome). Clin Endocrinol 30:57–63.
7. Gagel RF, Levy ML, Donovan DT, Alford BR, Wheeler T, Tschen JA. 1989. Multiple

endocrine neoplasia type 2a associated with cutaneous lichen amyloidosis. Ann Intern Med 111:802–806.

8. Erdheim J. 1903. Zur normalen und pathologischen Histologie der Glandula Thyreoidea, Parathyreoidea und Hypophysis. Beitr Pathol Anat 33:158–236.

9. Williams ED, Pollock DJ. 1966. Multiple mucosal neuromata with endocrine tumours: A syndrome allied to Von Recklinghausen's disease. J Pathol Bacteriol 91:71–80.

10. Rashid M, Khairi MR, Dexter RN, Burzynski NJ, Johnston CC Jr. 1975. Mucosal neuroma, pheochromocytoma and medullary thyroid carcinoma: Multiple endocrine neoplasia type 3. Medicine (Baltimore) 54:89–112.

11. Carney JA, Sizemore GW, Hayles AB. 1978. Multiple endocrine neoplasia, type 2b. Pathobiol Annu 8:105–153.

12. Vasen HFA, van der Feltz M, Raue F, Nieuwenhuyzen Krusemean A, Koppeschaar HPF, Pieters G, Seif FJ, Blum WF, Lips CJM. 1992. The natural course of multiple endocrine neoplasia type IIb: A study of 18 cases. Arch Intern Med 152:1250–1252.

13. Sizemore GW, Carney JA, Gharib H, Capen CC. 1992. Multiple endocrine neoplasia type 2B: Eighteen-year follow-up of a four-generation family. Henry Ford Hosp J 40:236–244.

14. Mathew CG, Chin KS, Easton DF, Thorpe K, Carter C, Liou GI, Fong SL, Bridges CD, Haak H, Kruseman AC, Schifter S, Hansen HH, Telenius H, Telenius-Berg M, Ponder BAJ. 1987. A linked genetic marker for multiple endocrine neoplasia type 2A on chromosome 10. Nature 328:527–528.

15. Simpson NE, Kidd KK, Goodfellow PJ, McDermid H, Myers S, Kidd JR, Jackson CE, Duncan AM, Farrer LA, Brasch K. 1987. Assignment of multiple endocrine neoplasia type 2A to chromosome 10 by linkage. Nature 328:528–530.

16. Mulligan LM, Kwok JBJ, Healey CS, Elsdon MJ, Eng C, Gardner E, Love DR, Mole SE, Moore JK, Papi L, Ponder MA, Telenius H, Tunnacliffe A, Ponder BAJ. 1993. Germline Mutations of the RET proto-oncogene in multiple endocrine neoplasia type 2A (MEN 2A). Nature 363:458–460.

17. Donis-Keller H, Shenshen D, Chi D, Carlson KM, Toshima K, Lairmore TC, Howe JR, Moley JF, Goodfellow P, Wells SA Jr. 1993. Mutations in the RET proto-oncogene are associated with MEN 2A and FMTV. Hum Mol Genet 2:851–856.

18. Takahashi M, Ritz J, Cooper GM. 1985. Activation of a novel human transforming gene, ret, by DNA rearrangement. Cell 42:581–588.

19. Takahashi M, Cooper GM. 1987. ret transforming gene encodes a fusion protein homologous to tyrosine kinases. Mol Cell Biol 7:1378–1385.

20. Lin LF, Doherty DH, Lile JD, Bektesh S, Colline F. 1993. GDNF: A glial cell line-derived neurotrophic factor for midbrain dopaminergic neurons. Science 260:1130–1132.

21. Trupp M, Arenas E, Falnzilber M, Nilsson AS, Sieber BA, Grigoriou M, Kilkenny C, Salazar-Grueso E, Pachnis V, Arumae U, Sarlola H, Saarma M, Ibanez CF. 1996. Functional receptor for GDNF encoded by the c-ret proto-oncogene. Nature 381:785–788.

22. Jinq S, Wen D, Yu Y, Holst PL, Luo Y, Fang M, Tamin R, Antonio L, Hu Z, Cupples R, Louis JC, Hu S, Altnock BW, Fox GM. 1996. GDNF-induced activation of the Ret tyrosine kinase is medicated by GDNFR-α, a novel receptor for GDNF. Cell 85:1113–1124.

23. Bongarzone I, Butti MG, Coronelli S, Borrello MG, Santoro M, Mondellini P, Pilotti S, Fusco A, Della Porta G, Pierotti MA. 1994. Frequent activation of RET protooncogene by fusion with a new activating gene in papillary thyroid carcinomas. Cancer Res 54:2979–2985.

24. Bongarzone I, Pierotti MA, Monzini N, Mondellini P, Manenti G, Donghi R, Pilotti S, Grieco M, Santoro M, Fusco A, Vecchio G, Della Porta G. 1989. High frequency of activation of tyrosine kinase oncogenes in human papillary thyroid carcinoma. Oncogene 4:1457–1462.

25. Jhiang S, Smanik P, Mazzaferri E. 1994. Development of a single-step duplex RT-PCR detecting different forms of ret activation, and identification of the third form of in vivo ret activation in human papillary thyroid carcinoma. Cancer Lett 78:69–76.

26. Wajjwalku W, Nakamura S, Hasegawa Y, Miyazaki K, Satoh Y, Funahashi H, Matsuyama M, Takahashi M. 1992. Low frequency of rearrangements of the ret and trk proto-oncogenes in Japanese thyroid papillary carcinomas. Jpn J Cancer Res 83:671–675.

438

27. Iwamoto T, Takahashi M, Ito M, Hamaguchi M, Isobe K, Misawa N, Asai J, Yoshida T, Nakashima I. 1990. Oncogenicity of the ret transforming gene in MMTV/ret transgenic mice. Oncogene 5:535–542.

28. Iwamoto T, Taniguchi M, Wajjwalku W, Nakashima I, Takahashi M. 1993. Neuroblastoma in a transgenic mouse carrying a metallothionein/ret fusion gene. Br J Cancer 67:504–507.

29. Schuchardt A, D'Agati V, Larsson-Blomberg L, Costantini F, Pachnis V. 1994. Defects in the kidney and enteric nervous system of mice lacking the tyrosine kinase receptor Ret. Nature 367:380–383.

30. Wohllk N, Cote GJ, Evans D, Goepfert H, Ordonez N, Gagel RF. 1996. Application of genetic screening information to the management of medullary thyroid carcinoma and multiple endocrine neoplasia. Endocri Metab Clin North Am 25:1–25.

31. Mulligan LM, Eng C, Healey CS, Clayton D, Kwok JB, Gardner E, Ponder MA, Frilling A, Jackson CE, Lehnert H, Neumann HPH, Thibodeau SN, Ponder BAJ. 1994. Specific mutations of the RET proto-oncogene are related to disease phenotype in MEN 2A and FMTC. Nature Genet 6:70–74.

32. Mulligan LM, Marsh DJ, Robinson BG, Lenoir G, Schuffenecker I, Zedenius J, Lips CJM, Gagel RF, Takai SI, Noll WW, Fink M, Raue F, LaCroix A, Thibodeau SN, Frilling A, Ponder BAJ, Eng C. 1995. Genotype-phenotype correlation in multiple endocrine neoplasia type 2: Report of the international RET mutation consortium. J Intern Med 238:343–346.

33. Mulligan LM, Eng C, Healey CS, Clayton D, Kwok JBJ, Gardner E, Ponder MA, Frilling A, Jackson CE, Lehnert H, Neumann HPH, Thibodeau SN, Ponder BAJ. 1994. Specific mutations of the RET proto-oncogene are related to disease phenotype in MEN 2A and FMTC. Nature Genet 6:70–74.

34. Donis-Keller H, Dou S, Chi D, Carlson KM, Toshima K, Lairmore TC, Howe JR, Moley JF, Goodfellow P, Wells SA Jr. 1993. Mutations in the RET proto-oncogene are associated with MEN 2A and FMTC. Hum Mol Genet 2:851–856.

35. Bolino A, Schuffenecker I, Luo Y, Seri M, Silengo M, Tocco T, Chabrier G, Houdent C, Murat A, Schlumberger M, Tourniaire J, Lenoir GM, Romeo G. 1995. RET mutations in exons 13 and 14 of FMTC patients. Oncogene 10:2415–2419.

36. Eng C, Smith DP, Mulligan LM, Healey CS, Zvelebil MJ, Stonehouse TJ, Ponder MA, Jackson CE, Waterfield MD, Ponder BA. 1995. A novel point mutation in the tyrosine kinase domain of the RET proto-oncogene in sporadic medullary thyroid carcinoma and in a family with FMTC. Oncogene 10:509–513.

37. Angrist M, Bolk S, Thiel B, Puffenberger EG, Hofstra RM, Buys CHCM, Cass DT, Chakravarti A, Chakravarti A. 1995. Mutation analysis of the RET receptor tyrosine kinase in Hirschsprung's disease. Hum Mol Genet 4:821–830.

38. Wohllk N, Cote GJ, Bugalho MMJ, Ordonez N, Evans DB, Goepfert H, Khorana S, Schultz PS, Richards CS, Gagel RF. 1996. Relevance of RET proto-oncogene mutations in sporadic medullary thyroid carcinoma. J Clin Endocrinol Metab 85:1113–1124.

39. Ceccherini I, Romei C, Barone V, Pacini F, Martino E, Loviselli A, Pinchera A, Romeo G. 1994. Identification of the Cys634–Tyr mutation of the RET proto-oncogene in a pedigree with multiple endocrine neoplasia type 2A and localized cutaneous lichen amyloidosis. J Endocrinol Invest 17:201–204.

40. Robinson MF, Cote CJ, Nunziata V, Brandi ML, Ferrer JP, Bugalho M, Almedia Ruas MM, Chik C, Colantuoni V, Gagel RF, Consortium MAC. 1994. Mutation of a specific condon of the ret proto-oncogene in the multiple endocrine neoplasia type 2A/cutaneous lichen amyloidosis syndrome. Abstract, presented at the Vth International Workshop on Multiple Endocrine Neoplasia, June 29–July 2, 1994 Stockholm, Sweden.

41. Hofstra RM, Landsvater RM, Ceccherini I, Stulp RP, Stelwagen T, Luo Y, Pasini B, Hoppener JW, van Amstel HK, Romeo G, Ponder BAJ. 1994. A mutation in the RET proto-oncogene associated with multiple endocrine neoplasia type 2B and sporadic medullary thyroid carcinoma. Nature 367:375–376.

42. Komminoth P, Kunz EK, Matias-Guiu X, Hiort O, Christiansen G, Colomer A, Roth J, Heitz

PU. 1995. Analysis of RET proto-oncogene point mutations distinguishes heritable from nonheritable medullary thyroid carcinomas. Cancer 76:479–489.

43. Zedenius J, Wallin G, Hamberger B, Nordenskjold M, Weber G, Larsson C. 1994. Somatic and MEN 2A de novo mutations identified in the RET proto-oncogene by screening of sporadic MTCs. Hum Mol Genet 3:1259–1262.

44. Zedenius J, Larsson C, Bergholm U, Bovee J, Svensson A, Hallengren B, Grimelius L, Backdahl M, Weber G, Wallin G. 1995. Mutations of codon 918 in the RET proto-oncogene correlate to poor prognosis in sporadic medullary thyroid carcinomas. J Clin Endocrinol Metab 80:3088–3090.

45. Komminoth P, Kunz E, Hiort O, Schroder S, Matias Guiu X, Christiansen G, Roth J, Heitz PU. 1994. Detection of RET proto-oncogene point mutations in paraffin-embedded pheochromocytoma specimens by nonradioactive single-strand conformation polymorphism analysis and direct sequencing. Am J Pathol 145:922–929.

46. Decker RA, Peacock ML, Borst MJ, Sweet JD, Thompson NW. 1995. Progress in genetic screening of multiple endocrine neoplasia type 2A: Is calcitonin testing obsolete? Surgery 118:257–264.

47. Martucciello EA. 1992. Chromosome 10 deletion in Hirschsprung's disease. Pediatr Surg Int 7:308–310.

48. Lyonnet S, Bolino A, Pelet A, Abel L, Nihoul-Fekete C, Briard ML, Mok-Siu V, Kaariainen H, Martucciello G, Lerone M, Puliti A, Yin Luo, Weissenbach J, Devoto M, Munnich A, Romeo G. 1993. A gene for Hirschsprung disease maps to the proximal long arm of chromosome 10. Nature Genet 4:346–350.

49. Romeo G, Ronchetto P, Luo Y, Barone V, Seri M, Ceccherini I, Pasini B, Bocciardi R, Lerone M, Kääriäinen H, Martucciello G. 1994. Point mutations affecting the tyrosine kinase domain of the RET proto-oncogene in Hirschsprung's disease. Nature 367:377–378.

50. Puffenberger E, Hosoda K, Washington S, Nakao K, deWit D, Yanagisawa M, Chakravarti A. 1994. A missense mutation of the endothelin-B receptor gene in multigenic Hirschsprung's disease. Cell 79:1257–1266.

51. Xing S, Smanik PA, Mazzaferri EL, Jhiang SM, Oglesbee MJ, Trosko JE. 1996. Characterization of RET oncogenic activation in MEN 2 inherited cancer syndromes. Endocrinology 137:1512–1519.

52. Asai N, Iwashita T, Matsuyama M, Takahashi M. 1995. Mechansims of activation of the ret proto-oncogene by multiple endocrine neoplasia 2A mutations. Mol Cell Biol 15:1613–1619.

53. Santoro M, Carlomagno F, Romano A, Bottaro DP, Dathan NA, Grieco M, Fusco A, Vecchio G, Matoskova B, Kraus MH, Di Fiiore PP. 1995. Activation of RET as a dominant transforming gene by germline mutations of MEN 2A and MEN 2B. Science 267:381–383.

54. Lorenzo MJ, Eng C, Mulligan LM, Stonehouse TJ, Healey CS, Ponder BA, Smith DP. 1995. Multiple mRNA isoforms of the human RET proto-oncogene generated by alternate splicing. Oncogene 10:1377–1383.

55. Handyside AH, Lesko JG, Tarin JJ, Winston RM, Hughes MR. 1992. Birth of a normal girl after in vitro fertilization and preimplantation diagnostic testing for cystic fibrosis. N Engl J Med 32:905–909.

56. Wells SA Jr, Donis-Keller H. 1994. Current perspectives on the diagnosis and management of patients with multiple endocrine neoplasia type 2 syndromes. Endocrinol Metab Clin North Am 23:215–228.

57. Gagel RF, Cote GJ, Martins Bugalho MJG, Boyd AE, Cummings T, Goepfert H, Evans DB, Cangir A, Khorana S, Schultz PN. 1995. Clinical use of molecular information in the management of multiple endocrine neoplasia type 2A. J Intern Med 238:333–341.

58. Khorana S, Gagel RF, Cote GJ. 1994. Direct sequencing of PCR products in agarose gel slices. Nucleic Acids Res 22:3425–3426.

59. Decker R, Borst M, Peacock M. 1994. Rapid screening for ret mutations in multiple endocrine neoplasia type 2 by denaturing gradient electrophoresis. Presented at the Vth International Workshop on Multiple Endocrine Neoplasia, Stockholm, Sweden, July, 1994.

60. Iitia A, Mikola M, Gregersen N, Hurskainen P, Lovgren T. 1994. Detection of a point

mutation using short oligonucleotide probes in allele-specific hybridization. Biotechniques 17:566–573.

61. Trupp M, Ryden M, Jornvall H, Funakoshi H, Timmusk T, Arenas E, Ibanez CF. 1995. Peripheral expression and biological activities of GDNF, a new neurotrophic factor for avian and mammalian peripheral neurons. J Cell Biol 130:137–148.

62. Lairmore TC, Ball DW, Baylin SB, Wells SA Jr. 1993. Management of pheochromocytomas in patients with multiple endocrine neoplasia type 2 syndromes. Ann Surg 217:595–601; discussion, 601–603.

63. Cance WG, Wells SA Jr. 1985. Multiple endocrine neoplasia Type IIa. Curr Probl Surg 22:1–56.

64. Telander RL, Zimmerman D, van Heerden JA, Sizemore GW. 1986. Results of early thyroidectomy for medullary thyroid carcinoma in children with multiple endocrine neoplasia type 2. J Pediatr Surg 21:1190–1194.

65. Lips CJ, Landsvater RM, Hoppener JW, Geerdink RA, Blijham G, van Veen JM, van Gils AP, de Wit MJ, Zewald RA, Berends MJ, Beemer FA, Brouwers-Smalbraak J, Jansen RPM, van Amstel HKP, van Vroonhoven TJMV, Vroom TM. 1994. Clinical screening as compared with DNA analysis in families with multiple endocrine neoplasia type 2A. N Engl J Med 331:828–835.

66. Wells SA, Chi DD, Toshima K, Dehner LP, Coffin CM, Dowton B, Ivanovich JL, DeBenedetti MK, Dilley WG, Moley JF, Norton JA, Donis-Keller H. 1994. Predictive DNA testing and prophylactic thyroidectomy in patients at risk for multiple endocrine neoplasia type 2A. Ann Surg 220:237–250.

67. Cote CJ, Wohllk N, Evans D, Goepfert H, Gagel RF. 1995. RET proto-oncogene mutations in multiple endocrine neoplasia type 2 and medullary thyroid carcinoma. Baillieres Clin Endocrinol Metab 9:609–630.

68. Graham SM, Genel M, Touloukian RJ, Barwick KW, Gertner JM, Torony C. 1987. Provocative testing for occult medullary carcinoma of the thyroid: Findings in seven children with multiple endocrine neoplasia type IIa. J Pediatr Surg 22:501–503.

69. Sisson JC, Shapiro B, Beierwaltes WH. 1984. Scintigraphy with I-131 MIBG as an aid to the treatment of pheochromocytomas in patients with the multiple endocrine neoplasia type 2 syndromes. Henry Ford Hosp Med J 32:254–261.

70. Telenius-Berg M, Adolfsson L, Berg B, Hamberger B, Nordenfelt I, Tibblin S, Welander G. 1987. Catecholamine release after physical exercise. A new provocative test for early diagnosis of pheochromocytoma in multiple endocrine neoplasia type 2. Acta Med Scand 222:351–359.

71. van der Vaart CH, Heringa MP, Dullaart RP, Aarnoudse JG. 1993. Multiple endocrine neoplasia presenting as phaeochromocytoma during pregnancy. Br J Obstet Gynaecol 100:1144–1145.

72. Wells SA Jr, Ellis GJ, Gunnells JC, Schneider AB, Sherwood LM. 1976. Parathyroid autotransplantation in primary parathyroid hyperplais. N Engl J Med 195:57–62.

73. Samaan NA, Draznin MB, Halpin RE, Bloss RS, Hawkins E, Lewis RA. 1991. Multiple endocrine syndrome type IIb in early childhood. Cancer 68:1832–1834.

74. Sciubba JJ, DAmico E, Attie JN. 1987. The occurrence of multiple endocrine neoplasia type IIb, in two children of an affected mother. J Oral Pathol 16:310–316.